TABLE 4-12
Prilocaine Hydrochloride

Proprietary Name	Manufacturer	Percent Local Anesthetic	Vasoconstrictor	Duration of Analgesia (min)		MRD-m and MRD-a
				Pulpal	*Soft-Tissue*	
Prilocaine HCl Citanest Plain	Generic Dentsply	4		10–15 (infiltration) 40–60 nerve block	90–120 (inf) 120–240 (nb)	6 mg/kg 2.7 mg/lb 400 mg absolute maximum
Prilocaine HCl + epinephrine 1:200,000 Citanest Forte	Generic Dentsply	4	Epinephrine 1:200,000	60–90	180–480	6 mg/kg 2.7 mg/lb 400 mg absolute maximum

MRD, Maximum recommended dose.

TABLE 4-14
Articaine Hydrochloride

Proprietary Name	Manufacturer	Percent Local Anesthetic	Vasoconstrictor	Duration of Analgesia (min)		MRD-m and MRD-a
				Pulpal	*Soft-Tissue*	
(United States) Septocaine	Septodont	4	Epinephrine 1:100,000	60–75	180–360	7 mg/kg
(Canada) Septanest SP Astracaine Ultracaine D-S forte	Septodont Dentsply Hoechst					3.2 mg/lb 500 mg absolute maximum
(Canada) Septanest N Astracaine Ultracaine D-S	Septodont Dentsply Hoechst	4	Epinephrine 1:200,000	45–60	120–300	7 mg/kg 3.2 mg/lb 500 mg absolute maximum

MRD, Maximum recommended dose.

TABLE 4-15
Bupivacaine Hydrochloride

Proprietary Name	Manufacturer	Percent Local Anesthetic	Vasoconstrictor	Duration of Analgesia (min)		MRD-m and MRD-a
				Pulpal	*Soft-Tissue*	
Marcaine	Kodak	0.5	Epinephrine 1:200,000	90–180	240–540 (reports up to 720)	1.3 mg/kg 0.6 mg/lb 90 mg absolute maximum

MRD, Maximum recommended dose.

Handbook *of*
LOCAL ANESTHESIA

Handbook *of* LOCAL ANESTHESIA

FIFTH EDITION

Stanley F. Malamed, DDS

Professor of Anesthesia and Medicine
School of Dentistry
University of Southern California
Los Angeles, California

With 400 illustrations

Selected illustrations by
Imagineering Scientific and Technical Artworks, Inc.

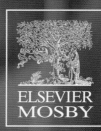

ELSEVIER
MOSBY

ELSEVIER
MOSBY

11830 Westline Industrial Drive
St. Louis, Missouri 63146

Notice

Dentistry is an ever-changing field. Standard safety precautions must be followed, but as new research and clinical experience broaden our knowledge, changes in treatment and drug therapy may become necessary or appropriate. Readers are advised to check the most current product information provided by the manufacturer of each drug to be administered to verify the recommended dose, the method and duration of administration, and contraindications. It is the responsibility of the licensed prescriber, relying on experience and knowledge of the patient, to determine dosages and the best treatment for each individual patient. Neither the Publisher nor the author assumes any liability for any injury and/or damage to persons or property arising from this publication.

Previous editions copyrighted 1980, 1986, 1990, 1997.

ISBN-13: 978–0–323–02449–5
ISBN-10: 0–323–02449–1

Publishing Director: *Linda L. Duncan*
Executive Editor: *Penny Rudolph*
Senior Developmental Editor: *Kimberly Alvis*
Publishing Services Manager: *Patricia Tannian*
Project Manager: *Sharon Corell*
Designer: *Julia Dummitt*

Printed in China

Last digit is the print number: 9   8   7   6   5   4

To Beverly, Heather, Jennifer, and Jeremy

CONTRIBUTOR

Daniel L. Orr II, DDS, MS (Anesthesiology), PhD, JD, MD
Clinical Professor
Oral and Maxillofacial Surgery and Anesthesiology for
  Dentistry
University of Nevada School of Medicine
Las Vegas, Nevada

PREFACE

It is difficult for me to comprehend that a quarter of a century has passed since I started writing the first edition of *Handbook of Local Anesthesia* (1978), but it has. Looking back at that first edition allows one a nostalgic visit to the (good?) "old days," when dentists were truly "wet fingered." No gloves, no masks, no face shields. The author sitting and administering local anesthetic injections, wearing a long-sleeved dress shirt and tie. An entirely different world indeed.

At that time (the late 1970s), the ability to provide a patient with clinically adequate pain control was a concern of dentists throughout the world. It remains so today.

Many changes have occurred over these years, most of a positive nature: changes in the local anesthetic drugs that are available for clinical use, changes in the armamentarium for delivering these drugs, and changes in the techniques for achieving pain control during dental therapies.

Dentistry in North America has seen the demise of the injectable ester-type local anesthetic (though esters [primarily benzocaine] are still widely employed successfully as topical anesthetics). The last of the esters available in dental cartridges, the combination of procaine HCl and propoxycaine HCl, was removed from the marketplace in 1996. The North American injectable local anesthetic armamentarium in 2004 consists exclusively of amides: articaine HCl, bupivacaine HCl, lidocaine HCl, mepivacaine HCl, and prilocaine HCl. These are the most used drugs in dentistry and represent the class of drugs that paved the way for the changes that enabled dentistry to evolve from what it was in the 1800s – a trade – to what it is today – a highly respected profession.

Local anesthetics are, in this author's opinion, *the safest* and *the most effective* drugs available in all of medicine for the prevention and the management of pain. Indeed, there are no other drugs that truly prevent pain; no other drugs which actually prevent a propagated nociceptive nerve impulse from reaching the patient's brain, where it would be interpreted as pain. Deposit a local anesthetic drug in close proximity to a sensory nerve and clinically adequate pain control will result in essentially all clinical situations.

Other drugs (analgesics, such as opioids and NSAIDs) and techniques (such as general anesthesia) affect pain by modifying the patient's response to the nociceptive stimulus through a drug-mediated depression of the central nervous system. The patient still feels the pain, but his or her response to it is minimized (opioids, NSAIDs) or prevented because the patient is unconscious (general anesthesia).

Find the nerve with the local anesthetic drug and pain control is virtually assured! Yet in certain clinical situations "finding the nerve" is anything but easy. This is especially so in the mandible, primarily mandibular molars. In my 30-plus years as a teacher of anesthesia in dentistry I have been invited by numerous dental societies to present seminars on "Trouble-shooting the Mandibular Block."* Previous editions of this text described "newer" approaches to effective mandibular anesthesia, such as the Gow-Gates mandibular nerve block and the Vazirani-Akinosi closed-mouth mandibular nerve block. These techniques have achieved a degree of clinical utility and as such have helped many doctors improve their success in obtaining mandibular anesthesia. Yet it wasn't until the rediscovery of intraosseous anesthesia in the early 1990s, coupled with the introduction in 2000 (in the USA) of articaine HCl, that the "problem" of the "hot" mandibular molar was essentially solved.

New local anesthetic delivery systems have been introduced over the years. The past decade has seen a significant increase in interest in computer-controlled local anesthetic delivery (CCLAD) systems. Designed to overcome the inherent clumsiness associated with the delivery of local anesthetic with the traditional hand-held dental syringe (whose hand hasn't shaken during injection, on occasion?), CCLAD systems have increased the ability of doctors to guarantee the pain-free delivery of local anesthesia to their patients. As a by-product of research into the efficacy of the CCLAD systems, several new techniques of maxillary anesthesia have been developed: the *anterior middle superior alveolar nerve block* (AMSA) and the *palatal approach – anterior superior alveolar nerve block* (P-ASA). These valuable nerve blocks have been well received and are fully discussed in Chapter 13.

As effective as our local anesthetics are, and as the likelihood of patients' experiencing truly pain-free dentistry increases, significant numbers of patients continue to fear intraoral injections. Fear of dentistry cannot be lightly dismissed by the doctor. Indeed, the overwhelming majority of medical emergencies that occur in dentistry happen during or immediately after local anesthetic administration. Anything a doctor can do to minimize stress at this time serves to prevent potential problems from developing. The seemingly basic review of local anesthetic injection technique (Chapter 11) should become periodic required reading to ensure that all that can be done *is* being done to minimize stress at this critical juncture during the dental appointment.

Two significant changes will be noted in this fifth edition. First is the inclusion of a new chapter on legal

---

*Though technically the term "mandibular block" is incorrect – the precise term is inferior alveolar nerve block – most doctors use the term mandibular block when describing any injection administered in the region of the mandibular ramus.

considerations associated with the administration of dental local anesthetics (Chapter 19). As safe and as effective as local anesthetic drugs and techniques are, unforeseen, unwanted, and undesirable events may still occur. These problems are discussed fully in Chapters 17 (Local Complications) and 18 (Systemic Complications). I have asked Dr. Dan Orr II to discuss the legal ramifications of local anesthetic administration in dentistry. As an oral and maxillofacial surgeon, dentist anesthesiologist, and attorney, Dr. Orr is well prepared to address this subject from both the dental and legal perspectives.

Second is the change from black and white to color photography. This represents to me a truly significant event in the evolution of this textbook. The ability to visualize intraoral landmarks as they actually appear, not in variegated shades of black and gray but in natural color, will greatly assist the student in the learning process. This change necessitated the reshooting of every photograph from prior editions, the end result of which, I hope, leads the reader to a clearer understanding of the concepts being presented.

Along with the use of color images in this fifth edition, and likely to be of even greater importance as a teaching and learning aid, is the third enhancement: an accompanying DVD. The DVD follows the structure of the textbook, providing live clinical demonstrations of the techniques and concepts presented in the text. Mechanisms of action and clinical anatomy are depicted through the use of animation to better illustrate these processes. It has oftentimes been difficult for me to describe adequately, in the written word and in diagrams, some of the concepts associated with the actions of local anesthetics. Through the use of animation we are now able to present these ideas in a manner that should help to clarify these concepts for the student. It is my feeling, as an educator for more than 30 years, that the combination of the written text plus the visual impact of the DVD will provide a more optimal learning experience for all who come to study this critically important subject.

ACKNOWLEDGMENTS

The people involved with the photography and video production cannot receive enough thanks: the still photographer, Mr. Reed Hutchinson; Dr. Joseph Massad and his excellent team at Millennium Productions (for the DVD); and the three models: Dr. Diane Conly (who gave the injections) and Drs. Corey Deeble and Hanann Tomeh (who sat and received the injections), enduring many hours of hot lights and needle sticks to produce the clinical components, both video and still, of this edition. Thanks, too, to the manufacturers of local anesthetic drugs and devices in North America, including Beutlich Pharmaceuticals; Dentsply; Kodak (Cook-Waite); Midwest; Milestone Scientific; Novocol; Septodont, Inc; and Sultan Safety, LLC, for their assistance in supplying photographs and graphics for use in this book.

I also want to thank Kimberly Alvis, Senior Developmental Editor, and Penny Rudolph, Executive Editor, from Mosby (an affiliate of Elsevier) who had the unenviable task of dealing with a frequently lazy, usually hard-to-reach author. Their perseverance has paid off with this fine fifth edition.

Finally, I wish to thank the many members of our profession, the dentists and dental hygienists, who have provided me with written and verbal input regarding prior editions of this textbook. Many of their suggestions for additions (e.g., the DVD), deletions, and corrections have been incorporated into this new text. Thanks to you all!

Stanley F. Malamed

CONTENTS

Handbook *of*

LOCAL ANESTHESIA

IN THIS PART

PART ONE

The Drugs

In the first section of this book the pharmacological and clinical properties of the classes of drugs known as local anesthetics (Chapter 2) and vasoconstrictors (Chapter 3) are discussed. Knowledge of both the pharmacological and clinical properties of these drugs, by all persons permitted to administer them, is absolutely essential for their safe use and for a better understanding of those potentially life-threatening systemic reactions associated with their administration. Emphasis is placed on those local anesthetic drug combinations currently used in anesthesia in dentistry (Chapter 4).

Chapter 1 provides a background for understanding how local anesthetics work to transiently block nerve conduction, thus preventing pain from being experienced. The anatomy and physiology of normal neurons and nerve conduction are reviewed as a background for the discussion, which, in subsequent chapters, takes up the pharmacology and clinical actions of various specific agents.

CHAPTER

1

DESIRABLE PROPERTIES OF LOCAL ANESTHETICS

Local anesthesia has been defined as a loss of sensation in a circumscribed area of the body caused by a depression of excitation in nerve endings or an inhibition of the conduction process in peripheral nerves.[1] An important feature of local anesthesia is that it produces this loss of sensation without inducing a loss of consciousness. In this one major area local anesthesia differs dramatically from general anesthesia.

There are many methods of inducing local anesthesia:
1. Mechanical trauma
2. Low temperature
3. Anoxia
4. Chemical irritants
5. Neurolytic agents such as alcohol and phenol
6. Chemical agents such as local anesthetics

However, only those methods or substances that induce a *transient* and *completely reversible* state of anesthesia have application in clinical practice. The following are those properties deemed most desirable for a local anesthetic:
1. It should not be irritating to the tissue to which it is applied.
2. It should not cause any permanent alteration of nerve structure.
3. Its systemic toxicity should be low.
4. It must be effective regardless of whether it is injected into the tissue or applied locally to mucous membranes.
5. The time of onset of anesthesia should be as short as possible.
6. The duration of action must be long enough to permit completion of the procedure yet not so long as to require an extended recovery.

Most local anesthetics discussed in this section meet the first two criteria: They are (relatively) *nonirritating* to tissues and *completely reversible*. Of paramount importance

is *systemic toxicity*, because all injectable and most topical local anesthetics are eventually absorbed from their site of administration into the cardiovascular system. The potential toxicity of a drug is an important factor in its consideration for use as a local anesthetic. Toxicity varies greatly among the local anesthetics currently in use. Toxicity is discussed more thoroughly in Chapter 2. Although it is a desirable characteristic, not all local anesthetics in clinical use today meet the criterion of being effective, *regardless of whether the drug is injected or applied topically*. Several of the more potent injectable local anesthetics (e.g., procaine or mepivacaine) prove to be relatively ineffective when applied topically to mucous membrane. To be effective as topical anesthetics, these drugs must be applied in concentrations that prove to be locally irritating to tissues and increase the risk of systemic toxicity. Dyclonine, a potent topical anesthetic, is not administered by injection because of its tissue-irritating properties. Lidocaine and tetracaine, on the other hand, are both effective anesthetics when administered by injection or topical application in clinically acceptable concentrations. The last factors, *rapid onset of action* and *adequate duration of clinical action*, are met satisfactorily by most of the clinically effective local anesthetics in use today. Clinical duration of action does vary considerably among drugs and also among different preparations of the same drug. The duration of anesthesia necessary to complete a procedure is a major consideration in the selection of a local anesthetic.

In addition to these qualities, Bennett[2] lists other desirable properties of an ideal local anesthetic:
7. It should have potency sufficient to give complete anesthesia without the use of harmful concentrated solutions.
8. It should be relatively free from producing allergic reactions.
9. It should be stable in solution and readily undergo biotransformation in the body.

10. It should either be sterile or capable of being sterilized by heat without deterioration.

No local anesthetic in use today satisfies all of these criteria; however, all anesthetics do meet a majority of them. Research is continuing in an effort to produce newer drugs that possess a maximum of desirable factors and a minimum of negative ones.

FUNDAMENTALS OF IMPULSE GENERATION AND TRANSMISSION

The discovery in the late 1800s of a group of chemicals with the ability to prevent pain without inducing a loss of consciousness was one of the major steps in the advancement of the medical and dental professions. Medical and dental procedures, for the first time, could be carried out easily and in the absence of pain, a fact that is virtually taken for granted by contemporary medical and dental professionals and their patients.

The concept behind the actions of local anesthetics is simple: They prevent both the generation and conduction of a nerve impulse. In effect, local anesthetics set up a chemical roadblock between the source of the impulse (e.g., the scalpel incision in soft tissues) and the brain. Therefore the aborted impulse, prevented from reaching the brain, is not interpreted as pain by the patient.

This is similar to the effect of lighting the fuse on a stick of dynamite. The fuse is the "nerve," whereas the dynamite is the "brain." If the fuse is lit and the flame reaches the dynamite, an explosion occurs (Fig. 1-1). When the nerve is stimulated, an impulse is propagated that is interpreted as pain when it reaches the brain. If the fuse is lit, but "water" is placed midway between the tip of the fuse and the dynamite, the fuse will burn up to the point of water application and then die. The dynamite does not explode. When a local anesthetic is placed at some point between the pain stimulus and the brain, the nerve impulse travels up to the point of local anesthetic application and then "dies," never reaching the brain, and pain does not occur (Fig. 1-2).

How, in fact, do local anesthetics, the most commonly used drugs in dentistry, function to abolish or prevent pain? The following is a discussion of current theories seeking to explain the mode of action of local anesthetic drugs. To understand their action better, however, the reader must have an acquaintance with the fundamentals of nerve conduction. A review of the relevant characteristics and properties of nerve anatomy and physiology follows.

The Neuron

The neuron, or nerve cell, is the structural unit of the nervous system. It is able to transmit messages between

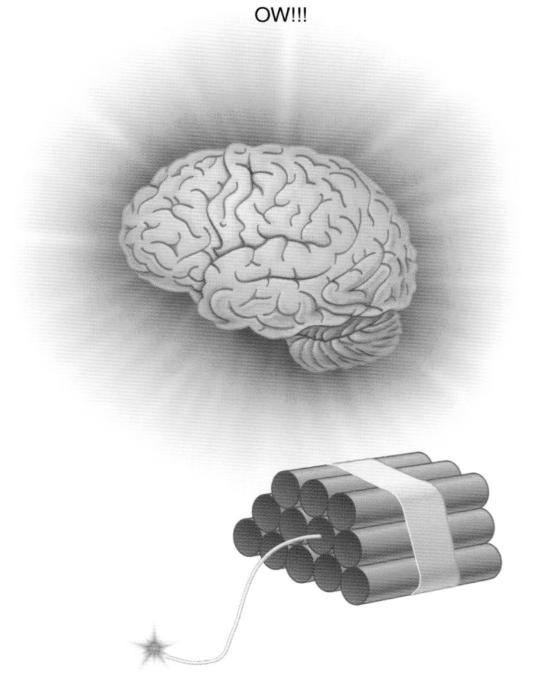

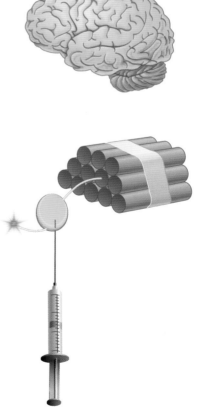

OW!!!

Figure 1-1. Fuse is lit and the flame reaches the dynamite; an explosion occurs, and the patient experiences pain.

Figure 1-2. Local anesthetic is placed at some point between the pain stimulus and the brain (dynamite). The nerve impulse travels up to the point of the local anesthetic application and then "dies," never reaching the brain, and pain does not occur.

the central nervous system (CNS) and all parts of the body. There are two basic types of neuron: the sensory (afferent) and motor (efferent). The basic structure of these two neuronal types differs significantly (Fig. 1-3).

Sensory neurons that are capable of transmitting the sensation of pain consist of three major portions.[3] The peripheral process (also known as the *dendritic zone)*, which is composed of an arborization of free nerve endings, is the most distal segment of the sensory neuron. These free nerve endings respond to stimulation produced in the tissues in which they lie, provoking an impulse that is transmitted centrally along the *axon*. The axon is a thin cable-like structure that may be quite long (the giant squid axon has been measured at 100 to 200 cm). At its mesial (or central) end there is an arborization similar to that seen in the peripheral process. However, in this case the arborizations form synapses with various nuclei in the CNS to distribute incoming (sensory) impulses to their appropriate sites within the CNS for interpretation. The *cell body* is the third part of the neuron. In the sensory neuron described here, the cell body is located at a distance from the axon, or the main pathway of impulse transmission in this nerve. The cell body of the sensory nerve therefore is not involved in the process of impulse transmission, its primary function being to provide the vital metabolic support for the entire neuron (see Fig. 1-3, *B*).

Nerve cells that conduct impulses from the CNS toward the periphery are termed *motor neurons* and are structurally different from the sensory neurons just described in that their cell body is interposed between the axon and dendrites. In motor neurons the cell body not only is an integral component of the impulse transmission system but also provides metabolic support for the cell. Near its termination the axon branches with each branch, ending as a bulbous axon terminal (or bouton). Axon terminals synapse with muscle cells (see Fig. 1-3, *A*).

The Axon

The single nerve fiber, the axon, is a long cylinder of neural cytoplasm (axoplasm) encased in a thin sheath, the nerve membrane, or axolemma. Neurons have a cell body and a nucleus, as do all other cells; however, neurons differ from other cells in that they have an axonal process from which the cell body may be at a considerable

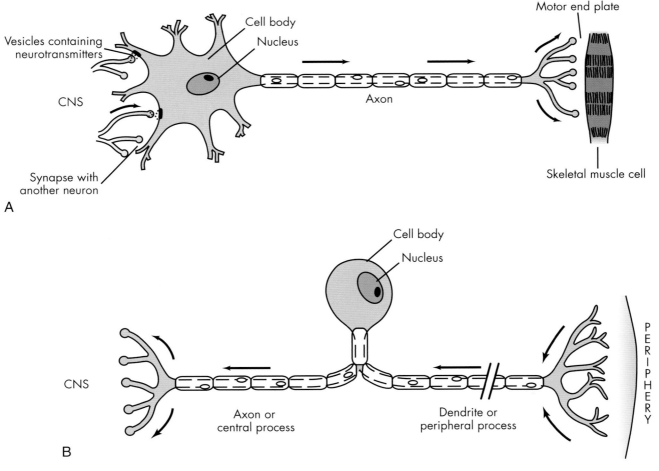

Figure 1-3. A, Multipolar motor neuron. **B,** Unipolar sensory neuron. (From Liebgott B: *Anatomical basis of dentistry*, ed 2, St Louis, 2001. Mosby.)

distance. The axoplasm, a gelatinous substance, is separated from extracellular fluids by a continuous nerve membrane. In some nerves this membrane is itself covered by an insulating lipid-rich layer of myelin.

Current thinking holds that sensory nerve excitability and conduction are both attributable to changes developing within the *nerve membrane*. The cell body and axoplasm are not essential for nerve conduction. They are important, however. The metabolic support of the membrane is probably derived from the axoplasm.

The nerve (cell) membrane itself is approximately 70 to 80 Å thick. (An angstrom unit is 1/10,000 of a micrometer.) Figure 1-4 represents a currently acceptable configuration. All biological membranes are organized[1] to block the diffusion of water-soluble molecules;[2] be selectively permeable to certain molecules via specialized pores or channels;[3] and transduce information by protein receptors responsive to chemical or physical stimulation by neurotransmitters or hormones (chemical) or light, vibrations, or pressure (physical).[4] The membrane is described as a flexible nonstretchable structure

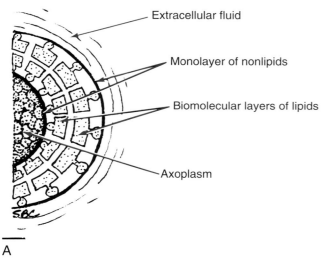

A

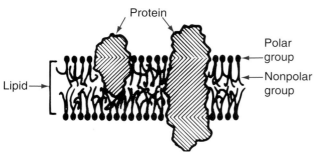

B

Figure 1-4. A, Configuration of a biological membrane. **B,** Heterogeneous lipoprotein membrane as suggested by Singer and Nicholson.[5] (Redrawn from Covino BG, Vassalo HG: *Local anesthetics: mechanisms of action and clinical use,* New York, 1976, Grune & Stratton.)

consisting of two layers of lipid molecules (bilipid layer of phospholipids) and associated proteins, lipids, and carbohydrates. The lipids are oriented with their hydrophilic (polar) ends facing the outer surface and the hydrophobic (nonpolar) ends projecting to the middle of the membrane (see Fig. 1-4, *A*). Proteins are visualized as the primary organizational elements of membranes (see Fig. 1-4, *B*).[5] Proteins are classified as *transport proteins* (channels, carriers, or pumps) and *receptor sites.* Channel proteins are thought to be continuous pores through the membrane, allowing some ions (Na⁺, K,⁺ Ca⁺⁺) to flow passively, whereas other channels are "gated," permitting ion flow only when the gate is "open."[4] The nerve membrane lies at the interface between the extracellular fluid and axoplasm. It separates highly diverse ionic concentrations within the axon from those outside. The *resting nerve membrane* has an electrical resistance about 50 times greater than that of the intracellular and extracellular fluids, thus preventing the passage of sodium, potassium, and chloride ions down their concentration gradients. However, when a nerve impulse passes, electrical conductivity of the nerve membrane increases approximately 100-fold. This increase in conductivity permits the passage of sodium and potassium ions along their concentration gradients through the nerve membrane. It is the movement of these ions that provides the immediate source of energy for impulse conduction along the nerve.

Some nerve fibers are covered by an insulating lipid layer of myelin. In vertebrates, myelinated nerve fibers include all but the smallest of axons (Table 1-1).[6] Myelinated nerve fibers (Fig. 1-5) are enclosed in spirally wrapped layers of lipoprotein myelin sheaths, which are actually a specialized form of Schwann cell. Although primarily (75%) lipid, the myelin sheath also contains some protein (20%) and carbohydrate (5%).[7] Each myelinated nerve fiber is enclosed in its own myelin sheath. The outermost layer of myelin consists of the Schwann cell cytoplasm and its nucleus. There are constrictions located at regular intervals (approximately every 0.5 to 3 mm) along the myelinated nerve fiber. These are *nodes of Ranvier,* and they form a gap between two adjoining Schwann cells and their myelin spirals.[8] At these nodes the nerve membrane is exposed directly to the extracellular medium.

Unmyelinated nerve fibers (Fig. 1-6) are also surrounded by a Schwann cell sheath. Groups of unmyelinated nerve fibers share the same sheath. The insulating properties of the myelin sheath enable a myelinated nerve to conduct impulses at a much faster rate than can an unmyelinated nerve of equal size.

Physiology of the Peripheral Nerves

The function of a nerve is to carry messages from one part of the body to another. These messages, in the form of electrical action potentials, are called *impulses.* Action potentials are transient depolarizations of the membrane

TABLE 1-1
Classification of Peripheral Nerves According to Fiber Size and Physiological Properties

Fiber Class	Subclass	Myelin	Diameter, μ	Conduction Velocity (m/s)	Location	Function
A	alpha	+	6–22	30–120	Afferent to and efferent from muscles and joints	Motor, proprioception
	beta	+	6–22	30–120	Afferent to and efferent from muscles and joints	Motor, proprioception
	gamma	+	3–6	15–35	Efferent to muscle spindles	Muscle tone
	delta	+	1–4	5–25	Afferent sensory nerves	Pain, temperature, touch
B		+	<3	3–15	Preganglionic sympathetic	Various autonomic functions
C	sC	–	0.3–1.3	0.7–1.3	Postganglionic sympathetic	Various autonomic functions
	d gammaC	–	0.4–1.2	0.1–2.0	Afferent sensory nerves	Various autonomic functions; pain, temperature, touch

(From Berde CB, Strichartz GR: *Local anesthetics.* In Miller RD, editor: *Anesthesia,* ed 5, Philadelphia, 2000, Churchill Livingstone, pp 491–521.)

that result from a brief increase in the permeability of the membrane to sodium, and usually also from a delayed increase in the permeability to potassium.[9] Impulses are initiated by chemical, thermal, mechanical, or electrical stimuli.

Once an impulse is initiated by a stimulus in any particular nerve fiber, the amplitude and shape of that impulse remain constant, regardless of changes in the quality of the stimulus or its strength. The impulse remains constant without losing strength as it passes along the nerve because the energy used for its propagation is derived from energy that is released by the nerve fiber along its length and not solely from the initial stimulus. de Jong has described impulse conduction as being like the active progress of a spark along a fuse of gunpowder.[10] Once lit, the fuse burns steadily along its length, one burning segment providing the energy necessary to ignite its neighbor. Such is the situation with impulse propagation along a nerve.

Electrophysiology of Nerve Conduction

The following is a description of electrical events that occur within a nerve during the conduction of an impulse. Subsequent sections describe the precise mechanisms for each of these steps:

A nerve possesses a resting potential (Fig. 1-7, *Step 1*). This is a negative electrical potential of −70 mV that exists across the nerve membrane, produced by differing concentrations of ions on either side of the membrane (Table 1-2). The interior of the nerve is negative relative to the exterior.

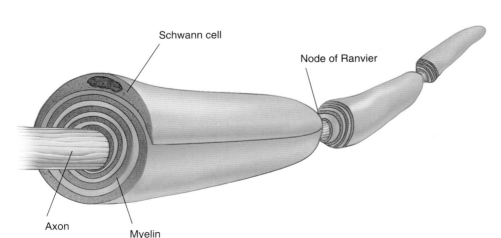

Schwann cell

Node of Ranvier

Axon

Myelin

Figure 1-5. Structure of a myelinated nerve fiber. (Redrawn from de Jong RH: *Local anesthetics,* St Louis, 1994, Mosby.)

UNMYELINATED

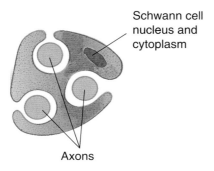

Schwann cell
nucleus and
cytoplasm

Axons

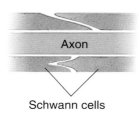

Axon

Schwann cells

Figure 1-6. Types of Schwann cell sheaths. (Redrawn from Wildsmith JAW: Peripheral nerve and anaesthetic drugs, *Br J Anaesthes* 58:692-700, 1986.)

Step 1. A stimulus *excites* the nerve, leading to the following sequence of events:
A. An initial phase of *slow depolarization*. The electrical potential within the nerve becomes slightly less negative (see Fig. 1-7, *Step 1A*).
B. When the falling electrical potential reaches a critical level, an extremely rapid phase of depolarization results. This is termed *threshold potential*, or *firing threshold* (see Fig. 1-7, *Step 1B*).
C. This phase of *rapid depolarization* results in a reversal of the electrical potential across the nerve membrane (see Fig. 1-7, *Step 1C*). The interior of the nerve is now electrically positive in relation to the exterior. An electrical potential of +40 mV exists on the interior of the nerve cell.[11]

Step 2. After these steps of depolarization, *repolarization* occurs (see Fig. 1-7, *Step 2*). The electrical potential gradually becomes more negative inside the nerve cell relative to outside until the original resting potential of −70 mV is again achieved.

The entire process (Steps 1 and 2) requires 1 millisecond (msec); depolarization (Step 1) takes 0.3 msec; repolarization (Step 2) takes 0.7 msec.

Electrochemistry of Nerve Conduction

The preceding sequence of events depends on two important factors: the concentrations of electrolytes in the axoplasm (interior of the nerve cell) and extracellular fluids[1] and the permeability of the nerve membrane to sodium and potassium ions.[2]

Table 1-2 shows the differing concentrations of ions found within neurons and in the extracellular fluids. Significant differences exist for ions between their intracellular and extracellular concentrations. These ionic gradients differ because the nerve membrane exhibits *selective permeability*.

Resting State. In its resting state the nerve membrane is
• Slightly permeable to sodium ions (Na+)
• Freely permeable to potassium ions (K+)
• Freely permeable to chloride ions (Cl−)

Potassium remains *within* the axoplasm, despite its ability to diffuse freely through the nerve membrane and its concentration gradient (passive diffusion usually occurs from a region of greater concentration to one of lesser concentration), because the negative charge of the nerve membrane restrains the positively charged ions by electrostatic attraction.

Chloride remains *outside* the nerve membrane instead of moving along its concentration gradient into the nerve cell because the opposing, nearly equal, electrostatic influence (electrostatic gradient from inside to outside) forces outward migration. The net result is no diffusion of chloride through the membrane.

Sodium migrates *inwardly* because both the concentration (greater outside) and the electrostatic gradient (positive ion attracted by negative intracellular potential) favor such migration. Only the fact that the resting nerve membrane is relatively impermeable to sodium prevents a massive influx of this ion.

Membrane Excitation.
Depolarization. Excitation of a nerve segment leads to an increase in permeability of the cell membrane to sodium ions. This is accomplished by a transient widening of transmembrane ion channels sufficient to permit the unhindered passage of hydrated sodium ions (p. 11). The rapid influx of sodium ions to the interior of the nerve cell causes depolarization of the nerve membrane from its resting level to its firing threshold of approximately −50 to −60 mV (see Fig. 1-7, *Steps 1A* and *B*).[12] The firing threshold is actually the *magnitude of the decrease in negative transmembrane potential that is necessary to initiate an action potential (impulse)*.

A decrease in negative transmembrane potential of 15 mV (e.g., from −70 to −55 mV) is necessary to reach the firing threshold; a voltage difference of less than 15 mV will not initiate an impulse. In a normal nerve the firing threshold remains constant. Exposure of the nerve to a local anesthetic *raises* its firing threshold. Elevating the firing threshold means that more sodium must pass through the membrane to decrease the negative transmembrane potential to a level where depolarization occurs.

When the firing threshold is reached, membrane permeability to sodium increases dramatically and sodium ions rapidly enter the axoplasm. At the end of depolarization

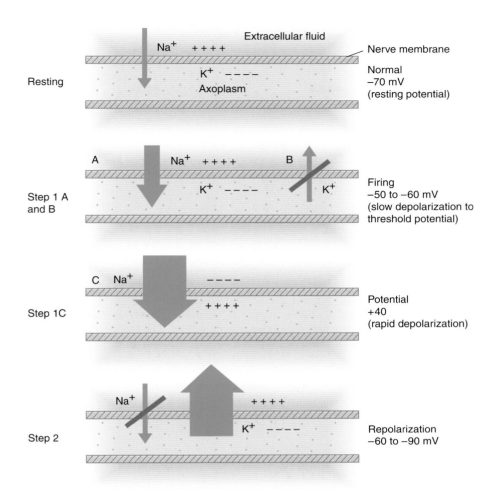

Figure 1-7. *Top,* Resting potential. *Step 1, A* and *B,* Slow depolarization to threshold. *Step 1, C,* Rapid depolarization. *Step 2,* Repolarization.

(the peak of the action potential), the electrical potential of the nerve is actually reversed; an electrical potential of +40 mV exists (see Fig. 1-7, *Step 1C*). The entire depolarization process requires approximately 0.3 msec.

Repolarization. The action potential is terminated when the membrane repolarizes. This is caused by the extinction ("inactivation") of increased permeability to sodium. In many cells permeability to potassium also increases, resulting in the efflux of K+, and leading to a more rapid membrane repolarization and return to its resting potential (see Fig. 1-7, *Step 2*).

TABLE **1-2**
Intracellular and Extracellular Ionic Concentrations

Ion	Intracellular (mEq/L)	Extracellular (mEq/L)	Ratio (approximate)
Potassium (K+)	110 to 170	3 to 5	27:1
Sodium (Na+)	5 to 10	140	1:14
Chloride (Cl−)	5 to 10	110	1:11

The movement of sodium ions into the cell during depolarization and the subsequent movement of potassium ions out of the cell during repolarization are passive (not requiring the expenditure of energy), because each ion moves along its concentration gradient (higher → lower). After the return of the membrane potential to its original level (−70 mV), a slight excess of sodium exists within the nerve cell, with a slight excess of potassium extracellularly. A period of metabolic activity then begins in which active transfer of sodium ions out of the cell occurs via the "sodium pump." An expenditure of energy is necessary to move sodium ions *out* of the nerve cell against their concentration gradient; this energy comes from the oxidative metabolism of adenosine triphosphate (ATP). The same pumping mechanism is thought to be responsible for the active transport of potassium ions *into* the cell against their concentration gradient. The entire process of repolarization requires 0.7 msec.

Immediately after a stimulus has initiated an action potential, a nerve is unable, for a time, to respond to another stimulus, regardless of its strength. This is termed the *absolute refractory period,* and it lasts for about the duration of

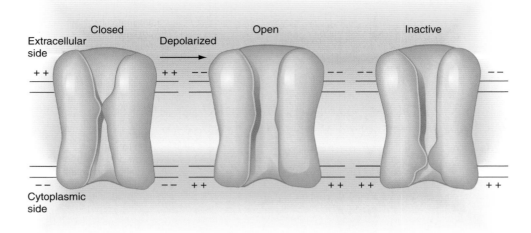

Figure 1-8. Sodium channel transition stages. Depolarization reverses resting membrane potential from interior negative *(left)* to interior positive *(center)*. The channel proteins undergo corresponding conformational changes from resting state (closed) to ion-conducting stage (open). State changes continue from open *(center)* to inactive *(right)*, where channel configuration assumes a different, but still impermeable, state. With repolarization the inactivated refractory channel reverts to the initial resting configuration *(left)*, ready for the next sequence. (Redrawn from Siegelbaum SA, Koester F: *Ion channels.* In Kandel ER, editor: *Principles of neural science*, ed 3, Norwalk, Conn, 1991, Appleton-Lange.)

the main part of the action potential. The absolute refractory period is followed by a *relative refractory period*, during which a new impulse can be initiated but only by a stronger than normal stimulus. The relative refractory period continues to decrease until the normal level of excitability returns, at which point the nerve is said to be repolarized.

During depolarization the major proportion of ionic sodium channels are found in their "open" (O) state (thus permitting the rapid influx of Na^+). This is followed by a slower decline into a state of "inactivation" (I) of the channels to a nonconducting state. Inactivation temporarily converts the channels to a state from which they cannot open in response to depolarization (absolute refractory period). This inactivated state is slowly converted back, so the majority of channels are found in their closed (C) resting form when the membrane is repolarized (–70 mV). Upon depolarization the channels change configuration, first to an open ion-conducting (O) state and then to an inactive nonconducting (I) state. Although both C and I states correspond to nonconducting channels, they differ in that depolarization can recruit channels to the conducting O state from C but not from I. Figure 1-8 describes the sodium channel transition stages.[13]

Membrane Channels. Discrete aqueous pores through the excitable nerve membrane, called sodium (or ion) channels, are molecular structures that mediate its sodium permeability. A channel seems to be a lipoglycoprotein firmly situated in the membrane (see Fig. 1-4). It consists of an aqueous pore spanning the membrane that is narrow enough at least at one point to discriminate between sodium ions and others; Na^+ passes through 12 times more easily than K^+. The channel also includes a portion that changes configuration in response to changes in membrane potential, thereby "gating" the passage of ions through the pore (C, O, and I states are described). The presence of these channels helps explain membrane permeability or impermeability to certain ions. Sodium channels have an internal diameter of approximately 0.3×0.5 nm.[14]

A sodium ion is "thinner" than either a potassium or chloride ion and therefore should diffuse freely down its concentration gradient through membrane channels into the nerve cell. However, this does not occur because all these ions attract water molecules and thus become hydrated. Hydrated sodium ions have a radius of 3.4 Å, which is approximately 50% greater than the 2.2 Å radius of potassium and chloride ions. Sodium ions therefore are too large to pass through the narrow channels when a nerve is at rest (Fig. 1-9). Potassium and chloride ions can pass through these channels. During *depolarization*, sodium ions readily pass through the nerve membrane because configurational changes that develop within the membrane produce a transient widening of these transmembrane channels to a size adequate to allow the unhindered passage of sodium ions down their concentration gradient into the axoplasm (transformation from the C to the O configuration). This concept can be visualized as the opening of a gate during depolarization that

Extracellular fluid

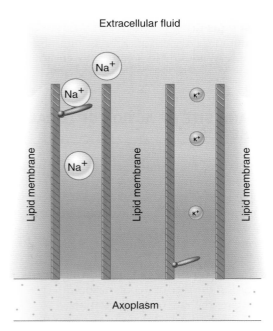

Figure 1-9. Membrane channels are partially occluded; the nerve is at rest. Hydrated sodium ions (*Na⁺*) are too large to pass through channels, although potassium ions (*K⁺*) can pass through unimpeded.

Extracellular fluid

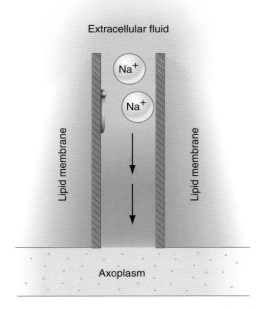

Figure 1-10. Membrane channels are open; depolarization occurs. Hydrated sodium ions (*Na⁺*) now pass unimpeded through the sodium channel.

is partially occluding the channel in the resting membrane (C) (Fig. 1-10).

Recent evidence indicates that *channel specificity* exists in that sodium channels differ from potassium channels.[15] The gates on the sodium channel are located near the external surface of the nerve membrane, whereas those on the potassium channel are located near the internal surface of the nerve membrane.

Impulse Propagation

After the initiation of an action potential by a stimulus, the impulse must move along the surface of the axon. Energy for impulse propagation is derived from the nerve membrane in the following manner:

The stimulus disrupts the resting equilibrium of the nerve membrane; the transmembrane potential is reversed momentarily, the interior of the cell changing from negative to positive, the exterior changing from positive to negative. This new electrical equilibrium in this segment of nerve produces local currents that begin flowing between the depolarized segment and the adjacent resting area. These local currents flow from positive to negative, extending for several millimeters along the nerve membrane.

As a result of this current flow, the interior of the adjacent area becomes less negative and its exterior less positive. Transmembrane potential decreases, approaching firing threshold for depolarization. When transmembrane potential is decreased by 15 mV from resting potential, firing threshold is reached and rapid

depolarization occurs. The newly depolarized segment sets up local currents in adjacent resting membrane, and the entire process starts anew.

Conditions in the segment that has just depolarized return to normal after the absolute and relative refractory periods. Because of this the wave of depolarization can spread in only one direction. Backward (retrograde) movement is prevented by the inexcitable, refractory segment.

Impulse Spread

The propagated impulse travels along the nerve membrane toward the CNS. The spread of this impulse differs depending on whether or not a nerve is myelinated.

Unmyelinated Nerves. An unmyelinated nerve fiber is basically a long cylinder with a high-electrical resistance cell membrane surrounding a low-resistance conducting core of axoplasm, all of which is bathed in low-resistance extracellular fluid.

The high-resistance cell membrane and low-resistance intracellular and extracellular media produce a rapid decrease in the density of current within a short distance of the depolarized segment. In areas immediately adjacent to this depolarized segment, local current flow may be adequate to initiate depolarization in the resting membrane. Farther away it will prove to be inadequate to achieve firing threshold.

The spread of an impulse in an unmyelinated nerve fiber is therefore characterized as a relatively slow

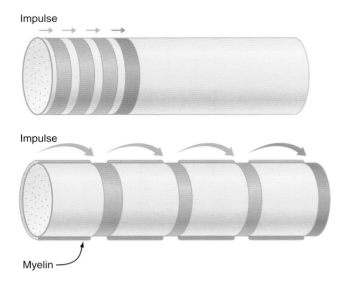

Impulse

Impulse

Myelin

Figure 1-11. Saltatory propagation. Comparing impulse propagation in nonmyelinated *(upper)* and myelinated *(lower)* axons. In nonmyelinated axons the impulse moves forward by sequential depolarization of short adjoining membrane segments. Depolarization in myelinated axons, on the other hand, is discontinuous; the impulse leaps forward from node to node. Note how much farther ahead the impulse is in the myelinated axon after four depolarization sequences. (Redrawn from de Jong RH: *Local anesthetics*, St Louis, 1994, Mosby.)

forward-creeping process (Fig. 1-11). Conduction rate in unmyelinated C fibers is 1.2 m/sec compared with 14.8 to 120 m/sec in myelinated A-alpha and A-delta fibers.[16]

Myelinated Nerves. Impulse spread within myelinated nerves differs from that in unmyelinated nerves because of the layer of insulating material separating the intracellular and extracellular charges. The farther apart the charges, the smaller is the current necessary to charge the membrane. Local currents thus can travel much farther in a myelinated nerve than in an unmyelinated nerve before becoming incapable of depolarizing the nerve membrane ahead of it.

Impulse conduction in myelinated nerves occurs by means of current leaps from node to node, a process termed *saltatory conduction* (see Fig. 1-11) (*saltare* is the Latin verb "to leap"). This form of impulse conduction proves to be much faster and more energy efficient than that employed in unmyelinated nerves. The thickness of the myelin sheath increases with increasing diameter of the axon. In addition, the distance between adjacent nodes of Ranvier increases with greater axonal diameter. Because of these two factors, saltatory conduction is more rapid in a thicker axon.

Saltatory conduction usually progresses from one node to the next in a stepwise manner. However, it can be demonstrated that the current flow at the next node still exceeds that necessary to reach the firing threshold of the nodal membrane. If conduction of an impulse is blocked at one node, the local current skips over that node and

proves adequate to raise the membrane potential at the next node to its firing potential and produce depolarization. A minimum of perhaps 8 to 10 mm of nerve must be covered by anesthetic solution to ensure thorough blockade.[17]

MODE AND SITE OF ACTION OF LOCAL ANESTHETICS

How and where local anesthetics alter the processes of impulse generation and transmission should be discussed. It is possible for local anesthetics to interfere with the excitation process in a nerve membrane in one or more of the following ways:
1. Altering the basic resting potential of the nerve membrane
2. Altering the threshold potential (firing level)
3. Decreasing the rate of depolarization
4. Prolonging the rate of repolarization

It has been established that the primary effects of local anesthetics occur during the depolarization phase of the action potential.[18] These effects include a decrease in the rate of depolarization, particularly in the phase of slow depolarization. Because of this, cellular depolarization is not sufficient to reduce the membrane potential of a nerve fiber to its firing level, and a propagated action potential does not develop. There is *no* accompanying change in the rate of repolarization.

Where Do Local Anesthetics Work?

The nerve membrane is the site at which local anesthetics exert their pharmacological actions. Many theories have been promulgated over the years to explain the mechanism of action of local anesthetics, including the acetylcholine, calcium displacement, and surface charge theories. The *acetylcholine theory* stated that acetylcholine was involved in nerve conduction in addition to its role as a neurotransmitter at nerve synapses.[19] There is no evidence that acetylcholine is involved in neural transmission along the body of the neuron. The *calcium displacement theory*, once popular, maintained that local anesthetic nerve block was produced by the displacement of calcium from some membrane site that controlled permeability to sodium.[20] Evidence that varying the concentration of calcium ions bathing a nerve does not affect local anesthetic potency has diminished the credibility of this theory. The *surface charge (repulsion) theory* proposed that local anesthetics acted by binding to the nerve membrane and changing the electrical potential at the membrane surface.[21] Cationic (RNH^+) (p. 6) drug molecules were aligned at the membrane–water interface, and because some of the local anesthetic molecules carried a net positive charge, they made the electrical potential at the membrane surface more positive, thus decreasing the excitability of the nerve by increasing the threshold potential. Current evidence indicates that the resting potential of the nerve membrane is unaltered by local anesthetics (they do not become hyperpolarized) and that conventional local anesthetics act within the membrane channels rather than at the membrane surface. Also, the surface charge theory cannot explain the activity of uncharged anesthetic molecules in blocking nerve impulses (e.g., benzocaine).

Two other theories, *membrane expansion* and *specific receptor*, are given some credence today. Of the two, the specific receptor theory is more widely held.

The *membrane expansion theory* states that local anesthetic molecules diffuse to hydrophobic regions of excitable membranes, producing a general disturbance of the bulk membrane structure, expanding some critical region(s) in the membrane, and preventing an increase in the permeability to sodium ions.[22,23] Local anesthetics that are highly lipid soluble can easily penetrate the lipid portion of the cell membrane, producing a change in configuration of the lipoprotein matrix of the nerve membrane. This results in a decreased diameter of sodium channels, which leads to an inhibition of both sodium conductance and neural excitation (Fig. 1-12). The membrane expansion theory serves as a possible explanation for the local anesthetic activity of a drug such as benzocaine,

which does not exist in cationic form yet still exhibits potent topical anesthetic activity. It has been demonstrated that nerve membranes, in fact, do expand and become more "fluid" when exposed to local anesthetics. However, there is no direct evidence that nerve conduction is entirely blocked by membrane expansion per se.

The *specific receptor theory*, the most favored today, proposes that local anesthetics act by binding to specific receptors on the sodium channel (Fig. 1-13).[24] The action of the drug is direct, not mediated by some change in the general properties of the cell membrane. Both biochemical and electrophysiological studies have indicated that a specific receptor site for local anesthetic agents exists in the sodium channel either on its external surface or on the internal axoplasmic surface.[25,26] Once the local anesthetic has gained access to the receptors, permeability to sodium ions is decreased or eliminated and nerve conduction is interrupted.

Local anesthetics are classified by their ability to react with specific receptor sites in the sodium channel. It appears that there are at least four sites within the sodium channel at which drugs can alter nerve conduction (see Fig. 1-13):

1. Within the sodium channel (tertiary amine local anesthetics)

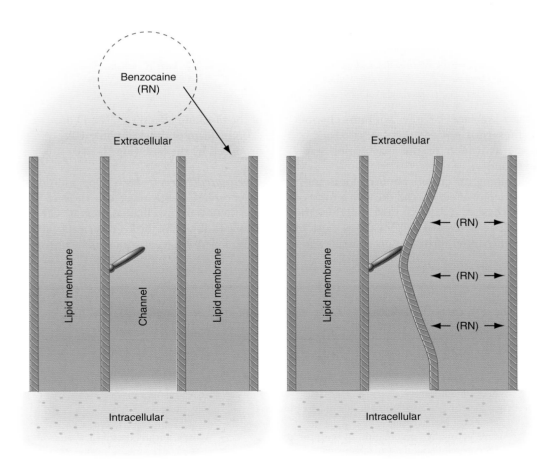

Figure 1-12. Membrane expansion theory.

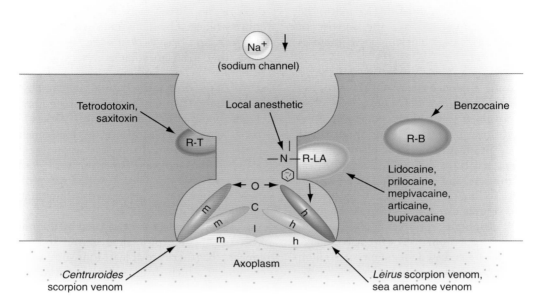

Figure 1-13. Tertiary amine local anesthetics inhibit the influx of sodium during nerve conduction by binding to a receptor within the sodium channel (*R-LA*). This blocks the normal activation mechanism (*O* gate configuration, depolarization) and also promotes movement of the activation and inactivation gates (*m* and *h*) to a position resembling that in the inactivated state (*I*). Biotoxins (*R-T*) block the influx of sodium at an outer surface receptor; various venoms do it by altering the activity of the activation and inactivation gates; and benzocaine (*R-B*) does it by expanding the membrane. *C*, Channel in the closed configuration. (Redrawn from Pallasch TJ: *Dent Drug Serv Newsletter* 4:25, 1983.)

2. At the outer surface of the sodium channel (tetrodotoxin, saxitoxin)

3–4. At either the activation or the inactivation gates (scorpion venom)

Table 1-3 is a biological classification of local anesthetics based on their site of action and the active form of the compound. Drugs in Class C exist only in the uncharged form (RN), whereas Class D drugs exist in both charged and uncharged forms. Approximately 90%

of the blocking effects of Class D drugs are caused by the cationic form of the drug; only 10% of blocking action is produced by the base (Fig. 1-14).

Myelinated Nerve Fibers. One additional factor should be considered with regard to the site of action of local anesthetics in myelinated nerves. The myelin sheath insulates the axon both electrically and pharmacologically. The only site at which molecules of local anesthetic

TABLE 1-3

Classification of Local Anesthetic Substances According to Biological Site and Mode of Action

Classification	Definition	Chemical Substance
Class A	Agents acting at receptor site on external surface of nerve membrane	Biotoxins (e.g., tetrodotoxin and saxitoxin)
Class B	Agents acting at receptor sites on internal surface of nerve membrane	Quaternary ammonium analogues of lidocaine Scorpion venom
Class C	Agents acting by a receptor-independent physico-chemical mechanism	Benzocaine
Class D	Agents acting by combination of receptor and receptor-independent mechanisms	Most clinically useful local anesthetic agents (e.g., articaine, lidocaine, mepivacaine, prilocaine)

(Modified from Covino BG, Vassallo HG: *Local anesthetics: mechanisms of action and clinical use*, New York, 1976, Grune & Stratton. Used by permission.)

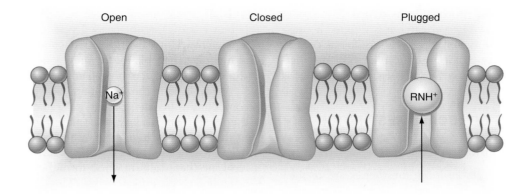

Figure 1-14. Channel entry. On the left is an open channel; inward permeant to sodium ion. The center channel is in the resting closed configuration; though impermeant to sodium ion here, the channel remains voltage responsive. The channel on the right, though in open configuration, is impermeant because it has local anesthetic cation bound to the gating receptor site. Note that the local anesthetic enters the channel from the axoplasmic (lower) side; the channel filter precludes direct entry via the external mouth. Local anesthetic renders the membrane impermeant to sodium ion; hence inexcitable by local action currents. (Redrawn from de Jong RH: *Local anesthetics*, St Louis, 1994, Mosby.)

have access to the nerve membrane is at the nodes of Ranvier where sodium channels are found in abundance. The ionic changes that develop during impulse conduction also arise only at the nodes.

Because an impulse may skip over or bypass one or two blocked nodes and continue on its way, it is necessary for at least two or three nodes immediately adjacent to the anesthetic solution to be blocked to ensure effective anesthesia, a length of approximately 8 to 10 mm.

Sodium channel densities differ in myelinated and unmyelinated nerves. In small unmyelinated nerves the density of sodium channels is about $35/\mu m,^2$ whereas at the nodes of Ranvier in myelinated fibers it may be as high as $20,000/\mu m.^2$ On an average nerve-length basis, there are relatively few sodium channels in unmyelinated nerve membranes. For example, in the garfish olfactory nerve the ratio of sodium channels to phospholipid molecules is 1:60,000, corresponding to a mean distance between channels of 0.2 μm, whereas at densely packed nodes of Ranvier the channels are separated by only 70 Å.[27,28]

How Local Anesthetics Work

The primary action of local anesthetics in producing a conduction block is to decrease the permeability of the ion channels to sodium ions (Na^+). Local anesthetics selectively inhibit the peak permeability of sodium, whose value is normally about five to six times greater than the minimum necessary for impulse conduction (e.g., there is a safety factor for conduction of 5× to 6×).[29] Local anesthetics reduce this safety factor, decreasing both the rate of rise of the action potential and its conduction velocity. When the safety factor falls below unity,[10] conduction fails and nerve block occurs.

Local anesthetics produce a very slight, virtually insignificant decrease in potassium (K^+) conductance through the nerve membrane.

Calcium ions (Ca^{++}), which exist in bound form within the cell membrane, are thought to exert a regulatory role on the movement of sodium ions across the nerve membrane. Release of bound calcium ions from the ion channel receptor site may be the primary factor responsible for the increased sodium permeability of the nerve membrane. This represents the first step in nerve membrane depolarization. Local anesthetic molecules may act by competitive antagonism with calcium for some site on the nerve membrane.

The following sequence is a proposed mechanism of action of local anesthetics:[1]

1. Displacement of calcium ions from the sodium channel receptor site, *which permits …*
2. Binding of the local anesthetic molecule to this receptor site, *which thus produces …*
3. Blockade of the sodium channel, *and a …*
4. Decrease in sodium conductance, *which leads to …*
5. Depression of the rate of electrical depolarization, *and a …*
6. Failure to achieve the threshold potential level, *along with a …*
7. Lack of development of propagated action potentials, *which is called …*
8. Conduction blockade.

The mechanism whereby sodium ions gain entry to the axoplasm of the nerve, thereby initiating an action potential, is altered by local anesthetics. The nerve membrane remains in a polarized state because the ionic movements responsible for the action potential fail to develop. Because the membrane's electrical potential remains unchanged, local currents do not develop and the self-perpetuating mechanism of impulse propagation is stalled. An impulse that arrives at a blocked nerve segment is stopped because it is unable to release the energy necessary for its continued propagation. Nerve block produced by local anesthetics is called a *nondepolarizing nerve block.*

ACTIVE FORMS OF LOCAL ANESTHETICS

Local Anesthetic Molecules

The majority of injectable local anesthetics are tertiary amines. Only a few (e.g., prilocaine and hexylcaine) are secondary amines. The typical local anesthetic structure is shown in Figures 1-15 and 1-16. The lipophilic part is the largest portion of the molecule. Aromatic in structure, it is derived from benzoic acid, aniline, or thiophene (articaine). All local anesthetics are amphipathic; that is, they possess both lipophilic and hydrophilic characteristics, generally at opposite ends of the molecule. The hydrophilic part is an amino derivative of ethyl alcohol or acetic acid. Local anesthetics without a hydrophilic part are not suited for injection but are good topical anesthetics (e.g., benzocaine). The anesthetic structure is completed by an intermediate hydrocarbon chain containing either an ester or an amide linkage. Other chemicals, especially histamine blockers and anticholinergics, share this basic structure with local anesthetics and commonly exhibit weak local anesthetic properties.

Local anesthetics are classified as either *amino esters* or *amino amides* according to their chemical linkages. The nature of the linkage is important in defining several properties of the local anesthetic, including the basic mode of biotransformation. Ester-linked local anesthetics (e.g., procaine) are readily hydrolyzed in aqueous solution. Amide-linked local anesthetics (e.g., lidocaine) are relatively resistant to hydrolysis. A greater percentage of an amide-linked drug is excreted unchanged in the urine than

of an ester-linked drug. Procainamide, which is procaine with an amide linkage replacing the ester linkage, is as potent a local anesthetic as procaine; yet, because of its amide linkage, it is hydrolyzed much more slowly. Procaine is hydrolyzed in plasma in only a few minutes, but just approximately 10% of procainamide is hydrolyzed in 1 day.

As prepared in the laboratory, local anesthetics are basic compounds, poorly soluble in water, and unstable on exposure to air.[30] Their pK_a values range from 7.5 to 10. In this form they have little or no clinical value. However, being weakly basic, they combine readily with acids to form local anesthetic salts, in which form they are quite soluble in water and comparatively stable. Thus local anesthetics used for injection are dispensed as salts, most commonly the hydrochloride salt, dissolved in either sterile water or saline.

It is well known that the pH of a local anesthetic solution (and the pH of the tissue into which it is injected) greatly influences its nerve-blocking action. *Acidification of tissue decreases local anesthetic effectiveness.* Inadequate anesthesia results when local anesthetics are injected into inflamed or infected areas. The inflammatory process produces acidic products: The pH of normal tissue is 7.4; the pH of an inflamed area is 5 to 6. Local anesthetics containing epinephrine or other vasopressors are acidified by the manufacturer to inhibit the oxidation of the vasopressor (p. 19). The pH of solutions without epinephrine is about 5.5; epinephrine-containing solutions have a pH of about 3.3. Clinically, this lower pH is more likely to produce a burning sensation on injection, as well as a slightly slower onset of anesthesia.

Increasing pH (alkalinization) of a local anesthetic solution speeds the onset of its action, increases its clinical effectiveness, and makes its injection more comfortable. However, the local anesthetic base, because it is unstable, precipitates out of alkalinized solutions, making these preparations ill suited for clinical use. Carbonated local anesthetics have received much attention in recent years. Sodium bicarbonate or carbon dioxide (CO_2) added to the anesthetic solution immediately before injection provides greater comfort and a more rapid onset of anesthesia (see Chapter 20).[31,32]

Despite wide pH variation of extracellular fluids, the pH at the interior of a nerve remains stable. Normal functioning of a nerve therefore is affected very little by changes in the extracellular environment. However, the ability of a local anesthetic to block nerve impulses is profoundly altered by changes in extracellular pH.

Dissociation of Local Anesthetics

As discussed, local anesthetics are available as salts (usually the hydrochloride) for clinical use. The local anesthetic salt, both water soluble and stable, is dissolved in either sterile water or saline. In this solution it exists simultaneously as uncharged molecules (RN),[1] also called the *base*, and positively charged molecules (RNH[+]),[2] called the *cation*.

$$RNH^+ \leftrightarrow RN + H^+$$

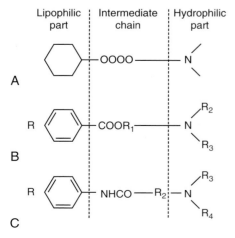

Figure 1-15. A, Typical local anesthetic. **B,** Ester type. **C,** Amide type.

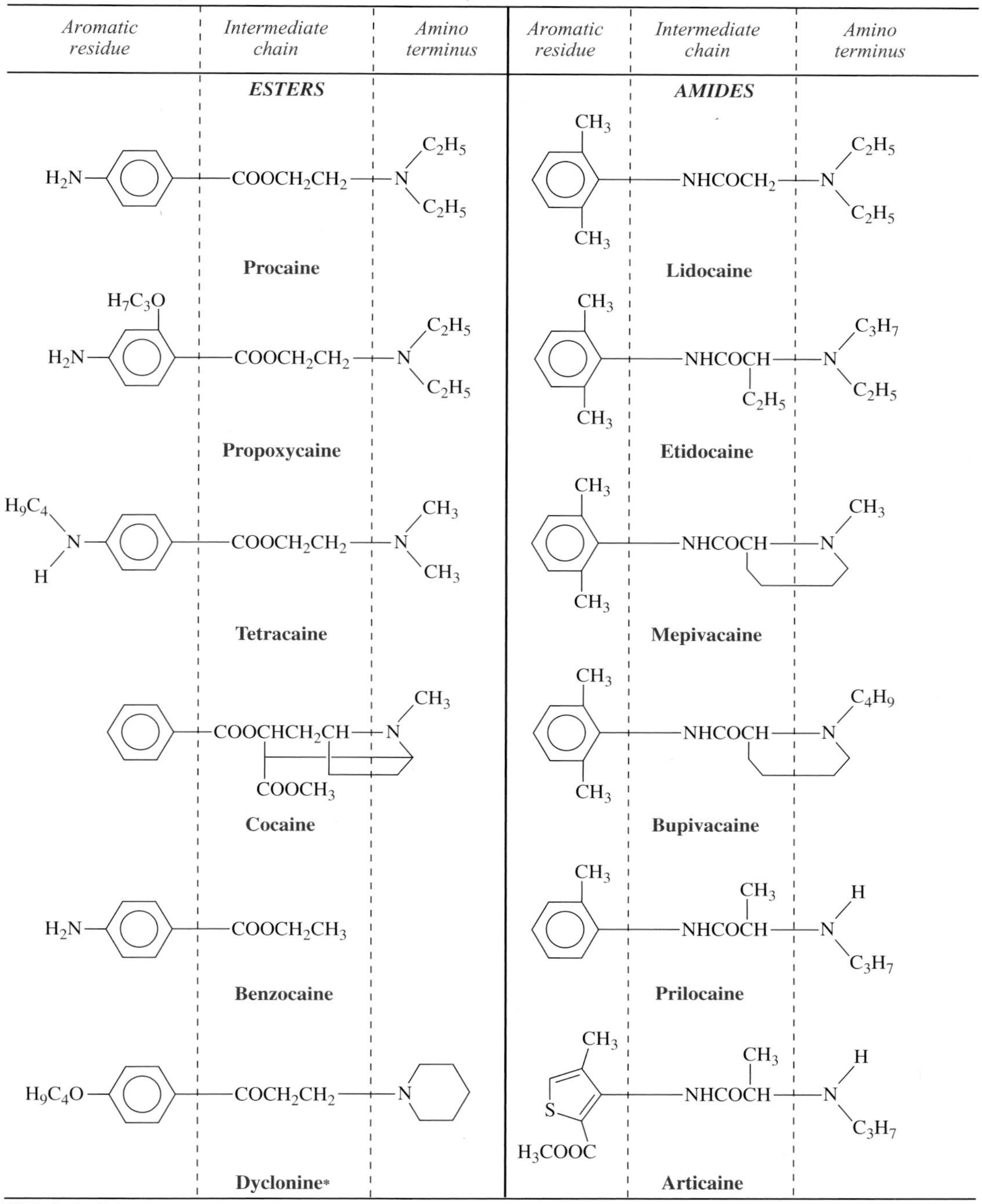
Aromatic residue
Intermediate chain
Amino terminus
Aromatic residue
Intermediate chain
Amino terminus
ESTERS
AMIDES
Procaine
Propoxycaine
Tetracaine
Cocaine
Benzocaine
Dyclonine*
Lidocaine
Etidocaine
Mepivacaine
Bupivacaine
Prilocaine
Articaine

*Dyclonine is a ketone.

Figure 1-16. Chemical configuration of local anesthetics. (From Yagiela JA, Neidle EA, Dowd FJ: *Pharmacology and therapeutics for dentistry*, ed 5, St Louis, in press, Mosby.)

The relative proportion of each ionic form in the solution varies with the pH of the solution or surrounding tissues. In the presence of a high concentration of hydrogen ions (low pH), the equilibrium shifts to the left and most of the anesthetic solution exists in cationic form:

$$RNH^+ > RN + H^+$$

As hydrogen ion concentration decreases (higher pH), the equilibrium shifts toward the free base form:

$$RNH^+ < RN + H^+$$

The relative proportion of ionic forms also depends on the pK_a, or dissociation constant, of the specific local anesthetic. The pK_a is a measure of a molecule's affinity for hydrogen ions (H^+). When the pH of the solution has the same value as the pK$_a$ of the local anesthetic, exactly 50% of the drug exists in the RNH$^+$ form and 50% in the RN form. The percentage of drug existing in either form can be determined from the Henderson-Hasselbalch equation:

$$\text{Log}\ \frac{\text{Base}}{\text{Acid}} = \text{pH} - \text{pK}_a$$

Table 1-4 lists the pK$_a$ values for the commonly used local anesthetics.

Actions on Nerve Membranes

The two factors involved in the action of a local anesthetic are *diffusion of the drug through the nerve sheath* and *binding at the receptor site* in the ion channel. The uncharged, lipid-soluble, free base form (RN) of the anesthetic is responsible for diffusion through the nerve sheath. This process is explained in the following example:

1. One thousand molecules of a local anesthetic with a pK$_a$ of 7.9 are injected in the tissues outside a nerve. The tissue pH is normal (7.4) (Fig. 1-17).
2. From Table 1-4 and the Henderson-Hasselbalch equation, it can be determined that at normal tissue pH, 75% of the local anesthetic molecules are present in the cationic form (RNH$^+$) and 25% in the free base form (RN).
3. Theoretically, all 250 lipophilic RN molecules diffuse through the nerve sheath to reach the interior (axoplasm) of the neuron.
4. Extracellularly, the equilibrium between RNH$^+$ and RN has been disrupted by the passage of the free base forms into the neuron. The remaining 750 extracellular RNH$^+$ molecules now reequilibrate according to the tissue pH and the drug pK$_a$.

$$\text{RNH}^+(570) \rightleftarrows \text{RN}(180) + \text{H}^+$$

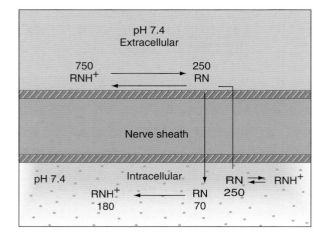

Figure 1-17. Mechanism of action of the local anesthetic molecule. Anesthetic pK$_a$ of 7.9; tissue pH of 7.4.

TABLE 1-4
Dissociation Constants (pK$_a$) of Local Anesthetics

Agent	pK$_a$	Percent Base (RN) at pH 7.4	Approximate Onset of Action (min)
Benzocaine	3.5	100	—
Mepivacaine	7.7	33	2 to 4
Lidocaine	7.7	29	2 to 4
Prilocaine	7.7	25	2 to 4
Articaine	7.8	29	2 to 4
Etidocaine	7.9	25	2 to 4
Ropivacaine	8.1	17	2 to 4
Bupivacaine	8.1	17	5 to 8
Tetracaine	8.6	7	10 to 15
Cocaine	8.6	7	—
Chloroprocaine	8.7	6	6 to 12
Propoxycaine	8.9	4	9 to 14
Procaine	9.1	2	14 to 18
Procainamide	9.3	1	—

5. The 180 newly created lipophilic RN molecules diffuse into the cell, starting the entire process (Step 4) again. Theoretically, this continues until all local anesthetic molecules diffuse into the axoplasm. In reality, however, not all the local anesthetic molecules reach the interior of the neuron because of the process of diffusion and because some are absorbed into local blood vessels and extracellular soft tissues at the injection site.
6. The inside of the nerve should be viewed next. After penetration of the nerve sheath and entry into the axoplasm by the lipophilic RN form of the anesthetic, a reequilibration takes place inside the nerve because the local anesthetic cannot exist in only the RN form at an intracellular pH of 7.4. Seventy-five percent of the RN molecules present within the axoplasm revert to the RNH$^+$ form; the remaining 25% of molecules remain in the uncharged RN form.
7. From the axoplasmic side the RNH$^+$ ions enter into the sodium channels and bind to the channel receptor site and are ultimately responsible for the conduction blockade that results (see Figs. 1-13 and 1-14).

Of the two factors, diffusibility and binding, responsible for local anesthetic effectiveness, the former is extremely important in actual practice. A local anesthetic's ability to diffuse through the tissues surrounding a nerve is of critical significance because in clinical situations the local anesthetic cannot be applied directly to the nerve membrane as it can in a laboratory setting. Local anesthetic solutions better able to diffuse through soft tissue are at an advantage in clinical practice.

A local anesthetic with a high pK$_a$ value has very few molecules available in the RN form at a tissue pH of 7.4. The onset of anesthetic action of this drug is slow because too few base molecules are available to diffuse through the nerve membrane (e.g., procaine, with a pK$_a$ of 9.1). *The rate of onset of anesthetic action is related to the pK$_a$ of the local anesthetic* (see Table 1-4).

A local anesthetic with a lower pK$_a$ (<7.5) has a very large number of lipophilic free base molecules that are able to diffuse through the nerve sheath; however, the anesthetic action of this drug is also inadequate because at an intracellular pH of 7.4, only a very small number of base molecules dissociate back to the cationic form necessary for binding at the receptor site.

In actual clinical situations with the local anesthetics currently available, the pH of the *extracellular fluid* determines the ease with which a local anesthetic moves from the site of its administration into the axoplasm of the nerve cell. The intracellular pH remains stable and independent of the extracellular pH. This is because hydrogen ions (H$^+$), like the local anesthetic cations (RNH$^+$), do not readily diffuse through tissues. The pH of extracellular fluid therefore may differ from that at the nerve membrane. The ratio of anesthetic cations to uncharged base molecules (RNH$^+$/RN) also may vary greatly at these sites. Differences in extracellular and intracellular pH are highly significant in pain control where there is inflammation or infection.[33] The effect of a decrease in tissue pH on the actions of a local anesthetic is described in Figure 1-18. This can be compared with the example in Figure 1-17, involving normal tissue pH.

1. Approximately 1000 molecules of a local anesthetic with a pK$_a$ of 7.9 are deposited outside a nerve. The tissue is inflamed and infected and has a pH of 6.
2. At this tissue pH, approximately 99% of the local anesthetic molecules are present in the charged cationic (RNH$^+$) form, with approximately 1% in the lipophilic free base (RN) form.
3. Approximately 10 RN molecules diffuse across the nerve sheath to reach the interior of the cell (contrasting with 250 RN molecules in the healthy example). The pH of the interior of the nerve cell remains normal (e.g., 7.4).

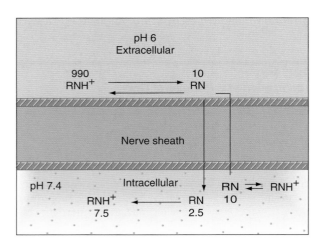

Figure 1-18. Effect of decreased tissue pH on the actions of a local anesthetic.

4. Extracellularly, the equilibrium between RNH$^+$ and RN, which has been disrupted, is reestablished. The relatively few newly created RN molecules diffuse into the cell, starting the entire process again. However, a sum total of fewer RN molecules succeed in eventually crossing the nerve sheath than would succeed at a normal pH because of the greatly increased absorption of anesthetic molecules into the blood vessels in the region (there is increased vascularity in the area of inflammation and infection).
5. After penetration of the nerve sheath by the base form, reequilibrium occurs. Approximately 75% of the molecules present intracellularly revert to the cationic form (RNH$^+$), 25% remaining in the uncharged free base form (RN).
6. The cationic molecules bind to receptor sites within the sodium channel, resulting in conduction blockade.

Adequate blockade of the nerve is more difficult to achieve in inflamed or infected tissues because of the relatively small number of molecules able to cross the nerve sheath (RN) and the increased absorption of the remaining anesthetic molecules into dilated blood vessels in this region. Although a potential problem in all aspects of dental practice, this situation is seen most often in endodontics. Possible remedies are described in Chapter 16.

Clinical Implications of pH and Local Anesthetic Activity

Most commercially prepared solutions of local anesthetics without a vasoconstrictor have a pH between 5.5 and 7. When injected into tissue, the vast buffering capacity of the tissue fluids rapidly returns the pH at the injection site to a normal 7.4. Local anesthetic solutions containing a vasopressor (e.g., epinephrine) are acidified by the manufacturer to retard oxidation of the vasoconstrictor, thereby prolonging the period of the drug's effectiveness. (See Chapter 3 for a discussion of the appropriate use of vasoconstrictors in local anesthetics.)

Epinephrine may be added to a local anesthetic solution immediately before its administration without the addition of antioxidants; however, if the solution is not used in a short time it will oxidize, turning a reddish brown.

Rapid oxidation of the vasopressor may be delayed, thereby increasing the shelf life of the product, through the addition of antioxidants. Sodium bisulfite is commonly used, in a concentration between 0.05% and 0.1%. A 2% solution of lidocaine HCl, with a pH of 6.8, is acidified to 4.2 by the addition of sodium bisulfite.

Even in this situation, the large buffering capacity of the tissues tends to maintain a normal tissue pH; however, it does require a longer time to do so after injection of a pH 4.2 solution than with a pH 6.8 solution. During this time the local anesthetic is not able to function at its full effectiveness, resulting in a slower onset of clinical action for local anesthetics with vasoconstrictors compared with their "plain" counterparts.

Local anesthetics are clinically effective on both axons and free nerve endings. Free nerve endings lying below intact skin may be reached only by the injection of anesthetic beneath the skin. Intact skin forms an impenetrable barrier to the diffusion of local anesthetics. The recently formulated EMLA (eutectic mixture of local anesthetics) enables local anesthetics to penetrate intact skin, albeit slowly.[34]

Mucous membranes and injured skin (e.g., burns and abrasions) lack the protection afforded by intact skin, permitting topically applied local anesthetics to diffuse through to reach free nerve endings. Topical anesthetics can be employed effectively wherever skin is no longer intact because of injury, as well as on mucous membranes (e.g., cornea, gingiva, pharynx, trachea, larynx, esophagus, rectum, vagina, and bladder).[35]

The buffering capacity of mucous membrane is poor; thus the topical application of a local anesthetic with a pH between 5.5 and 6.5 lowers the regional pH to below normal, and less local anesthetic base is formed. Diffusion of the drug across the mucous membrane to free nerve endings is limited and nerve block is ineffective. Increasing the pH of the drug provides more RN form, thereby increasing potency of the topical anesthetic; however, the drug in this form is more rapidly oxidized. The effective shelf life of the local anesthetic decreases as the drug's pH increases.[30]

To increase the clinical efficacy of topical anesthetics, a more concentrated form of the drug commonly is used (5% or 10% lidocaine) than for injection (2% lidocaine). Although only a small percentage of the drug is available in the base form, raising the concentration provides more RN molecules for diffusion and dissociation to the active cation form at free nerve endings.

Some topical anesthetics (e.g., benzocaine) are not ionized in solution; thus their anesthetic effectiveness is unaffected by pH. Because of benzocaine's poor water solubility, its absorption from the site of application is minimal, and systemic reactions (e.g., overdoses) are rarely encountered.

KINETICS OF LOCAL ANESTHETIC ONSET AND DURATION OF ACTION

Barriers to Diffusion of the Solution

A peripheral nerve is composed of hundreds to thousands of tightly packed axons. These axons are protected, supported, and nourished by several layers of fibrous and elastic tissues. Nutrient blood vessels and lymphatics course throughout the layers.

Individual nerve fibers (axons) are covered with, and also separated from each other by, the *endoneurium*. The *perineurium* then binds these nerve fibers together into

bundles called *fasciculi*. The radial nerve, located in the wrist, contains between 5 and 10 fasciculi. Each fasciculus contains between 500 and 1000 individual nerve fibers. Five thousand nerve fibers occupy approximately 1 mm^2 of space.

The thickness of the perineurium varies with the diameter of the fasciculus it surrounds. The thicker the perineurium, the slower the rate of local anesthetic diffusion across it.[36] The innermost layer of perineurium is the perilemma. It is covered with a smooth mesothelial membrane. The perilemma represents the main barrier to diffusion into a nerve.

Fasciculi are contained within a loose network of areolar connective tissue called the *epineurium*. The epineurium constitutes between 30% and 75% of the total cross-section of a nerve. Local anesthetics are readily able to diffuse through the epineurium because of its loose consistency. Nutrient blood vessels and lymphatics traverse the epineurium. These vessels absorb local anesthetic molecules, thus removing them from the site of injection.

The outer layer of the epineurium surrounding the nerve is denser and thickened, forming what is termed the *epineural sheath* or *nerve sheath*. The epineural sheath does not constitute a barrier to diffusion of local anesthetic into a nerve.

Table 1-5 summarizes the layers of a typical peripheral nerve.

Induction of Local Anesthesia

After the administration of a local anesthetic into the soft tissues near a nerve, molecules of the local anesthetic traverse the distance from one site to another according to their concentration gradient. During the induction phase of anesthesia, the local anesthetic moves from its extraneural site of deposition toward the nerve (as well as in all other possible directions). This process is termed *diffusion*. It is the unhindered migration of molecules or ions through a fluid medium under the influence of the concentration gradient. *Penetration* of an anatomical barrier

TABLE 1-5	
Organization of a Peripheral Nerve	
Structure	**Description**
Nerve fiber	Single nerve cell
Endoneurium	Covers each nerve fiber
Fasciculi	Bundles of 500 to 1000 nerve fibers
Perineurium*	Covers fasciculi
Perilemma*	Innermost layer of perineurium
Epineurium	Alveolar connective tissue supporting fasciculi and carrying nutrient vessels
Epineural sheath	Outer layer of epineurium

*The perineurium and perilemma constitute the greatest anatomical barriers to diffusion in a peripheral nerve.

to diffusion occurs when a drug passes through a tissue that tends to restrict free molecular movement. The perineurium is the greatest barrier to penetration of local anesthetics.

Diffusion. The rate of diffusion is governed by several factors, the most significant of which is the *concentration gradient*. The greater the initial concentration of the local anesthetic, the faster is the diffusion of its molecules and the more rapid its onset of action.

Fasciculi that are located near the surface of the nerve are termed *mantle bundles* (Fig. 1-19, *A*). Mantle bundles are the first ones reached by the local anesthetic and are exposed to a higher concentration of it. Mantle bundles usually are blocked completely shortly after the injection of a local anesthetic (Fig. 1-19, *B*).

Fasciculi found closer to the center of the nerve are called *core bundles*. Core bundles are contacted by a local anesthetic only after much delay and by a lower anesthetic concentration because of the greater distance that the solution must traverse and the greater number of barriers it must cross.

As the local anesthetic diffuses into the nerve, it becomes increasingly diluted by tissue fluids with some being absorbed by capillaries and lymphatics. Ester anesthetics undergo almost immediate enzymatic hydrolysis. Thus core fibers are exposed to a decreased concentration of local anesthetic, a fact that may explain the clinical situation of inadequate pulpal anesthesia developing in the presence of subjective symptoms of adequate soft-tissue anesthesia. Complete conduction blockade of all nerve fibers in a peripheral nerve requires that an adequate *volume*, as well as an adequate *concentration* of the local anesthetic be deposited. In no clinical situation are 100% of the fibers within a peripheral nerve blocked, even in cases of clinically excellent pain control.[37] Fibers near the surface of the nerve (mantle fibers) tend to innervate more proximal regions (e.g., the molar area with an inferior alveolar nerve block), whereas fibers in the core bundles innervate the more distal points of nerve distribution (e.g., the incisors and canine with an inferior alveolar block).

Blocking Process. After deposition of the local anesthetic as close to the nerve as possible, the solution diffuses in all directions according to prevailing concentration gradients. A portion of the injected local anesthetic diffuses toward the nerve and into the nerve. However, a significant portion of the injected drug also diffuses away from the nerve. The following reactions then occur:

1. Some of the drug is absorbed by nonneural tissues (e.g., muscle and fat).
2. Some is diluted by interstitial fluid.
3. Some is removed by capillaries and lymphatics from the injection site.
4. Ester-type anesthetics are hydrolyzed.

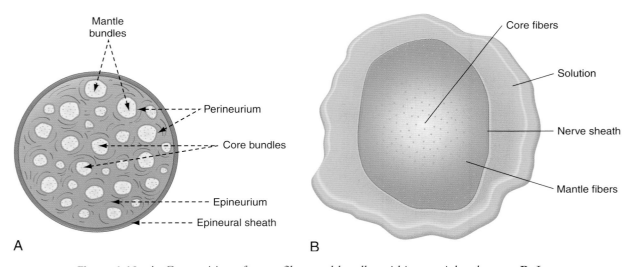

A   **B**

Figure 1-19. A, Composition of nerve fibers and bundles within a peripheral nerve. **B,** In a large peripheral nerve (containing hundreds or thousands of axons), local anesthetic solution must diffuse inward toward the nerve core from the extraneural site of injection. Local anesthetic molecules are removed by tissue uptake while tissue fluid mixes with the carrier solvent. This results in a gradual dilution of the local anesthetic solution as it penetrates the nerve toward the core. A concentration gradient occurs during induction so that the outer mantle fibers are solidly blocked, whereas the inner core fibers are not yet blocked. Core fibers are not only exposed to a lower local anesthetic concentration, but the drug also arrives later. Delay depends on the tissue mass to be penetrated and the diffusivity of the local anesthetic. (Redrawn from **B,** de Jong RH: *Local anesthetics,* St Louis, 1994, Mosby.)

TABLE 1-6
Chemical Structure, Physicochemical Properties, and Pharmacological Properties of Local Anesthetic Agents

Agent	Chemical Configuration			Physicochemical Properties				Pharmacological Properties		
	Aromatic (lipophilic)	Intermediate Chain	Amine (hydrophilic)	Molecular Weight (base)	pKa (36°C)	Onset	Approx. Lipid Solubility	Usual Effective Concentration %	Protein Binding	Duration
ESTERS										
Procaine				236	9.1	Slow	1.0	2 to 4	5	Short
Chloroprocaine				271	8.7	Fast	NA	2	NA	Short
Tetracaine				264	8.4	Slow	80	0.15	85	Long
AMIDES										
Mepivacaine				246	7.9	Fast	1.0	2 to 3	75	Moderate
Prilocaine				220	7.7	Fast	1.5	4	55	Moderate

Drug							
Lidocaine		234	7.7	Fast	4.0	2	65	Moderate
Ropivacaine		274	8.1	Moderate	2.8	0.2 to 0.5	94	Long
Bupivacaine		288	8.1	Moderate	NA	0.5 to 0.75	95	Long
Etidocaine		276	7.9	Fast	140	0.5 to 1.5	94	Long
Articaine		320	7.8	Fast	17	4	95	Moderate

(Modified from Rogers MC, et al, editors: *Principles and practice of anesthesiology*, St Louis, 1993, Mosby.)
NA, Not available.

The sum total of these factors is to decrease the local anesthetic concentration outside the nerve; however, the concentration of local anesthetic within the nerve continues to rise as diffusion progresses. These processes continue until an equilibrium results between the intraneural and extraneural concentrations of anesthetic solution.

Induction Time. *Induction time* is defined as the period from deposition of the anesthetic solution to complete conduction blockade. Several factors control the induction time of a given drug. Those under the operator's control are the concentration of the drug and the pH of the local anesthetic solution. Factors not under the clinician's control are the diffusion constant of the anesthetic drug and the anatomical diffusion barriers of the nerve.

Physical Properties and Clinical Actions. There are other physicochemical factors of a local anesthetic that influence its clinical characteristics.

The effect of the *dissociation constant* (pK$_a$) on the rate of onset of anesthesia has been described. Although both molecular forms of the anesthetic are important in neural blockade, drugs with a lower pK$_a$ possess a more rapid onset of action than do those with a higher pK$_a$.[38]

Lipid solubility of a local anesthetic appears to be related to its intrinsic potency. The estimated lipid solubilities of various local anesthetics are presented in Table 1-6. Increased lipid solubility permits the anesthetic to penetrate the nerve membrane (which itself is 90% lipid) more easily. This is reflected biologically in the increased potency of the anesthetic. Local anesthetics with greater lipid solubility produce more effective conduction blockade at lower concentrations (lower percentage solutions or smaller volumes deposited) than do the less lipid-soluble local anesthetics.

The degree of *protein binding* of the local anesthetic molecule is responsible for the duration of anesthetic activity. After penetration of the nerve sheath, a reequilibrium occurs between the base and cationic forms of the local anesthetic. Now, in the sodium channel itself, the RNH$^+$ ions bind at the receptor site. Proteins constitute approximately 10% of the nerve membrane, and local anesthetics (e.g., etidocaine, ropivacaine, and bupivacaine) possessing a greater degree of protein binding (see Table 1-6) than others (e.g., procaine) appear to attach more securely to the protein receptor sites and to possess a longer duration of clinical activity.[39]

Vasoactivity affects both the anesthetic potency and the duration of anesthesia provided by a drug. Injection of local anesthetics, such as procaine, with greater vasodilating properties increases perfusion of the local site with blood. The injected local anesthetic is absorbed into the cardiovascular compartment more rapidly and carried away from the injection site and from the nerve, thus providing for a shortened duration of anesthesia, as well as decreased potency of the drug. Table 1-7 summarizes the influence of various factors on local anesthetic action.

Recovery from Local Anesthetic Block

Emergence from a local anesthetic nerve block follows the same diffusion patterns as induction does; however, it does so in the *reverse order.*

The extraneural concentration of local anesthetic is continually depleted by diffusion, dispersion, and uptake of the drug, whereas the intraneural concentration of the local anesthetic remains relatively stable. The concentration gradient thus is reversed, the intraneural concentration exceeding the extraneural concentration, and the anesthetic molecules begin to diffuse out of the nerve.

Fasciculi in the mantle begin to lose the local anesthetic much earlier than do the core bundles. Recovery from block anesthesia appears first in the proximally innervated regions (e.g., third molars before the central incisors). Core fibers gradually lose their local anesthetic concentration. Recovery is usually a slower process than induction because the local anesthetic is bound to the drug receptor site in the sodium channel and therefore is released more slowly than it is absorbed.

Reinjection of Local Anesthetic

Frequently a dental procedure outlasts the duration of clinically effective pain control and a repeat injection of local anesthetic is necessary. Usually this repeat injection immediately results in a return of profound anesthesia; on some occasions, however, the clinician may encounter greater difficulty in reestablishing adequate pain control.

Recurrence of Immediate Profound Anesthesia. At the time of reinjection, the concentration of local anesthetic in the mantle fibers is below that in the more centrally located core fibers. The partially recovered mantle fibers still contain some local anesthetic, although not enough to provide complete anesthesia. After deposition of a new high concentration of anesthetic near the nerve, the mantle fibers are once again exposed to a concentration gradient directed inward toward the nerve. This combination of residual local anesthetic (in the nerve) and the newly deposited supply results in a rapid onset of profound anesthesia with a smaller volume of local anesthetic drug being administered.

Difficulty Reachieving Profound Anesthesia. In this second situation, as in the first, the dental procedure has outlasted the clinical effectiveness of the local anesthetic drug and the patient is experiencing pain. The doctor readministers a volume of local anesthetic but, unlike the first scenario, effective control of pain does not occur.

Tachyphylaxis. In this second clinical situation a process known as tachyphylaxis occurs. *Tachyphylaxis* is defined as an increasing tolerance to a drug that is administered repeatedly. It is much more likely to develop if nerve function is allowed to return before reinjection (e.g., if the patient complains of pain). The duration,

TABLE **1-7**

Factors Affecting Local Anesthetic Action

Factor	Action Affected	Description
pK_a	Onset	Lower pK_a = More rapid onset of action, more RN molecules present to diffuse through nerve sheath; thus onset time is decreased
Lipid solubility	Anesthetic potency	Increased lipid solubility = Increased potency (example: procaine = 1; etidocaine = 140)
		Etidocaine produces conduction blockade at very low concentrations, whereas procaine poorly suppresses nerve conduction, even at higher concentrations
Protein binding	Duration	Increased protein binding allows anesthetic cations (RNH^+) to be more firmly attached to proteins located at receptor sites; thus duration of action is increased
Nonnervous tissue diffusibility	Onset	Increased diffusibility = Decreased time of onset
Vasodilator activity	Anesthetic potency and duration	Greater vasodilator activity = Increased blood flow to region = Rapid removal of anesthetic molecules from injection site; thus decreased anesthetic potency and decreased duration

(From Cohen S, Burns RC: *Pathways of the pulp*, ed 6, St Louis, 1994, Mosby.)

intensity, and spread of anesthesia with reinjection are greatly reduced.[40]

Although difficult to explain, tachyphylaxis is probably brought about through some or all of the following factors: edema, localized hemorrhage, clot formation, transudation, hypernatremia, and decreased pH of tissues. The first four factors isolate the nerve from contact with the local anesthetic solution. The fifth, hypernatremia, raises the sodium ion gradient, thus counteracting the decrease in sodium ion conduction brought about by the local anesthetic. The last factor, a decrease in pH of the tissues, is brought about by the first injection of the acidic local anesthetic. The ambient pH in the area of injection may be somewhat lower, so that fewer local anesthetic molecules are transformed into the free base (RN) on reinjection.

Duration of Anesthesia

As the local anesthetic is removed from the nerve, the function of the nerve returns rapidly at first but then gradually slows. Compared with the onset of the nerve block, which is rapid, recovery from nerve block is much slower because the local anesthetic is bound to the nerve membrane. Longer-acting local anesthetics (e.g., bupivacaine, ropivacaine, and tetracaine) are more firmly bound in the nerve membrane (increased protein binding) than are shorter-acting drugs (e.g., procaine and lidocaine), and therefore are released from the receptor sites in the sodium channels more slowly. The rate at which an anesthetic is removed from a nerve has an effect on the duration of neural blockade; in addition to increased *protein binding*, other factors that influence the rate of a drug's removal from the injection site are the *vascularity of the injection site* and the *presence or absence of a vasoactive substance*. Anesthetic duration is increased in areas of decreased vascularity, and the addition of a vasopressor decreases tissue perfusion to a local area, thus increasing the duration of the block.

REFERENCES

1. Covino BG, Vassallo HG: *Local anesthetics: mechanisms of action and clinical use*, New York, 1976, Grune & Stratton.
2. Bennett CR: *Monheim's local anesthesia and pain control in dental practice*, ed 5, St Louis, 1974, Mosby.
3. Fitzgerald MJT: *Neuroanatomy: basic and clinical*, London, 1992, Baillière Tyndall.
4. Noback CR, Strominger NL, Demarest RJ: *The human nervous system: introduction and review*, ed 4, Philadelphia, 1991, Lea & Febiger.
5. Singer SJ, Nicholson GL: The fluid mosaic model of the structure of cell membranes, *Science* 175:720-731, 1972.
6. Guyton AC: *Basic neuroscience: anatomy and physiology*, ed 2, Philadelphia, 1991, WB Saunders.
7. Guidotti G: The composition of biological membranes, *Arch Intern Med* 129:194-201, 1972.
8. Denson DD, Maziot JX: *Physiology, pharmacology, and toxicity of local anesthetics: adult and pediatric considerations*. In Raj PP, editor: *Clinical practice of regional anesthesia*, New York, 1991, Churchill Livingstone.
9. Heavner JE: *Molecular action of local anesthetics*. In Raj PP, editor: *Clinical practice of regional anesthesia*, New York, 1991, Churchill Livingstone.
10. de Jong RH: *Local anesthetics*, ed 2, Springfield, Ill, 1977, Charles C Thomas.
11. Hodgkin AL, Huxley AF: A quantitative description of membrane current and its application to conduction and excitation in nerve, *J Physiol (London)* 117:500-544, 1954.
12. Noback CR, Demarest RJ: *The human nervous system: basic principles of neurobiology*, ed 3, New York, 1981, McGraw-Hill, pp 44-45.
13. Keynes RD: Ion channels in the nerve-cell membrane, *Sci Am* 240:326-135, 1979.
14. Cattarall WA: Structure and function of voltage-sensitive ion channels, *Science* 242:50-61, 1988.
15. Hille B: Ionic selectivity, saturation, and block in sodium channels: a four-barrier model, *J Gen Physiol* 66:535-560, 1975.

16. Ritchie JM: *Physiological basis for conduction in myelinated nerve fibers.* In Morell P, editor: *Myelin,* ed 2, New York, 1984, Plenum Press, pp 117-145.

17. Franz DN, Perry RS: Mechanisms for differential block among single myelinated and non-myelinated axons by procaine, *J Physiol* 235:193-210, 1974.

18. de Jong RH, Wagman IH: Physiological mechanisms of peripheral nerve block by local anesthetics, *Anesthesiology* 24:684-727, 1963.

19. Dettbarn WD: The acetylcholine system in peripheral nerve, *Ann NY Acad Sci* 144:483-503, 1967.

20. Goldman DE, Blaustein MP: Ions, drugs and the axon membrane, *Ann NY Acad Sci* 137:967-981, 1966.

21. Wei LY: Role of surface dipoles on axon membrane, *Science* 163:280-282, 1969.

22. Lee AG: Model for action of local anesthetics, *Nature* 262:545-548, 1976.

23. Seeman P: The membrane actions of anesthetics and tranquilizers, *Pharmacol Rev* 24:583-655, 1972.

24. Strichartz GR, Ritchie JM: *The action of local anesthetics on ion channels of excitable tissues.* In Strichartz GR, editor: *Local anesthetics,* New York, 1987, Springer-Verlag.

25. Butterworth JF IV, Strichartz GR: Molecular mechanisms of local anesthesia: a review, *Anesthesiology* 72:711-734, 1990.

26. Ritchie JM: Mechanisms of action of local anesthetic agents and biotoxins, *Br J Anaesthes* 47:191-198, 1975.

27. Rasminsky M: *Conduction in normal and pathological nerve fibers.* In Swash M, Kennard C, editors: *Scientific basis of clinical neurology,* Edinburgh, 1985, Churchill Livingstone.

28. Ritchie JM: *The distribution of sodium and potassium channels in mammalian myelinated nerve.* In Ritchie JM, Keyes RD, Bolis L, editors: *Ion channels in neural membranes,* New York, 1986, Alan R Liss.

29. Hille B, Courtney K, Dum R: *Rate and site of action of local anesthetics in myelinated nerve fibers.* In Fink BR, editor: *Molecular mechanisms of anesthesia,* New York, 1975, Raven Press, pp 13-20.

30. Setnikar I: Ionization of bases with limited solubility: investigation of substances with local anesthetic activity, *J Pharm Sci* 55:1190-1195, 1990.

31. Stewart JH, Chinn SE, Cole GW, Klein JA: Neutralized lidocaine with epinephrine for local anesthesia-II, *J Dermatol Surg Oncol* 16:942-845, 1990.

32. Bokesch PM, Raymond SA, Strichartz GR: Dependence of lidocaine potency on pH and pCO_2, *Anesth Analg* 66:9-17, 1987.

33. Bieter RN: Applied pharmacology of local anesthetics, *Am J Surg* 34:500-510, 1936.

34. Buckley MM, Benfield P: Eutectic lidocaine/prilocaine cream: a review of the topical anesthetic/analgesic efficacy of a eutectic mixture of local anesthetics (EMLA), *Drugs* 46:126-151, 1993.

35. Campbell AH, Stasse JA, Lord GH, Willson JE: In vivo evaluation of local anesthetics applied topically, *J Pharm Sci* 57:2045-2048, 1968.

36. Noback CR, Demarest RJ: *The human nervous system: basic principles of neurobiology,* ed 3, New York, 1981, McGraw-Hill.

37. de Jong RH: *Local anesthetics,* ed 2, Springfield, Ill, 1977, Charles C Thomas, pp 66-68.

38. Ritchie JM, Ritchie B, Greengard P: The active structure of local anesthetics, *J Pharmacol Exp Ther* 150:152, 1965.

39. Tucker GT: Plasma binding and disposition of local anesthetics, *Int Anesthesiol Clin* 13:33, 1975.

40. Cohen EN, Levine DA, Colliss JE, Gunther RE: The role of pH in the development of tachyphylaxis to local anesthetic agents, *Anesthesiology* 29:994-1001, 1968.

Pharmacology of Local Anesthetics

CHAPTER

2

Local anesthetics, when used for the management of pain, differ from most other drugs commonly used in medicine and dentistry in one important manner. Virtually all other drugs, regardless of the route through which they are administered, must ultimately enter into the circulatory system in sufficiently high concentrations (e.g., attain therapeutic blood levels) *before* they can begin to exert a clinical action. Local anesthetics, however, when used for pain control, *cease* to provide a clinical effect when they are absorbed from the site of administration into the circulation. One prime factor involved in the termination of action of local anesthetics used for pain control is their redistribution from the nerve fiber into the cardiovascular system.

The presence of a local anesthetic in the circulatory system means that the drug will be transported to every part of the body. Local anesthetics have the ability to alter the functioning of some of these cells. In this chapter the actions of local anesthetics, other than their ability to block conduction in nerve axons of the peripheral nervous system, are reviewed. A classification of local anesthetics is shown in Box 2-1.

PHARMACOKINETICS OF LOCAL ANESTHETICS

Uptake

When injected into soft tissues, local anesthetics exert a pharmacological action on the blood vessels in the area. All local anesthetics possess a degree of vasoactivity, most producing dilation of the vascular bed into which they are deposited, although the degree of vasodilation may vary, and some may produce vasoconstriction. To some degree these effects may be concentration dependent.[1] Relative vasodilating values of amide local anesthetics are shown in Table 2-1.

Ester local anesthetics are also potent vasodilating drugs. *Procaine*, probably the most potent vasodilator, is used clinically for vasodilation when peripheral blood flow has been compromised because of (accidental) intraarterial (IA) injection of a drug (e.g., thiopental).[2] IA administration of an irritating drug such as thiopental may produce arteriospasm with an attendant decrease in tissue perfusion that if prolonged could lead to tissue death, gangrene, and loss of the limb. In this situation procaine is administered IA in an attempt to break the arteriospasm and reestablish blood flow to the affected limb. *Tetracaine*, *chloroprocaine*, and *propoxycaine* also possess vasodilating properties to varying degrees but not to the degree of procaine.

Cocaine is the only local anesthetic consistently producing vasoconstriction.[3] The initial action of cocaine is vasodilation, which is followed by an intense and prolonged vasoconstriction. It is produced by an inhibition of the uptake of catecholamines (especially norepinephrine) into tissue binding sites. This results in an excess of free norepinephrine, leading to a prolonged and intense state of vasoconstriction. This inhibition of the reuptake of norepinephrine has not been demonstrated with other local anesthetics, such as lidocaine and bupivacaine.

A significant clinical effect of vasodilation is an increase in the rate of absorption of the local anesthetic into the blood, thus decreasing the duration and quality (e.g., depth) of pain control while increasing the anesthetic blood (or plasma) concentration and the potential for overdose (toxic reaction). The rates at which local anesthetics are absorbed into the bloodstream and reach their peak blood level vary according to their route of administration (Table 2-2).

Oral Route. With the exception of cocaine, local anesthetics are absorbed poorly, if at all, from the gastrointestinal tract after oral administration. In addition, most local anesthetics (especially lidocaine) undergo a significant

BOX 2-1

Classification of Local Anesthetics

ESTERS
Esters of benzoic acid:
   Butacaine
   Cocaine
   Ethyl aminobenzoate (benzocaine)
   Hexylcaine
   Piperocaine
   Tetracaine
Esters of paraaminobenzoic acid:
   Chloroprocaine
   Procaine
   Propoxycaine

AMIDES
   Articaine
   Bupivacaine
   Dibucaine
   Etidocaine
   Lidocaine
   Mepivacaine
   Prilocaine
   Ropivacaine

QUINOLINE
   Centbucridine

TABLE 2-1
Relative Vasodilating Values of Amide-Type Local Anesthetics

	Vasodilating Activity	Mean % Increase in Femoral Artery Blood Flow in Dogs After Intraarterial Injection*	
		1 min	5 min
Articaine	1 (approx)	NA	NA
Bupivacaine	2.5	45.4	30
Etidocaine	2.5	44.3	26.6
Lidocaine	1	25.8	7.5
Mepivacaine	0.8	35.7	9.5
Prilocaine	0.5	42.1	6.3
Tetracaine	NA	37.6	14

(Modified from Blair MR: Cardiovascular pharmacology of local anaesthetics, *Br J Anaesth* 47(suppl):247–252, 1975.)
*Each agent injected rapidly in a dose of 1 mg/0.1 ml saline.
NA, Not available.

TABLE 2-2
Time to Achieve Peak Blood Level

Route	Time (min)
Intravenous	1
Topical	5 (approximately)
Intramuscular	5–10
Subcutaneous	30–90

hepatic first-pass effect after oral administration. After absorption of lidocaine from the gastrointestinal tract into the enterohepatic circulation, a fraction of the drug dose is carried to the liver, where approximately 72% of the dose is biotransformed into inactive metabolites.[4] This has seriously hampered the use of lidocaine as an oral antidysrhythmic drug. In 1984 Astra Pharmaceuticals and Merck Sharp & Dohme introduced an analogue of lidocaine, tocainide hydrochloride, which is effective orally.[5] The chemical structures of tocainide and lidocaine are presented in Figure 2-1.

Topical Route. Local anesthetics are absorbed at differing rates after application to mucous membrane: In the *tracheal mucosa,* absorption is almost as rapid as with intravenous (IV) administration (indeed, intratracheal drug administration [epinephrine, lidocaine, atropine, naloxone, and flumazenil] is used in certain emergency situations); in *the pharyngeal mucosa,* absorption is slower; and in the *esophageal* or *bladder mucosa,* uptake is even slower than occurs through the pharynx. Wherever there is no layer of intact skin present, topically applied local anesthetics can produce an anesthetic effect. Sunburn remedies (e.g., Solarcaine) usually contain lidocaine, benzocaine, or other anesthetics in an ointment formulation. Applied to intact skin, they will not provide an anesthetic action, but with skin damaged by sunburn they bring rapid relief of pain. A eutectic mixture of local anesthetics (EMLA) has been developed that is able to provide surface anesthesia of intact skin.[6] (EMLA is discussed in Chapter 19.)

Injection. The rate of uptake (absorption) of local anesthetics after parenteral administration (subcutaneous, intramuscular, or IV) is related to both the vascularity of the injection site and the vasoactivity of the drug.

IV administration of local anesthetics provides the most rapid elevation of blood levels and is used clinically in the primary management of ventricular dysrhythmias.[7] Rapid IV administration can lead to significantly high

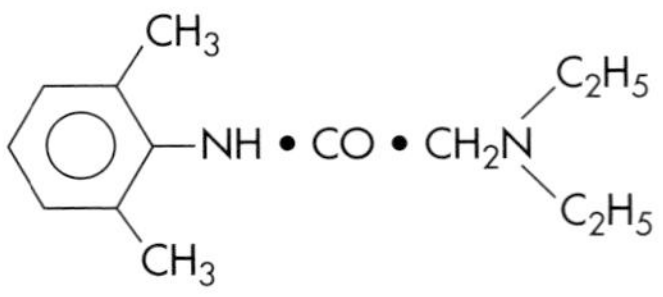

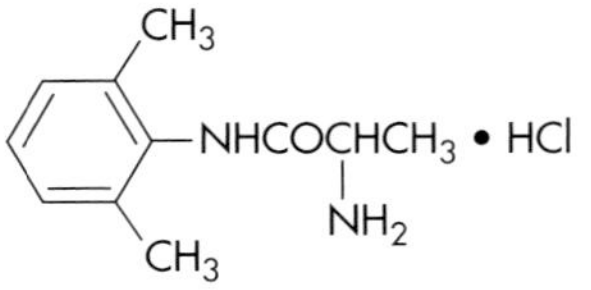

Figure 2-1. Tocainide. **A,** Represents a modification of a lidocaine, **B,** that is able to pass through the liver after oral administration with minimal hepatic first-pass effect.

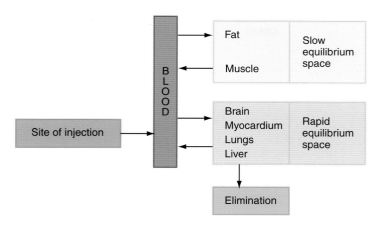

Figure 2-2. Pattern of distribution of local anesthetics after absorption. (Redrawn from Wildsmith JAW, Armitage EN, McClure JH: *Principles and practice of regional anesthesia*, ed 3, Edinburgh, 2003, Churchill Livingstone.)

local anesthetic blood levels, which can induce serious toxic reactions. The benefits to be accrued from IV drug administration always must be carefully weighed against any risks associated with IV administration. Only when the benefits clearly outweigh the risks should the drug be administered, as is the case with ventricular dysrhythmias such as premature ventricular contractions (PVCs).[8]

Distribution

Once absorbed into the blood, local anesthetics are distributed throughout the body to all tissues (Fig. 2-2). Highly perfused organs (and areas), such as the brain, head, liver, kidneys, lungs, and spleen, initially have higher blood levels of the anesthetic than do less highly perfused organs. Skeletal muscle, although not as highly perfused as these areas, contains the greatest percentage of local anesthetic of any tissue or organ in the body because it constitutes the largest mass of tissue in the body (Table 2-3).

The plasma concentration of a local anesthetic in certain "target" organs has a significant bearing on the potential toxicity of the drug. The blood level of the local anesthetic is influenced by the following factors:

1. Rate at which the drug is absorbed into the cardiovascular system
2. Rate of distribution of the drug from the vascular compartment to the tissues (more rapid in healthy patients than in those who are medically compromised [e.g., congestive heart failure], thus leading to lower blood levels in healthier patients)
3. Elimination of the drug through metabolic or excretory pathways

The latter two factors serve to decrease the blood level of the local anesthetic.

The rate at which a local anesthetic is removed from the blood is described as its *elimination half-life*. Simply stated, the elimination half-life is the time necessary for a 50% reduction in the blood level (one half-life = 50% reduction; two half-lives = 75% reduction; three half-lives = 87.5% reduction; four half-lives = 94% reduction; five half-lives = 97% reduction; six half-lives = 98.5% reduction) (Table 2-4).

TABLE 2-3
Percentages of Cardiac Output Distributed to Different Organ Systems

Region	Percent of Cardiac Output Received
Kidney	22
Gastrointestinal system, spleen	21
Skeletal muscle	15
Brain	14
Skin	6
Liver	6
Bone	5
Heart muscle	3
Other	8

(From Mohrman DE, Heller LJ: *Cardiovascular physiology,* ed 5, New York, 2003, Lange Medical Books/McGraw-Hill.)

TABLE 2-4
Half-life of Local Anesthetics

Drug	Half-life (hours)
Chloroprocaine*	0.1
Procaine*	0.1
Tetracaine*	0.3
Articaine†	0.5
Cocaine*	0.7
Prilocaine†	1.6
Lidocaine†	1.6
Mepivacaine†	1.9
Ropivacaine†	1.9
Etidocaine†	2.6
Bupivacaine†	3.5
Propoxycaine*	NA

*Ester.
†Amide.
NA, Not available.

All local anesthetics readily cross the blood–brain barrier. They also readily cross the placenta and enter the circulatory system of the developing fetus.

Metabolism (Biotransformation)

A significant difference between the two major groups of local anesthetics, the esters and the amides, is the means by which the body biologically transforms the active drug into one that is pharmacologically inactive. Metabolism (or biotransformation) of local anesthetics is important because the overall toxicity of a drug depends on a balance between its rate of absorption into the bloodstream at the site of injection and its rate of removal from the blood through the processes of tissue uptake and metabolism.

Ester Local Anesthetics. Ester local anesthetics are hydrolyzed in the plasma by the enzyme pseudo-cholinesterase.[9] The rate at which hydrolysis of different esters occurs varies considerably (Table 2-5).

The rate of hydrolysis has an impact on the potential toxicity of a local anesthetic. *Chloroprocaine*, the most rapidly hydrolyzed, is the least toxic, whereas *tetracaine*, hydrolyzed 16 times more slowly than chloroprocaine, has the greatest potential toxicity. Procaine undergoes hydrolysis to paraaminobenzoic acid (PABA), which is excreted unchanged in the urine, and to diethylamine alcohol, which undergoes further biotransformation before excretion (Fig. 2-3). *Allergic reactions* that occur in response to ester local anesthetics usually are *not* related to the parent compound (e.g., procaine) but rather to PABA, which is a major metabolic product of ester local anesthetics.

Approximately 1 of every 2800 persons has an *atypical form of pseudocholinesterase*, which causes an inability to hydrolyze ester local anesthetics and other chemically related drugs (e.g., succinylcholine).[10] Its presence leads to a prolongation of higher local anesthetic blood levels and an increased potential for toxicity.

Succinylcholine is a short-acting muscle relaxant commonly employed during the induction phase of general anesthesia. It produces respiratory arrest (apnea) for a period of approximately 2 to 3 minutes. Then plasma pseudocholinesterase hydrolyzes succinylcholine, blood levels fall, and spontaneous respiration resumes. Persons with atypical pseudocholinesterase are unable to hydrolyze succinylcholine at a normal rate; therefore the duration of apnea is prolonged. Atypical

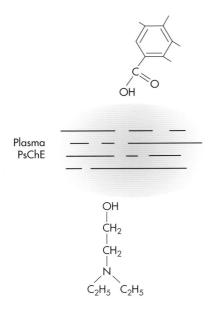

Figure 2-3. Metabolic hydrolysis of procaine. *PsChE*, pseudocholinesterase. (From Tucker GT: Biotransformation and toxicity of local anesthetics, *Acta Anaesthesiol Belg* 26(suppl): 123, 1975.)

pseudocholinesterase is a *hereditary* trait. Any familial history of "difficulty" during general anesthesia should be carefully evaluated by the doctor before any dental care. A confirmed or strongly suspected history, in the patient or biological family, of atypical pseudo-cholinesterase represents a relative contraindication to the use of ester local anesthetics.

There are absolute and relative contraindications to drug administration. An *absolute contraindication* implies that under no circumstance should this drug be administered to this patient because the possibility of potentially toxic or lethal reactions is increased. A *relative contraindication* means that the drug in question may be administered to the patient after carefully weighing the risk of using the drug to its potential benefit, and if an acceptable alternative drug is not available. However, the smallest clinically effective dose always should be used. There is an *increased* likelihood of adverse reaction to this drug in this patient.

Amide Local Anesthetics. The biotransformation of amide local anesthetics is more complex than that of the esters. The primary site of biotransformation of amide drugs is the *liver*. Virtually the entire metabolic process occurs in the liver for lidocaine, mepivacaine, articaine, etidocaine, and bupivacaine. *Prilocaine* undergoes primary metabolism in the liver, with some also possibly occurring in the lung.[11,12]

The rates of biotransformation of lidocaine, mepivacaine, etidocaine, ravocaine, and bupivacaine are similar. Therefore liver function and hepatic perfusion significantly influence the rate of biotransformation of an amide local anesthetic. Approximately 70% of a dose of injected lidocaine undergoes biotransformation in

TABLE 2-5	
Hydrolysis Rate of Esters	
Drug	**Rate of Hydrolysis (μmol/ml/hr)**
Chloroprocaine	4.7
Procaine	1.1
Tetracaine	0.3

TABLE 2-6
Lidocaine Disposition in Various Groups of Patients

Group	Lidocaine Half-life (hr)	Mean Total Body Clearance (ml/kg/min)
Normal	1.8	10
Heart failure	1.9	6.3
Hepatic disease	4.9	6
Renal disease	1.3	13.7

(Data from Thomson PD, et al: Lidocaine pharmacokinetics in advanced heart failure, liver disease, and renal failure in humans, *Ann Intern Med* 78:499–513, 1973.)

patients with normal liver function.[4] Patients with lower than usual hepatic blood flow (hypotension, congestive heart failure) or poor liver function (cirrhosis) are unable to biotransform amide local anesthetics at a normal rate.[13,14] This slower than normal biotransformation rate leads to increased anesthetic blood levels and a potential increase in toxicity. Significant liver dysfunction (ASA IV to V) or heart failure (ASA IV to V) represents a *relative contraindication* to the administration of amide local anesthetic drugs (Table 2-6). Articaine has a shorter half-life than other amides because a portion of its biotransformation occurs in the blood by the enzyme plasma cholinesterase.[15]

The biotransformation products of certain local anesthetics can possess significant clinical activity if they are permitted to accumulate in the blood. This may be seen in renal or cardiac failure and during periods of prolonged drug administration. A clinical example is the production of *methemoglobinemia* in patients receiving large doses of prilocaine.[16,17] Prilocaine, the parent compound, does not produce methemoglobinemia; but orthotoluidine, a primary metabolite of prilocaine, does induce the formation of methemoglobin, which is responsible for methemoglobinemia. When methemoglobin blood levels become elevated, clinical signs and symptoms are observed. Methemoglobinemia is discussed more fully in Chapter 10. Another example of pharmacologically active metabolites is the sedative effect occasionally observed after lidocaine administration. Lidocaine does not produce sedation; however, two metabolites—monoethylglycinexylidide and glycine

xylidide—currently are thought to be responsible for this clinical action.[18]

The metabolic pathways of lidocaine and prilocaine are shown in Figures 2-4 and 2-5.

Excretion

The kidneys are the primary excretory organ for both the local anesthetic and its metabolites. A percentage of a given dose of local anesthetic is excreted unchanged in the urine. This percentage varies according to the drug. *Esters* appear in only very small concentrations as the parent compound in the urine. This is because they are hydrolyzed almost completely in the plasma. Procaine appears in the urine as PABA (90%) and 2% unchanged. Ten percent of a cocaine dose is found in the urine unchanged. *Amides* usually are present in the urine as the parent compound in a greater percentage than the esters, primarily because of their more complex process of biotransformation. Although the percentages of parent drug found in urine vary from study to study, less than 3% lidocaine, 1% mepivacaine, and 1% etidocaine are found unchanged in the urine.

Patients with *significant renal impairment* may be unable to eliminate the parent local anesthetic compound or its major metabolites from the blood, resulting in slightly elevated blood levels and an increased potential for toxicity. This may occur with either the esters or the amides and is especially likely with cocaine. Thus significant renal disease (ASA IV to V) represents a *relative contraindication* to the administration of local anesthetics. This includes patients undergoing renal dialysis and those with chronic glomerulonephritis or pyelonephritis.

SYSTEMIC ACTIONS OF LOCAL ANESTHETICS

Local anesthetics are chemicals that reversibly block action potentials in all excitable membranes. The central nervous system (CNS) and the cardiovascular system (CVS) therefore are especially susceptible to their actions. Most of the systemic actions of local anesthetics are related to their *blood* or *plasma* level. The higher the level, the greater will be the clinical action.

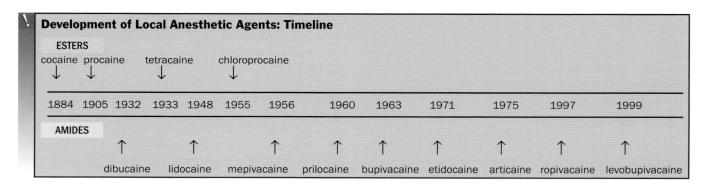

Development of Local Anesthetic Agents: Timeline

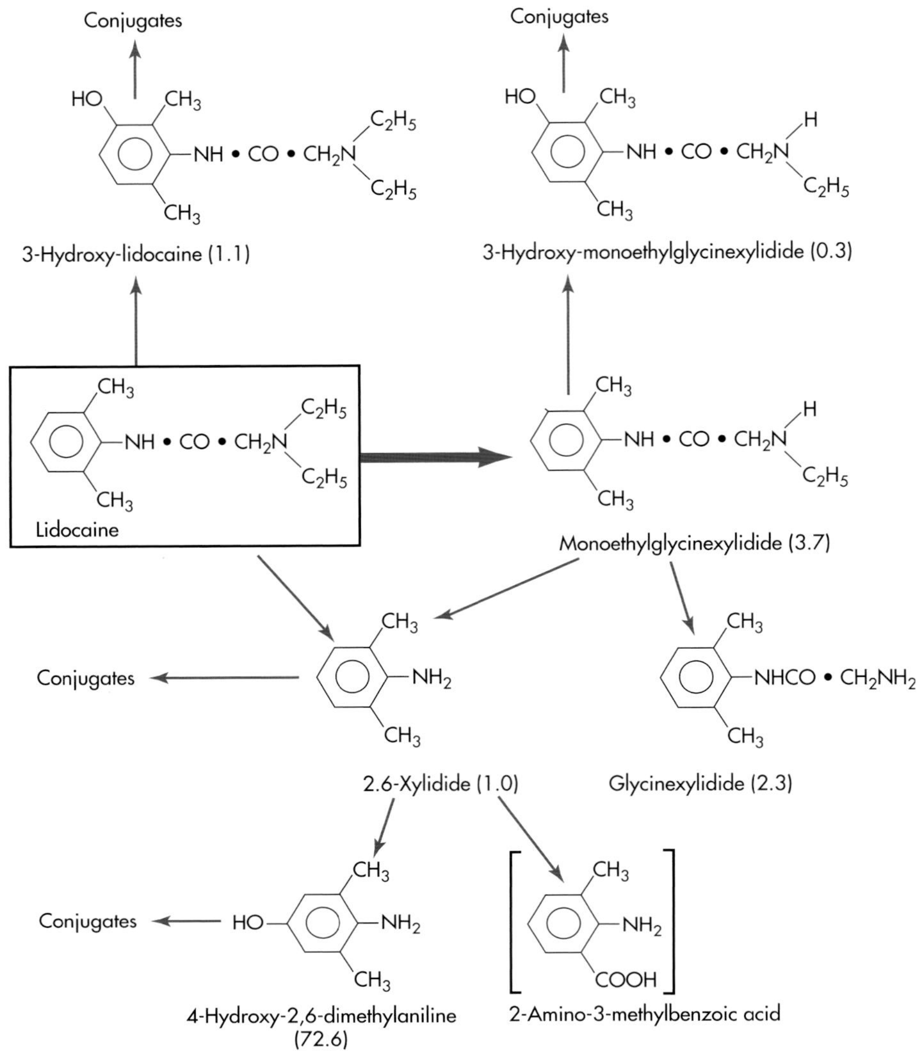

Figure 2-4. Metabolic pathways of lidocaine. Percentages of dose found in urine are indicated in parentheses. (From Cousins JM, Bridenbaugh PO, editors: *Neural blockade*, Philadelphia, 1980, JB Lippincott.)

Centbucridine (a quinoline derivative) has proved to be five to eight times as potent a local anesthetic as lidocaine, with an equally rapid onset of action and an equivalent duration.[19,20] Of potentially great importance is the finding that it does not affect the CNS or CVS adversely except in very high doses. (Centbucridine is discussed more fully in Chapter 19.)

Local anesthetics are absorbed from their site of administration into the circulatory system, which effectively dilutes them and carries them to all cells of the body. The blood level of the anesthetic depends on its rate of uptake from its site of administration *into* the circulatory system (increasing the blood level) and on the rates of distribution in tissue and biotransformation (in the liver), which remove the drug *from* the blood (decreasing the blood level) (see Fig. 2-3).

Central Nervous System

Local anesthetics readily cross the blood–brain barrier. Their pharmacological action on the CNS is depression.

At low (therapeutic, nontoxic) blood levels, there are no CNS effects of any clinical significance. At higher (toxic, overdose) levels, the primary clinical manifestation is a generalized tonic–clonic convulsion. Between these two extremes there exists a spectrum of other clinical signs and symptoms. (See "Preconvulsive Signs and Symptoms," Box 2-2.)

Anticonvulsant Properties. Some local anesthetics (e.g., procaine, lidocaine, mepivacaine, prilocaine, and even cocaine) have demonstrated *anticonvulsant* properties.[21,22] These occur at a blood level considerably *below* that at which the same drugs produce seizure activity. Values for anticonvulsive blood levels of lidocaine are shown in Table 2-7.[23]

Procaine, mepivacaine, and lidocaine have been used intravenously to terminate or decrease the duration of both grand mal and petit mal seizures.[21,24] The anticonvulsant blood level of lidocaine (about 0.5 to 4 μg/ml) is very close to its cardiotherapeutic range (see the following). It has been demonstrated to be effective in

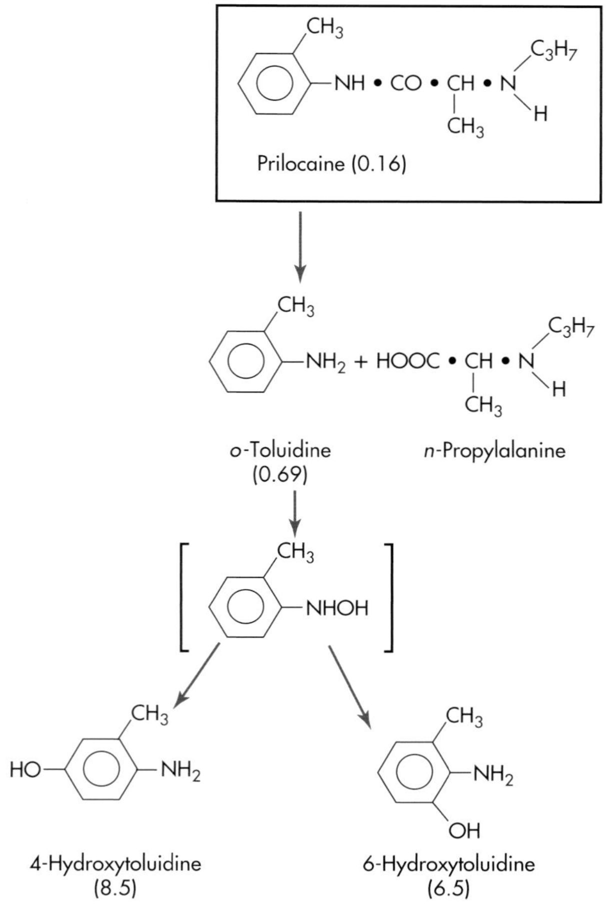

Figure 2-5. Metabolic pathways of prilocaine. Percentages of dose found in urine are indicated in parentheses. (From Ackerman B, Astrom A, Ross S, et al: Studies on the absorption, distribution, and metabolism of labeled prilocaine and lidocaine in some animal species, *Acta Pharmacol [Kobenhavn]* 24:389-403, 1966.)

BOX 2-2

Preconvulsive Signs and Symptoms of Central Nervous System Toxicity

SIGNS (Objectively Observable)	SYMPTOMS (Subjectively Felt)
Slurred speech	Numbness of tongue and circumoral region
Shivering	Warm, flushed feeling of skin
Muscular twitching	Pleasant dreamlike state
Tremor of muscles of face and distal extremities	
Generalized lightheadedness	
Dizziness	
Visual disturbances (inability to focus)	
Auditory disturbance (tinnitus)	
Drowsiness	
Disorientation	

TABLE 2-7

Anticonvulsive Blood Levels of Lidocaine

Clinical Situation	Lidocaine Blood Level (μg/ml)
Anticonvulsive level	0.5 to 4
Preseizure signs and symptoms	4.5 to 7
Tonic–clonic seizure	>7.5

---

temporarily arresting seizure activity in a majority of human epileptics.[25] It was especially effective in interrupting status epilepticus at therapeutic doses of 2 to 3 mg/kg given at a rate of 40 to 50 mg/min.

Mechanism of anticonvulsant properties. Epileptic patients possess hyperexcitable cortical neurons at a site within the brain where the convulsive episode originates (epileptic focus). Local anesthetics, by virtue of their depressant actions on the CNS, raise the seizure threshold by decreasing the excitability of these neurons, thereby preventing or terminating seizures.

Preconvulsive Signs and Symptoms. With a further increase in the blood level of the local anesthetic above its "therapeutic" level, adverse actions may be observed. Because the CNS is much more susceptible to the actions of local anesthetics than other systems, it is not surprising that the initial clinical signs and symptoms of overdose (toxicity) are CNS in origin. With lidocaine this second phase is observed at a level between 4.5 and 7 μg/ml in the average normal healthy patient.* Initial clinical signs and symptoms of CNS toxicity are usually *excitatory* in nature (Box 2-2).

These signs and symptoms, except for the sensation of circumoral and lingual numbness, are all related to the direct depressant action of the local anesthetic on the CNS. Numbness of the tongue and circumoral regions is *not* caused by the CNS effects of the local anesthetic.[26] Rather it is the result of a direct anesthetic action of the local anesthetic, which is present in high concentrations in these highly vascular tissues, on free nerve endings. The anesthetic has been transported to these tissues by the CVS. A dentist treating a patient might have difficulty conceptualizing why anesthesia of the tongue is considered to be a sign of a toxic reaction when lingual anesthesia is commonly produced after mandibular nerve blocks. Consider for a moment a physician administering a local anesthetic into the patient's foot. Overly high blood levels would produce a *bilateral* numbing of the tongue, as contrasted to the usual *unilateral* anesthesia seen after dental nerve blocks.

---

*Individual variation in response to drugs, as depicted in the normal distribution curve, may produce clinical symptoms at levels lower than these (in hyperresponders) or may fail to produce them at higher levels (in hyporesponders).

Lidocaine and procaine differ somewhat from other local anesthetics in that the usual progression of signs and symptoms just noted may *not* be seen. Lidocaine and procaine frequently produce an initial *mild sedation* or *drowsiness* (more common with lidocaine).[27] Because of this potential, the United States Air Force and the Navy ground airplane pilots for 24 hours after the receipt of a local anesthetic.[28]

Sedation may develop *in place of* the excitatory signs. If either excitation or sedation is observed in the initial 5 to 10 minutes after the intraoral administration of a local anesthetic, it should serve as a warning to the clinician of a rising local anesthetic blood level and the possibility (if the blood level continues to rise) of a more serious reaction, possibly a generalized convulsive episode.

Convulsive Phase. Further elevation of the local anesthetic blood level produces clinical signs and symptoms consistent with a generalized tonic–clonic convulsive episode. The duration of seizure activity is related to the local anesthetic blood level and inversely related to the arterial P_{CO_2} level.[29] At a normal pCO_2 a lidocaine blood level between 7.5 and 10 $\mu g/ml$ usually results in a convulsive episode. When CO_2 levels are increased, the blood level of local anesthetic necessary for seizures decreases while the duration of the seizure increases.[29] Seizure activity is generally self-limiting, because cardiovascular activity usually is not significantly impaired and biotransformation and redistribution of the local anesthetic continue throughout the episode. This results in a decrease of the anesthetic blood level and termination of seizure activity, usually in less than 1 minute.

However, several other mechanisms are also at work that unfortunately act to prolong the convulsive episode. Both cerebral blood flow and cerebral metabolism increase during local anesthetic-induced convulsions. *Increased blood flow* to the brain leads to an increase in the volume of local anesthetic being delivered to the brain, tending to prolong the seizure. *Increased cerebral metabolism* leads to a progressive metabolic acidosis as the seizure continues, and this tends to *prolong* the seizure activity (by *lowering* the blood level of anesthetic necessary to provoke a seizure), even in the presence of a declining local anesthetic level in the blood. As noted in Tables 2-8 and 2-9, the dose of local anesthetic necessary to induce seizures is markedly diminished in the presence of hypercarbia (Table 2-8) or acidosis (Table 2-9).[29,30]

Further increases in local anesthetic blood level result in a cessation of seizure activity as electroencephalographic (EEG) tracings become flattened, indicative of a generalized CNS depression. Respiratory depression occurs at this time, eventually leading to respiratory arrest if the anesthetic blood levels continue to rise. Respiratory effects are a result of the depressant action of the local anesthetic drug on the CNS.

Mechanism of preconvulsant and convulsant actions. It is known that local anesthetics exert a *depressant* action on excitable membranes, yet the primary clinical manifestation associated with high local anesthetic blood levels is related to varying degrees of *stimulation*. How can a drug that depresses the CNS be responsible for the production of varying degrees of stimulation, including tonic–clonic seizure activity? It is thought that local anesthetics produce clinical signs and symptoms of CNS excitation (including convulsions) through a selective blockade of inhibitory pathways in the cerebral cortex.[31–33] de Jong states that "inhibition of inhibition thus is a presynaptic event that follows local anesthetic blockade of impulses traveling along inhibitory pathways."[34]

The cerebral cortex has pathways of neurons that are essentially inhibitory and others that are facilitatory (excitatory). A state of balance normally is maintained between the degrees of effect exerted by these neuronal paths (Fig. 2-6). At *preconvulsant* local anesthetic blood levels, the observed clinical signs and symptoms are produced because the local anesthetic selectively *depresses* the action of inhibitory neurons (Fig. 2-7). Balance then is tipped slightly in favor of excessive facilitatory (excitatory) input, leading to the symptoms of tremor and slight agitation.

TABLE **2-8**

Effects of pCO_2 on the Convulsive Threshold (CD_{100}) of Various Local Anesthetics in Cats

Agent	CD_{100} (mg/kg)		Percent Change in CD_{100}
	pCO_2 (25–40 torr)	pCO_2 (65–81 torr)	
Procaine	35	17	51
Mepivacaine	18	10	44
Prilocaine	22	12	45
Lidocaine	15	7	53
Bupivacaine	5	2.5	50

(Data from Englesson S, Grevsten S, Olin A: Some numerical methods of estimating acid-base variables in normal human blood with a haemoglobin concentration of 5 g/100 cm^3, *Scand J Lab Clin Invest* 32: 289–295, 1973.)

TABLE **2-9**

Convulsant Dose (CD_{100}) and Acid-Base Status*

	pH 7.10	pH 7.20	pH 7.30	pH 7.40
pCO_2 30	—	—	27.5	26.6
pCO_2 40	—	20.6	21.4	22.0
pCO_2 60	13.1	15.4	17.5	—
pCO_2 80	11.3	14.3	—	—

(From Englesson S: The influence of acid-base changes on central nervous toxicity of local anaesthetic agents, *Acta Anaesth Scand* 18: 88-103, 1974.)

*Intravenous lidocaine 5 mg/kg/min, cats; doses in mg/kg.

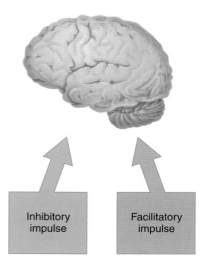

Figure 2-6. Balance between inhibitory and facilitatory impulses in a normal cerebral cortex.

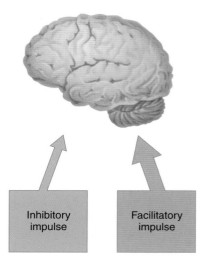

Figure 2-7. In the preconvulsive stage of local anesthetic action, the inhibitory impulse is more profoundly depressed than the facilitatory impulse.

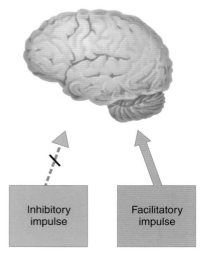

Figure 2-8. In the convulsive stage of local anesthetic action, the inhibitory impulse is totally depressed, permitting unopposed facilitatory impulse activity.

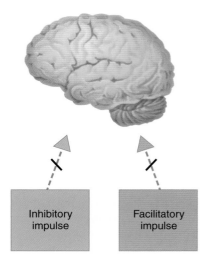

Figure 2-9. In the final stage of local anesthetic action, both inhibitory and facilitatory impulses are totally depressed, producing generalized central nervous system depression.

At higher *(convulsive)* blood levels, inhibitory neuron function is completely depressed, allowing unopposed function of facilitatory neurons (Fig. 2-8). Pure facilitatory input without inhibition produces the tonic–clonic activity observed at these levels.

Further increases in anesthetic blood level lead to depression of the facilitatory and inhibitory pathways, producing generalized CNS depression (Fig. 2-9). The precise site of action of the local anesthetic within the CNS is not known but is thought to be either at the inhibitory cortical synapses or directly on the inhibitory cortical neurons.

Analgesia. There is a second action that local anesthetics possess in relation to the CNS. Administered intravenously,

they increase the pain reaction threshold and also produce a degree of analgesia.

In the 1940s and 1950s procaine was administered intravenously for the management of chronic pain and arthritis.[35] The *procaine unit* was commonly used for this purpose; it consisted of 4 mg/kg of body weight administered over 20 minutes. The technique was ineffective for acute pain. Because of the relatively narrow safety margin between procaine's analgesic actions and the occurrence of signs and symptoms of overdose, this technique is no longer in use today.

Mood Elevation. The use of local anesthetic drugs for mood elevation and rejuvenation has persisted for centuries, despite documentation of both catastrophic events (mood elevation) and a lack of effect (rejuvenation).

Cocaine has long been used for both its euphoria-inducing and fatigue-lessening actions, dating back to the chewing of coca leaves by Incas and other South American natives.[36,37] Unfortunately, as is well known today, the prolonged use of cocaine leads to habituation. William Stewart Halsted (1852–1922) the father of American surgery, cocaine researcher, and the first person to administer a local anesthetic by injection, suffered greatly because of an addiction to cocaine.[38] In more recent times the sudden, unexpected deaths of several prominent professional athletes caused by cocaine, and the addiction of many others, clearly demonstrate the dangers involved in the casual use of potent drugs.[39,40]

More benign, but totally unsubstantiated, is the use of procaine (Novocain) as a rejuvenating drug. Clinics professing to "restore youthful vigor" claim that procaine is a literal Fountain of Youth. These clinics operate primarily in central Europe and Mexico, where procaine is used under the proprietary name "Gerovital." de Jong states that "whatever the retarding effect on aging, it probably is relegated most charitably to mood elevation."[41]

Cardiovascular System

Local anesthetics have a *direct* action on the myocardium and peripheral vasculature. In general, however, the cardiovascular system appears to be more resistant to the effects of local anesthetic drugs than the CNS (Table 2-10).[42]

Direct Action on the Myocardium. Local anesthetics modify electrophysiological events in the myocardium in a manner similar to their actions on peripheral nerves. As the local anesthetic blood level increases, the rate of rise of various phases of myocardial depolarization is reduced. There is no significant change in resting membrane potential, and no significant prolongation of the phases of repolarization.[43]

Local anesthetics produce a myocardial *depression* that is related to the local anesthetic blood level. Local anesthetics decrease electrical excitability of the myocardium, decrease the conduction rate, and decrease the force of contraction.[44–46]

TABLE **2-10**

Intravenous Dose of Local Anesthetic Agents Required for Convulsive Activity (CD$_{100}$) and Irreversible Cardiovascular Collapse (LD$_{100}$) in Dogs

Agent	CD$_{100}$ (mg/kg)	LD$_{100}$ (mg/kg)	LD$_{100}$/CD$_{100}$ Ratio
Lidocaine	22	76	3.5
Etidocaine	8	40	5.0
Bupivacaine	4	20	5.0
Tetracaine	5	27	5.4

(Data from Liu P, et al: Acute cardiovascular toxicity of intravenous amide local anesthetics in anesthetized ventilated dogs, *Anesth Analg* 61:317-322, 1982.)

Therapeutic advantage is taken of this depressant action in managing the hyperexcitable myocardium, which manifests itself as various cardiac dysrhythmias. Although many local anesthetics have demonstrated anti-dysrhythmic actions in animals, only *procaine* and *lidocaine* have gained significant clinical reliability in humans. Lidocaine is the most widely used and intensively studied local anesthetic in this regard.[8,27,47,48] *Procainamide* is the procaine molecule with an amide linkage replacing the ester linkage. Because of this, it is hydrolyzed much more slowly than procaine.[49] Tocainide, a chemical analogue of lidocaine, was introduced in 1984 as an oral antidysrhythmic drug, since lidocaine is ineffective after oral administration.[50] Tocainide also is effective in managing ventricular dysrhythmias but is associated with a 40% incidence of adverse effects, including nausea, vomiting, tremor, paresthesias, agranulocytosis, and pulmonary fibrosis.[51,52] Tocainide worsens symptoms of congestive heart failure in about 5% of patients and may provoke dysrhythmias (is prodysrhythmic) in 1% to 8%.[53]

Blood levels of lidocaine that normally develop after intraoral injection of one or two dental cartridges, 0.5 to 2 μg/ml, are not associated with cardiodepressant activity. Increasing lidocaine blood levels slightly is still nontoxic and is associated with antidysrhythmic actions. Therapeutic blood levels of lidocaine for antidysrhythmic activity range from 1.8 to 6 μg/ml.[46,54]

Lidocaine is usually administered intravenously in a bolus of 50 to 100 mg at a rate of 25 to 50 mg/min. This dose is based on 1 to 1.5 mg/kg of body weight every 3 to 5 minutes and is frequently followed by a continuous IV infusion of 1 to 4 mg/min. Signs and symptoms of local anesthetic overdose will be noted if the blood level rises beyond 6 μg/ml of blood.[54]

Lidocaine is used clinically primarily in the management of PVCs and ventricular tachycardia. It is also used as a (class-indeterminate) drug in advanced cardiovascular life support and in managing cardiac arrest caused by ventricular fibrillation.[55]

Direct cardiac actions of local anesthetics at blood levels greater than the therapeutic (antidysrhythmic) level include a decrease in myocardial contractility and decreased cardiac output, both of which lead to circulatory collapse (see Table 2-10).

Box 2-3 summarizes the CNS and cardiovascular effects of increasing local anesthetic blood levels.

Direct Action on the Peripheral Vasculature. Cocaine is the only local anesthetic drug that consistently produces *vasoconstriction* at commonly employed dosages.[3] Ropivacaine causes cutaneous vasoconstriction, whereas its congener bupivacaine produces vasodilation.[56] All other local anesthetics produce a peripheral *vasodilation*, through relaxation of the smooth muscle in the walls of blood vessels. This results in an increase in blood flow to and from the site of local anesthetic deposition (see Table 2-1). Increase in local blood flow increases the rate of

BOX 2-3

Minimal to Moderate Overdose Levels

SIGNS	SYMPTOMS
(Progressive with increasing blood levels)	
Talkativeness	Lightheadedness and dizziness
Apprehension	Restlessness
Excitability	Nervousness
Slurred speech	Sensation of twitching before
Generalized stutter,	actual twitching is observed
leading to muscular	(see "Generalized stutter"
twitching and tremor	under "SIGNS")
in the face and	Metallic taste
distal extremities	Visual disturbances
Euphoria	(inability to focus)
Dysarthria	Auditory disturbances
Nystagmus	(tinnitus)
Sweating	Drowsiness and
Vomiting	disorientation
Failure to follow commands	Loss of consciousness
or be reasoned with	
Elevated blood pressure	
Elevated heart rate	
Elevated respiratory rate	

Moderate to High Overdose Levels

Tonic–clonic seizure activity followed by:
   Generalized central nervous system depression
   Depressed blood pressure, heart rate, and respiratory rate

(From Malamed SF: *Medical emergencies in the dental office,* ed 4, St Louis, 1993, Mosby.)

drug absorption, in turn leading to a decreased depth and duration of local anesthetic action, increased bleeding in the treatment area, and increased local anesthetic blood levels.

Table 2-11 provides examples of peak blood levels achieved after local anesthetic injection with and without the presence of a vasopressor.[56–58]

The primary effect of local anesthetics on blood pressure is *hypotension*. Procaine produces hypotension more frequently and significantly than does lidocaine: 50% of patients in one study receiving procaine became hypotensive, compared with 6% of those receiving lidocaine.[59] This action is produced by a direct depression of the myocardium and smooth muscle relaxation in the vessel walls by the local anesthetic.

In summary, negative effects on the cardiovascular system are not noted until significantly elevated local anesthetic blood levels are reached. The usual sequence of local anesthetic-induced actions on the cardiovascular system is as follows:

At nonoverdose levels there is a slight increase or no change in blood pressure because of increased cardiac output and heart rate, as a result of enhanced sympathetic activity; also there is direct vasoconstriction of certain peripheral vascular beds.

At levels approaching, yet still below, overdose level a mild degree of hypotension is noted; this is produced by a direct relaxant action on the vascular smooth muscle.

At overdose levels there is profound hypotension caused by decreased myocardial contractility, cardiac output, and peripheral resistance.

At lethal levels cardiovascular collapse is noted. This is caused by massive peripheral vasodilation, and decreased myocardial contractility and heart rate (sinus bradycardia).

Certain local anesthetics such as bupivacaine (and to a lesser degree ropivacaine and etidocaine) may precipitate potentially fatal ventricular fibrillation.[60,61]

Local Tissue Toxicity

Skeletal muscle appears to be more sensitive to the local irritant properties of local anesthetics than other tissues. Intramuscular and intraoral injection of articaine, lidocaine, mepivacaine, prilocaine, bupivacaine, and etidocaine can produce skeletal muscle alterations.[62–65] It appears that the longer-acting local anesthetics cause more localized skeletal muscle damage than shorter-acting drugs. The changes occurring in skeletal muscle are reversible, with muscle regeneration being complete within 2 weeks after local anesthetic administration. These muscle changes have not been associated with any overt clinical signs of local irritation.

TABLE 2-11
Peak Plasma Levels Following Local Anesthetic Administration with and without Vasopressor

Injection Site	Anesthetic	Dose (mg)	Epinephrine Dilution	Peak Level (μg/ml)
Infiltration	Lidocaine	400	None	2.0
Infiltration	Lidocaine	400	1:200,000	1.0
Intercostal	Lidocaine	400	None	6.5
Intercostal	Lidocaine	400	1:200,000	5.3
Intercostal	Lidocaine	400	1:80,000	4.9
Infiltration	Mepivacaine	5 mg/kg	None	1.2
Infiltration	Mepivacaine	5 mg/kg	1:200,000	0.7

(Data from Kopacz DJ, Carpenter RL, Mackay DL: Effect of ropivacaine on cutaneous capillary flow in pigs, *Anesthesiology* 71:69, 1989; Scott DB, et al: Factors affecting plasma levels of lignocaine and prilocaine, *Br J Anaesth* 44:1040-1049, 1972; Duhner KG, et al: Blood levels of mepivacaine after regional anaesthesia, *Br J Anaesth* 37:746-752, 1965.)

Respiratory System

Local anesthetics exert a dual effect on respiration. At nonoverdose levels they have a direct relaxant action on bronchial smooth muscle, whereas at overdose levels they may produce respiratory arrest as a result of generalized CNS depression. In general, respiratory function is unaffected by local anesthetics until near-overdose levels are achieved.

Miscellaneous Actions

Neuromuscular Blockade. Many local anesthetics have been demonstrated to block neuromuscular transmission in humans. This is a result of the inhibition of sodium diffusion through a blockade of sodium channels in the cell membrane. This action is normally slight and usually clinically insignificant. On occasion, however, it can be additive to that produced by both depolarizing (e.g., succinylcholine) and nondepolarizing (e.g., atracurium, vecuronium) muscle relaxants, and this may lead to abnormally prolonged periods of muscle paralysis. Such actions are unlikely to occur in the dental outpatient.

Drug Interactions. In general, CNS depressants (e.g., opioids, antianxiety drugs, phenothiazines, and barbiturates), when administered in conjunction with local anesthetics, lead to potentiation of the CNS-depressant actions of the local anesthetic. The conjoint use of local anesthetics and drugs that share a common metabolic pathway can produce adverse reactions. Both ester local anesthetics and the depolarizing muscle relaxant succinylcholine require plasma pseudocholinesterase for hydrolysis. Prolonged apnea may result from the concomitant use of these drugs.

Drugs that induce the production of hepatic microsomal enzymes (e.g., barbiturates) may alter the rate at which amide local anesthetics are metabolized. Increased hepatic microsomal enzyme induction *increases* the rate of metabolism of the local anesthetic.

Specific drug–drug interactions relating to the administration of local anesthetics are reviewed in Chapter 10.

Malignant Hyperthermia. Malignant hyperthermia (MH; hyperpyrexia) is a pharmacogenic disorder in which a genetic variant in the individual alters that person's response to certain drugs. Acute clinical manifestations of MH include tachycardia, tachypnea, unstable blood pressure, cyanosis, respiratory and metabolic acidosis, fever (as high as 108° F [42° C] or more), muscle rigidity, and death. Mortality ranges from 63% to 73%. Many commonly used anesthetic drugs can trigger MH in certain individuals.

Until recently the amide local anesthetics were thought to be capable of provoking MH and were considered to be absolutely contraindicated in MH-susceptible patients.[66] The Malignant Hyperthermia Association of the United States (MHAUS), after evaluating recent clinical research, has concluded that there are in fact *no documented cases* in the medical or dental literature (over the past 25 years) supporting the concept of amide anesthetics triggering malignant hyperthermia.[67-71]

MHAUS maintains a website with information for both healthcare providers and patients: *www.mhaus.org*.

REFERENCES

1. Aps C, Reynolds F: The effect of concentration in vasoactivity of bupivacaine and lignocaine, *Br J Anaesth* 48:1171-1174, 1976.
2. Covino BG: Pharmacology of local anaesthetic agents, *Br J Anaesth* 58:701-716, 1986.
3. Benowitz NL: Clinical pharmacology and toxicology of cocaine, *Pharmacol Toxicol* 72:1-12, 1993.
4. Arthur GR: *Pharmacokinetics of local anesthetics.* In Strichartz GR, editor: *Local anesthetics: handbook of experimental pharmacology,* vol 81, Berlin, 1987, Springer-Verlag.
5. Hohnloser SH, Lange HW, Raeder E, et al: Short- and long-term therapy with tocainide for malignant ventricular tachyarrhythmias, *Circulation* 73:143, 1986.
6. Soliman IE, Broadman LM, Hannallah RS, et al: Comparison of the analgesic effects of EMLA (eutectic mixture of local anesthetics) to intradermal lidocaine infiltration prior to venous cannulation in unpremedicated children, *Anesthesiology* 68:804, 1988.
7. American Heart Association: *ACLS provider manual*, Dallas, 2001, American Heart Association, pp 83-84.
8. Haugh KH: Antidysrhythmic agents at the turn of the twenty-first century: a current review, *Crit Care Nursing Clin North Am* 14:13-69, 2002.
9. Kalow W: Hydrolysis of local anesthetics by human serum cholinesterase, *J Pharmacol Exp Ther* 104:122-134, 1952.
10. Watson CB: Respiratory complications associated with anesthesia, *Anesth Clin North Am* 20:375-399, 2002.
11. Harris WH, Cole DW, Mital M, Laver MB: Methemoglobin formation and oxygen transport following intravenous regional anesthesia using prilocaine, *Anesthesiology* 29:65, 1968.
12. Arthur GR: *Distribution and elimination of local anesthetic agents: the role of the lung, liver, and kidneys*, PhD thesis, Edinburgh, 1981, University of Edinburgh.
13. Nation RL, Triggs EJ: Lidocaine kinetics in cardiac patients and aged subjects, *Br J Clin Pharmacol* 4:439-448, 1977.
14. Thompson P, Melmon K, Richardson J, et al: Lidocaine pharmacokinetics in advanced heart failure, liver disease, and renal failure in humans, *Ann Intern Med* 78:499, 1973.
15. Oertel R, Rahn R, Kirch W: Clinical pharmacokinetics of articaine. *Clin Pharmacokinet* 33:617-625, 1997.
16. Prilocaine-induced methemoglobinemia—Wisconsin, 1993, *MMWR Morb Mortal Wkly Rep* 43:3555-35657, 1994.
17. Wilburn-Goo D, Lloyd LM: When patients become cyanotic: acquired methemoglobinemia, *J Am Dent Assoc* 130:626-631, 1999.
18. Strong JM, Parker M, Atkinson AJ Jr: Identification of glycinexylidide in patients treated with intravenous lidocaine, *Clin Pharmacol Ther* 14:67-72, 1973.

19. Gupta PP, Tangri AN, Saxena RC, Dhawan BN: Clinical pharmacology studies on 4-N-butylamino-1,2,3,4,-tetrahydroacridine hydrochloride (Centbucridine), a new local anaesthetic agent, *Indian J Exp Biol* 20:344-346, 1982.

20. Vacharajani GN, Parikh N, Paul T, Satoskar RS: A comparative study of Centbucridine and lidocaine in dental extraction, *Int J Clin Pharmacol Res* 3:251-255, 1983.

21. Bernhard CG, Bohm E: *Local anaesthetics as anticonvulsants: a study on experimental and clinical epilepsy*, Stockholm, 1965, Almqvist & Wiksell.

22. Bernhard CG, Bohm E, Wiesel T: On the evaluation of the anticonvulsive effect of different local anesthetics, *Arch Int Pharmacodyn Ther* 108:392-407, 1956.

23. Julien RM: Lidocaine in experimental epilepsy: correlation of anticonvulsant effect with blood concentrations, *Electroencephalogr Clin Neurophysiol* 34:639-645, 1973.

24. Berry CA, Sanner JH, Keasling HH: A comparison of the anticonvulsant activity of mepivacaine and lidocaine, *J Pharmacol Exp Ther* 133:357-363, 1961.

25. Walker IA, Slovis CM: Lidocaine in the treatment of status epilepticus, *Acad Emer Med* 4:918-922, 1997.

26. Chen AH: Toxicity and allergy to local anesthesia, *J Calif Dent Assoc* 26:983-992, 1998.

27. Katz J, Feldman MA, Bass EB, et al: Injectable versus topical anesthesia for cataract surgery: patient perceptions of pain and side effects. The Study of Medical Testing for Cataract Surgery study team, *Ophthalmology* 107:11054-11060, 2000.

28. Bureau of Medicine and Surgery: 2300 E Street N.W, Washington DC, 20372-5300, *http://navymedicine.med.navy.mil/*.

29. Englesson S: The influence of acid-base changes on central nervous system toxicity of local anesthetic agents. I. An experimental study in cats, *Acta Anaesthesiol Scand* 18:79, 1974.

30. Englesson S, Grevsten S, Olin A: Some numerical methods of estimating acid-base variables in normal human blood with a haemoglobin concentration of 5 g-100 cm,[3] *Scand J Lab Clin Invest* 32:289-295, 1973.

31. de Jong RH, Robles R, Corbin RW: Central actions of lidocaine-synaptic transmission, *Anesthesiology* 30:19, 1969.

32. Huffman RD, Yim GKW: Effects of diphenylaminoethanol and lidocaine on central inhibition, *Int J Neuropharmacol* 8:217, 1969.

33. Tanaka K, Yamasaki M: Blocking of cortical inhibitory synapses by intravenous lidocaine, *Nature* 209:207, 1966.

34. de Jong RH: *Local anesthetics*, St Louis, 1994, Mosby.

35. Graubard DJ, Peterson MC: *Clinical uses of intravenous procaine*, Springfield, Ill, 1950, Charles C Thomas.

36. Garcilasso de la Vega: *Commentarios reales de los Incas (1609–1617)*. In Freud S: *Uber Coca*, Wien, 1884, Verlag von Moritz Perles.

37. *Disertacion sobre el aspecto, cultivo, comercio y virtudes de la famosa planta del Peru nombrado Coca. Lima, 1794*. In Freud S: *Uber Coca*, Wien, 1884, Verlag von Moritz Perles.

38. Olch PD, William S: Halsted and local anesthesia: contributions and complications, *Anesthesiology* 42:479-486, 1975.

39. Preboth M: Cocaine abuse among athletes, *Amer Family Phys* 62:1850-2000 (15 October).

40. Harriston K, Jenkins S: Maryland basketball star Len Bias is dead at 22, *Washington Post*, 20 June 1986.

41. de Jong RH: *Local anesthetics*, ed 2, Springfield, Ill, 1977, Charles C Thomas, p 89.

42. Scott DB: Toxicity caused by local anaesthetic drugs, *Br J Anaesth* 53:553-554, 1981.

43. Pinter A, Dorian P: Intravenous antiarrhythmic agents, *Curr Opin Cardiol* 16:17-22, 2001.

44. Sugi K: Pharmacological restoration and maintenance of sinus rhythm by antiarrhythmic agents, *J Cardiol* 33(suppl)1:59-64, 1999.

45. Alexander JH, Granger CB, Sadowski Z, et al: Prophylactic lidocaine use in acute myocardial infarction: incidence and outcomes from two international trials. The GUSTO-I and GUSTO-IIb Investigators, *Am Heart J* 137:599-805, 1999.

46. Cannom DS, Prystowsky EN: Management of ventricular arrhythmias: detection, drugs, and devices, *JAMA* 281:272-279, 1999.

47. Tan HL, Lie KI: Prophylactic lidocaine use in acute myocardial infarction revisited in the thrombolytic era, *Am Heart J* 137:570-573, 1999.

48. Kowey PR: An overview of antiarrhythmic drug management of electrical storm, *Can J Cardiol* 12(suppl B):3B-8B; discussion 27B-28B, 1996.

49. Slavik RS, Tisdale JE, Borzak S: Pharmacologic conversion of atrial fibrillation: a systematic review of available evidence, *Prog Cardiovasc Dis* 44:221-252, 2001.

50. Lalka D, Meyer MB, Duce BR, et al: Kinetics of the oral antiarrhythmic lidocaine congener, tocainide, *Clin Pharmacol Ther* 19:757, 1976.

51. Perlow GM, Jain BP, Pauker SC, et al: Tocainide-associated interstitial pneumonitis, *Ann Intern Med* 94:489, 1981.

52. Volosin K, Greenberg RM, Greenspon AJ: Tocainide associated agranulocytosis, *Am Heart J* 109:1392, 1985.

53. Bronheim D, Thys DM: *Cardiovascular drugs*. In Longnecker DE, Tinker JH, Morgan GE Jr, editors: *Principles and practice of anesthesiology*, ed 2, St Louis, 1998, Mosby.

54. Kudenchuk PJ: Advanced cardiac life support antiarrhythmic drugs, *Cardiol Clin* 20:19-87, 2002.

55. American Heart Association: Guidelines 2000 for cardiopulmonary resuscitation and emergency cardiovascular care, *Circulation* 102:8-149, 2000.

56. Kopacz DJ, Carpenter RL, MacKay DL: Effect of ropivacaine on cutaneous capillary flow in pigs, *Anesthesiology* 71:69, 1989.

57. Scott DB, Jebson PJR, Braid DP, et al: Factors affecting plasma levels of lignocaine and prilocaine, *Br J Anaesth* 44:1040-1049, 1972.

58. Duhner KG, Harthon JGL, Hebring BG, Lie T: Blood levels of mepivacaine after regional anaesthesia, *Br J Anaesth* 37:746-752, 1965.

59. Kimmey JR, Steinhaus JE: Cardiovascular effects of procaine and lidocaine (Xylocaine) during general anesthesia, *Acta Anaesthesiol Scand* 3:9-15, 1959.

60. de Jong RH, Ronfeld R, DeRosa R: Cardiovascular effects of convulsant and supraconvulsant doses of amide local anesthetics, *Anesth Analg* 61:3, 1982.

61. Feldman HS, Arthur GR, Covino BG: Comparative systemic toxicity of convulsant and supraconvulsant doses of intravenous ropivacaine, bupivacaine and lidocaine in the conscious dog, *Anesth Analg* 69:794, 1989.

62. Zink W, Graf BM, Sinner B, et al: Differential effects of bupivacaine on intracellular Ca^{2+} regulation: potential

mechanisms of its myotoxicity, *Anesthesiology* 97:310-316, 2002.

63. Irwin W, Fontaine E, Agnolucci L, et al: Bupivacaine myotoxicity is mediated by mitochondria, *J Biol Chem* 277:142221-142227, 2002.

64. Benoit PW, Yagiela JA, Fort NF: Pharmacologic correlation between local anesthetic-induced myotoxicity and disturbances of intracellular calcium distribution, *Toxicol Appl Pharmacol* 52:187-198, 1980.

65. Hinton RJ, Dechow PC, Carlson DS: Recovery of jaw muscle function following injection of a myotoxic agent (lidocaine-epinephrine), *Oral Surg Oral Med Oral Pathol* 59:247-251, 1986.

66. Denborough MA, Forster JF, Lovell RR, et al: Anaesthetic deaths in a family, *Br J Anaesth* 34:395-396, 1962.

67. Gielen M, Viering W: 3-in-1 lumbar plexus block for muscle biopsy in malignant hyperthermia patients: amide local anaesthetics may be used safely, *Acta Anaesthesiol Scand* 30:581-583, 1986.

68. Ording H: Incidence of malignant hyperthermia in Denmark, *Anesth Analg* 64:700-704, 1985.

69. Paasuke PT, Brownell AKW: Amine local anaesthetics and malignant hyperthermia (editorial), *Can Anaesth Soc J* 33:126-129, 1986.

70. Jastak JT, Yagiela JA, Donaldson D: *Local anesthesia of the oral cavity*, Philadelphia, 1995, WB Saunders, pp. 141-142.

71. Malignant Hyperthermia Association of the United States: *www.mhaus.org*.

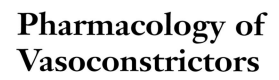

Pharmacology of Vasoconstrictors

CHAPTER

3

All clinically effective injectable local anesthetics possess some degree of vasodilating activity. The degree of vasodilation varies from significant (procaine) to minimal (prilocaine, mepivacaine) and also may vary with both the injection site and individual patient response. After local anesthetic injection into tissues, blood vessels in the area dilate, resulting in an increased perfusion at the site, leading to the following reactions:

1. An increased rate of absorption of the local anesthetic into the cardiovascular system, which in turn removes it from the injection site (redistribution)
2. Higher plasma levels of the local anesthetic, with an attendant increase in the risk of local anesthetic toxicity
3. Decreased depth of anesthesia and a decreased duration of action because the local anesthetic diffuses away from the injection site more rapidly
4. Increased bleeding at the site of treatment because of increased perfusion

Vasoconstrictors are drugs that constrict blood vessels and thereby control tissue perfusion. They are added to local anesthetic solutions to oppose the vasodilatory actions of the local anesthetics. Vasoconstrictors are important additions to a local anesthetic solution for the following reasons:

1. By constricting blood vessels, vasoconstrictors decrease blood flow (perfusion) to the site of administration.
2. Absorption of the local anesthetic into the cardiovascular system is slowed, resulting in lower anesthetic blood levels.[1,2] Table 3-1 illustrates levels of local anesthetic in the blood with and without a vasoconstrictor.[1]
3. Local anesthetic blood levels are lowered, thereby minimizing the risk of local anesthetic toxicity.
4. Increased amounts of the local anesthetic remain in and around the nerve for longer periods, thereby increasing (in some cases significantly,[3] in others minimally)[4] the duration of action of most local anesthetics.

5. Vasoconstrictors decrease bleeding at the site of administration; therefore they are useful when increased bleeding is anticipated (e.g., during a surgical procedure).[5,6]

The vasoconstrictors commonly used in conjunction with injected local anesthetics are chemically identical or similar to the sympathetic nervous system mediators epinephrine and norepinephrine. The actions of the vasoconstrictors so resemble the response of adrenergic nerves to stimulation that they are classified as *sympathomimetic*, or *adrenergic*, drugs. These drugs have many clinical actions besides vasoconstriction.

Sympathomimetic drugs also may be classified according to their chemical structure and mode of action.

CHEMICAL STRUCTURE

Classification of sympathomimetic drugs by chemical structure is related to the presence or absence of a catechol nucleus. Catechol is orthodihydroxybenzene.

TABLE 3-1			
Effect of Vasoconstrictor (Epinephrine 1:200,000) on Peak Local Anesthetic Level in Blood			
		Peak Level (μg/ml)	
Local Anesthetic	**Dose (mg)**	**Without Vasoconstrictor**	**With Vasoconstrictor**
Mepivacaine	500	4.7	3
Lidocaine	400	4.3	3
Prilocaine	400	2.8	2.6
Etidocaine	300	1.4	1.3

(Data from: Cannall H, Walters H, Beckett AH, Saunders A: Circulating blood levels of lignocaine after peri-oral injections, *Br Dent J* 138:87-93, 1975.)

Sympathomimetic drugs that have hydroxyl (OH) substitutions in the third and fourth positions of the aromatic ring are termed *catechols*.

	①	②
Epinephrine	H	CH_3
Levonordefrin	CH_3	H
Norepinephrine	H	H

If they also contain an amine group (NH_2) attached to the aliphatic side chain, they are then called *catecholamines*. Epinephrine, norepinephrine, and dopamine are the naturally occurring catecholamines of the sympathetic nervous system. Isoproterenol and levonordefrin are synthetic catecholamines.

Vasoconstrictors that do not possess OH groups in the third and fourth positions of the aromatic molecule are not catechols but are amines because they have an NH_2 group attached to the aliphatic side chain.

Catecholamines	Noncatecholamines
Epinephrine	Amphetamine
Norepinephrine	Methamphetamine
Levonordefrin	Ephedrine
Isoproterenol	Mephentermine
Dopamine	Hydroxyamphetamine
	Metaraminol
	Methoxamine
	Phenylephrine

Felypressin, a synthetic analogue of the polypeptide vasopressin (antidiuretic hormone), is available in many countries as a vasoconstrictor. At present (June 2004) felypressin is not available in the United States.

MODES OF ACTION

There are three categories of sympathomimetic amines: *direct-acting drugs*, which exert their action directly on adrenergic receptors; *indirect-acting drugs*, which act by releasing norepinephrine from adrenergic nerve terminals; and *mixed-acting drugs*, with both direct and indirect actions (Box 3-1).[1-3]

Adrenergic Receptors

Adrenergic receptors are found in most tissues of the body. The concept of adrenergic receptors was proposed

---

BOX 3-1

Categories of Sympathomimetic Amines

DIRECT-ACTING	INDIRECT-ACTING	MIXED-ACTING
Epinephrine	Tyramine	Metaraminol
Norepinephrine	Amphetamine	Ephedrine
Levonordefrin	Methamphetamine	
Isoproterenol	Hydroxyamphetamine	
Dopamine		
Methoxamine		
Phenylephrine		

---

by Ahlquist in 1948 and is well accepted today.[7] Ahlquist recognized two types of adrenergic receptors, termed *alpha* (α) and *beta* (β) based on the inhibitory or excitatory actions of the catecholamines on smooth muscle.

Activation of α receptors by a sympathomimetic drug usually produces a response that includes contraction of smooth muscle in blood vessels (vasoconstriction). Based on differences in their function and location, α receptors have since been subcategorized. Whereas α_1 receptors are excitatory-postsynaptic, α_2 receptors are inhibitory-postsynaptic.[8]

Activation of β receptors produces smooth muscle relaxation (vasodilation and bronchodilation) and cardiac stimulation (increased heart rate and strength of contraction).

Beta receptors are further divided into β_1 and β_2: The former are found in the heart and small intestines and are responsible for cardiac stimulation and lipolysis; the latter, found in the bronchi, vascular beds, and uterus, produce bronchodilation and vasodilation.[9]

Table 3-2 illustrates the differences in the varying degrees of α and β receptor activity of three commonly used vasoconstrictors.

Table 3-3 lists the systemic effects, based on α and β receptor activity, of epinephrine and norepinephrine.

Release of Catecholamines

Other sympathomimetic drugs, such as tyramine and amphetamine, act *indirectly* by causing the release of the catecholamine norepinephrine from storage sites in adrenergic nerve terminals. In addition, these drugs also may exert a direct action on α and β receptors.

TABLE 3-2
Adrenergic Receptor Activity of Vasoconstrictors

Drug	α_1	α_2	β_1	β_2
Epinephrine	+++	+++	+++	+++
Norepinephrine	++	++	++	+
Levonordefrin	+	++	++	+

(From Jastak JT, Yagiela JA, Donaldson D: *Local anesthesia of the oral cavity*, Philadelphia, 1995, WB Saunders.)
Relative potency of drugs is indicated as follows: +++ = high, ++ = intermediate, and + = low.

TABLE 3-3
Systemic Effects of Sympathomimetic Amines

Effector Organ or Function	Epinephrine	Norepinephrine
CARDIOVASCULAR SYSTEM		
Heart rate	+	–
Stroke volume	++	++
Cardiac output	+++	0,–
Arrhythmias	++++	++++
Coronary blood flow	++	++
BLOOD PRESSURE		
Systolic arterial	+++	+++
Mean arterial	+	++
Diastolic arterial	+,0,–	++
PERIPHERAL CIRCULATION		
Total peripheral resistance	–	++
Cerebral blood flow	+	0,–
Cutaneous blood flow	–	–
Splanchnic blood flow	+++	0,+
RESPIRATORY SYSTEM		
Bronchodilation	+++	0
GENITOURINARY SYSTEM		
Renal blood flow	–	–
SKELETAL MUSCLE		
Muscle blood flow	+++	0,–
METABOLIC EFFECTS		
Oxygen consumption	++	0,+
Blood glucose	+++	0,+
Blood lactic acid	+++	0,+

(After Goldenberg M, Aranow H Jr, Smith AA, Faber M: Pheochromocytoma and essential hypertensive vascular disease, *Arch Intern Med* 86:823-836, 1950.)

The clinical actions of this group of drugs therefore are quite similar to the actions of norepinephrine. Successively repeated doses of these drugs will prove to be less effective than those given previously because of the depletion of norepinephrine from storage sites. This phenomenon is termed *tachyphylaxis* and is *not* seen with drugs that act directly on adrenergic receptors.

DILUTIONS OF VASOCONSTRICTORS

The dilution of vasoconstrictors is commonly referred to as a ratio (e.g., 1 to 1000 [written 1:1000]). Because maximum doses of vasoconstrictors are presented in milligrams, or more commonly today as micrograms (μg), the following interpretations should enable the reader to convert these terms readily:

- A concentration of 1:1000 means that there is 1 gram (or 1000 mg) of solute (drug) contained in 1000 ml of solution.

- Therefore a 1:1000 dilution contains 1000 mg in 1000 ml or 1.0 mg/ml of solution (1000 μg/ml).

Vasoconstrictors, as used in dental local anesthetic solutions, are much less concentrated than the 1:1000 described in the preceding. To produce these more dilute, clinically safer, yet effective concentrations, the 1:1000 dilution must be diluted further. This process is described in the following:

- To produce a 1:10,000 concentration, 1 ml of a 1:1000 solution is added to 9 ml of solvent (e.g., sterile water); therefore 1:10,000 = 0.1 mg/ml.

- To produce a 1:100,000 concentration, 1 ml of a 1:10,000 concentration is added to 9 ml of solvent; therefore 1:100,000 = 0.01 mg/ml.

The milligram per milliliter and μg per milliliter values of the various vasoconstrictor dilutions used in medicine and dentistry are shown in Table 3-4.

The genesis of vasoconstrictor dilutions in local anesthetics began with the discovery of adrenalin in 1897 by Abel. In 1903 Braun suggested using adrenalin as a "chemical tourniquet" to prolong the duration of local anesthetics.[10] Braun recommended the use of a 1:10,000 dilution of epinephrine, ranging to as dilute as 1:100,000, for use with cocaine when used for nasal surgery. It appears at present that an epinephrine concentration of 1:200,000 provides comparable results, with fewer systemic side effects. The 1:200,000 dilution, which contains 5 μg/ml (or 0.005 mg/ml), has become widely used in both medicine and dentistry and is currently found in articaine, prilocaine, lidocaine, etidocaine, and bupivacaine. In several European and Asian countries, lidocaine with epinephrine concentrations as low as 1:300,000 and 1:400,000 are available in dental cartridges.

Although it is the most used vasoconstrictor in local anesthetics in both medicine and dentistry, epinephrine is not an ideal drug. The benefits to be gained from adding epinephrine (or any vasoconstrictor, for that matter) to a local anesthetic solution must be weighed against any risks that might be present. Epinephrine is absorbed from the site of injection, just as is the local anesthetic. Measurable epinephrine blood levels are obtained, which influence the heart and blood vessels. Resting plasma epinephrine levels (39 pg/ml) are doubled after the administration of one cartridge of lidocaine with 1:100,000 epinephrine.[11] The elevation of epinephrine plasma levels is linearly dose dependent and persists from several minutes to half an hour.[12] Contrary to a previously held position that the intraoral administration of "usual" volumes of epinephrine produced no cardiovascular response and that patients were more at risk from endogenously released epinephrine than they were from exogenously administered epinephrine,[13,14] recent evidence demonstrates that epinephrine plasma levels equivalent to those achieved during moderate to heavy exercise may occur after intraoral injection.[15,16] These are associated with moderate increases in cardiac output and stroke volume (see the following section). Blood

TABLE **3-4**
Concentrations of Clinically Used Vasoconstrictors

Concentration (Dilution)	Milligrams per Milliliter (mg/ml)	Micrograms per Milliliter (μg/ml)	μg per Cartridge (1.8 ml)	Therapeutic Use
1:1,000	1.0	1000		Epinephrine—Emergency medicine (IM/SC anaphylaxis)
1:2,500	0.4	400		Phenylephrine
1:10,000	0.1	100		Epinephrine—Emergency medicine (IV/ET cardiac arrest)
1:20,000	0.05	50	90	Levonordefrin—Local anesthetic
1:30,000	0.033	33.3	73 (2.2-ml cartridge)	Norepinephrine—Local anesthetic
1:50,000	0.02	20	36	Epinephrine—Local anesthetic
1:80,000	0.0125	12.5	27.5 (2.2-ml cartridge)	Epinephrine—Local anesthetic (United Kingdom)
1:100,000	0.01	10	18	Epinephrine—Local anesthetic
1:200,000	0.005	5	9	Epinephrine—Local anesthetic

pressure and heart rate, however, are minimally affected at these dosages.[17]

In patients with preexisting cardiovascular or thyroid disease, the side effects of absorbed epinephrine must be weighed against those of elevated local anesthetic blood levels. It is currently thought that the cardiovascular effects of conventional epinephrine doses are of little practical concern, even in patients with heart disease.[12] However, even following usual precautions (e.g., aspiration, slow injection), sufficient epinephrine can be absorbed to cause sympathomimetic reactions such as apprehension, tachycardia, sweating, and pounding in the chest (palpitation): the so-called "epinephrine reaction."[18]

Intravascular administration of vasoconstrictors and their administration to "sensitive" individuals (hyperresponders), or the occurrence of unanticipated drug–drug interactions can, however, produce significant clinical manifestations. Intravenous administration of 0.015 mg of epinephrine with lidocaine results in increase in the heart rate ranging from 25 to 70 beats per minute, with elevations in the systolic blood from 20 to 70 mm Hg.[12,19,20] Occasional rhythm disturbances may also be observed, premature ventricular contractions (PVCs) being the most often noted.

Other vasoconstrictors used in medicine and dentistry include norepinephrine, phenylephrine, levonordefrin, and octapressin. *Norepinephrine*, lacking significant β_2 actions, produces intense peripheral vasoconstriction with possible dramatic elevation of blood pressure, and is associated with a side effect ratio nine times higher than that of epinephrine.[21] Although it is currently available in many countries in local anesthetic solutions, norepinephrine's use as a vasopressor in dentistry is diminishing and is not recommended. The use of a mixture of epinephrine and norepinephrine is to be absolutely avoided.[22] *Phenylephrine*, a pure α-adrenergic

agonist, theoretically possesses advantages over other vasoconstrictors. However, in clinical trials peak blood levels of lidocaine were actually higher with phenylephrine 1:20,000 (lidocaine blood level = 2.4 μg/ml) than with epinephrine 1:200,000 (1.4 μg/ml).[23] The cardiovascular effects of *levonordefrin* most closely resemble those of norepinephrine.[24] *Octapressin* was shown to be about as effective as epinephrine in reducing cutaneous blood flow.[5]

Epinephrine remains the most effective and used vasoconstrictor in medicine and dentistry.

PHARMACOLOGY OF SPECIFIC AGENTS

The pharmacological properties of the sympathomimetic amines commonly used as vasoconstrictors in local anesthetics are reviewed. *Epinephrine* is the most useful and represents the best example of a drug mimicking the activity of sympathetic discharge. Its clinical actions are reviewed in depth. The actions of other drugs are compared with those of epinephrine.

Epinephrine

Proprietary name. Adrenalin.

Chemical structure. Epinephrine as the acid salt is highly soluble in water. Slightly acid solutions are relatively stable if they are protected from air. Deterioration (through oxidation) is hastened by heat and the presence of heavy metal ions. *Sodium bisulfite* usually is added to epinephrine solutions to delay this deterioration. The shelf life of a local anesthetic cartridge containing a vasoconstrictor is somewhat shorter (18 months) than that of a cartridge containing no vasoconstrictor (36 months).

OH H   H
| | |
C—C—N
| | |
H H   CH₃

HO
OH

Source. Epinephrine is available as a synthetic and is also obtained from the adrenal medulla of animals (approximately 80% of adrenal medullary secretions being epinephrine). It exists in both levorotatory and dextrorotatory forms; the levorotatory form is approximately 15 times as potent as the dextrorotatory.

Mode of action. Epinephrine acts directly on both α- and β-adrenergic receptors; β effects predominate.

Systemic Actions.
Myocardium. Epinephrine stimulates the β_1 receptors of the myocardium. There is a positive inotropic (force of contraction) and positive chronotropic (rate of contraction) effect. Both cardiac output and heart rate are increased.

Pacemaker cells. Epinephrine stimulates β_1 receptors and increases the irritability of pacemaker cells, leading to an increased incidence of dysrhythmias. Ventricular tachycardia and premature ventricular contractions are common.

Coronary arteries. Epinephrine produces dilation of the coronary arteries, increasing coronary artery blood flow.

Blood pressure. Systolic blood pressure is *increased.* Diastolic pressure is *decreased* when small doses are administered because of the greater sensitivity to epinephrine of β_2 receptors than of α receptors in vessels supplying the skeletal muscles. Diastolic pressure is *increased* with larger epinephrine doses because of constriction of blood vessels supplying the skeletal muscles caused by α-receptor stimulation.

Cardiovascular dynamics. The overall action of epinephrine on the heart and cardiovascular system is direct stimulation:
• Increased systolic and diastolic pressures
• Increased cardiac output
• Increased stroke volume
• Increased heart rate
• Increased strength of contraction
• Increased myocardial oxygen consumption
These actions lead to an overall *decrease* in cardiac efficiency.

The cardiovascular responses of increased systolic blood pressure and increased heart rate develop with the administration of one to two dental cartridges of a 1:100,000 epinephrine dilution.[25] Administration of four cartridges of 1:100,000 epinephrine will bring about a slight decrease in diastolic blood pressure.

Vasculature. The primary action of epinephrine is on smaller arterioles and precapillary sphincters. Blood vessels supplying the skin, mucous membranes, and kidneys primarily contain α receptors. Epinephrine produces constriction in these vessels. Vessels supplying the skeletal muscles contain both α and β_2 receptors, with β_2 predominating. Small doses of epinephrine produce dilation of these vessels as a result of β_2 actions. β_2 receptors are more sensitive to epinephrine than are α receptors. Larger doses produce vasoconstriction because the α receptors are stimulated.

Hemostasis. Clinically, epinephrine is used frequently as a vasoconstrictor for hemostasis during surgical procedures. The injection of epinephrine directly into surgical sites rapidly produces high tissue concentrations, a predominant α-receptor stimulation, and hemostasis. As epinephrine tissue levels decrease over time, its primary action on blood vessels reverts to vasodilation because β_2 actions predominate; therefore it is common for some bleeding to be noted at about 6 hours after a surgical procedure. In a clinical trial involving extraction of third molars, postsurgical bleeding occurred in 13 of 16 patients receiving epinephrine with their local anesthetic for hemostasis, whereas 0 of 16 patients receiving local anesthetic without vasoconstrictor (mepivacaine plain) had bleeding 6 hours postsurgery.[26] Additional findings of increased postsurgical pain and delayed wound healing in the epinephrine-receiving group also were noted.[26]

Respiratory system. Epinephrine is a potent dilator (β_2 effect) of bronchiole smooth muscle. It is the drug of choice for management of acute asthmatic episodes (bronchospasm).

Central nervous system. In usual therapeutic dosages epinephrine is *not* a potent CNS stimulant. Its CNS-stimulating actions become prominent when an excessive dose is administered.

Metabolism. Epinephrine increases oxygen consumption in all tissues. Through a β action it stimulates glycogenolysis in the liver and skeletal muscle, producing an elevation of blood sugar levels at plasma epinephrine concentrations of 150 to 200 pg/ml.[25] The equivalent of four dental local anesthetic cartridges of 1:100,000 epinephrine must be administered to elicit this response.[27]

Termination of action and elimination. The action of epinephrine is terminated primarily by its reuptake by adrenergic nerves. Epinephrine that escapes reuptake is rapidly inactivated in the blood by the enzymes catechol-O-methyltransferase (COMT) and monoamine oxidase (MAO), both of which are present in the liver.[28] Only small amounts (approximately 1%) of epinephrine are excreted unchanged in the urine.

Side effects and overdose. The clinical manifestations of epinephrine overdose relate to CNS stimulation and include increasing fear and anxiety, tension, restlessness, throbbing headache, tremor, weakness, dizziness, pallor, respiratory difficulty, and palpitation.

With increasing levels of epinephrine in the blood, cardiac dysrhythmias (especially ventricular) become more common; ventricular fibrillation is a rare but possible consequence. Dramatic increases in both systolic (>300 mm Hg) and diastolic (>200 mm Hg) pressures may be noted, which have led to cerebral hemorrhage.[29] Anginal episodes may be precipitated in patients with coronary insufficiency. Because of the rapid inactivation of epinephrine, the stimulatory phase of the overdose (toxic) reaction usually is brief. Vasoconstrictor overdose is discussed in greater depth in Chapter 18.

Clinical Applications.
- Management of acute allergic reactions
- Management of bronchospasm
- Management of cardiac arrest
- As a vasoconstrictor, for hemostasis
- As a vasoconstrictor in local anesthetics, to decrease absorption into the cardiovascular system
- As a vasoconstrictor in local anesthetics, to increase depth of anesthesia
- As a vasoconstrictor in local anesthetics, to increase duration of anesthesia
- To produce mydriasis

Availability in dentistry. Epinephrine is the most potent and widely used vasoconstrictor in dentistry. It is available in the following dilutions and drugs:

Epinephrine Dilution	Local Anesthetic (generic)
1:50,000	Lidocaine
1:80,000	Lidocaine [lignocaine] (United Kingdom)
1:100,000	Articaine
	Lidocaine
1:200,000	Articaine*
	Bupivacaine
	Etidocaine†
	Lidocaine
	Mepivacaine*
	Prilocaine
1:300,000	Lidocaine*

*Not available in the United States (June 2004).
†No longer marketed in the United States (2002).

Maximum Doses. *The least concentrated solution that produces effective pain control should be used.* Lidocaine is available with two dilutions of epinephrine—1:50,000 and 1:100,000 in the United States and Canada—and with 1:80,000, 1:200,000, and 1:300,000 in other countries. The duration of effective pulpal and soft-tissue anesthesia is equivalent with all forms. Therefore it is recommended (in North America) that the 1:100,000 epinephrine concentration be used with lidocaine when extended pain control is necessary. Where 1:200,000 or 1:300,000 epinephrine is available with lidocaine, these are preferred for pain control.[30]

The dosages in Table 3-5 represent recommended maximums as suggested by this author and others.[31] They are conservative figures but still provide the dental practitioner with adequate volumes to produce clinically acceptable anesthesia. The American Heart Association (1964) has stated that "the typical concentrations of vasoconstrictors contained in local anesthetics are not contraindicated in patients with cardiovascular disease so long as preliminary aspiration is practiced, the agent is injected slowly, and the smallest effective dose is administered."[32] In 1954 the New York Heart Association recommended that maximal epinephrine doses be limited to 0.2 mg per appointment.[33] In following years, the American Heart Association recommended the restriction of epinephrine in local anesthetics when administered to patients with ischemic heart disease.[34]

More recently, the Agency for Healthcare Research and Quality (AHRQ) reviewed the published literature on the subject of the effects of epinephrine in dental patients with high blood pressure.[35]

The report reviewed six studies that evaluated the effect of dental treatment (extraction of teeth) in hypertensive patients when they received local anesthetics with and without epinephrine. The results suggest that hypertensive subjects undergoing an extraction experience small increases in systolic blood pressure and heart rate associated with the use of a local anesthetic containing epinephrine. These increases associated with the use of

TABLE 3-5
Recommended Maximum Dosages of Epinephrine

Epinephrine Concentration (μg/Cartridge)	Cartridges (Rounded Off)	
	Normal, Healthy Patient (ASA I)*	Patient with Clinically Significant Cardiovascular Disease (ASA III or IV)†
1:50,000 (36)	5.5	1
1:100,000 (18)	11‡	2
1:200,000 (9)	22‡	4

*Maximum epinephrine dose of 0.2 mg or 200 μg per appointment.
†Maximum recommended dose of 0.04 or 40 μg per appointment.
‡Actual maximum volume of administration is limited by the dosage of local anesthetic drug.

epinephrine occur in addition to increases in systolic and diastolic blood pressure and heart rate associated with undergoing the procedure without epinephrine that are larger for hypertensive than for normotensive patients. No adverse outcomes were reported among any of the subjects in the studies included in the review, and only one report of an adverse event associated with the use of epinephrine in local anesthetic in a hypertensive patient was identified in the literature (Table 3-6).[35]

In cardiovascularly compromised patients it seems prudent to limit or avoid exposure to vasoconstrictors, if possible. These include poorly controlled ASA III, and all ASA IV and greater, cardiovascular risk patients. However, as stated, the risk of epinephrine administration must be weighed against the benefits to be gained from its inclusion in the local anesthetic solution. Can clinically adequate pain control be provided for this patient without a vasoconstrictor in the solution? What is the potential negative effect of poor anesthesia on endogenous release of catecholamines in response to sudden, unexpected pain?

The use of vasoconstrictors for cardiovascularly compromised patients is reviewed in greater depth in Chapter 20.

Hemostasis. Epinephrine-containing local anesthetic solutions are used, via infiltration into the surgical site, to prevent or to minimize hemorrhage during surgical and other procedures. The 1:50,000 dilution of epinephrine is more effective in this regard than less concentrated 1:100,000 or 1:200,000 solutions.[36] Epinephrine dilutions of 1:50,000 and 1:100,000 are considerably more

effective in restricting surgical blood loss than local anesthetics without vasoconstrictor additives.[26]

Clinical experience has shown that effective hemostasis can be obtained with concentrations of 1:100,000 epinephrine. Although the small volume of 1:50,000 epinephrine required for hemostasis does not increase a patient's risk, consideration always should be given to use of the 1:100,000 dilution, especially in patients known to be more sensitive to catecholamines. These include the ASA III or IV risk cardiovascularly compromised individuals and geriatric patients.

Norepinephrine (Levarterenol)

Proprietary names. Levophed, Noradrenalin; levarterenol is the official name of norepinephrine.

Chemical structure. Norepinephrine (as the bitartrate) in dental cartridges is relatively stable in acid solutions, deteriorating on exposure to light and air. The shelf life of a cartridge containing norepinephrine bitartrate is 18 months. Acetone-sodium bisulfite is added to the cartridge to retard deterioration.

Source. Norepinephrine is available in both synthetic and natural forms. The natural form constitutes approximately 20% of the catecholamine production of the adrenal medulla. In patients with pheochromocytoma, a tumor of the adrenal medulla, norepinephrine may comprise up to 80% of adrenal medullary secretions. It exists in both levorotatory and dextrorotatory forms; the levorotatory form is 40 times as potent as the dextrorotatory form. Norepinephrine is synthesized and is stored at postganglionic adrenergic nerve terminals.

Mode of action. The actions of norepinephrine are almost exclusively on α receptors (90%). It also stimulates β actions in the heart (10%). Norepinephrine is one fourth as potent as epinephrine.

Systemic Actions.
   Myocardium. Norepinephrine has a positive inotropic action on the myocardium through β_1 stimulation.

   Pacemaker cells. Norepinephrine stimulates pacemaker cells and increases their irritability, leading to a greater incidence of cardiac dysrhythmias (β_1 action).

   Coronary arteries. Norepinephrine produces an increase in coronary artery blood flow through a vasodilatory effect.

TABLE **3-6**
Means of Maximum Changes from Baseline for Blood Pressure and Heart Rate*

	max Δ SBP (mm)	max Δ DBP (mm)	max Δ HR (bpm)
HYPERTENSIVES			
Anesthesia with epinephrine	15.3	2.3	9.3
Anesthesia without epinephrine	11.7	3.3	4.7
NORMOTENSIVES			
Anesthesia with epinephrine	5.0	−0.7	6.3
Anesthesia without epinephrine*	5.0	4.0	0.7

*Unweighted mean of subject means reported in three studies. *DBP,* Diastolic blood pressure; *HR,* heart rate; *SBP,* systolic blood pressure. (Data from *Cardiovascular effects of epinephrine in hypertensive dental patients: Summary, evidence report/technology assessment number 48.* AHRQ Publication Number 02-E005, March 2002. Agency for Healthcare Research and Quality, Rockville, MD. http://www.ahrq.gov/clinic/epcsums/ephypsum.htm.)

Heart rate. It produces a *decrease* in heart rate caused by reflex action of the carotid and aortic baroreceptors and the vagus nerve after a marked increase in both systolic and diastolic pressures.

Blood pressure. Both systolic and diastolic pressures are increased, the systolic to a greater extent. This is produced through the α-stimulating actions of norepinephrine, which lead to peripheral vasoconstriction and a concomitant increase in peripheral vascular resistance.

Cardiovascular dynamics. The overall action of norepinephrine on the heart and cardiovascular system is as follows:
- Increased systolic pressure
- Increased diastolic pressure
- Decreased heart rate
- Unchanged or slightly decreased cardiac output
- Increased stroke volume
- Increased total peripheral resistance

Vasculature. Norepinephrine, through α stimulation, produces constriction of cutaneous blood vessels. This leads to increased total peripheral resistance and increased systolic and diastolic blood pressures.

The degree and duration of ischemia noted after norepinephrine infiltration into the palate have led to soft-tissue necrosis (Fig. 3-1).

Respiratory system. Norepinephrine does not relax bronchial smooth muscle, as does epinephrine. It does, however, produce α-induced constriction of lung arterioles, which reduces airway resistance to a small degree. Norepinephrine is *not* clinically effective in the management of bronchospasm.

Central nervous system. Like epinephrine, norepinephrine does *not* exhibit CNS-stimulating actions at usual therapeutic doses; its CNS-stimulating properties are most prominent after overdose. Clinical manifestations are similar to those of epinephrine overdose (p. 41) but are less frequent and usually not as severe.

Metabolism. Norepinephrine increases basal metabolic rate. Tissue oxygen consumption is also increased in the area of injection. Norepinephrine produces an elevation in the blood sugar level in the same manner as epinephrine, but to a lesser degree.

Termination of action and elimination. The action of norepinephrine is terminated through its reuptake at adrenergic nerve terminals and its oxidation by MAO. Exogenous norepinephrine is inactivated by COMT.

Side effects and overdose. Clinical manifestations of norepinephrine overdose are similar to but less frequent and less severe than those of epinephrine. They normally involve CNS stimulation. Excessive levels of norepinephrine in the blood produce markedly elevated systolic and diastolic pressures with an increased risk of hemorrhagic "stroke," headache, anginal episodes in susceptible patients, and cardiac dysrhythmias.

The extravascular injection of norepinephrine into tissues may produce necrosis and sloughing because of intense α stimulation. In the oral cavity the most likely site to encounter this phenomenon is the hard palate (see Fig. 3-1). Norepinephrine should be avoided for vasoconstricting purposes (e.g., hemostasis), especially on the palate. Several authorities have stated that norepinephrine should not be used at all with local anesthetics.[30,37]

Clinical applications. Norepinephrine is used as a vasoconstrictor in local anesthetics and for the management of hypotension.

Availability in dentistry. In the United States norepinephrine is no longer available in local anesthetic solutions used in dentistry. In the past it was included with the local anesthetics propoxycaine and procaine in a 1:30,000 concentration. In other countries norepinephrine is included with lidocaine (Germany) and mepivacaine (Germany) or as the combination of norepinephrine and epinephrine with lidocaine (Germany) or tolycaine (Japan).[21]

Maximum doses. When used, norepinephrine should be used for *pain control only,* there being no justification for its use in obtaining hemostasis. It is approximately 25% as potent a vasopressor as epinephrine and therefore is used clinically as a 1:30,000 dilution.

Recent recommendations of the International Federation of Dental Anesthesiology Societies (IFDAS)

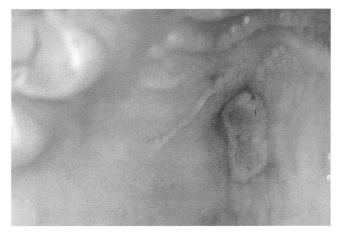

Figure 3-1. Sterile abscess on the palate produced by excessive use of a vasoconstrictor (norepinephrine).

suggest that norepinephrine be eliminated as a vasoconstrictor in dental local anesthetics.[30]

Normal healthy patient: 0.34 mg per appointment; 10 ml of a 1:30,000 solution

Patient with clinically significant cardiovascular disease (ASA III or IV): 0.14 mg per appointment; approximately 4 ml of a 1:30,000 solution

Levonordefrin*

Proprietary name. Neo-Cobefrin.

Chemical structure. Levonordefrin is freely soluble in dilute acidic solutions. Sodium bisulfite is added to the solution to delay its deterioration. The shelf life of a cartridge containing levonordefrin-sodium bisulfite is 18 months.

Source. Levonordefrin, a synthetic vasoconstrictor, is prepared by the resolution of nordefrin into its optically active isomers. The dextrorotatory form of nordefrin is virtually inert.

Mode of action. It appears to act through direct α receptor stimulation (75%) with some β activity (25%), but to a lesser degree than epinephrine. Levonordefrin is 15% as potent a vasopressor as epinephrine.

Systemic Actions. Levonordefrin produces less cardiac and CNS stimulation than does epinephrine.

Myocardium. There is the same action as epinephrine, but to a lesser degree.

Pacemaker cells. There is the same action as epinephrine, but to a lesser degree.

Coronary arteries. There is the same action as epinephrine, but to a lesser degree.

Heart rate. There is the same action as epinephrine, but to a lesser degree.

Vasculature. There is the same action as epinephrine, but to a lesser degree.

Respiratory system. There is some bronchodilation, but to a much smaller degree than with epinephrine.

Central nervous system. There is the same action as epinephrine, but to a lesser degree.

Metabolism. There is the same action as epinephrine, but to a lesser degree.

Termination of action and elimination. Levonordefrin is eliminated through the actions of COMT and MAO.

Side effects and overdose. These are the same as with epinephrine, but to a lesser extent. In higher doses additional side effects include hypertension, ventricular tachycardia, and anginal episodes in patients with coronary insufficiency.

Clinical applications. Levonordefrin is used as a vasoconstrictor in local anesthetics.

Availability in dentistry. It can be obtained with mepivacaine in a 1:20,000 dilution.

Maximum doses. Levonordefrin is considered one sixth (15%) as effective a vasopressor as epinephrine; therefore it is used in a higher concentration (1:20,000).

For all patients the maximum dose should be 1 mg per appointment; 20 ml of a 1:20,000 dilution (11 cartridges)[†]

In the concentration at which it is available, levonordefrin has the same effect on clinical activity of local anesthetics as does epinephrine in 1:50,000 or 1:100,000 concentrations.

Phenylephrine Hydrochloride

Proprietary name. Neo-Synephrine.

Chemical structure. Phenylephrine is quite soluble in water. It is the most stable and the weakest vasoconstrictor employed in dentistry.

Source. Phenylephrine is a synthetic sympathomimetic amine.

Mode of action. There is direct α receptor stimulation (95%). Although the effect is less than with epinephrine, its duration is longer. Phenylephrine exerts little or no β action on the heart. Only a small portion of its activity results from its ability to release norepinephrine. Phenylephrine is only 5% as potent as epinephrine.

---

*In mid-2003 levonordefrin became unavailable in the United States and Canada. Local anesthetics containing levonordefrin have been withdrawn from the market in these countries.

[†]Maximum volume for administration may be limited by the dose of the local anesthetic.

Systemic Actions.

Myocardium. It has little chronotropic or inotropic effect on the heart.

Pacemaker cells. There is little effect.

Coronary arteries. There is increased blood flow, caused by dilation.

Blood pressure. α action produces increases in both systolic and diastolic pressures.

Heart rate. Bradycardia is produced by reflex actions of the carotid–aortic baroreceptors and the vagus nerve. Cardiac dysrhythmias are rarely noted, even after large doses of phenylephrine.

Cardiovascular dynamics. Overall, the cardiovascular actions of phenylephrine are as follows:
- Increased systolic and diastolic pressures
- Reflex bradycardia
- Slightly decreased cardiac output (resulting from increased blood pressure and bradycardia)
- Powerful vasoconstriction (most vascular beds constricted, peripheral resistance increased significantly) but without marked venous congestion
- Rarely associated with provoking cardiac dysrhythmias

Respiratory system. Bronchi are dilated but to a lesser degree than with epinephrine. Phenylephrine is not effective in treating bronchospasm.

Central nervous system. There is a minimum effect on CNS activity.

Metabolism. Some increase in the metabolic rate is noted. Other actions (e.g., glycogenolysis) are similar to those produced by epinephrine.

Termination of action and elimination. Phenylephrine undergoes hydroxylation to epinephrine, then oxidation to metanephrine, after which it is eliminated in the same manner as epinephrine.

Side effects and overdose. CNS effects are minimal with phenylephrine. Headache and ventricular dysrhythmias have been noted after overdose. Tachyphylaxis is observed with chronic use.

Clinical applications. Phenylephrine is used as a vasoconstrictor in local anesthetics, for the management of hypotension, as a nasal decongestant, and in ophthalmic solutions to produce mydriasis.

Availability in dentistry. Phenylephrine was used with 4% procaine in a 1:2500 dilution (no longer available in dental cartridges).

Maximum doses. Phenylephrine is considered only one twentieth as potent as epinephrine, hence its use in a 1:2500 dilution (equivalent to a 1:50,000 epinephrine concentration). It is an excellent vasoconstrictor, with few significant side effects.

Normal healthy patient: 4 mg per appointment; 10 ml of a 1:2500 solution

Patient with clinically significant cardiovascular impairment (ASA III or IV): 1.6 mg per appointment, equivalent to 4 ml of a 1:2500 solution

Felypressin

Proprietary name. Octapressin.

Chemical structure

$$\text{Cys-Phe-Phe-Gly-Asn-Cys-Pro-Lys-GlyNH}_2$$

Source. Felypressin is a synthetic analogue of the antidiuretic hormone vasopressin. It is a non-sympathomimetic amine, categorized as a vasoconstrictor.

Mode of action. It acts as a direct stimulant of vascular smooth muscle. Its actions appear to be more pronounced on the venous than on the arteriolar microcirculation.[37]

Systemic Actions.

Myocardium. There are no direct effects.

Pacemaker cells. Felypressin is nondysrhythmogenic, in contradistinction to the sympathomimetic amines (e.g., epinephrine and norepinephrine).

Coronary arteries. When administered in high doses (greater than therapeutic), it may impair blood flow through the coronary arteries.

Vasculature. In high doses (greater than therapeutic), felypressin-induced constriction of cutaneous blood vessels may produce facial pallor.

Central nervous system. Felypressin has no effect on adrenergic nerve transmission; thus it may be safely administered to hyperthyroid patients and to anyone receiving MAO inhibitors or tricyclic antidepressants.

Uterus. It has both antidiuretic and oxytocic actions, the latter contraindicating its use in pregnant patients.

Side effects and overdose. Laboratory and clinical studies with felypressin in animals and humans have demonstrated a wide margin of safety.[38] The drug is well tolerated by tissues into which it is deposited, with little irritation developing. The incidence of systemic reactions to felypressin is minimal.

Clinical applications. Felypressin is used as a vasoconstrictor in local anesthetics to decrease their absorption and increase their duration of action.

Availability in dentistry. Felypressin is employed in a dilution of 0.03 IU/ml (International Units) with 3% prilocaine in Japan, Germany, and other countries. It is not available as a vasoconstrictor in local anesthetics in the United States.

Maximum doses. Felypressin-containing solutions are *not recommended for use when hemostasis is necessary* because of their predominant effect on the venous rather than the arterial circulation.[39]

For *patients with clinically significant cardiovascular impairment* (ASA III or IV), the maximum recommended dose is 0.27 IU; 9 ml of 0.03 IU/ml.

SELECTION OF A VASOCONSTRICTOR

Two vasoconstrictors are available in local anesthetic solutions in North America, epinephrine and levonordefrin. Levonordefrin has become impossible to obtain in North America (as of June 2004, it was still unobtainable). The three major North American manufacturers of local anesthetics containing levonordefrin—Dentsply, Kodak, and Septodont—have ceased marketing their version of the drug. It is expected that levonordefrin will again be available in North America by early 2005.

In the selection of an appropriate vasoconstrictor, if any, for use with a local anesthetic, several factors must be considered: the length of the dental procedure, the need for hemostasis during and after the procedure, the requirement for postoperative pain control, and the medical status of the patient.[1-4]

Length of the Dental Procedure

The addition of any vasoactive drug to a local anesthetic prolongs the duration (and depth) of pulpal and soft-tissue anesthesia of most local anesthetics. For example, pulpal and hard-tissue anesthesia with 2% lidocaine lasts approximately 10 minutes; the addition of 1:50,000, 1:80,000, 1:100,000, or 1:200,000 epinephrine increases this to approximately 60 minutes. The addition of a vasoconstrictor to prilocaine, on the other hand, does not significantly increase the duration of clinically effective pain control. Prilocaine 4%, after nerve block injection, provides pulpal anesthesia of about 40 to 60 minutes duration. (Infiltration injection with prilocaine 4% provides approximately 10 to 15 minutes of pulpal anesthesia.) The addition of a 1:200,000 epinephrine concentration to prilocaine increases this slightly (to about 60 to 90 minutes).[40,41]

Average durations of pulpal and hard-tissue anesthesia expected from commonly used local anesthetics with and without vasoconstrictors are shown in Table 3-7.

TABLE 3-7
Average Durations of Pulpal and Hard-tissue Anesthesia

Local Anesthetic	Infiltration (minutes)	Nerve Block (minutes)
LIDOCAINE HCL		
2% – no vasoconstrictor	5–10*	~10–20*
2% + epinephrine 1:50,000	~60	≥60
2% + epinephrine 1:100,000	~60	≥60
2% + epinephrine 1:200,000	~60	≥60
MEPIVACAINE HCL		
3% – no vasoconstrictor	5–10*	20–40*
2% + levonordefrin 1:20,000	≤60	≥60
2% + epinephrine 1:100,000	≤60	≥60
PRILOCAINE HCL		
4% – no vasoconstrictor	10–15*	40–60*
4% + epinephrine 1:200,000	≤60	60–90
ARTICAINE HCL		
4% + epinephrine 1:100,000	≤60	≥60

The typical dental patient is scheduled for a 1-hour appointment. Duration of actual treatment (and the desirable duration of profound pulpal anesthesia) is 47.9 minutes (standard deviation [SD] 14.7 minutes) in a general dentistry office, whereas in the offices of dental specialists treatment time is 39.1 minutes (SD 19.4 minutes).[42]

For routine restorative procedures it might be estimated that pulpal anesthesia will be required for approximately 40 to 50 minutes. As can be seen in Table 3-7, it is difficult to achieve consistently reliable pulpal anesthesia without the inclusion of a vasoconstrictor (see minutes marked with asterisks in Table 3-7).

Requirement for Hemostasis

Epinephrine is effective in preventing or minimizing blood loss during surgical procedures. However, epinephrine also produces a rebound vasodilatory effect as the tissue level of epinephrine declines. This leads to possible bleeding postoperatively, which potentially interferes with wound healing.[26]

Epinephrine, which possesses both α and β actions, produces vasoconstriction through its α effects. Used in a 1:50,000 concentration, and even at 1:100,000 (but to a lesser extent), epinephrine produces a definite rebound β effect once the α-induced vasoconstriction has ceased. This leads to increased postoperative blood loss, which if significant (usually in dentistry it is not), could compromise a patient's cardiovascular status.

Phenylephrine, a longer-acting, almost pure α-stimulating vasoconstrictor, does not produce a rebound β effect because its β actions are minimal. Therefore because it is not as potent a vasoconstrictor as epinephrine, hemostasis *during* the procedure is not as effective; however, because of the long duration of action of phenylephrine compared with that of epinephrine, the postoperative period passes with less bleeding. Total blood loss is usually lower when phenylephrine is used. Phenylephrine is *not* included in any dental local anesthetic cartridge.

Norepinephrine is a potent α stimulator and vasoconstrictor that has produced documented cases of tissue necrosis and slough. It cannot be recommended as a vasoconstrictor in dentistry because its disadvantages outweigh its advantages. Other more or equally effective vasoconstrictors are available that do not possess norepinephrine's disadvantages.[43,44]

Felypressin constricts the venous circulation more than the arteriolar circulation and therefore is of minimum value for hemostasis.

Vasoconstrictors used to achieve hemostasis must be deposited locally into the surgical site (area of bleeding) to be effective. They act directly on α receptors in the vascular smooth muscle. Only small volumes of local anesthetic solutions with vasoconstrictor are required to achieve hemostasis.

Medical Status of the Patient

There are few contraindications to vasoconstrictor administration in the concentrations in which they are found in dental local anesthetics. For all patients, and for some in particular, the benefits and risks of including the vasopressor in the local anesthetic solution must be weighed against the benefits and risks of using a "plain" anesthetic solution.[45–47] In general, these groups are:

- Patients with more significant cardiovascular disease (ASA III and IV)*
- Patients with certain noncardiovascular diseases (e.g., thyroid dysfunction, diabetes, and sulfite sensitivity)
- Patients receiving MAO inhibitors, tricyclic antidepressants, and phenothiazines

In each of these situations it is necessary to determine the degree of severity of the underlying disorder to determine whether a vasoconstrictor may be included safely or should be excluded from the local anesthetic solution. It is not uncommon for medical consultation to be sought to aid in determining this information.

Management of these patients is discussed in depth in Chapters 10 and 20. Briefly, however, it may be stated that local anesthetics with vasoconstrictors are not absolutely contraindicated for the patient whose medical condition has been diagnosed and is under control through medical or surgical means (ASA II or III risk) and if the vasoconstrictor is administered slowly, in minimal doses, after negative aspiration has been ensured.

Patients with a resting blood pressure (minimum 5-minute rest) of either greater than 200 mm Hg systolic

or greater than 115 mm Hg diastolic should not receive elective dental care until their more significant medical problem of high blood pressure is corrected. Patients with severe cardiovascular disease (ASA IV+ risk) may be at too great a risk for elective dental therapy; for example, a patient who has had an acute myocardial infarction within the past 6 months, a patient who has been experiencing anginal episodes at rest on a daily basis or whose signs and symptoms are increasing in severity (preinfarction or unstable angina), or a patient whose cardiac dysrhythmias are refractory to antiarrhythmic drug therapy.[45] Epinephrine and other vasoconstrictors can be administered, within limits, to patients with mild to moderate cardiovascular disease (ASA II or III). Felypressin has minimum cardiovascular stimulatory actions and is nondysrhythmogenic; it is the recommended drug for ASA III and IV cardiovascular risk patients. Epinephrine also is contraindicated in patients exhibiting clinical evidence of the hyperthyroid state.[46] Signs and symptoms include exophthalmos, hyperhydrosis, tremor, irritability and nervousness, increased body temperature, inability to tolerate heat, increased heart rate, and increased blood pressure. Minimal dosages of epinephrine are recommended as a vasoconstrictor during general anesthesia when a patient (in any ASA category) is receiving a halogenated anesthetic (halothane, isoflurane, sevoflurane, or enflurane). These inhalation (general) anesthetics sensitize the myocardium such that epinephrine administration is frequently associated with the occurrence of ventricular dysrhythmias (PVCs or ventricular fibrillation). Felypressin is recommended in these situations; however, because of its potential oxytocic actions, felypressin is not recommended for pregnant patients. Once the impaired medical status of the patient is improved (e.g., ASA IV becomes ASA III), routine dental care involving the administration of local anesthetics with vasoconstrictors is indicated.

Patients being treated with MAO inhibitors may receive vasoconstrictors within the usual dental dosage parameters without increased risk.[47,48] Patients receiving tricyclic antidepressants are at greater risk for development of dysrhythmias with epinephrine administration. It is recommended that when epinephrine is administered, its dose be minimal. The administration of either levonordefrin or norepinephrine is absolutely contraindicated in patients receiving tricyclic antidepressants.[49] Large doses of vasoconstrictor may induce severe (exaggerated) responses.

Local anesthetic solutions containing a vasoconstrictor also contain an antioxidant (to delay the oxidation of the vasoconstrictor). *Sodium bisulfite* is the most frequently used antioxidant in dental cartridges. It prolongs the shelf life of the anesthetic solution with vasoconstrictor to approximately 18 months. However, sodium bisulfite renders the local anesthetic considerably more *acidic* than the same solution without a vasoconstrictor. Acidic solutions of local anesthetics contain a greater proportion of charged cation molecules (RNH^+)

---

*The ASA Physical Evaluation System is discussed in depth in Chapter 10.

than of uncharged base molecules (RN). Because of this, the diffusion of the local anesthetic solution into the axoplasm is slower, resulting in a (slightly) delayed onset of anesthesia when local anesthetics containing sodium bisulfite (and vasoconstrictors) are injected.

Vasoconstrictors are important additions to local anesthetic solutions. Numerous studies have demonstrated conclusively that epinephrine, added to short- or medium-duration local anesthetic solutions, slows the rate of absorption, lowers the systemic blood level, delays cresting of the peak blood level, prolongs duration of anesthesia, intensifies "depth" of anesthesia, and reduces the incidence of systemic reactions.[18] In modern dentistry, adequate pain control of sufficient clinical duration and depth is difficult to achieve without the inclusion of vasoconstrictors in the local anesthetic solution. Unless specifically contraindicated by a patient's medical status (ASA IV or above) or by the required duration of treatment (short), the inclusion of a vasoconstrictor should be considered. Whenever these drugs are used, however, care always must be taken to avoid unintended intravascular administration of the vasoconstrictor (and the local anesthetic) through multiple aspirations and the slow administration of minimum concentrations of both the vasoconstrictor and the local anesthetic.

REFERENCES

1. Cannall H, Walters H, Beckett AH, Saunders A: Circulating blood levels of lignocaine after peri-oral injections, *Br Dent J* 138:87-93, 1975.
2. Finder RL. Moore PA: Adverse drug reactions to local anesthesia, *Dent Clin N Am* 46:447-457, 2002.
3. Brown G: The influence of adrenaline, noradrenaline vasoconstrictors on the efficacy of lidocaine, *J Oral Ther Pharmacol* 4:398-405, 1968.
4. Cowan A: Further clinical evaluation of prilocaine (Citanest), with and without epinephrine, *Oral Surg Oral Med Oral Pathol* 26:304-311, 1968.
5. Carpenter RL, Kopacz DJ, Mackey DC: Accuracy of Doppler capillary flow measurements for predicting blood loss from skin incisions in pigs, *Anesth Analg* 68:308-311, 1989.
6. Myers RR, Heckman HM: Effects of local anesthesia on nerve blood flow: studies using lidocaine with and without epinephrine, *Anesthesiology* 71:757-762, 1989.
7. Ahlquist RP: A study of adrenotropic receptors, *Am J Physiol* 153:586-600, 1948.
8. Hieble JP: Adrenoceptor subclassification: an approach to improved cardiovascular therapeutics, *Pharmaceut Acta Helvetiae* 74:63-71, 2000.
9. Smiley RM, Kwatra MM, Schwinn DA: New developments in cardiovascular adrenergic receptor pharmacology: molecular mechanisms and clinical relevance, *J Cardiothor Vasc Anesth* 12:10-95, 1998.
10. Braun H: Uber den Einfluss der Vitalitat der Gewebe auf die ortlichen und allgemeinen Giftwirkungen local-abaesthesierender Mittel, und uber die Bedeutung des Adrerenalins fur die Lokalanasthesie, *Arch Klin Chir* 69:541-591, 1903.
11. Tolas AG, Pflug AE, Halter JB: Arterial plasma epinephrine concentrations and hemodynamic responses after dental injection of local anesthetic with epinephrine, *J Am Dent Assoc* 104:41-43, 1982.
12. Jastak JT, Yagiela JA, Donaldson D, editors: *Local anesthesia of the oral cavity*, Philadelphia, 1995, WB Saunders.
13. Holroyd SV, Requa-Clark B: *Local anesthetics*. In Holroyd SV, Wynn RL, editors: *Clinical pharmacology in dental practice*, ed 3, St Louis, 1983, Mosby.
14. Malamed SF: *Handbook of local anesthesia*, ed 4, St Louis, 1997, Mosby.
15. Cryer PE: Physiology and pathophysiology of the human sympathoadrenal neuroendocrine system, *N Engl J Med* 303:436-444, 1980.
16. Yagiela JA: Epinephrine and the compromised heart, *Orofac Pain Manage* 1:5-8, 1991.
17. Kaneko Y, Ichinohe T, Sakurai M, et al: Relationship between changes in circulation due to epinephrine oral injection and its plasma concentration, *Anesth Prog* 36: 188-190, 1989.
18. de Jong RH: *Uptake, distribution, and elimination*. In de Jong RH: *Local anesthetics*, St Louis, 1994, Mosby.
19. Huang KC: Effect of intravenous epinephrine on heart rate as monitored with a computerized tachometer, *Anesthesiology* 73:A762, 1990.
20. Narchi P, Mazoit J-X, Cohen S, Samii K: Heart rate response to an IV test dose of adrenaline and lignocaine with and without atropine pretreatment, *Br J Anaesth* 66:583-586, 1991.
21. Malamed SF, Sykes P, Kubota Y, et al: Local anesthesia: a review, *Anesth Pain Control Dent* 1:11-24, 1992.
22. Lipp M, Dick W, Daublander M: Examination of the central venous epinephrine level during local dental infiltration and block anesthesia using tritium marked epinephrine as vasoconstrictor, *Anesthesiology* 69:371, 1988.
23. Stanton-Hicks Md'A, Berges PU, Bonica JJ: Circulatory effects of peridural block: IV. Comparison of the effects of epinephrine and phenylephrine, *Anesthesiology* 39:308-314, 1973.
24. Robertson VJ, Taylor SE, Gage TW: Quantitative and qualitative analysis of the pressor effects of levonordefrin, *J Cardiovasc Pharmacol* 6:529-935, 1984.
25. Clutter WE, Bier DM, Shah SD, Cryer PE: Epinephrine plasma metabolic clearance rates and physiologic thresholds for metabolic and hemodynamic actions in man, *J Clin Invest* 66:94-101, 1980.
26. Sveen K: Effect of the addition of a vasoconstrictor to local anesthetic solution on operative and postoperative bleeding, analgesia, and wound healing, *Int J Oral Surg* 8: 301-306, 1979.
27. Meechan JG: The effects of dental local anaesthetics on blood glucose concentration in healthy volunteers and in patients having third molar surgery, *Br Dent J* 170:373-376, 1991.
28. Lefkowitz RJ, Hoffman BB, Taylor P: *Neurohumoral transmission: the autonomic and somatic motor nervous system*. In Gilman AG, et al, editors: *Goodman and Gilman's the pharmacological basis of therapeutics*, ed 8, New York, 1990, Pergamon Press.
29. Campbell RL: Cardiovascular effects of epinephrine overdose: case report, *Anesth Prog* 24:190-193, 1977.
30. Jakob W: Local anaesthesia and vasoconstrictive additional components, *Newslett Int Fed Dent Anesthesiol Soc* 2:1, 1989.
31. Bennett CR: *Monheim's local anesthesia and pain control in dental practice*, ed 7, St Louis, 1983, Mosby.

32. Management of dental problems in patients with cardiovascular disease: report of a working conference jointly sponsored by the American Dental Association and American Heart Association, *J Am Dent Assoc* 68:333-342, 1964.

33. Use of epinephrine in connection with procaine in dental procedures: report of the Special Committee of the New York Heart Association, Inc., on the use of epinephrine in connection with procaine in dental procedures, *J Am Dent Assoc* 50:108, 1955.

34. Kaplan EL, editor: *Cardiovascular disease in dental practice*, Dallas, 1986, American Heart Association.

35. *Cardiovascular effects of epinephrine in hypertensive dental patients: summary, evidence report/technology assessment number 48*. AHRQ Publication Number 02-E005, March 2002. Agency for Healthcare Research and Quality, Rockville, MD. *http://www.ahrq.gov/clinic/epcsums/ephypsum.htm*.

36. Buckley JA, Ciancio SG, McMullen JA: Efficacy of epinephrine concentration in local anesthesia during periodontal surgery, *J Periodontol* 55:653-657, 1984.

37. Holroyd SV, Wynn RL, Requa-Clark B, eds.: *Clinical pharmacology in dental practice*, ed 4, St Louis, 1988, Mosby.

38. Altura BM, Hershey SG, Zweifach BW: Effects of a synthetic analogue of vasopressin on vascular smooth muscle, *Proc Soc Exp Biol Med* 119:258-261, 1965.

39. Sunada K, Nakamura K, Yamashiro M, et al: Clinically safe dosage of felypressin for patients with essential hypertension, *Anesth Prog* 43:408-415, 1996.

40. Newcomb GM, Waite IM: The effectiveness of local analgesic preparations in reducing haemorrhage during periodontal surgery, *J Dent* 1:37-42, 1972.

41. Epstein S: Clinical study of prilocaine with varying concentrations of epinephrine, *J Am Dent Assoc* 78:85-90, 1969.

42. American Dental Association: *1999 Survey of dental practice*, Chicago, American Dental Association, February 2001.

43. van der Bijl P, Victor AM: Adverse reactions associated with norepinephrine in dental local anesthesia, *Anesth Prog* 39: 37-89, 1992.

44. Hirota Y, Hori T, Kay K, Matsuura H: Effects of epinephrine and norepinephrine contained in 2% lidocaine on hemodynamics of the carotid and cerebral circulation in older and younger adults, *Anesth Pain Control Dent* 1:343-151, 1992.

45. Goulet JP, Perusse R, Turcotte JY: Contraindications to vasoconstrictors in dentistry: Part I. Cardiovascular diseases, *Oral Surg Oral Med Oral Pathol* 74:579-686, 1992.

46. Goulet JP, Perusse R, Turcotte JY: Contraindications to vasoconstrictors in dentistry: Part II. Hyperthyroidism, diabetes, sulfite sensitivity, cortico-dependent asthma, and pheochromocytoma, *Oral Surg Oral Med Oral Pathol* 74: 587-691, 1992.

47. Goulet JP, Perusse R, Turcotte JY: Contraindications to vasoconstrictors in dentistry: Part III. Pharmacologic interactions, *Oral Surg Oral Med Oral Pathol* 74:592-697, 1992.

48. Verrill PJ: Adverse reactions to local anaesthetics and vasoconstrictor drugs, *Practitioner* 214:380-387, 1975.

49. Jastak JT, Yagiela JA, Donaldson D, editors: *Local anesthesia of the oral cavity*, Philadelphia, 1995, WB Saunders.

Clinical Action of Specific Agents

CHAPTER 4

Although many drugs are classified as local anesthetics and find use within the health professions, only a handful are currently used in dentistry. In 1980, when the first edition of this text was published, five local anesthetics were available in dental cartridge form in the United States: *lidocaine, mepivacaine, prilocaine,* and the combination of *procaine* and *propoxycaine*.[1] In the years since that first edition, increased demand for longer-acting local anesthetics led to the introduction, in dental cartridges, of *bupivacaine* (1982 Canada, 1983 United States) and *etidocaine* (1985). In 1975 *articaine* became available in Germany, and then throughout Europe. Articaine came to North America in 1983 (Canada) and the United States in 2000. Articaine is classified as an intermediate-duration local anesthetic.

The combination of procaine and propoxycaine was withdrawn from the United States market in January 1996. Etidocaine was removed from the United States market in 2002. Local anesthetics containing the vasoconstrictor levonordefrin (Neo-Cobefrin) have become impossible to obtain (June 2004).

As this fifth edition of *Handbook of Local Anesthesia* goes to press the local anesthetic armamentarium in North American dentistry includes: articaine, bupivacaine, lidocaine, mepivacaine, and prilocaine.

With the availability of these local anesthetics, in various combinations with and without vasoconstrictors, it is now possible for a doctor to select a drug possessing the specific pain controlling properties necessary for the patient for a given dental procedure. Table 4-1 lists local anesthetics and the various combinations in which they are currently available in the United States and Canada, and Box 4-1 lists these combinations by their expected duration of clinical action.

In this chapter, each of the available local anesthetics in its various combinations is described. In addition, the rationale for the selection of an appropriate local anesthetic for a given patient at a given appointment is presented. It is strongly suggested that the reader, who

TABLE **4-1**

Local Anesthetics Available in North America (June 2004)

Local Anesthetic (+ Vasoconstrictor)	Duration of Action*
Articaine HCl	
4% + epinephrine 1:100,000	Intermediate
4% + epinephrine 1:200,000[†]	Intermediate
Bupivacaine HCl	
0.5% + epinephrine 1:200,000	Long
Lidocaine HCl	
2%	Short
2% + epinephrine 1:50,000	Intermediate
2% + epinephrine 1:100,000	Intermediate
Mepivacaine HCl	
3%	Short
2% + levonordefrin 1:20,000[†]	Intermediate
2% + epinephrine 1:100,000[†]	Intermediate
Prilocaine HCl	
4%	Short (infiltration); intermediate (nerve block)
4% + epinephrine 1:200,000	Intermediate

*The classification of duration of action is approximate, for extreme variations may be noted among patients. Short-duration drugs provide pulpal or deep anesthesia for less than 30 minutes; intermediate-duration drugs for about 60 minutes; and long-duration drugs for longer than 90 minutes.

[†]Not available in the United States (June 2004).

BOX 4-1

Approximate Duration of Action of Local Anesthetics

SHORT DURATION (pulpal anesthesia approximately
30 minutes)
Lidocaine HCl 2%
Mepivacaine HCl 3%
Prilocaine HCl 4% (by infiltration)

INTERMEDIATE DURATION (pulpal anesthesia approximately
60 minutes)
Articaine HCl 4% + epinephrine 1:100,000
Articaine HCl 4% + epinephrine 1:200,000
Lidocaine HCl 2% + epinephrine 1:50,000
Lidocaine HCl 2% + epinephrine 1:100,000
Mepivacaine HCl 2% + levonordefrin 1:20,000
Mepivacaine HCl 2% + epinephrine 1:100,000
Prilocaine HCl 4% (via nerve block only)
Prilocaine HCl 4% + epinephrine 1:200,000

LONG DURATION (pulpal anesthesia approximately
90+ minutes)
Bupivacaine HCl 0.5% + epinephrine 1:200,000

is the potential administrator of these drugs, become familiar with this material, including the contraindications to the administration of certain local anesthetic agents (Table 4-2).

In the following discussion of the clinical properties of specific local anesthetic combinations, several concepts

are presented that require some explanation. These are the *duration of action* of the drug and the determination of the *maximum recommended dose*.

DURATION

The duration of pulpal (hard tissue) and soft tissue (total) anesthesia cited for each drug is an approximation. Factors exist that affect both the depth and the duration of a drug's anesthetic action, either prolonging or (much more commonly) decreasing it. These factors include:
1. Individual response to drug (the "bell-shaped" curve)
2. Accuracy in deposition of the local anesthetic
3. Status of the tissues at the site of drug deposition (vascularity, pH)
4. Anatomical variation
5. Type of injection administered (supraperiosteal ["infiltration"] or nerve block)

In the subsequent discussion of individual local anesthetics the durations of anesthesia (pulpal and soft tissue) are presented as a range (e.g., 40 to 60 minutes). This attempts to take into account the factors mentioned that can influence drug action.

Variation in individual response to a drug is common and is depicted in the so-called bell or normal distribution curve (Fig. 4-1). A majority of patients respond in a predictable manner to a drug's actions (e.g., 40 to 60 minutes). However, some patients (with none of the other factors that influence drug action obviously present) have either

TABLE **4-2**
Contraindications for Local Anesthetics

Medical Problem	Drugs to Avoid	Type of Contraindication	Alternative Drug
Local anesthetic allergy, documented	All local anesthetics in same chemical class (e.g., esters)	Absolute	Local anesthetics in different chemical class (e.g., amides)
Bisulfite allergy	Vasoconstrictor-containing local anesthetics	Absolute	Any local anesthetic without vasoconstrictor
Atypical plasma cholinesterase	Esters	Relative	Amides
Methemoglobinemia, idiopathic or congenital	Prilocaine	Relative	Other amides or esters
Significant liver dysfunction (ASA III-IV)	Amides	Relative	Amides or esters, but judiciously
Significant renal dysfunction (ASA III-IV)	Amides or esters	Relative	Amides or esters, but judiciously
Significant cardiovascular disease (ASA III-IV)	High concentrations of vasoconstrictors (as in racemic epinephrine gingival retraction cords)	Relative	Local anesthetics with epinephrine concentrations of 1:200,000 or 1:100,000 or mepivacaine 3% or prilocaine 4% (nerve blocks)
Clinical hyperthyroidism (ASA III-IV)	High concentrations of vasoconstrictors (as in racemic epinephrine gingival retraction cords)	Relative	Local anesthetics with epinephrine concentrations of 1:200,000 or 1:100,000 or mepivacaine 3% or prilocaine 4% (nerve blocks)

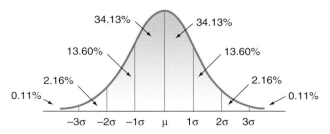

Figure 4-1. "Bell-shaped" curve.

a shorter or a longer duration of anesthesia. *This is to be expected and is entirely normal.*

For example, if 100 persons are administered an appropriate dose of 2% lidocaine HCl with epinephrine 1:100,000 via supraperiosteal injection over a maxillary lateral incisor, and a pulp-tester is used to assess the duration of anesthesia, approximately 70% (68.26%) would have pulpal anesthesia for approximately 60 minutes. These represent the *normal responders.* Approximately 15% would have pulpal anesthesia that lasts beyond the expected 60 minutes—perhaps 70 or 80 minutes, or even longer. These persons are termed *hyper-responders.* No dentist complains about these patients because their dental treatment proceeds without any pain or need for repeated injection of local anesthetic. However, it is the final 15%, the *hypo-responders,* who are well-remembered by the dentist. These patients, given lidocaine with epinephrine, are anesthetized for 45 minutes, 30 minutes, 15 minutes, or even less. These are the patients about whom the doctor states (incorrectly): "They metabolize the drug rapidly." As was mentioned in Chapter 2, metabolism (biotransformation, detoxification) has nothing to do with the clinical actions of the dissipation of a local anesthetic. The duration of anesthetization is simply based on the way some persons respond to this drug (or group of drugs).

Accuracy in the administration of the injected local anesthetic is the second factor influencing drug action. Although not as significant in certain techniques (e.g., supraperiosteal), or with certain drugs (e.g., articaine), accuracy in deposition is a major factor in many nerve blocks in which a considerable thickness of soft tissue must be penetrated to access the nerve to be blocked. The inferior alveolar nerve block (IANB) is the prime example of a technique in which the depth and duration of anesthesia is greatly influenced by accuracy of injection. Deposition of the local anesthetic close to the nerve provides greater depth and duration of anesthesia compared with an anesthetic deposited at a greater distance from the nerve to be blocked.

The *status of the tissues* into which a local anesthetic is deposited influences the observed duration of anesthetic action. The presence of normal healthy tissue at the site of drug deposition is assumed. Inflammation, infection, or pain (either acute or chronic) usually decreases depth and anticipated duration of anesthesia. Increased vascularity

at the site of drug deposition results in a more rapid absorption of the local anesthetic and a decreased duration of anesthesia. This is most notable in areas of inflammation and infection but is also a consideration in "normal" anatomy. The neck of the mandibular condyle, the target for local anesthetic deposition in the Gow-Gates mandibular nerve block, is considerably less vascular than the target area for the IANB. The expected duration of anesthesia for any local anesthetic is greater in the less vascular region.

Anatomical variation also influences clinical anesthesia. The normal anatomy of the maxilla and mandible is described in Chapter 12. The most notable aspect of "normal" anatomy is the presence of extreme variation (e.g., in size and shape of the head or thickness of bone) from person to person. The techniques presented in later chapters are based on the middle of the bell curve, the so-called "normal responders." Anatomical variations away from this "norm" adversely influence the duration of clinical drug action. Although most obvious in the mandible (height of the mandibular foramen, width of the ramus), such variation also may be noted in the maxilla. Supraperiosteal infiltration, usually effective in providing pulpal anesthesia for all maxillary teeth, provides a shorter duration than expected or inadequate depth of anesthesia when alveolar bone is more dense than usual. Where the zygomatic arch is lower (primarily in children, but occasionally in adults), infiltration anesthesia of the maxillary first and second molars may provide a shorter duration or even fail to provide adequate depth of pulpal anesthesia. In other cases the palatal root of maxillary molars may not be adequately anesthetized, even in the presence of normal thickness of the buccal alveolar bone, when that root flares greatly toward the midline of the palate.

Finally, the duration of clinical anesthesia is influenced by the *type of injection administered.* For all the drugs presented, administration of a nerve block provides a longer duration of both pulpal and soft-tissue anesthesia than supraperiosteal injection (e.g., infiltration). This assumes that the recommended minimum volume of anesthetic is injected. Smaller than recommended volumes decrease the duration of action. Larger than recommended doses do *not* provide increased duration. For example, a duration of pulpal anesthesia of 10 to 15 minutes may be expected to follow a supraperiosteal injection with prilocaine 4% (no vasoconstrictor), whereas a 40- to 60-minute duration is normal with a nerve block (Table 4-3).

MAXIMUM DOSES OF LOCAL ANESTHETICS

The doses of local anesthetic drugs are presented in terms of milligrams of drug per unit of body weight, either milligrams per kilogram (mg/kg) or milligrams per pound (mg/lb). These numbers, like the ones presented for duration, reflect estimated values because there is a wide range in patient response to blood levels of local anesthetics (or of any drug).

TABLE 4-3
Duration of Clinical Anesthesia by Type of Injection

Local Anesthetic	Infiltration (Minutes)	Nerve Block (Minutes)
Lidocaine HCl		
2%: no vasoconstrictor	5–10	~10–20
Mepivacaine HCl		
3%: no vasoconstrictor	5–10	20–40
Prilocaine HCl		
4%: no vasoconstrictor	10–15	40–60
Etidocaine HCl*		
1.5% + epinephrine 1:200,000	15	90–180

*Etidocaine is no longer available in dental cartridges in the United States (June 2004).

In patients whose responses to anesthetic blood levels lie in the middle of the normal distribution curve, the administration of a maximum dose based on body weight produces a local anesthetic blood level just below the threshold for an overdose (toxic) reaction. The response observed if an overdose reaction develops is mild (e.g., tremor of the arms and legs, drowsiness). Patients who are hypo-responders to elevated local anesthetic blood levels may not experience adverse reactions until their local anesthetic blood level is above this "normal" threshold. These patients represent little or no increased risk when local anesthetics are administered in "usual" dental doses. However, hyper-responders may demonstrate clinical signs and symptoms of local anesthetic overdose at blood levels that are somewhat lower than those normally necessary to produce such reactions. To increase safety during the administration of local anesthetics for all patients, but especially in this latter group, one should *always minimize drug doses and use the smallest clinically effective dose.* Recommended volumes of local anesthetics are presented for each injection technique in Chapters 13, 14, and 15.

Maximum doses for many of the local anesthetics have been modified since the first edition of this book. The Council on Dental Therapeutics of the American Dental Association and the United States Pharmacopeial (USP) Convention reviewed (independently) the maximum recommended doses (MRDs) for local anesthetics and no longer adjust them for inclusion of a vasoconstrictor.[2,3] The doses recommended by this author represent the more conservative of those recommended by either the Council, the USP, or the drug's manufacturer.[4,5] To avoid potential confusion, the manufacturers' recommended maximum dosages have been included in all charts discussing MRDs. They are listed as author's MRD (MRD-a) and manufacturers' MRD (MRD-m) (Table 4-4).

Before this change the maximum recommended adult dose of lidocaine, for example, without a vasoconstrictor was 300 mg, whereas if epinephrine was included in the

TABLE 4-4
Maximum Recommended Dosages (MRDs) of Local Anesthetics Available in North America

Local Anesthetic	Manufacturer's (MRD-m)			Author's (MRD-a)		
	mg/kg	mg/lb	MRD (mg)	mg/kg	mg/lb	MRD (mg)
Articaine						
With vasoconstrictor	7.0	3.2	500	7.0	3.2	500
Bupivacaine						
With vasoconstrictor	1.3	0.6	90	1.3	0.6	90
Lidocaine						
No vasoconstrictor	4.4	2.0	300	4.4	2.0	300
With vasoconstrictor	6.6	3.0	500	4.4	2.0	300
Mepivacaine						
No vasoconstrictor	6.6	3.0	400	4.4	2.0	300
With vasoconstrictor	6.6	3.0	400	4.4	2.0	300
Prilocaine						
No vasoconstrictor	6.0	2.7	400	6.0	2.7	400
With vasoconstrictor	6.0	2.7	400	6.0	2.7	400

Calculation of Milligrams of Local Anesthetic per Dental Cartridge (1.8 ml Cartridge)

Local Anesthetic	Percent Concentration	mg/ml	× 1.8 ml = mg/Cartridge
Articaine	4	40	72*
Bupivacaine	0.5	5	9
Lidocaine	2	20	36
Mepivacaine	2	20	36
	3	30	54
Prilocaine	4	40	72

*Cartridges of articaine HCl in the United States read: "minimum content of each cartridge is 1.7 ml."

solution the maximum dose was 500 mg.[4] Such distinctions are no longer made.

Maximum doses are unlikely to be reached in most dental patients, especially adults of normal body weight for most dental procedures. Two groups of patients, however, constitute a potentially increased risk from overly high local anesthetic blood levels: the smaller (well-behaved) child and the debilitated elderly individual. Considerable attention must be given to drug administration in these two groups.

The maximum calculated drug dose always should be decreased in medically compromised, debilitated, or elderly persons.

Changes in liver function, plasma protein binding, blood volume, and other important physiological functions influence the manner in which local anesthetics are distributed and biotransformed in the body.[6] The net result of these changes is to increase plasma blood levels of the drug, thereby increasing the relative risk of overdose reaction. The half-lives of the amide local anesthetics are significantly increased in the presence of decreased liver function or perfusion.[7] Peak plasma local anesthetic blood levels tend to be higher and to remain so longer in these situations. The calculated drug dose (based on body weight) should be decreased in all "at risk" individuals. Unfortunately, there is no guaranteed formula to aid in determining the degree of dose reduction for a given patient. It is suggested that the doctor evaluate each patient's dental care needs and then devise a treatment plan that takes into account that person's requirement for smaller doses of local anesthetic at every treatment appointment.

A point that has come up in several medicolegal situations related to overdosage (OD) of local anesthetics related to the maximum number of milligrams administered and the effect on the patient. Assume, for example, that the MRD for a local anesthetic in a given patient is 270 mg and the patient is administered 271 mg. The thinking among lay persons (and unfortunately some healthcare professionals) is that an overdose will definitely occur. However, such may not be the case. As mentioned, many factors interact to determine how a patient will respond to a given drug. When the MRD is exceeded, there is no guarantee that an OD will occur, only that there is a greater likelihood of it arising. Indeed, in certain individuals an OD may arise with dosages below the calculated MRD (hyper-responders). Another factor in determining whether an OD will occur is the time factor over which the local anesthetic dose was administered. If all 271 mg are administered within a brief time frame, the resulting local anesthetic blood level will be greater than in a situation in which the same dose was administered a little at a time over several hours. These points are discussed in greater detail in Chapter 18.

Box 4-2 provides examples of how to calculate maximum dosages and numbers of local anesthetic cartridges to be administered to various patients.

A commonly asked question is, *"How do I determine the dose of each local anesthetic administered in clinical situations where more than one drug is necessary?"* The answer is again that no guaranteed formula exists for determining this number. One method is simply to ensure that *the total dose of both local anesthetics not exceed the lower of the two maximum doses for the individual agents.*

For example, a 100-lb (45-kg) patient receiving 4% prilocaine with epinephrine may be given 2.7 mg/lb (or 270 mg) during a 90-minute procedure (the estimated half-life of prilocaine). She receives two cartridges (144 mg), but anesthesia is inadequate for the treatment to proceed. As is commonly the case, the doctor believes that the lack of anesthesia is caused by the anesthetic drug ("I've got a bad batch of local," but not by technique or patient anatomy, as is more likely to be the case) and elects to change to lidocaine 2% with epinephrine 1:100,000 to provide anesthesia. How does one determine the maximum dose of lidocaine that may be used?

BOX 4-2

Calculation of Maximum Dosages and Number of Cartridges (Single Drug)

PATIENT: 22 YEARS OLD, HEALTHY, FEMALE, 110 LBS
Lidocaine 2% = 36 mg/cartridge

Number of cartridges: Author: 220/36 = ~6
Manufacturer: 330/36 = ~9

LOCAL ANESTHETIC: LIDOCAINE HCL + EPINEPHRINE 1:100,000
Lidocaine: 2.0 mg/lb = 220 mg (MRD-a)
3.0 mg/lb = 330 mg (MRD-m)

PATIENT: 40 YEARS OLD, HEALTHY, MALE, 200 LBS
Prilocaine 4% = 72 mg/cartridge

Number of cartridges: Author and manufacturer: 400/72 = 5.5

LOCAL ANESTHETIC: PRILOCAINE HCL + EPINEPHRINE 1:200,000
Prilocaine: 2.7 mg/lb = 540 mg (MRD-a and MRD-m)
ABSOLUTE maximum = 400 mg

PATIENT: 6 YEARS OLD, HEALTHY, MALE, 40 LBS
Mepivacaine 3% = 54 mg/cartridge

Number of cartridges: Author: 80/54 = ~1.5
Manufacturer: 120/54 = 2

LOCAL ANESTHETIC: MEPIVACAINE HCL, NO VASOCONSTRICTOR
Mepivacaine: 2.0 mg/lb = 80 mg (MRD-a)
3.0 mg/lb = 120 mg (MRD-m)

BOX 4-3

Calculation of Maximum Dosages and Number of Cartridges (Multiple Drugs)

PATIENT: 100-LB FEMALE, HEALTHY
Prilocaine 4% = 72 mg/cartridge
Patient receives 2 cartridges = 144 mg, but anesthesia is inadequate;
Doctor wishes to change to lidocaine 2% + epinephrine 1:100,000

LOCAL ANESTHETIC: PRILOCAINE 4% + EPINEPHRINE 1:200,000
Prilocaine: 2.7 mg/lb = 270 mg (MRD-a and MRD-m)

HOW MUCH LIDOCAINE CAN THIS PATIENT RECEIVE?
Lidocaine 2% = 36 mg/cartridge

Lidocaine: 2.0 mg/lb = 200 mg (MRD-a)

Total dose of BOTH local anesthetics should not exceed the lower of the two calculated doses, or 200 mg
Patient has received 144 mg (prilocaine); thus can still receive 56 mg of lidocaine
Therefore: 56 mg/36 mg per cartridge = 1.5 cartridges of lidocaine 2% + epinephrine 1:100,000 (MRD-a)

If lidocaine were being administered alone to this patient, its maximum dose (MRD-a) would be 100 (lb) × 2 (mg/lb), or 200 mg. However, she has already received 144 mg of prilocaine in the past few minutes. The amount of lidocaine permitted thus is the smaller total maximum dose (which in this case is 200 mg [lidocaine] versus 270 mg [prilocaine]) minus the dose of prilocaine already administered (144 mg), which permits a dose of 56 mg of lidocaine, or 1.5 cartridges, to be administered to this patient (Box 4-3).

As already discussed, it is highly unlikely that a "bad batch" of local anesthetic has been distributed to the doctor. The most common causes for failure to achieve adequate anesthesia are anatomical variation and faulty technique. (However, blaming the failure to obtain adequate pain control on the local anesthetic drug serves to soothe the doctor's ego.)

The concept of maximum dose is discussed more fully in Chapter 18.

Clinically available local anesthetics (the amides: articaine, bupivacaine, lidocaine, mepivacaine, and prilocaine) are discussed in detail. Esters (procaine and propoxycaine) are mentioned in passing, more as a matter of historical interest than necessity. Agents available for topical application (topical anesthetics) also are discussed.

ESTER-TYPE LOCAL ANESTHETICS

Procaine HCl

Pertinent Information

Classification. Ester

Chemical formula. 2-Diethylaminoethyl 4-aminobenzoate hydrochloride

Prepared by. Alfred Einhorn, 1904 to 1905

Potency. 1 (procaine = 1)

Toxicity. 1 (procaine = 1)

Metabolism. Hydrolyzed rapidly in plasma by plasma pseudocholinesterase

Excretion. More than 2% unchanged in the urine (90% as paraaminobenzoic acid [PABA], 8% as diethylaminoethanol)

Vasodilating properties. Produces the greatest vasodilation of all currently used local anesthetics

pK_a. 9.1

pH of plain solution. 5.0 to 6.5

pH of vasoconstrictor-containing solution. 3.5 to 5.5

Onset of action. 6 to 10 minutes

Effective dental concentration. 2% to 4%

Anesthetic half-life. 0.1 hour (6 minutes)

Topical anesthetic action. Not in clinically acceptable concentration

Comments. Procaine HCl, the first synthetic injectable local anesthetic, is no longer available in North America in dental cartridges. However, its proprietary name, Novocain, is synonymous throughout the world with dental local anesthesia. Procaine was found until 1996 in dental cartridges in combination with a second ester anesthetic, propoxycaine.

Used as the sole local anesthetic agent for pain control in dentistry, as it was from its introduction in 1904 until the introduction of the amide local anesthetic lidocaine in the mid-1940s, 2% procaine (plain) provides essentially *no* pulpal anesthesia and from 15 to 30 minutes of soft-tissue anesthesia. This is a result of its profound vasodilating properties. Procaine produces the most vasodilation of all clinically used local anesthetics.[9] Thus a clean surgical field is more difficult to maintain with procaine because of increased bleeding.

Procaine is of importance in the immediate management of inadvertent intraarterial (IA) injection of a drug; its vasodilating properties are used to aid in breaking arteriospasm.[10]

Although not extremely common, the incidence of allergy to both procaine and other ester local anesthetics is significantly greater than that to amide local anesthetics.[11]

Metabolized in the blood by plasma cholinesterase, procaine does not exhibit increased toxicity in patients with hepatic dysfunction.

The maximum recommended dose of procaine, used for peripheral nerve blocks, is 1000 mg.[12]

With a pK$_a$ of 9.1, procaine has a slow clinical onset of anesthesia (6 to 10 minutes), a reason for the inclusion of propoxycaine in the anesthetic cartridge.

Propoxycaine HCl

Pertinent Information

Classification. Ester

Chemical formula. 2-Diethylaminoethyl-4-amino-2-propoxybenzoate hydrochloride

Prepared by. Clinton and Laskowski, 1952

Potency. 7 to 8 (procaine = 1)

Toxicity. 7 to 8 (procaine = 1)

Metabolism. Hydrolyzed in both plasma and the liver

Excretion. Via the kidneys; almost entirely hydrolyzed

Vasodilating properties. Yes, but not as profound as those of procaine

pK$_a$. Not available

pH of plain solution. Not available

Onset of action. Rapid (2 to 3 minutes)

Effective dental concentration. 0.4%

Anesthetic half-life. Not available

Topical anesthetic action. Not in clinically acceptable concentrations

Comments. Propoxycaine was combined with procaine in solution to provide a more rapid onset and more profound and longer-lasting anesthesia than could be obtained with procaine alone. Propoxycaine was not available alone because its higher toxicity (7 to 8 times that of procaine) limited its usefulness as a sole agent.

Procaine HCl + Propoxycaine HCl

Although seldom used as the local anesthetic of choice in contemporary dental practice, the combination of two ester anesthetics, propoxycaine + procaine, was worthy of consideration for inclusion in a dentist's armamentarium of local anesthetics. It was useful when the amides were absolutely contraindicated (e.g., because of documented allergy [although this is an extremely unlikely occurrence]) or when several amide local anesthetics failed to provide clinically adequate anesthesia. Until its removal from the United States market in January 1996, the combination of procaine and propoxycaine was the only ester local anesthetic available in dental cartridge form.

0.4% Propoxycaine/2% procaine with 1:20,000 levonordefrin (United States) or *with 1:30,000 norepinephrine* (Canada) provided approximately 40 minutes of pulpal anesthesia and 2 to 3 hours of soft-tissue anesthesia. The use of norepinephrine in local anesthetic solutions is not recommended, especially in areas where prolonged ischemia can lead to tissue necrosis. In the oral cavity this is most likely to develop in the palate.

Maximum Recommended Dose. The manufacturer's maximum recommended dose was 3.0 mg/lb or 6.6 mg/kg of body weight for the adult patient.[13] For children a dose of 3.0 mg/lb is recommended up to a maximum of five cartridges.

AMIDE-TYPE LOCAL ANESTHETICS

Lidocaine HCl

Pertinent Information

Classification. Amide

Chemical formula. 2-Diethylamino 2′,6-acetoxylidide hydrochloride

Prepared by. Nils Löfgren, 1943

FDA Approved. November 1948

Potency. 2 (compared with procaine) (procaine = 1; today lidocaine is used as the standard of comparison [lidocaine = 1] for all local anesthetics)

Toxicity. 2 (compared with procaine)

Metabolism. In the liver, by the microsomal fixed-function oxidases, to monoethylglyceine and xylidide; xylidide is a local anesthetic and potentially toxic[14] (see Fig. 2-3).

Excretion. Via the kidneys; less than 10% unchanged, more than 80% various metabolites

Vasodilating properties. Considerably less than that of procaine; however, more than that of prilocaine or mepivacaine

pK$_a$. 7.9

pH of plain solution. 6.5

pH of vasoconstrictor-containing solution. 5.0 to 5.5

Onset of action. Rapid (2 to 3 minutes)

Effective dental concentration. 2%

Anesthetic half-life. 1.6 hours (~90 minutes)

Topical anesthetic action. Yes (in clinically acceptable concentrations [5%])

Pregnancy classification. B

Safety during lactation. S

Maximum Recommended Dose. The *manufacturer's* maximum recommended dose of lidocaine with epinephrine is 3.2 mg/lb or 7.0 mg/kg of body weight for the adult patient, not to exceed a dose of 500 mg. For children, the same dose for lidocaine with epinephrine of 3.2 mg/lb is recommended by the manufacturer.[15] The manufacturer also recommends a dose of 2.0 mg/lb (4.4 mg/kg), not to exceed 300 mg for lidocaine without a vasoconstrictor. This author recommends the more conservative dosage regimen for lidocaine suggested by the Council on Dental Therapeutics of the American Dental Association and the USP Convention.[2,3] This dose is 2.0 mg/lb (4.4 mg/kg) for lidocaine with or without a vasoconstrictor additive. This dose still allows for a significant volume of drug to be used to achieve profound clinical anesthesia with a somewhat diminished risk of development of toxic (overdose) reactions (Table 4-5).

Comments. Lidocaine HCl was synthesized in 1943 and, in 1948, became the first amide local anesthetic to be marketed. Its entry into clinical practice transformed dentistry, replacing procaine (Novocain) as the drug of choice for pain control. Compared with procaine, lidocaine possesses a significantly more rapid onset of action (2 to 3 minutes versus 6 to 10 minutes), produces more profound anesthesia, has a longer duration of action, and has a greater potency.

Allergy to amide local anesthetics is virtually nonexistent; true, documented, and reproducible allergic reactions are extremely rare, although possible.[16–22] This is a major clinical advantage of lidocaine (and all amides) over the ester-type local anesthetics.[11]

Within a few years of its introduction, lidocaine replaced procaine as the most widely used local anesthetic in both

---

TABLE **4-5**
Lidocaine Hydrochloride

Proprietary Name	Manufacturer	Percent Local Anesthetic	Vasoconstrictor	Duration of Analgesia (min)		MRD-m	MRD-a
				Pulpal	Soft-Tissue		
Lidocaine HCl Alphacaine Xylocaine	Many generics Carlisle Labs Dentsply	2	—	5–10	60–120	4.4 mg/kg 2.0 mg/lb 300 mg absolute maximum	
Lidocaine HCl Alphacaine Lignospan Octocaine Xylocaine	Many generics Carlisle Labs Septodont Novocol Chemical Dentsply	2	Epinephrine 1:50,000	60	180–300	6.6 mg/kg 3.0 mg/lb 500 mg absolute maximum	4.4 mg/kg 2.0 mg/lb 300 mg absolute maximum
Lidocaine HCl Alphacaine Lignospan Octocaine Xylocaine	Many generics Carlisle Labs Septodont Novocol Chemical Dentsply	2	Epinephrine 1:100,000	60	180–300	6.6 mg/kg 3.0 mg/lb 500 mg absolute maximum	4.4 mg/kg 2.0 mg/lb 300 mg absolute maximum

MRD, Maximum recommended dose.

medicine and dentistry, a position it maintains today in most countries. It represents the "gold standard," the drug to which all new local anesthetics are compared.

Lidocaine HCl is available in three formulations in North America: 2% without a vasoconstrictor, 2% with epinephrine 1:50,000, and 2% with epinephrine 1:100,000 (Fig. 4-2). Recently, 2% lidocaine with epinephrine 1:300,000 became available in several countries (although not in North America as of September 2003).

Two percent lidocaine HCl without a vasoconstrictor (lidocaine plain) (Table 4-6). Its vasodilating effect limits pulpal anesthesia to only 5 to 10 minutes. This vasodilatory effect leads to higher blood levels of the lidocaine, with a consequent increase in the risk of adverse reaction along with an increase in perfusion in the region of drug deposition. There are very few clinical indications for the use of 2% lidocaine without a vasoconstrictor in the typical dental practice. Indeed, several major manufacturers

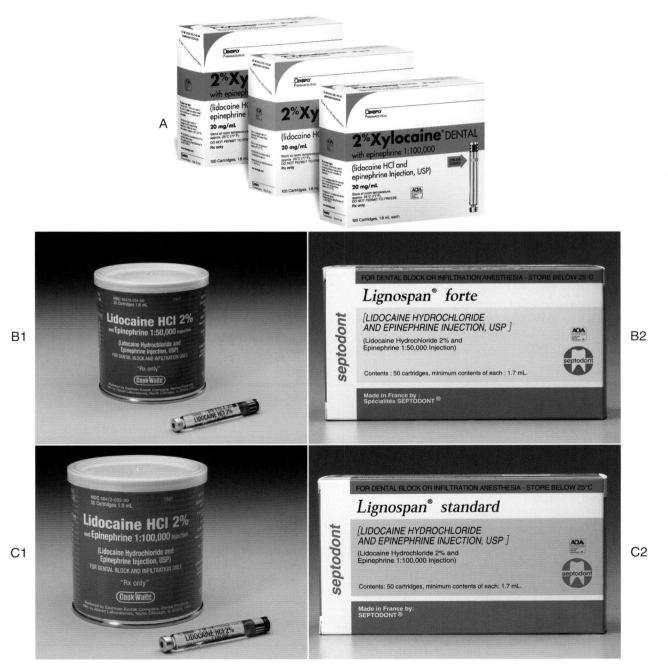

Figure 4-2. A, Lidocaine 2%. **B,** Lidocaine 2% with epinephrine 1:50,000. **C,** Lidocaine with epinephrine 1:100,000. (**A,** Courtesy Dentsply, York, Pa. **B** and **C,** Courtesy Eastman Kodak, N.Y.; and Septodont, New Castle, Del.)

TABLE 4-6
Lidocaine Without Vasoconstrictor

Concentration: 2% Max dose: 4.4 mg/kg			Cartridge contains: 36 mg Max dose: 2 mg/lb		
Weight (kg)	mg	Cartridges*	Weight (kg)	mg	Cartridges*
10	44	1	20	40	1
20	88	2	40	80	2
30	132	3.5	60	120	3
40	176	4.5	80	160	4
50	220	6	100	200	5.5
60	264	7	120	240	6.5
70	300	8	140	280	7.5
80	300	8	160	300	8
90	300	8	180	300	8
100	300	8	200	300	8

1. As with all local anesthetics, the dose varies and depends on the area to be anesthetized, the vascularity of the tissues, individual tolerance, and the technique of anesthesia. The lowest dose needed to provide effective anesthesia should be administered.
2. Doses indicated are the maximum suggested for normal healthy individuals (ASAI); they should be decreased for debilitated or elderly patients.
*Rounded to the nearest half-cartridge.

of local anesthetics in North America have ceased marketing lidocaine plain in dental cartridges.[23,24]

Two percent lidocaine with epinephrine 1:50,000 (Table 4-7). The inclusion of epinephrine produces a decrease in blood flow (perfusion) leading to a decrease in bleeding in the area of injection because of the α-stimulating actions of the epinephrine. Because of this decrease in perfusion, the local anesthetic is absorbed into the cardiovascular system more slowly (thereby remaining at the site of administration longer, hopefully near the nerve), leading to an increased duration (and depth) of action: approximately 60 minutes of pulpal anesthesia and 3 to 5 hours of soft-tissue anesthesia. The blood level of the local anesthetic also is decreased. The 1:50,000 epinephrine concentration is equal to 20 μg/ml, or 36 μg per cartridge. For patients weighing more than 45 kg (100 lb), the limiting factor in determining the MRD of this local anesthetic combination is the maximum epinephrine dose of 200 μg for the healthy patient. The MRD for epinephrine-sensitive individuals (e.g., certain cardiovascularly compromised patients and clinically hyperthyroid patients) is 40 μg per appointment. This is equivalent to about *one* cartridge of 1:50,000 epinephrine (see Chapter 20).

The only recommended use of 2% lidocaine with a 1:50,000 epinephrine concentration is for hemostasis (where only small volumes are infiltrated directly into the surgical site).

Two percent lidocaine with epinephrine 1:100,000 (Table 4-8) decreases blood flow into the area of injection. There is also an increased duration of action: approximately 60 minutes of pulpal anesthesia and 3 to 5 hours of soft-tissue anesthesia. In addition to the lower blood level of lidocaine, less bleeding occurs in the area of injection. The epinephrine dilution is 10 μg/ml, or 18 μg per cartridge. Epinephrine-sensitive patients should be limited to *two* cartridges of 1:100,000 epinephrine per appointment.

The duration and depth of pulpal anesthesia obtained with both lidocaine–epinephrine solutions (1:50,000 and 1:100,000) are equivalent. Each may provide 60 minutes of pulpal anesthesia in ideal circumstances and soft-tissue anesthesia of 3 to 5 hours' duration. Indeed, 2% lidocaine

TABLE 4-7
Lidocaine HCl + Epinephrine 1:50,000

Concentration: 2%						Cartridge contains: 36 mg					
MRD-a 4.4 mg/kg			MRD-a 2.0 mg/lb			MRD-m 6.6 mg/kg			MRD-m 3.0 mg/lb		
Weight (kg)	mg	Cartridges*	Weight (lb)	mg	Cartridges*	Weight (kg)	mg	Cartridges*	Weight (lb)	mg	Cartridges*
10	44	1	20	40	1	10	66	2	20	60	1.5
20	88	2	40	80	2	20	132	3.5	40	120	3.0
30	132	3.5	60	120	3	30	198	5.5	60	180	5
40	176	4.5	80	160	4	40	264	7	80	240	6.5
50	220	6	100	200	5.5	50	330	9	100	300	8
60	220	6[†]	120	200	5.5[†]	60	396	11	120	360	10
70	220	6[†]	140	200	5.5[†]	70	462	13	140	420	11.5
80	220	6[†]	160	200	5.5[†]	80	500	13.5	160	480	13
90	220	6[†]	180	200	5.5[†]	90	500	13.5	180	500	13.5
100	220	6[†]	200	200	5.5[†]	100	500	13.5	200	500	13.5

1. As with all local anesthetics, the dose varies and depends on the area to be anesthetized, the vascularity of the tissues, individual tolerance, and the technique of anesthesia. The lowest dose needed to provide clinically effective anesthesia should be administered.
2. Doses indicated are the maximum suggested for normal, healthy individuals (ASA I); they should be decreased for debilitated or elderly patients.
*Rounded to the nearest half-cartridge.
[†]200 μg of epinephrine is the dose-limiting factor.

TABLE **4-8**
Lidocaine HCl + Epinephrine 1:100,000

Concentration: 2%						Cartridge contains: 36 mg					
MRD-a 4.4 mg/kg			MRD-a 2.0 mg/lb			MRD-m 6.6 mg/kg			MRD-m 3.0 mg/lb		
Weight (kg)	mg	Cartridges*	Weight (lb)	mg	Cartridges*	Weight (kg)	mg	Cartridges*	Weight (lb)	mg	Cartridges*
10	44	1	20	40	1	10	66	2	20	60	1.5
20	88	2	40	80	2	20	132	3.5	40	120	3.0
30	132	3.5	60	120	3	30	198	5.5	60	180	5
40	176	4.5	80	160	4	40	264	7	80	240	6.5
50	220	6	100	200	5.5	50	330	9	100	300	8
60	264	7	120	240	6.5	60	396	11	120	360	10
70	300	8	140	280	7.5	70	462	13	140	420	11.5
80	300	8	160	300	8	80	500	13.5	160	480	13
90	300	8	180	300	8	90	500	13.5	180	500	13.5
100	300	8	200	300	8	100	500	13.5	200	500	13.5

1. As with all local anesthetics, the dose varies and depends on the area to be anesthetized, the vascularity of the tissues, individual tolerance, and the technique of anesthesia. The lowest dose needed to provide clinically effective anesthesia should be administered.
2. Doses indicated are the maximum suggested for normal, healthy individuals (ASA I); they should be decreased for debilitated or elderly patients.
*Rounded to the nearest half-cartridge

with 1:200,000 or 1:250,000 epinephrine provides the same duration of pulpal and soft-tissue anesthesia, although not the same level of hemostasis.[25]

For *duration* and *depth* of pain control for most dental procedures in a typical dental patient, 2% lidocaine with 1:100,000 epinephrine is preferred to 2% lidocaine with 1:50,000 epinephrine. Both provide equal duration and depth, but the 1:100,000 solution contains only half as much epinephrine as the 1:50,000. Although the dose of epinephrine in the 1:50,000 is not dangerous to most patients, ASA III and IV risks with histories of cardiovascular problems might prove overly sensitive to these concentrations. Also, an elderly patient is likely to be more hyper-responsive to vasoconstrictors. In these individuals the greater dilution (1:100,000 or 1:200,000) should be used.

For *hemostasis* in procedures in which bleeding is definitely or potentially a problem, 2% lidocaine with 1:50,000 epinephrine is recommended because it decreases bleeding (during periodontal surgery) by 50% compared with a 1:100,000 epinephrine dilution.[26] Vasoconstrictors act directly at the site of administration to decrease tissue perfusion, and the 1:50,000 provides excellent hemostatic action. The 1:100,000 dilution also may be used for hemostasis, but is not as effective. Rebound vasodilation occurs with both 1:50,000 and 1:100,000 epinephrine concentrations. Minimum volumes should be administered to provide excellent hemostasis.

Signs and symptoms of lidocaine toxicity (overdose) may be the same (central nervous system [CNS] stimulation followed by CNS depression) as described in Chapter 2. However, the stimulatory phase may be brief or may not develop at all.[27] The first signs and symptoms of lidocaine overdose may be drowsiness, leading to a loss of consciousness and respiratory arrest.

Mepivacaine HCl

Pertinent Information

Classification. Amide

Chemical formula. 1-methyl 2',6'-pipecoloxylidide hydrochloride

Prepared by. A.F. Ekenstam, 1957, and introduced into dentistry in 1960 as a 2% solution containing the synthetic vasopressor levonordefrin, and in 1961 as a 3% solution without a vasoconstrictor

FDA Approved. April 1960

Potency. 2 (procaine = 1; lidocaine = 2)

Toxicity. 1.5 to 2 (procaine = 1; lidocaine = 2)

Metabolism. In the liver, by microsomal fixed-function oxidases. Hydroxylation and *N*-demethylation play important roles in the metabolism of mepivacaine.

Excretion. Via the kidneys; approximately 1% to 16% of anesthetic dose is excreted unchanged

Vasodilating properties. Mepivacaine produces only slight vasodilation. The duration of pulpal anesthesia with mepivacaine without a vasoconstrictor is 20 to 40 minutes (that with lidocaine without a vasoconstrictor is

5 minutes; that with procaine without a vasoconstrictor is up to 2 minutes).

pK$_a$. 7.6

pH of plain solution. 4.5

pH of vasoconstrictor-containing solution. 3.0 to 3.5

Onset of action. Rapid (1 ½ to 2 minutes)

Effective dental concentration. 3% without a vasoconstrictor; 2% with a vasoconstrictor

Anesthetic half-life. 1.9 hours

Topical anesthetic action. Not in clinically acceptable concentrations

Pregnancy classification. C

Safety during lactation. S?

Maximum Recommended Dose. MRD-m is 3.0 mg/lb or 6.6 mg/kg of body weight, not to exceed 400 mg for the adult patient.[24] For children a dose of 3.0 mg/lb is recommended up to a maximum of five cartridges of either the 2% or 3% form of the drug. MRD-a for mepivacaine is 2.0 mg/lb (4.4 mg/kg), not to exceed 300 mg for either adult or child (Table 4-9).

Comments. The mild vasodilating properties of mepivacaine provide a longer duration of anesthesia than most other local anesthetics when the drug is administered without a vasoconstrictor. Mepivacaine 3% plain provides 20 to 40 minutes of pulpal anesthesia (20 minutes via infiltration; 40 minutes via nerve block) and 2 to 3 hours of soft-tissue anesthesia.

Three percent mepivacaine without a vasoconstrictor (Fig. 4-3 and Table 4-10) is recommended for patients in whom a vasoconstrictor is not indicated and for minor dental procedures requiring neither lengthy nor profound pulpal anesthesia. Mepivacaine plain is the most used local anesthetic in pediatric patients when the treating doctor is not a pediatric dentist (is a general practitioner) and is often quite appropriate in the management of geriatric patients.

Two percent mepivacaine with a vasoconstrictor (Table 4-11) provides a depth and duration of both pulpal (hard-tissue)

TABLE 4-9
Mepivacaine Hydrochloride

Proprietary Name	Manufacturer	Percent Local Anesthetic	Vasoconstrictor	Duration of Analgesia (min)		MRD-m	MRD-a
				Pulpal	Soft-Tissue		
Mepivacaine HCl Arestocaine Carbocaine Isocaine Polocaine Scandonest	Many generics Carlisle Labs Kodak Novocol Dentsply Septodont	3	—	20–40 (20 for infiltration; 40 for nerve block)	120–180	6.6 mg/kg 3.0 mg/lb 400 mg absolute maximum	4.4 mg/kg 2.0 mg/lb 300 mg absolute maximum
Mepivacaine HCl Arestocaine Isocaine Polocaine Scandonest Carbocaine	Many generics Carlisle Labs Dentsply Kodak Septodont Novocol	2	Levonordefrin 1:20,000 Neo-Cobefrin 1:20,000	60	180–300	6.6 mg/kg 3.0 mg/lb 400 mg absolute maximum	4.4 mg/kg 2.0 mg/lb 300 mg absolute maximum
Carbocaine	Kodak	2	Epinephrine 1:200,000	45–60	120–240	6.6 mg/kg 3.0 mg/lb 400 mg absolute maximum	4.4 mg/kg 2.0 mg/lb 300 mg absolute maximum
Scandonest 2% Special	Septodont	2	Epinephrine 1:200,000	60	120–300	6.6 mg/kg 3.0 mg/lb 400 mg absolute maximum	4.4 mg/kg 2.0 mg/lb 300 mg absolute maximum

*In mid-2003, local anesthetics containing levonordefrin (Neo-Cobefrin) were removed from the market in North America because of difficulties in obtaining the product. It is thought that levonordefrin will become available again in 2004–2005.
MRD, Maximum recommended dose.

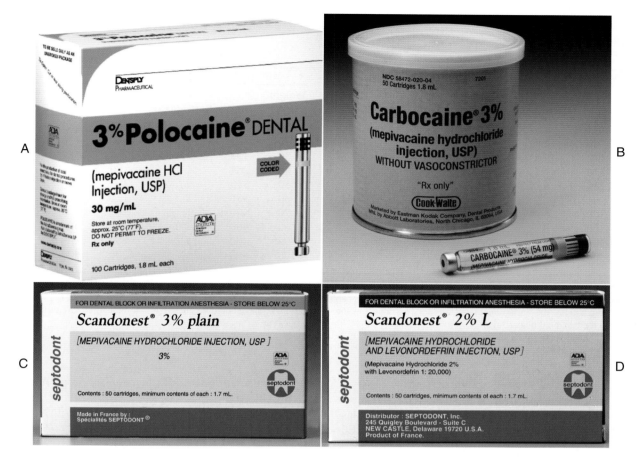

Figure 4-3. A-C, Mepivacaine 3%. **D,** Mepivacaine 2% with levonordefrin 1:20,000. (**A,** Courtesy Dentsply, York, Pa. **B,** Courtesy Eastman Kodak, N.Y. **C** and **D,** Courtesy Septodont, New Castle, Del.*)*

TABLE **4-10**

Mepivacaine HCl Without Vasoconstrictor

Concentration: 3%						Cartridge contains: 54 mg					
MRD-a 4.4 mg/kg			MRD-a 2.0 mg/lb			MRD-m 6.6 mg/kg			MRD-m 3.0 mg/lb		
Weight (kg)	mg	Cartridges*	Weight (lb)	mg	Cartridges*	Weight (kg)	mg	Cartridges*	Weight (lb)	mg	Cartridges*
10	44	1	20	40	1	10	66	1	20	60	1
20	88	1.5	40	80	1.5	20	132	1.5	40	120	2
30	132	3	60	120	2	30	198	3.5	60	180	3
40	176	4	80	160	3	40	264	5	80	240	4.5
50	220	4.5	100	200	3.5	50	330	6.5	100	300	5
60	264	5.5	120	240	4	60	396	8	120	360	6.5
70	300	5.5	140	280	5	70	400	8	140	400	7.5
80	300	5.5	160	300	5.5	80	400	8	160	400	7.5
90	300	5.5	180	300	5.5	90	400	8	180	400	7.5
100	300	5.5	200	300	5.5	100	400	8	200	400	7.5

1. As with all local anesthetics, the dose varies and depends on the area to be anesthetized, the vascularity of the tissues, individual tolerance, and the technique of anesthesia. The lowest dose needed to provide clinically effective anesthesia should be administered.
2. Doses indicated are the maximum suggested for normal, healthy individuals (ASA I); they should be decreased for debilitated or elderly patients.

*Rounded to the nearest half-cartridge.

TABLE 4-11
Mepivacaine HCl With Vasoconstrictor

Concentration: 2%						Cartridge contains: 36 mg					
MRD-a 4.4 mg/kg			MRD-a 2.0 mg/lb			MRD-m 6.6 mg/kg			MRD-m 3.0 mg/lb		
Weight (kg)	mg	Cartridges*	Weight (lb)	mg	Cartridges*	Weight (kg)	mg	Cartridges*	Weight (lb)	mg	Cartridges*
10	44	1	20	40	1	10	66	2	20	60	1.5
20	88	2	40	80	2	20	132	3.5	40	120	3
30	132	3.5	60	120	3	30	198	5.5	60	180	5
40	176	4.5	80	160	4	40	264	7	80	240	6.5
50	220	6	100	200	5.5	50	330	9	100	300	8
60	264	7	120	240	6.5	60	396	11	120	360	10
70	300	8	140	280	7.5	70	400	11	140	400	11
80	300	8	160	300	8	80	400	11	160	400	11
90	300	8	180	300	8	90	400	11	180	400	11
100	300	8	200	300	8	100	400	11	200	400	11

1. As with all local anesthetics, the dose varies and depends on the area to be anesthetized, the vascularity of the tissues, individual tolerance, and the technique of anesthesia. The lowest dose needed to provide clinically effective anesthesia should be administered.
2. Doses indicated are the maximum suggested for normal, healthy individuals (ASA I); they should be decreased for debilitated or elderly patients.
*Rounded to the nearest half-cartridge.

and total (soft-tissue) anesthesia similar to those observed with the lidocaine–epinephrine solutions. Pulpal anesthesia of approximately 60 minutes' duration and soft-tissue anesthesia of 3 to 5 hours are to be expected. Two vasoconstrictors, levonordefrin (1:20,000) and epinephrine (1:100,000), are available with mepivacaine. Although hemostasis is present, levonordefrin does not provide the intensity of hemostasis noted with epinephrine 1:100,000.

Mepivacaine 2% with levonordefrin 1:20,000 has become impossible to obtain (June 2004). Levonordefrin is manufactured in Europe and imported into North America, where local anesthetic manufacturers prepare the finished solution. A lack of supply of levonordefrin made 2% mepivacaine with levonordefrin extremely difficult to obtain. It is expected that levonordefrin will again be available in North America by early 2005.

The incidence of true, documented, and reproducible allergy to mepivacaine, an amide local anesthetic, is virtually nonexistent.

Signs and symptoms of mepivacaine overdose usually follow the more typical pattern of CNS stimulation followed by depression. Although possible, the absence of stimulation with immediate CNS depression (e.g., drowsiness and unconsciousness, as is seen with lidocaine) is rare with mepivacaine.

Prilocaine HCl

Pertinent Information

Classification. Amide

Other chemical name. Propitocaine

Chemical formula. 2-Propylamino-o-propionotoluidide hydrochloride

Prepared by. Löfgren and Tegnér, 1953; reported in 1960

FDA Approved. November 1965

Potency. 2 (procaine = 1; lidocaine = 2)

Toxicity. 1 (procaine = 1; lidocaine = 2); 40% less toxic than lidocaine

Metabolism. Differs significantly from that of lidocaine and mepivacaine. Being a secondary amine, prilocaine is hydrolyzed straightforwardly by hepatic amidases into orthotoluidine and N-propylalanine. Carbon dioxide is a major end-product of prilocaine biotransformation. The efficiency of the body's degradation of prilocaine is demonstrated by the extremely small fraction of intact prilocaine recoverable in the urine.[28] Orthotoluidine can induce the formation of methemoglobin, producing methemoglobinemia if large doses are administered. Minor degrees of methemoglobinemia also have been observed with both benzocaine and lidocaine administration,[29,30] but prilocaine consistently reduces the blood's oxygen-carrying capacity, at times sufficiently to cause observable cyanosis.[31,32] Limiting the total prilocaine dose to 600 mg (as recommended by the manufacturer) avoids symptomatic cyanosis. Methemoglobin levels of less than 20% usually do not produce clinical signs or symptoms (which are grayish or slate blue cyanosis of the lips, mucous membranes, and nail beds and [infrequently] respiratory and circulatory distress). Methemoglobinemia may be reversed within 15 minutes with administration of 1 to 2 mg/kg body weight of 1% methylene blue solution intravenously over a 5-minute period.[30] The mechanism of methemoglobin production is discussed in Chapter 10. Prilocaine undergoes biotransformation more rapidly and completely than lidocaine, taking place not only in the liver, but also to a smaller degree in the kidney and lung.[32] Plasma levels of prilocaine decrease more rapidly than lidocaine.[33] Prilocaine is thus considered to be less toxic systemically than comparably potent local anesthetic amides.[34] Signs of CNS toxicity after prilocaine administration in humans are briefer and less severe than after the same intravenous (IV) dose of lidocaine.[35]

Excretion. Prilocaine and its metabolites are excreted primarily via the kidneys. Renal clearance of prilocaine is faster than that for other amides, resulting in its faster removal from the circulation.[36]

Vasodilating properties. Prilocaine is a vasodilator. It produces greater vasodilation than does mepivacaine but less than lidocaine and significantly less than procaine.

pK_a. 7.9

pH of plain solution. 4.5

pH of vasoconstrictor-containing solution. 3.0 to 4.0

Onset of action. Slightly slower than that of lidocaine (2 to 4 minutes)

Effective dental concentration. 4%

Anesthetic half-life. 1.6 hours

Topical anesthetic action. Not in clinically acceptable concentrations

Prilocaine, in its uncharged base form, is an integral part of EMLA (eutectic mixture of local anesthetics) cream, which permits the anesthetics (lidocaine–prilocaine) to penetrate the imposing anatomic barrier of intact skin. EMLA cream is used to provide topical anesthesia of skin before venipuncture.[37]

Pregnancy classification. B

Safety during lactation. Unknown

Maximum Recommended Dose. Both the MRD-m and MRD-a for prilocaine is 2.7 mg/lb or 6.0 mg/kg of body weight for the adult patient, to a maximum recommended dose of 400 mg (Table 4-12).[36]

Comments. Clinical actions of *prilocaine plain* (Fig. 4-4) vary significantly with the type of injection technique used. Although true for all anesthetics, the variation between supraperiosteal (infiltration) and nerve block is more pronounced with prilocaine plain. Infiltration provides short durations of pulpal (10 to 15 minutes) and soft-tissue (1½ to 2 hours) anesthesia, whereas regional nerve block (e.g., inferior alveolar nerve block) provides pulpal anesthesia for up to 60 minutes (most often between 40 and 60 minutes) and soft-tissue anesthesia for 2 to 4 hours. Thus prilocaine plain frequently is able to provide anesthesia that is equal in duration to that obtained from lidocaine or mepivacaine with a vasoconstrictor.

Clinical actions of *prilocaine with 1:200,000 epinephrine* are not as dependent on anesthetic technique. Prilocaine with epinephrine provides lengthy anesthesia while

TABLE **4-12**
Prilocaine Hydrochloride

Proprietary Name	Manufacturer	Percent Local Anesthetic	Vasoconstrictor	Duration of Analgesia (min)		MRD-m and MRD-a
				Pulpal	*Soft-Tissue*	
Prilocaine HCl Citanest Plain	Generic Dentsply	4		10–15 (infiltration) 40–60 nerve block	90–120 (inf) 120–240 (nb)	6 mg/kg 2.7 mg/lb 400 mg absolute maximum
Prilocaine HCl + epinephrine 1:200,000 Citanest Forte	Generic Dentsply	4	Epinephrine 1:200,000	60–90	180–480	6 mg/kg 2.7 mg/lb 400 mg absolute maximum

MRD, Maximum recommended dose.

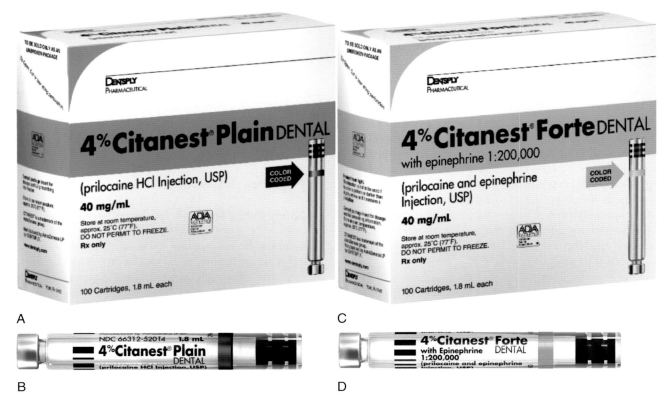

Figure 4-4. A and **B,** Prilocaine 4%. **C** and **D,** Prilocaine 4% with epinephrine 1:200,000. (Courtesy Dentsply, York, Pa.)

offering the least concentrated epinephrine dilution currently available: 1:200,000. Pulpal anesthesia of 60 to 90 minutes' duration and soft-tissue anesthesia of 3 to 8 hours may be obtained. The cartridge contains 9 μg of epinephrine; therefore epinephrine-sensitive individuals, such as the ASA III cardiovascular disease patient, may receive up to four cartridges (36 μg) of prilocaine with epinephrine.

In epinephrine-sensitive patients requiring prolonged pulpal anesthesia (≥60 minutes), prilocaine plain or with 1:200,000 epinephrine is strongly recommended. It is rapidly biotransformed and, for this reason, is considered a safe local anesthetic (e.g., lower toxicity).[33]

Prilocaine is *relatively contraindicated* in patients with idiopathic or congenital methemoglobinemia, hemoglobinopathies (sickle cell anemia), anemia, or cardiac or respiratory failure evidenced by hypoxia, because methemoglobin levels are increased, decreasing oxygen-carrying capacity. Prilocaine administration is also *relatively contraindicated* in patients receiving *acetaminophen* or *phenacetin*, both of which produce elevations in methemoglobin levels (Table 4-13).

TABLE 4-13

Prilocaine With and Without Vasoconstrictor

Concentration: 4% Max dose: 6 mg/kg			Cartridge contains: 72 mg Max dose: 2.7 mg/lb		
Weight (kg)	mg	Cartridges*	Weight (kg)	mg	Cartridges*
10	60	1	20	54	1
20	120	1.5	40	108	1.5
30	180	2.5	60	162	2
40	240	3	80	216	3
50	300	4	100	270	3.5
60	360	5	120	324	4.5
70	400	5.5	140	378	5
80	400	5.5	160	400	5.5
90	400	5.5	180	400	5.5
100	400	5.5	200	400	5.5

1. As with all local anesthetics, the dose varies and depends on the area to be anesthetized, the vascularity of the tissues, individual tolerance, and the technique of anesthesia. The lowest dose needed to provide effective anesthesia should be administered.
2. Doses indicated are the maximum suggested for normal healthy individuals (ASAI); they should be decreased for debilitated or elderly patients.

*Rounded to the nearest half-cartridge.

Articaine HCl

Pertinent Information

Classification. Amide

Chemical formula. 3-*N*-Propylamino-proprionylamino-2-carbomethoxy-4-methylthiophene hydrochloride

Prepared by. H. Rusching et al., 1969

FDA Approved. April 2000

Introduced. 1976 in Germany and Switzerland, 1983 in Canada, 2000 in the United States.

Potency. 1.5 times that of lidocaine and 1.9 times that of procaine

Toxicity. Similar to lidocaine and procaine

Metabolism. Articaine is the only amide-type local anesthetic that contains a thiophene group. In addition, because articaine HCl is the only widely used amide-type local anesthetic that also contains an ester group, biotransformation of articaine HCl occurs in both the plasma (hydrolysis by plasma esterase) and liver (hepatic microsomal enzymes). Degradation of articaine HCl is initiated by hydrolysis of the carboxylic acid ester groups to give free carboxylic acid.[39] Its primary metabolite, articainic acid, is pharmacologically inactive, undergoing additional biotransformation to form articainic acid glucuronide.[39] Additional metabolites have been detected in animal studies.[40] From that point the reaction can follow several pathways: cleavage of the carboxylic acid, formation of an acid amino group by internal cyclization, and oxidation.

Excretion. Via the kidneys; approximately 5% to 10% unchanged, approximately 90% metabolites (M_1 at 87%, M_2 at 2%).

Vasodilating properties. Articaine has a vasodilating effect equal to that of lidocaine. Procaine is slightly more vasoactive.

pKₐ. 7.8

pH of plain solution. Not available

pH of vasoconstrictor-containing solution. 4.4 to 5.2 for 1:100,000; 4.6 to 5.4 for 1:200,000

Onset of action. Articaine 1:200,000, infiltration 1 to 2 minutes, mandibular block 2 to 3 minutes; articaine 1:100,000, infiltration 1 to 2 minutes, mandibular block 2 to 2 ½ minutes

Effective dental concentration. 4% with 1:100,000 or 1:200,000 epinephrine

Anesthetic half-life. 0.5 hours[41]

Topical anesthetic action. Not in clinically acceptable concentration

Pregnancy classification. Unknown

Safety during lactation. Unknown

Maximum Recommended Dose. Manufacturer's maximum recommended dose is 3.2 mg/lb or 7.0 mg/kg of body weight for the adult patient (Table 4-14).[5,42]

Comments. Originally known as "carticaine," the generic nomenclature of this local anesthetic was changed in 1984 to articaine. Literature appearing before 1984 should be reviewed under the original name.

Articaine is the only anesthetic of the amide type to possess a thiophene ring as its lipophilic moiety. It has many of the physicochemical properties of other local anesthetics, with the exception of the aromatic moiety and the degree of protein binding.

Articaine has been available in Europe since 1976 and in Canada since 1984 in two formulations: *4% with 1:100,000 epinephrine* and *4% with 1:200,000 epinephrine* (Fig. 4-5). In 2000 the Food and Drug Administration approved articaine HCl with epinephrine 1:100,000 for marketing in the United States.[43–45] The formulation with 1:100:000 epinephrine provides between 60 and 75 minutes of pulpal anesthesia; the 1:200,000 formulation, approximately 45 to 60 minutes.[46,47]

As a relatively new drug in the United States, articaine has been the subject of much discussion and of many claims made by dentists, some good (faster onset, increased success rates; "don't miss as often"); some bad (increased risk of paresthesia).

It has been claimed that articaine is able to diffuse through soft and hard tissues more reliably than other local anesthetics.[48,49] Clinically it is claimed that maxillary buccal infiltration of articaine, on occasion, provides palatal soft-tissue anesthesia, obviating the need for a palatal injection which, in many hands, is traumatic.[49] Furthermore, it is claimed that articaine can provide pulpal and lingual anesthesia when administered by infiltration in the adult mandible.[49] However, controlled comparisons between articaine and standard local anesthetics, such as lidocaine and prilocaine, have failed to corroborate these claims.[45,50,51]

TABLE **4-14**
Articaine Hydrochloride

Proprietary Name	Manufacturer	Percent Local Anesthetic	Vasoconstrictor	Duration of Analgesia (min)		MRD-m and MRD-a
				Pulpal	*Soft-Tissue*	
(United States) Septocaine	Septodont	4	Epinephrine 1:100,000	60–75	180–360	7 mg/kg
(Canada) Septanest SP Astracaine Ultracaine D-S forte	Septodont Dentsply Hoechst					3.2 mg/lb 500 mg absolute maximum
(Canada) Septanest N Astracaine Ultracaine D-S	Septodont Dentsply Hoechst	4	Epinephrine 1:200,000	45–60	120–300	7 mg/kg 3.2 mg/lb 500 mg absolute maximum

MRD, Maximum recommended dose.

Yet in other countries in which articaine is available, it has become an extremely popular local anesthetic in dentistry. In Germany, which acquired the drug in 1976, articaine in 1989 was used by 71.7% of German dentists[52] and by 2002 commanded 92% of the dental local anesthetic market.[53] Articaine has become the leading local anesthetic in Canada, which acquired it in 1983; in the United States, where articaine has been available since June of 2000, it presently (March 2004) holds 26% of the local anesthetic market.[54]

Reports of paresthesia (usually in the mandible) have become more frequent since the introduction of articaine in the United States.[55,56] It is interesting that prilocaine is also associated with more frequent reports of paresthesia than other local anesthetics and that articaine and prilocaine are the only local anesthetics presently employed in a 4% concentration. Prilocaine is available in some countries as a 3% solution (with the vasoconstrictor felypressin). Reports of increased incidences of paresthesia are not heard in these areas. The problem of paresthesia related

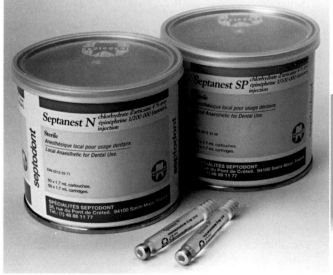
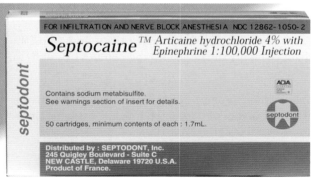

Figure 4-5. Articaine 4% with epinephrine 1:100,000 and 1:200,000. (Courtesy Septodont, New Castle, Del.)

to local anesthetic drug administration is addressed in depth in Chapter 17.

Methemoglobinemia was listed in previous editions of this textbook as a potential side effect of the administration of large doses of articaine.[57] Such reactions had been noted after the IV administration of articaine for regional anesthetic purposes; however, no cases have ever been reported when articaine was administered in the usual manner and volume for dental procedures.

Articaine HCl with epinephrine is contraindicated in persons with known sensitivity to amide-type local anesthetics (few to none) and persons with sulfite sensitivity (such as some asthmatics with allergic-type asthma). Articaine HCl should be used with caution in persons with hepatic disease and significant impairments in cardiovascular function because amide-type local anesthetics undergo biotransformation in the liver and possess myocardial depressant properties. Safe use during pregnancy and lactation has not been established. Use in children under 4 years of age is not recommended because no data exist to support such usage.

As originally marketed in Canada, cartridges of articaine contained the preservative methylparaben. Although the incidence of allergy to paraben-type preservatives is low, methylparaben has been removed from all other available local anesthetic cartridges in North America. All formulations of articaine now marketed in the United States and Canada are paraben-free.

Cartridges of articaine marketed in the United States are listed as containing "minimum contents of each 1.7 ml" (Fig. 4-6). Some might interpret this to mean that there are 68 mg in the cartridge. This is incorrect. Articaine HCl cartridges do indeed contain 1.8 ml or 72 mg of the drug. Food and Drug Administration regulations dictate that cartridges must state the preceding if it cannot be guaranteed that *all* cartridges of the drug contain minimally 1.8 ml or greater. Because local anesthetic cartridges are filled by machine on a conveyor belt, it cannot be guaranteed that all cartridges contain at least 1.8 ml; thus the labeling is used.

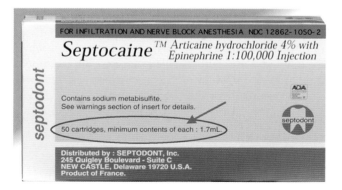

Figure 4-6. Articaine box showing "minimum content of each 1.7 ml."

Bupivacaine HCl

Pertinent Information

Classification. Amide

Chemical formula. 1-Butyl-2′,6′-pipecoloxylidide hydrochloride; structurally related to mepivacaine except for a butyl group replacing a methyl group

Prepared by. A.F. Ekenstam, 1957

FDA Approved. October 1972

Potency. Four times that of lidocaine, mepivacaine, and prilocaine

Toxicity. Less than four times that of lidocaine and mepivacaine

Metabolism. Metabolized in the liver by amidases

Excretion. Via the kidney; 16% unchanged bupivacaine has been recovered from human urine

Vasodilating properties. Relatively significant: greater than those of lidocaine, prilocaine, and mepivacaine, yet considerably less than those of procaine

pK$_a$. 8.1

pH of plain solution. 4.5 to 6.0

pH of vasoconstrictor-containing solution. 3.0 to 4.5

Onset of action. Occasionally similar to that of lidocaine, mepivacaine, and prilocaine, but usually requires longer onset time (e.g., 6 to 10 minutes)

Effective dental concentration. 0.5%

Anesthetic half-life. 2.7 hours

Topical anesthetic action. Not in clinically acceptable concentrations

Pregnancy classification. C

Safety during lactation. S?

Maximum Recommended Dose. The manufacturer's maximum recommended dose is 0.6 mg/lb or 1.3 mg/kg

TABLE **4-15**
Bupivacaine Hydrochloride

Proprietary Name	Manufacturer	Percent Local Anesthetic	Vasoconstrictor	Duration of Analgesia (min)		MRD-m and MRD-a
				Pulpal	*Soft-Tissue*	
Marcaine	Kodak	0.5	Epinephrine 1:200,000	90–180	240–540 (reports up to 720)	1.3 mg/kg 0.6 mg/lb 90 mg absolute maximum

MRD, Maximum recommended dose.

of body weight for the adult patient, with a maximum dose not to exceed 90 mg (Table 4-15).[53]

Comments. Bupivacaine has been available in cartridge form since February 1982 in Canada and July 1983 in the United States. Available as a 0.5% solution with 1:200,000 epinephrine (Fig. 4-7), there are two primary indications for its utilization in dentistry:

1. Lengthy dental procedures for which pulpal (deep) anesthesia in excess of 90 minutes is necessary (e.g., full mouth reconstruction, implant surgery, and extensive periodontal procedures)
2. Management of postoperative pain (e.g., endodontic, periodontal, postimplant, and surgical)

The patient's requirement for postoperative opioid analgesics is considerably lessened when bupivacaine is administered for pain control.[58] For postoperative pain control after a short surgical procedure (<30 minutes), bupivacaine may be administered at the start of the procedure; however, for postoperative pain control after lengthy surgical procedures, it might be reasonable to administer bupivacaine at the conclusion of the procedure, immediately before the patient's discharge from the office.

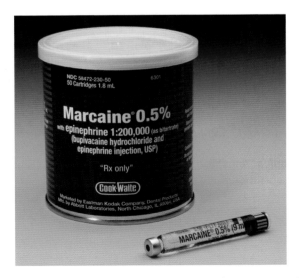

Figure 4-7. Bupivacaine 0.5% with epinephrine 1:200,000. (Courtesy Eastman Kodak, N.Y.)

A regimen for management of postsurgical pain has been developed that is clinically quite effective.[59,60] It suggests the pretreatment administration of one or two oral doses of a nonsteroidal antiinflammatory drug (NSAID), followed by the administration of any suitable (e.g., intermediate-duration) local anesthetic to manage the periprocedural pain. A long-duration local anesthetic (bupivacaine) is administered immediately before patient discharge (if deemed necessary), with the patient continuing to take the oral dose of NSAID every "x" hours as indicated (not "prn pain") for "y" number of days. The requirement for opioid agonist analgesics is significantly diminished with this protocol. Hargreaves demonstrated that the preoperative oral dose of NSAID is not necessary as long as the initial oral dose can be ingested within 1 hour of the start of the surgical procedure.[61]

For many patients receiving bupivacaine the onset of anesthesia is similar to that observed with other amide anesthetics (2 to 4 minutes); however, in many patients the onset of anesthesia is delayed for from 6 to 10 minutes, understandable in view of bupivacaine's pK_a of 8.1. If this occurs it may be advisable, at subsequent appointments, to initiate procedural pain control with a more rapid-acting amide (e.g., articaine, mepivacaine, lidocaine, or prilocaine), which provides clinically acceptable pain control within a few moments, allowing the procedure to commence more promptly. Follow this with an injection of bupivacaine for long-duration anesthesia.

Bupivacaine is not recommended in younger patients or in those for whom the risk of postoperative soft-tissue injury produced by self-mutilation is increased, such as physically and mentally disabled persons. Bupivacaine is rarely indicated in children because pediatric dental procedures are usually of short duration.

Etidocaine HCl

Pertinent Information

Classification. Amide

Chemical formula. 2-(*N*-Ethylpropylamino) butyro-2, 6-xylidide hydrochloride; structurally similar to lidocaine

The chemical structure diagram at top left showing a 2,6-xylidine ring with CH₃ groups, NH·CO, and an amino group with C₂H₅, C₂H₅, and C₃H₇ substituents.

Prepared by. Takman, 1971

FDA Approved. August 1976

Potency. Four times that of lidocaine

Toxicity. Two times as toxic as lidocaine after subcutaneous administration; four times as toxic as lidocaine after rapid IV administration

Metabolism. Undergoes *N*-dealkylation; can also be hydroxylated on the aromatic ring. Hydrolytic metabolism appears less important than for lidocaine and prilocaine, with less than 10% of the dose appearing in the urine as both 2,6-xylidine and its hydroxylated product, as opposed to more than 70% for lidocaine.[62]

Excretion. Etidocaine and its metabolites are excreted primarily via the kidneys

Vasodilating properties. Relatively significant: greater than those of lidocaine, prilocaine, and mepivacaine yet considerably less than those of procaine

pK$_a$. 7.7

pH of plain solution. 4.5

pH of vasoconstrictor-containing solution. 3.0 to 3.5

Onset of action. Equivalent to that of lidocaine, mepivacaine, and prilocaine (1 ½ to 3 minutes)

Effective dental concentration. 1.5%

Anesthetic half-life. 2.6 hours

Topical anesthetic action. Not in clinically acceptable concentrations

Maximum Recommended Dose. Manufacturer's maximum recommended dose is 3.6 mg/lb or 8.0 mg/kg of body weight for the adult patient, with an absolute maximum dose of 400 mg.[63]

Comments. Etidocaine is a long-acting local anesthetic, chemically related to lidocaine. Its clinical indications are identical to those of bupivacaine. The primary differences in clinical activity between the two are their onset of anesthetic action and duration for infiltration anesthesia. Etidocaine (with a pK$_a$ of 7.7) has an onset of action of about 3 minutes, whereas bupivacaine (with a pK$_a$ of 8.1) has an onset of 6 to 10 minutes. In addition, the duration of

clinical action of etidocaine is extremely dependent on the type of injection administered. After infiltration (supraperiosteal) administration, pulpal anesthesia is extremely variable in duration and depth, whereas after nerve block the duration of pulpal anesthesia is considerably longer, ranging from 90 to 180 minutes.[64]

Dental cartridges of etidocaine HCl with epinephrine 1:200,000 were withdrawn from the North American market in 2002.

ANESTHETICS FOR TOPICAL APPLICATION

The use of topically applied local anesthetics is an important component of the atraumatic administration of intraoral local anesthesia (see Chapter 11). Conventional topical anesthetics are unable to penetrate intact skin but do diffuse through abraded skin (e.g., sunburn) or any mucous membranes.

The concentration of a local anesthetic applied topically is typically greater than that same local anesthetic administered by injection. The higher concentration facilitates diffusion of the drug through the mucous membrane. Higher concentration also increases the risk of toxicity, both locally to the tissues and systemically.[65] Because topical anesthetics do not contain vasoconstrictors and local anesthetics are inherently vasodilators, vascular absorption of some topical formulations is rapid, and blood levels may quickly reach those achieved by direct IV administration.[65]

Many local anesthetics used effectively via injection prove to be ineffective when applied topically (e.g., articaine, mepivacaine, prilocaine, and procaine) because the concentrations necessary to produce anesthesia via topical application are high, with significantly increased overdose and local tissue toxicity potential (Table 4-16).

As a rule, topical anesthesia is effective only on surface tissues (2 to 3 mm). Tissues deep to the area of application are poorly anesthetized. However, surface anesthesia does allow for atraumatic needle penetration of the mucous membrane.[22,66]

The topical anesthetics benzocaine and lidocaine base are insoluble in water. However, they are soluble in alcohol, propylene glycol, polyethylene glycol, and

TABLE 4-16
Effective Concentrations for Injection and Topical Application of Local Anesthetics

	Effective Concentration		
Agent	**Injection (%)**	**Topical (%)**	**Useful as Topical**
Lidocaine	2	2 to 5	Yes
Mepivacaine	2 to 3	12 to 15	No
Procaine	2 to 4	10 to 20	No
Tetracaine	0.25 to 1	0.2 to 1	Yes

other vehicles suitable for surface application. The base forms of benzocaine and lidocaine are slowly absorbed into the cardiovascular system and therefore are less likely to produce an overdose reaction.

Some topical anesthetics are marketed in pressurized spray containers. Although they are no more effective than other forms, it is difficult to control the amount of anesthetic expelled and confine it to the desired site of application. Spray devices that do not deliver *measured doses* should not be used intraorally.

Benzocaine

Benzocaine (ethyl *p*-aminobenzoate) is an ester local anesthetic.
1. Poor solubility in water.

$$H_2N-\langle\bigcirc\rangle-CO \bullet OC_2H_5$$

2. Poor absorption into cardiovascular system.
3. Systemic toxic (overdose) reactions virtually unknown.
4. Remains at the site of application longer, providing a prolonged duration of action.
5. Not suitable for injection.
6. Localized allergic reactions may occur after prolonged or repeated use. Although allergic reaction to ester anesthetics is rare, ester local anesthetics are more allergenic than amide local anesthetics.[67]
7. Reported to inhibit the antibacterial action of sulfonamides.[68]
8. Availability (Fig. 4-8)
   a. Aerosol:
      1. Americaine
      2. Hurricaine
      3. Super-Dent
      4. Topex
   b. Gel: contain benzocaine in doses varying from 63, 75, 100, 150, 180, to 200 mg/ml
      1. Americaine Anesthetic Lubricant
      2. Anbesol
      3. Anbocaine
      4. Baby Orabase
      5. ComfortCaine
      6. Gingicaine
      7. Hurricaine
      8. Numzident
      9. Num-Zit
      10. Orajel
      11. Rid-A-Pain Dental
      12. SensoGARD Canker Sore Relief
      13. Super-Dent
      14. Topex
      15. Topicale
      16. Xylonor
      17. Zilactin-Baby
      18. Topicaine (Canada)

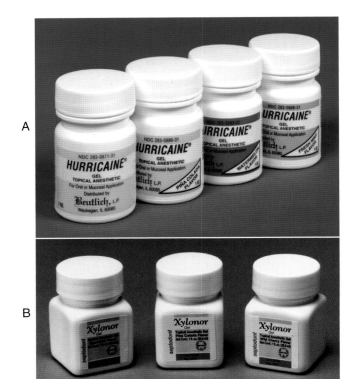

Figure 4-8. **A** and **B,** Topical anesthetics containing benzocaine. (**A,** Courtesy Beautlich Pharmaceuticals, Waukegan, Ill. **B,** Courtesy Septodont, New Castle, Del.)

   c. Gel patch: (2 cm long × 1 cm wide × 1 mm thick): 36 mg/patch
      1. Topicale GelPatch
   d. Ointment: 161, 200 mg/ml
      1. Benzodent
      2. Cora-Caine
      3. Dentapaine
      4. Topicale
   e. Solution: 2, 50, 200 mg/ml; 65 and 75 mg/ml (Canada)
      1. Anbesol Maximum Strength
      2. Dent-Zel-Ite
      3. Gingicaine
      4. Hurricaine
      5. Kank-a
      6. Num-Zit Lotion
      7. Topex
      8. Topicale
      9. Baby Oragel (Canada)
      10. Dentocaine (Canada)
      11. Oragel (Canada)

Benzocaine, Butamben, and Tetracaine HCl

Aerosol, gel, ointment, and solution: Benzocaine 140 mg/ml; butamben 20 mg/ml; tetracaine HCl, 20 mg/ml

Cocaine Hydrochloride

Cocaine hydrochloride (benzoylmethylecgonine hydrochloride) occurs naturally as a white crystalline solid that is *highly soluble in water*.

1. Used exclusively via topical application. Injection contraindicated because of the ready availability of more effective and less toxic local anesthetics. Cocaine is an ester local anesthetic.
2. Onset of topical anesthetic action is quite rapid, usually developing within 1 minute.
3. Duration of anesthetic action may be as long as 2 hours.
4. Absorbed rapidly but eliminated slowly.
5. Undergoes metabolism in the liver. The liver is able to detoxify one minimal lethal dose of cocaine per hour.
6. Unchanged cocaine may be found in the urine.
7. Only local anesthetic consistently demonstrated to produce vasoconstriction, which develops as a result of its ability to potentiate the actions of endogenous epinephrine and norepinephrine.[32] Addition of vasoconstrictors to cocaine is therefore unnecessary, and also potentially dangerous, increasing the likelihood of dysrhythmias, including ventricular fibrillation.
8. Classified as a Schedule II drug under the Controlled Substances Act. Repeated use results in psychological dependence and tolerance.
9. Overdose of cocaine is not uncommon, primarily because the drug is readily absorbed and its dosage is not carefully monitored.
10. Clinical manifestations of mild overdose: euphoria, excitement, restlessness, tremor, hypertension, tachycardia, and tachypnea.
11. Clinical manifestations of acute cocaine overdose: excitement, restlessness, confusion, tremor, hypertension, tachycardia, tachypnea, nausea and vomiting, abdominal pain, exophthalmos, and mydriasis; followed by depression (CNS, cardiovascular, respiratory) and death from respiratory arrest.
12. Available in concentrations ranging from 2% to 10%.
13. It is recommended that the concentration of cocaine not exceed 4% for topical application to oral mucous membranes.
14. Solutions of cocaine are unstable and deteriorate on standing.
15. Because of the extreme abuse potential of cocaine, its use as a topical anesthetic in dentistry is not recommended.

Dyclonine Hydrochloride

Dyclonine hydrochloride (4'-butoxy-3-piperidinopropiophenone hydrochloride) is chemically unique from all other local anesthetics in that it is a ketone.

1. Cross-sensitization with other local anesthetics does not occur; therefore dyclonine may be used in patients with known sensitivities to local anesthetics of other chemical groups.
2. Slightly soluble in water.
3. Potency equal to that of cocaine.
4. Onset of anesthesia slow, requiring up to 10 minutes.
5. Duration of anesthesia may be as long as 1 hour.
6. Systemic toxicity extremely low, primarily because of the agent's poor water solubility.
7. Not indicated for use by injection or infiltration; irritating to tissues at the site of application.
8. A 0.5% solution is used in dentistry. Maximum recommended dose is 200 mg (40 ml of a 0.5% solution).
9. Dyclonine was available as *Dyclone*. A 0.5% solution (Astra Pharmaceutical Products, Inc.): each 100 ml of solution contained 500 mg of dyclonine HCl, 300 mg of chlorobutanol as a preservative, sodium chloride for isotonicity, and hydrochloric acid, as needed, to adjust pH. Dyclone brand was withdrawn from the North American market in 2001.

EMLA (<u>E</u>utectic <u>M</u>ixture of <u>L</u>ocal <u>A</u>nesthetics)

EMLA cream (composed of lidocaine 2.5% and prilocaine 2.5%) is an emulsion in which the oil phase is a eutectic mixture of lidocaine and prilocaine in a ratio of 1:1 by weight. It was designed as a topical anesthetic able to provide surface anesthesia of intact skin (other topical anesthetics *do not* produce a clinical action on intact skin, only abraded skin), and as such is used primarily before painful procedures, such as venipuncture and other needle insertions. Originally marketed for use in pediatrics, EMLA has gained popularity among needle-phobic adults and persons having other superficial, but painful, procedures performed (e.g., hair removal).

EMLA use has become almost routine during circumcision,[69] leg ulcer débridement,[70] and in gynecological procedures.[71] Because intact skin is a barrier to drug diffusion, EMLA must be applied 1 hour before the procedure. Satisfactory numbing of the skin occurs 1 hour after application, reaches a maximum at 2 to 3 hours, and lasts for 1 to 2 hours after removal.

EMLA is supplied in a 5-g or 30-g tube or as an EMLA anesthetic disc. The EMLA disc is a white, round, cellulose disc preloaded with EMLA, packaged in a protective laminate foil surrounded with adhesive tape.

EMLA is contraindicated for use in patients with congenital or idiopathic methemoglobinemia, infants under the age of 12 months who are receiving treatment with methemoglobin-inducing agents, or patients with a known sensitivity to amide-type local anesthetics or any other component of the product.[72]

On November 15, 2002, AstraZeneca ceased distributing EMLA cream to drug wholesalers and direct buying retail pharmacies.[73] The product is being redesigned into child-resistant closure (CRC) tubes. EMLA with CRC is now available.

Because EMLA is effective in penetrating intact skin, its ability to produce effective topical anesthesia in the oral cavity seems obvious. Although the drug package insert[72] stated originally that "EMLA is not recommended for use on mucous membranes," several clinical trials have been published that demonstrated satisfactory results.[74,75]

Bernardi and associates demonstrated statistically significant analgesia in 52 dental patients requiring removal of metal maxillary or mandibular splints used to contain fractures.[74] The authors concluded that, "the analgesic effect of EMLA cream on oral mucosa allow the application of contact anesthesia to be broadened to oral surgery and dentistry, limiting it to those procedures that do not involve deep tissues and only require short-term anesthesia."[74]

Munshi and associates reported on the use of EMLA cream in 30 pediatric patients undergoing a variety of clinical procedures, including extraction of mobile primary teeth, root stumps, and pulpal therapy procedures in the primary teeth using EMLA as the sole anesthetic agent.[75] Results showed that the use of EMLA could to some extent eliminate the use of the needle in procedures performed in pediatric dentistry.

Lidocaine

Lidocaine is available in two forms for topical application: *lidocaine base*,[1] which is poorly soluble in water, used as a 5% concentration, indicated for use on ulcerated, abraded, or lacerated tissue; and *lidocaine hydrochloride*,[2] which is a water-soluble preparation used in a 2% concentration. This water-soluble form of lidocaine penetrates tissue more efficiently than the base form. However, systemic absorption also is greater, providing a greater risk of toxicity than the base form.

1. Lidocaine is an amide local anesthetic with an *exceptionally low* incidence of allergic reactions.

2. Maximum recommended dose is 200 mg.
3. Availability: lidocaine (base)
   a. Aerosol: 10 mg/metered spray
      1. Xylocaine
   b. Ointment: 50 mg/ml
      1. Octocaine (Fig. 4-9, *A*)
   c. Patch: (2 cm long × 1 cm wide × 2 mm thick): 46.1 mg/patch
      1. DentiPatch (Fig. 4-9, *B*)
   d. Solution: 25, 50 mg/ml
      1. Xylocaine
4. Availability: lidocaine hydrochloride (HCl)
   a. Oral topical solution: 20 mg/ml
      1. Xylocaine Viscous
   b. Solution: 40 mg/ml
      1. Xylocaine

Tetracaine Hydrochloride

Tetracaine hydrochloride (2-dimethylaminoethyl-4-butylaminobenzoate hydrochloride) is a long-duration ester local anesthetic that can be injected or applied topically.

1. Highly soluble in water.
2. Applied topically, five to eight times more potent than cocaine.
3. Onset of action after topical application is slow.
4. Duration of action is approximately 45 minutes after topical application.
5. Metabolized in plasma and the liver by plasma pseudocholinesterase at a slower rate than procaine.
6. Used for injection, available as a 0.15% concentration.
7. A 2% concentration is used for topical application.
8. Rapidly absorbed through mucous membranes. Use should be limited to small areas to avoid rapid absorption. Other, more slowly or poorly absorbed agents should be used in lieu of tetracaine when larger areas of topical anesthesia are necessary.

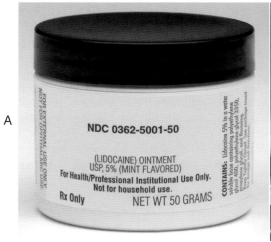
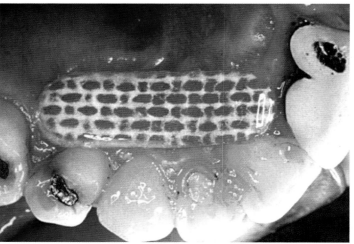

Figure 4-9. Topical anesthetics—Lidocaine. **A,** Octocaine ointment. **B,** Dentipatch. (**A,** Courtesy Septodent, New Castle, Del.)

9. Maximum recommended dose of 20 mg when used for topical application. This is 1 ml of a 2% solution.
10. Extreme caution urged because of the great potential for systemic toxicity.
11. Availability (Canada):
    a. Aerosol: 0.7 mg/metered spray
        1. Supracaine

SELECTION OF A LOCAL ANESTHETIC

With many local anesthetic combinations available for injection, it becomes difficult to select an ideal drug for a given patient. Many dentists simply deal with this by using one local anesthetic for all procedures, regardless of their duration. For example, the dentist may elect to use 2% lidocaine with 1:100,000 epinephrine for procedures lasting 5 to 10 minutes and for procedures involving 90 minutes of treatment time. Although the duration of pulpal anesthesia achievable with this drug in ideal circumstances *may* permit pain-free treatment in both these instances, the patient requiring only 10 minutes of pulpal anesthesia will remain anesthetized unnecessarily for an additional 3 to 5 hours (soft tissues), whereas the patient requiring 90 minutes of pulpal anesthesia will likely experience pain toward the end of the procedure.

A rational approach to the selection of an appropriate local anesthetic for a patient includes a consideration of several factors: *the length of time for which pain control is necessary; the need for posttreatment pain control; the need for hemostasis; and whether any contraindications exist to the administration of the selected local anesthetic.*[1-4] Table 4-17 lists the currently available local anesthetics according to their expected duration of both pulpal and soft-tissue anesthesia. Again it should be noted that these numbers are approximations, and the actual duration of clinical anesthesia may be somewhat longer or shorter than indicated.

A second consideration in the selection of a local anesthetic must be the *requirement for pain control after treatment.* A long-duration local anesthetic can be administered when postoperative pain is thought to be a factor. Local anesthetics providing a shorter duration of soft-tissue anesthesia can be used for nontraumatic procedures.

When postoperative pain is considered likely, 0.5% bupivacaine (for 8 to 12 hours of soft-tissue anesthesia) or 4% prilocaine with 1:200,000 epinephrine (for 5 to 8 hours of soft-tissue anesthesia) are suggested.

For patients in whom postoperative anesthesia is a potential hazard, shorter-duration anesthetics should be considered. These include younger children and the physically or mentally disabled, who might accidentally bite or chew their lips or tongue. For these patients 3% mepivacaine or 4% prilocaine (for infiltration) is recommended for use in short procedures.

A third factor is the need for *hemostasis* during the procedure. Anesthetic solutions containing epinephrine in a 1:50,000 or 1:100,000 concentration are recommended,

TABLE 4-17
Duration of Pulpal and Soft-tissue Anesthesia for Available Local Anesthetics

Drug Combination	Duration (Approximate Minutes)	
	Pulpal	*Soft-tissue*
Lidocaine 2%	<10	30–45
Mepivacaine 3%	5–10	90–120
Prilocaine 4% (infiltration)	10–15	60–120
Prilocaine 4% (nerve block)	40–60	120–240
Articaine 4% + epinephrine 1:200,000	45–60	180–240
Mepivacaine 2% + epinephrine 1:200,000	45–60	120–240
Lidocaine 2% + epinephrine 1:50,000	60	180–300
Lidocaine 2% + epinephrine 1:100,000	60	180–300
Mepivacaine 2% + levonordefrin 1:20,000	60	180–300
Articaine 4% + epinephrine 1:100,000	60–75	180–300
Prilocaine 4% + epinephrine 1:200,000	60–90	180–480
Bupivacaine 0.5% + epinephrine 1:200,000	>90	240–720

via local infiltration into the surgical site, when hemostasis is considered necessary.

A fourth factor in the selection of a local anesthetic involves the *presence of any contraindications to use of the selected local anesthetic* (see Table 4-2).

Absolute contraindications require that the offending drug(s) not be administered to the patient under any condition. The risk that a life-threatening situation will arise is increased. One absolute contraindication to local anesthetic administration exists: *true, documented reproducible allergy.* Fortunately this is an extremely rare occurrence with the amide local anesthetics, although the incidence of *alleged* local anesthetic allergy is high. Management of *alleged* and documented allergy to local anesthetics is discussed in Chapter 18.

In cases of a *relative contraindication* it is preferable to avoid administration of the drug in question because of an increased risk that an adverse reaction will develop. An alternative drug that is not contraindicated is recommended. However, if such an acceptable alternative is not available, the drug in question may be used, but

BOX 4-4

Factors in Selection of a Local Anesthetic for a Patient

1. Length of time pain control is necessary
2. Potential need for posttreatment pain control
3. Possibility of self-mutilation in the postoperative period
4. Requirement for hemostasis
5. Presence of any contraindications (absolute or relative) to the local anesthetic solution selected for administration

judiciously, with use of the minimum dose that will provide adequate pain control. One example of a relative contraindication is the presence of atypical plasma (pseudo) cholinesterase, which decreases the rate of biotransformation of ester local anesthetics. The amides may be used with no increase in risk in these patients. Relative contraindications are reviewed in Chapter 10.

Box 4-4 summarizes the criteria used in the selection of a local anesthetic for administration to a given patient at a given dental appointment.

The local anesthetic armamentarium for a dentist or dental hygienist therefore should include drugs of varying durations of action, such as the selection that follows. A minimum of two drugs is recommended for most offices. Amides are preferred to esters whenever possible.

1. Short-duration pulpal anesthesia (30 minutes)
2. Intermediate-duration pulpal anesthesia (approximately 60 minutes)
3. Long-duration pulpal anesthesia (90 or more minutes)
4. Topical anesthetic for tissue preparation before injection of local anesthetic

REFERENCES

1. Malamed SF: *Handbook of local anesthesia*, St Louis, 1980, Mosby.
2. ADA Council on Scientific Affairs: *ADA guide to dental therapeutics*, ed 2, Chicago, 2000, American Dental Association.
3. USP DI Updates On-line, United States Pharmacopeial Convention, Inc., *www.usp.org.*
4. Prescribing information: Scandanest, Septodont, Inc., *www.septodontusa.com.*
5. Prescribing information: Carbocaine, Eastman Kodak Company, *www.kodak.com.*
6. Iwatsubo T, Hirota N, Ooie T, et al: Prediction of in vivo drug metabolism in the human liver from in vitro metabolism data, *Pharmacol Ther* 73:247-271, 1997.
7. Thompson P, Melmon K, Richardson J, et al: Lidocaine pharmacokinetics in advanced heart failure, liver disease, and renal failure in humans, *Ann Intern Med* 78:499, 1973.
8. Haas DA, Lennon D: Local anesthetic use by dentists in Ontario, *J Can Dent Assoc* 61:497-304, 1995.
9. Kao FF, Jalar UH: The central action of lignocaine and its effects on cardiac output, *Br J Pharmacol* 14:522-526, 1959.
10. Malamed SF: *Sedation: a guide to patient management*, ed 4, St Louis, 2003, Mosby.
11. Wilson AW, Deacock S, Downie IP, Zaki G: Allergy to local anesthetic: the importance of thorough investigation, *Br Dent J* 188:320-322, 2000.
12. Covino BG: *Clinical pharmacology of local anesthetic agents.* In Cousins MJ, Bridenbaugh PO, editors: *Neural blockade in clinical anesthesia and management of pain*, ed 2, Philadelphia, 1988, JB Lippincott.
13. Prescribing information: Ravocaine and Novocain with Levophed, New York, 1993, Cook-Waite, Sterling Winthrop.
14. *Astra standard times*, Westborough, Mass, 1988, Astra Pharmaceutical Products.
15. Prescribing information: Xylocaine hydrochloride, Westborough, Mass, 1992, Astra Pharmaceutical Products.
16. Brown RS, Paluvoi S, Choksi S, Burgess CM, Reece ER: Evaluating a dental patient for local anesthesia allergy, *Comp Contin Educ Dent* 23:225-228, 131-132, 134; 140, 2002.
17. Jackson D, Chen AH, Bennett CR: Identifying true lidocaine allergy, *J Am Dent Assoc* 125:1362-1366, 1994.
18. Sindel LJ, deShazo RD: Accidents resulting from local anesthetics. True or false allergy? *Clin Rev Allergy* 9:379-395, 1991.
19. Ball IA: Allergic reactions to lignocaine, *Br Dent J* 186:524-526, 1999.
20. Baluga JC, Casamayou R, Carozzi E, et al: Allergy to local anaesthetics in dentistry. Myth or reality? *Allergologia et Immunopathologia* 30:14-19, 2002.
21. Shojaei AR, Haas DA: Local anesthetic cartridges and latex allergy: a literature review, *J Can Dent Assoc* 68:122-626, 2002.
22. Jeske AH, Blanton PL: Misconceptions involving dental local anesthesia. Part 2: Pharmacology, *Texas Dent J* 119:310-314, 2002.
23. *Astra dental anesthetics: times to count on*, Mississauga, Ontario, 1995, Astra Pharmaceutical Products.
24. Kodak Dental Products: Prescribing information, Rochester, NY, 1993, Eastman Kodak Company Dental Products.
25. Young ER, Mason DR, Saso MA, Albert BS: Some clinical properties of Octocaine 200 (2 percent lidocaine with epinephrine 1:200,000), *J Can Dent Assoc* 55:987-991, 1989.
26. Buckley JA, Ciancio SG, McMullen JA: Efficacy of epinephrine concentration in local anesthesia during periodontal surgery, *J Periodontol* 55:653-657, 1984.
27. DeToledo JC: Lidocaine and seizures, *Ther Drug Monit* 22:320-322, 2000.
28. Geddes IC: Metabolism of local anesthetic agents, *Int Anesthesiol Clin* 5:525-549, 1967.
29. Severinghaus JW, Xu F-D, Spellman MJ: Benzocaine and methemoglobin: recommended actions, *Anesthesiology* 74:385-386, 1991.
30. Schroeder TH, Dieterich HJ, Muhlbauer B: Methemoglobinemia after maxillary block with bupivacaine and additional injection of lidocaine in the operative field, *Acta Anaesthes Scand* 43:480-482, 1999.
31. Wilburn-Goo D, Lloyd LM: When patients become cyanotic: acquired methemoglobinemia, *J Am Dent Assoc* 130:626-631, 1999.
32. de Jong RH: *Local anesthetics*, St Louis, 1994, Mosby.
33. Akerman B, Astrom A, Ross S, et al: Studies on the absorption, distribution, and metabolism of labeled prilocaine and lidocaine in some animal species, *Acta Pharmacol Toxicol* 24:389-403, 1966.
34. Foldes FF, Molloy R, McNall PG, et al: Comparison of toxicity of intravenously given local anesthetic agents in man, *JAMA* 172:1493-1498, 1960.
35. Englesson S, Eriksson E, Wahlqvist S, et al: Differences in tolerance to intravenous Xylocaine and Citanest (L67), a

new local anesthetic: a double blind study in man, *Proc 1st Eur Congr Anesthesiol* 2:206-209, 1962.

36. Deriksson E, Granberg PO: Studies on the renal excretion of Citanest and Xylocaine, *Acta Anaesth Scand Suppl* 16: 79-85, 1985.

37. Smith DW, Peterson MR, DeBerard SC: Local anesthesia. Topical application, local infiltration, and field block, *Postgrad Med* 106:27-60, 64-66, 1999.

38. *Citanest and Citanest Forte: drug prescribing information,* Westborough, Mass, 1994, Astra Pharmaceutical Products.

39. van Oss GE, Vree TB, Baars AM, Termond EF, Booji LH: Pharmacokinetics, metabolism, and renal excretion of articaine and its metabolite articainic acid in patients after epidural administration, *Eur J Anaesthesiol* 6:19-56, 1989.

40. van Oss GE, Vree TB, Baars AM, Termond EF, Booji LH: Clinical effects and pharmacokinetics of articainic acid in one volunteer after intravenous administration, *Pharm Weekbl (Sc)* 10:284-286, 1988.

41. Vree TB, et al: High performance liquid chromatography and preliminary pharmacokinetics of articaine and its 2-carboxy metabolite in human serum and urine, *J Chromatogr* 424:240-444, 1988.

42. Prescribing information: Septocaine, Septodont, Inc., *www.septodontusa.com.*

43. Malamed SF, Gagnon S, Leblanc D: Safety of articaine: a new amide local anesthetic, *J Am Dent Assoc* 132:177-185, 2001.

44. Malamed SF, Gagnon S, Leblanc D: Articaine hydrochloride in pediatric dentistry: safety and efficacy of a new amide-type local anesthetic, *Pediatr Dent* 22:307-311, 2000.

45. Malamed SF, Gagnon S, Leblanc D: Efficacy of articaine: a new amide local anesthetic, *J Am Dent Assoc* 131:535-642, 2000.

46. Donaldson D, James-Perdok L, Craig BJ, Derkson GD, Richardson AS: A comparison of Ultracaine DS (articaine HCl) and Citanest Forte (prilocaine HCl) in maxillary infiltration and mandibular nerve block, *J Can Dent Assoc* 53:38-42, 1987.

47. Knoll-Kohler E, Rupprecht S: Articaine for local anaesthesia in dentistry: a lidocaine controlled double blind crossover study, *Eur J Pain* 13:59-63, 1992.

48. Schulze-Husmann M: *Experimental evaluation of the new local anesthetic Ultracaine in dental practice,* doctoral dissertation, Bonn, 1974, University of Bonn.

49. Clinicians guide to dental products and techniques. Septocaine. *CRA Newsletter.* June 2001.

50. Haas DA, Harper DG, Saso MA, Young ER: Comparison of articaine and prilocaine anesthesia by infiltration in maxillary and mandibular arches, *Anesth Prog* 37:230-237, 1990.

51. Haas DA, Harper DG, Saso MA, Young ER: Lack of differential effect by Ultracaine (articaine HCl) and Citanest (prilocaine HCl) in infiltration anesthesia, *J Can Dent Assoc* 57:217-223, 1991.

52. Jakobs W: Status of dental anesthesia in Germany, *Anesth Prog* 36:10-212, 1989.

53. Jakobs W: Actual aspects of dental anesthesia in Germany, presented at the 10(th) International Dental Congress on Modern Pain Control, IFDAS, Edinburgh, Scotland, UK, June 2003.

54. Personal communications with Septodont, Inc., Newark, Delaware, March 2004.

55. van Eden SP, Patel MF: Prolonged paraesthesia following inferior alveolar nerve block using articaine, *Br J Oral Maxillofac Surg* 40:519-520, 2002.

56. Dower JS Jr: A review of paresthesia in association with administration of local anesthesia, *Dent Today* 22:24-69, 2003.

57. Malamed SF: *Handbook of local anesthesia,* ed 4, St Louis, 1997, Mosby, pp 63-64.

58. *Marcaine HCl: drug prescribing information,* New York, 1990, Winthrop Pharmaceuticals.

59. Moore PA: Bupivacaine: a long-lasting local anesthetic for dentistry, *Oral Surg* 58:369, 1984.

60. Acute Pain Management Guideline Panel: *Acute pain management: operative or medical procedures and trauma. Clinical practice guideline,* AHCPR Pub. No. 92-0032, Rockville, Md, 1992, Agency for Health Care Policy and Research, Public Health Service, US Department of Health and Human Services.

61. Hargreaves KM, Keiser K: Development of new pain management strategies, *J Dent Educ* 66:113-121, 2002.

62. Vine J, Morgan D, Thomas D: The identification of eight hydroxylated metabolites of etidocaine by chemical ionization mass spectrometry, *Xenobiotica* 8:509-513, 1978.

63. Duranest HCl: drug prescribing information, Westborough, Mass, 1989, Astra Pharmaceutical Products.

64. Moore PA: Long-acting local anesthetics: a review of clinical efficacy in dentistry, *Compendium* 11:12, 24-26, 28-30, 1990.

65. Adriani J, Campbell D: Fatalities following topical application of local anesthetics to mucous membranes, *JAMA* 162:1527, 1956.

66. Rosivack RG, Koenigsberg SR, Maxwell KC: An analysis of the effectiveness of two topical anesthetics, *Anesth Prog* 37:290-292, 1990.

67. Patterson RP, Anderson J: Allergic reactions to drugs and biologic agents, *JAMA* 248:2637-2645, 1982.

68. Alston TA: Antagonism of sulfonamides by benzocaine and chloroprocaine, *Anesthesiology* 76:375-476, 1992.

69. Taddio A: Pain management for neonatal circumcision, *Paediatric Drugs* 3:101-111, 2001.

70. Vanscheidt W, Sadjadi Z, Lillieborg S: EMLA anaesthetic cream for sharp leg ulcer debridement: a review of the clinical evidence for analgesic efficacy and tolerability, *Eur J Dermatol* 11:20-96, 2001.

71. Wright VC: Vulvar biopsy: techniques for reducing patient discomfort, *Adv Nurse Pract* 9:17-60, 2001.

72. AstraZeneca LP: EMLA drug information sheet, 2000.

73. Letter to Health Care Providers: "Restricted availability of EMLA-Cream (lidocaine 2.5% and prilocaine 2.5%) effective November 15, 2002," AstraZeneca.

74. Bernardi M, Secco F, Benech A: Anesthetic efficacy of a eutectic mixture of lidocaine and prilocaine (EMLA) on the oral mucosa: prospective double-blind study with a placebo, *Minerva Stomatol* 48:9-43, 1999.

75. Munshi AK, Hegde AM, Latha R: Use of EMLA: is it an injection free alternative? *J Clin Pediatr Dent* 25:215-219, 2001.

IN THIS PART

PART TWO

The Armamentarium

The equipment necessary for the administration of local anesthetics is introduced and discussed in this section. This includes the syringe, the needle, the local anesthetic cartridge, and additional items of equipment. In addition to a description of the armamentarium, each chapter reviews the proper care and handling of the equipment and problems that may be encountered with its use. A discussion of the proper technique for assembling the equipment follows.

The introduction of computer-controlled local anesthetic delivery (CCLAD) systems has enhanced the delivery of local anesthetic for many dentists and their patients. Two CCLAD devices, "The Wand" and "The Comfort Control Syringe System," are described.

The Syringe

The syringe is one of three essential components of the local anesthetic armamentarium (others are the needle and the cartridge). It is the vehicle whereby the contents of the anesthetic cartridge are delivered through the needle to the patient.

TYPES OF SYRINGES

Eight types of syringes for local anesthetic administration are in use in dentistry today. They represent a considerable improvement over the local anesthetic syringes formerly used. The various types of syringes are listed in Box 5-1.

Syringes that do not permit easy aspiration (e.g., nonaspirating syringes) are not discussed because their use unacceptably increases the risk of inadvertent intravascular drug administration. Use of aspirating dental syringes (capable of the aspiration of blood) represents the standard of care.

American Dental Association criteria for acceptance of local anesthetic syringes include the following:[1,2]

1. They must be durable and able to withstand repeated sterilization without damage. (If the unit is disposable, it should be packaged in a sterile container.)

BOX 5-1

Syringe Types Available in Dentistry

1. Nondisposable syringes:
   a. Breech-loading, metallic, cartridge-type, aspirating
   b. Breech-loading, plastic, cartridge-type, aspirating
   c. Breech-loading, metallic, cartridge-type, self-aspirating
   d. Pressure syringe for periodontal ligament injection
   e. Jet injector ("needleless" syringe)
2. Disposable syringes
3. "Safety" syringes
4. Computer-controlled local anesthetic delivery systems

---

2. They should be capable of accepting a wide variety of cartridges and needles of different manufacture, and permit repeated use.
3. They should be inexpensive, self-contained, lightweight, and simple to use with one hand.
4. They should provide for effective aspiration and be constructed so that blood may be easily observed in the cartridge.

Nondisposable Syringes

Breech-loading, Metallic, Cartridge-type, Aspirating. The breech-loading, metallic, cartridge-type syringe (Fig. 5-1) is the most commonly used in dentistry. The term *breech-loading* implies that the cartridge is inserted into the syringe from the side. A needle is attached to the barrel of the syringe at the needle adaptor. The needle passes into the barrel and penetrates the diaphragm of the local anesthetic cartridge. The needle adaptor (screw hub or convertible tip) is removable and sometimes is discarded inadvertently along with the disposable needle.

The *aspirating* syringe has a device, such as a sharp tip (called the *harpoon*) that is attached to the piston and is used to penetrate the thick silicone rubber stopper (bung) at the opposite end of the cartridge (from the needle). Provided the needle is of adequate gauge, when a *negative pressure* is exerted on the thumb ring by the administrator, blood enters into the needle and is visible in the cartridge if the needle tip rests within the lumen of a blood vessel. *Positive pressure* applied to the thumb ring forces local anesthetic into the needle lumen and the patient's tissues wherever the needle tip lies. The thumb ring and finger grips give the administrator added control over the syringe.

Most metallic, breech-loading, aspirating syringes are constructed of chrome-plated brass and stainless steel (Fig. 5-2).

Advantages and disadvantages of the metallic, breech-loading, aspirating syringe are listed in Box 5-2.

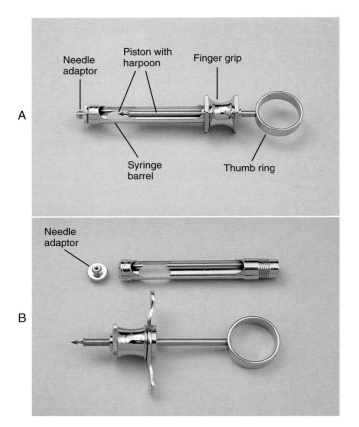

Figure 5-1. **A,** Breech-loading, metallic, cartridge-type syringe; assembled. **B,** Disassembled local anesthetic syringe.

Breech-loading, Plastic, Cartridge-type, Aspirating. A *plastic*, reusable, dental aspirating syringe is available. Because of recent advances in plastics, this syringe is both autoclavable and chemically sterilizable. With proper care and handling, multiple uses may be obtained from this syringe before it is discarded. Advantages and disadvantages of the plastic, reusable, aspirating syringe are listed in Box 5-3.

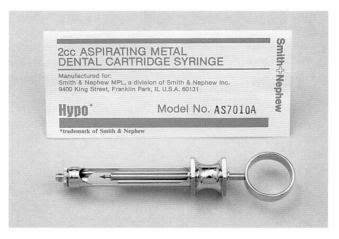

Figure 5-2. Harpoon-type aspirating syringe.

BOX 5-2

Advantages and Disadvantages of the Metallic, Breech-loading, Aspirating Syringe

ADVANTAGES	DISADVANTAGES
Visible cartridge	Weight (heavier than plastic syringe)
Aspiration with one hand	Syringe may be too big for small operators
Autoclavable	
Rust resistant	Possibility of infection with improper care
Long lasting with proper maintenance	

Breech-loading, Metallic, Cartridge-type, Self-aspirating. The potential hazards of intravascular administration of local anesthetics are great and are discussed more fully in Chapter 18. The incidence of positive aspiration may be as high as 10% to 15% in some injection techniques.[3] It is accepted by the dental profession that an aspiration test before administration of a local anesthetic drug is of great importance. Unfortunately, it is abundantly clear that in actual clinical practice too little attention is paid to this procedure (Table 5-1).

With the commonly used breech-loading, metallic, cartridge-type syringes, an aspiration test must be carried out purposefully by the administrator either before or during drug deposition. The key word here is *purposefully*. However, as demonstrated in Table 5-1, many dentists knowingly do not perform an aspiration test before injection of the anesthetic drug.[4]

To increase the ease of aspiration, several self-aspirating syringes have been developed (Fig. 5-3). These syringes use the elasticity of the rubber diaphragm in the anesthetic cartridge to obtain the necessary negative pressure for aspiration. The diaphragm rests on a metal projection inside the syringe that directs the needle into the cartridge (Fig. 5-4). Pressure acting directly on the cartridge

---

BOX 5-3

Advantages and Disadvantages of the Plastic, Reusable, Aspirating Syringe

ADVANTAGES	DISADVANTAGES
Plastic eliminates metallic, clinical look	Size (may be too big for small operators)
Lightweight: provides better "feel" during injection	Possibility of infection with improper care
Cartridge is visible	Deterioration of plastic with repeated autoclaving
Aspiration with one hand	
Rust resistant	
Long lasting with proper maintenance	
Lower cost	

TABLE **5-1**
Percentages of Dentists Who Aspirate Before Injection

Frequency	Inferior Alveolar Nerve Block		Maxillary Infiltration	
	Percent	*Cumulative*	*Percent*	*Cumulative*
Always	63.2		40.2	
Sometimes	14.7	77.9	24.1	64.3
Rarely	9.2	87.1	18.4	82.7
Never	12.9		17.3	

through the thumb disk (Fig. 5-5) or indirectly through the plunger shaft, distorts (stretches) the rubber diaphragm, producing a positive pressure within the anesthetic cartridge. When that pressure is released, sufficient negative pressure develops within the cartridge to permit aspiration. The thumb ring produces twice as much negative pressure as the plunger shaft. The use of a self-aspirating dental syringe permits multiple aspirations to be performed easily throughout the period of local anesthetic deposition.

The self-aspirating syringe was introduced into the United States in 1981. After an initial period of enthusiasm, the popularity of this syringe decreased. Some doctors felt that the self-aspirating syringe did not provide the same reliable degree of aspiration as what was possible with the harpoon-aspirating syringe. It has been demonstrated, however, that this syringe does in fact aspirate as reliably as the harpoon-aspirating syringe.[5-7] The notion can occur that aspiration may not be as reliable with the self-aspirating syringe because the administrator only has to depress and release the thumb ring to aspirate, rather than pulling back on the thumb ring. Moving the thumb off the thumb ring and onto the thumb disk for aspiration also has been mentioned by many doctors as being uncomfortable for them. Although this is the preferred means of obtaining a satisfactory aspiration test with these syringes, pressure adequate for aspiration also may be obtained by simply releasing pressure of the thumb on the thumb ring. The second generation of the self-aspirating syringe has eliminated the thumb disk.

The major factor influencing ability to aspirate is the *gauge of the needle* being used.[7] In addition, most doctors using the harpoon-aspirating syringe tend to overaspirate; that is, they retract the thumb ring back too far and with excessive force (frequently disengaging the harpoon from the stopper). These doctors especially feel insecure with the self-aspirating syringe. Proper technique of aspiration is discussed in Chapter 11. Advantages and disadvantages of the metallic, self-aspirating syringe are listed in Box 5-4.

Pressure Syringes. Introduced in the late 1970s, pressure syringes brought about a renewed interest in the periodontal ligament (PDL) injection (also known as the *intraligamentary injection* [ILI]). Discussed in Chapter 16, the PDL injection, though usable for any tooth, helped make it possible to achieve consistently reliable pulpal anesthesia of one isolated tooth in the mandibular arch where, in the past, nerve block anesthesia (e.g., inferior alveolar nerve block [IANB], Gow-Gates mandibular nerve block), with its attendant prolonged soft-tissue (e.g., lingual) anesthesia, was necessary.

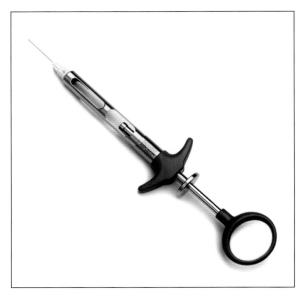

Figure 5-3. Self-aspirating syringe.

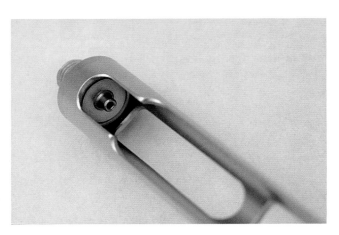

Figure 5-4. A metal projection within the barrel depresses the diaphragm of the local anesthetic cartridge.

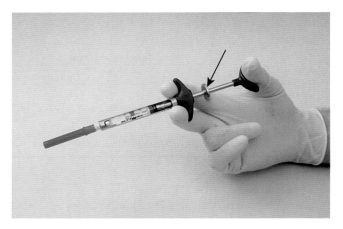

Figure 5-5. Pressure on the thumb disk *(arrow)* increases the pressure within the cartridge. Release of pressure on thumb disk produces self-aspiration test.

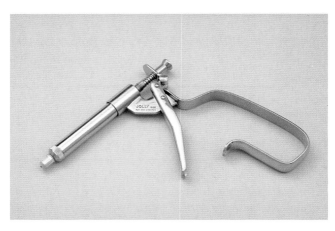

Figure 5-6. Original design of pressure syringe for periodontal ligament injection (PDL) or intraligamentary injection (ILI).

The original pressure devices, Peripress (Universal Dental Implements, Edison, N.J.) and Ligmaject (IMA Associates) (Fig. 5-6), were modeled after a device that was available in dentistry in 1905—the Wilcox-Jewett Obtunder (Fig. 5-7). These first-generation devices, using a pistol-grip, are somewhat larger than the newer, pen-grip devices (Fig. 5-8). Although "special" syringes such as these are not necessary for a successful PDL injection, there are several advantages attendant to their use, not the least of which is the mechanical advantage they give the administrator, making the local anesthetic somewhat easier to administer. This same mechanical advantage, however, makes the injection somewhat "too easy" to administer, leading to a "too-rapid" injection of the anesthetic solution and patient discomfort both during the injection and when the anesthesia has worn off. However, when used slowly, as recommended by the manufacturers, pressure syringes are of some benefit in the administration of this valuable technique of anesthesia.

Pressure syringes offer advantages over the conventional syringe when used for PDL injections because the trigger permits measured dose administration and enables a relatively weak (muscularly) administrator to overcome the significant tissue resistance that is encountered when the technique is administered properly. This mechanical advantage also may prove to be detrimental if the administrator deposits the anesthetic solution too quickly (<20 sec/0.2 ml dose). All of the pressure syringes completely encase the glass dental cartridge with plastic or metal, thereby protecting the patient in the unlikely event that the cartridge cracks or shatters during injection. The original pressure syringes looked somewhat threatening, having the appearance of a gun. Newer devices are smaller and considerably less intimidating.

Probably the greatest disadvantage to the use of the pressure syringe is the cost; most are priced at considerably more than US $200 (June 2004). For this reason among others, it is recommended that pressure devices be considered for use only after the PDL injection has been

---

BOX 5-4

Advantages and Disadvantages of the Metallic, Self-aspirating Syringe

ADVANTAGES	DISADVANTAGES
Cartridge visible	Weight
Easier to aspirate with small hands	Feeling of "insecurity" for doctors accustomed to harpoon-type syringe
Autoclavable	
Rust resistant	Finger must be moved from thumb ring to thumbdisk to aspirate
Long lasting with proper maintenance	
Piston is scored (indicates volume of local anesthetic administered)	Possibility of infection with improper care

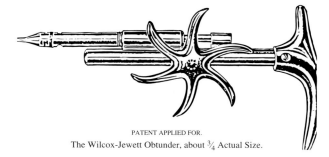

THE WILCOX-JEWETT OBTUNDER.

LEE S. SMITH & SON, PITTSBURG.

PATENT APPLIED FOR.

The Wilcox-Jewett Obtunder, about ¾ Actual Size.

Figure 5-7. Pressure syringe (1905) designed for a peridental injection.

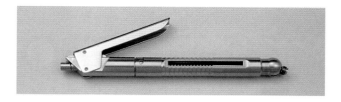

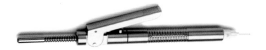

Figure 5-8. Second-generation syringe for PDL injection.

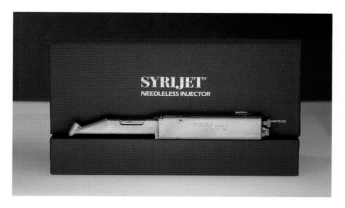

Figure 5-9. SyriJet needleless injector.

found to be ineffective after several attempts with a conventional syringe and needle. Box 5-5 lists the advantages and disadvantages of the pressure syringe.

Jet Injector. In 1947 Figge and Scherer introduced a new approach to parenteral injection, the jet or needle-less injection.[8] This represented the first fundamental change in the basic principles of injection since 1853, when Alexander Wood introduced the hypodermic syringe. The first report of the use of jet injections in dentistry was in 1958 by Margetis and associates.[9] Jet injection is based on the principle that liquids forced through very small openings, called jets, at very high pressure can penetrate intact skin or mucous membrane (visualize water flowing through a garden hose that is being crimped). The most used jet injectors in dentistry are the SyriJet Mark II (Mizzy, Inc.; *www.syrijet.com*) (Fig. 5-9) and the MadaJet (Mada Medical Products, Inc.; *www.madainternational.com*). The SyriJet holds any 1.8 ml dental cartridge of local anesthetic. It is calibrated to deliver 0.05 to 0.2 ml of solution at 2000 psi.

The primary use of the jet injector is to obtain topical anesthesia before the insertion of a needle. In addition, it may be used to obtain mucosal anesthesia of the palate. Regional nerve blocks or supraperiosteal injections still are necessary for complete anesthesia. The jet injector is not an adequate substitute for the more traditional needle and syringe in obtaining pulpal or regional block anesthesia. Additionally, many patients dislike the feeling accompanying use of the jet injector, as well as the possible postinjection soreness of soft tissue that may develop even with proper use of the device. Topical anesthetics, applied properly, serve the same purpose as jet injectors at a fraction of the cost (SyriJet Mark II, US $1595

[December 2003];* MadaJet XL Dental, US $630 [March 2003]) and with minimum risk. Advantages and disadvantages of this method are listed in Box 5-6.

Disposable Syringes

Plastic disposable syringes are available in a variety of sizes with an assortment of needle gauges. Most often they are used for intramuscular or intravenous drug administration but also may be used for intraoral injections.

These syringes contain a Luer-Lok screw-on needle attachment but no aspirating tip. Aspiration can be accomplished by pulling back on the plunger of the syringe before or during injection. Because there is no thumb ring, aspiration with the plastic disposable syringe requires the use of both hands. In addition, these syringes do not accept dental cartridges. The needle, attached to the syringe, must be inserted into a vial or cartridge of local anesthetic drug and an appropriate volume of solution withdrawn. Care must be taken to avoid contaminating the vial during this procedure. Two- and three-milliliter syringes with 23- or 25-gauge needles are recommended when the system is used for intraoral local anesthetic administration.

---

*Mizzy Inc. 616 Hollywood Ave., Cherry Hill, N.J. 08002, 1-800-663-4700, *www.keystoneind.com*.

BOX 5-5

Advantages and Disadvantages of the Pressure Syringe

ADVANTAGES	DISADVANTAGES
Measured dose	Cost
Overcomes tissue resistance	Easy to inject too rapidly
Nonthreatening (new devices)	Threatening (original devices)
Cartridges protected	

BOX 5-6

Advantages and Disadvantages of the Jet Injector

ADVANTAGES	DISADVANTAGES
Does not require use of needle (recommended for needle phobics)	Inadequate for pulpal anesthesia or for regional block
Delivers very small volumes of local anesthetic (0.01 to 0.2 ml)	Some patients are disturbed by the "jolt" of the injection
Used in lieu of topical anesthetics	Cost
	May damage periodontal tissues

Use of the plastic, disposable, non–cartridge-containing syringe is not recommended for routine use. Its use should be considered only when a traditional syringe is not available or cannot be used, such as in situations of severe latex allergy where glass ampules of local anesthetics must be used in medical syringes. This system is also practical when diphenhydramine is used as a local anesthetic in cases of presumed local anesthetic allergy (see Chapter 18). Box 5-7 lists the advantages and disadvantages of the disposable syringe.

Safety Syringes

In recent years there has been a move toward the development and introduction of "safety" syringes in both medicine and dentistry.* Use of a safety syringe minimizes the risk of accidental needle-stick injury occurring to a dental health provider with a contaminated needle after the administration of a local anesthetic. These syringes possess a sheath that "locks" over the needle when it is removed from the patient's tissues, preventing accidental needle stick.

Devices, such as the UltraSafety Plus XL,* the Hypo Safety Syringe,[†] and the 1 Shot Safety Syringe,[‡] were available as of July 2004.

The UltraSafety Plus XL aspirating syringe system contains a syringe body assembly and plunger assembly (Fig. 5-10). Once the syringe is properly assembled and the injection administered, the syringe may be made "safe" with one hand by gently moving the index and middle fingers against the front collar of the guard (Fig. 5-11). Once "guarded," the now-contaminated needle is "safe," so that it is virtually impossible to be injured with the needle. The entire syringe is discarded into the proper receptacle (e.g., sharps container).

Safety Plus is similar although somewhat different in design. It consists of an autoclavable syringe handle and a disposable self-contained injection unit. The dental anesthetic cartridge is clearly visible because the clear plastic design of the injection unit makes the result of

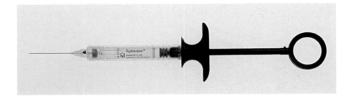

Figure 5-10. UltraSafety Plus XL aspirating syringe, ready for injection.

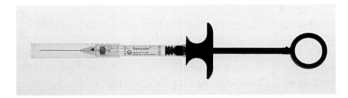

Figure 5-11. UltraSafety Plus XL aspirating syringe; needle sheathed to prevent needle-stick injury.

aspiration easy to discern. The cartridge also incorporates a self-aspiration system similar to those described previously. After the injection is completed the autoprotective system is used, markedly diminishing the risk of accidental needle-stick injury. The system provides two options after the injection. The protective sheath can be slid forward to an intermediate locking position, if multiple injections are necessary, or to the final locking position for safe disposal.

All dental safety syringes are designed to be single-use items (changed after each injection), although they both permit reinjection. Reloading the syringe with a second anesthetic cartridge and reinjecting with the same syringe is discouraged because this obviates the important safety aspect of the device.

Almost a year's clinical experience with safety syringe systems has demonstrated the ease with which these systems may be learned, their simplicity, and the importance of the safety syringe. Use of a safety syringe system is strongly recommended.

The advantages and disadvantages of the safety syringe are listed in Box 5-8.

Computer-Controlled Local Anesthetic Delivery Systems

The standard dental syringe described previously is a simple mechanical instrument that dates back to 1853 when Charles Pravaz patented the first syringe.[10] The dental syringe is a drug delivery device requiring that the operator simultaneously attempt to control the variables of drug infusion and the movement of a penetrating needle. The operator's inability to precisely control both of these activities during an injection can compromise an injection technique. In addition, a traditional syringe is handled with a palm-thumb grasp, which is not designed for ideal ergonomics or needle control during the injection. For certain practitioners—those with small hands—just

*UltraSafety Plus XL—Septodont, Inc. 245C Quigley Blvd., New Castle, Del. 19720, 1-800-872-8305, *www.septodontinc.com.*

[†]Hypo Safety Syringe—Dentsply MPL Technologies, 9400 King St., Franklin Park, Ill. 60131, 1-800-621-6421, *www.dentsply.com.*

[†]1 Shot Safety Syringe – Sultan Chemists, Englewood, N.J., 1-800-637-8582, www.sultanintl.com.

holding a syringe with a full cartridge of anesthetic may be difficult.

In 1997 the first computer controlled local anesthetic delivery (CCLAD) system was introduced into dentistry. The Wand (recently renamed: *The Wand/CompuDent*; Milestone Scientific, Inc., Livingston, NJ) was designed to improve on the ergonomics and precision of the dental syringe (Fig. 5-12). The system enables a dentist or hygienist to accurately manipulate needle placement with fingertip accuracy and deliver the local anesthetic with a foot-activated control (Fig. 5-13). The lightweight handpiece (Fig. 5-14) is held in a penlike grasp that provides increased tactile sensation and control compared with the traditional syringe. The available flow rates of local anesthetic delivery are computer controlled and thus remain consistent from one injection to the next. The CCLAD system represents a significant change in the manner in

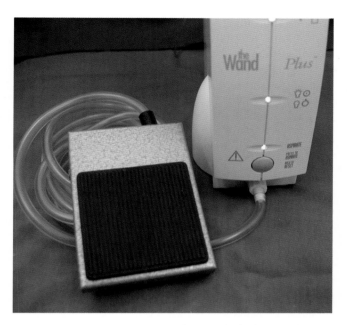

Figure 5-13. Foot-activated control of The Wand.

which a local anesthetic injection is administered. The operator focuses attention on needle insertion and positioning, allowing the motor in the device to administer the drug at a preprogrammed rate of flow. It is likely that the greater ergonomic control coupled with the fixed flow rates are responsible for an improved injection experience, as demonstrated in many clinical studies conducted with this device in dentistry.[11-15] Several clinical trials in medicine also have demonstrated measurable benefits of this technology.[16,17]

Hochman and associates were the first to demonstrate a marked reduction in pain perception for injections using CCLADs.[11] Fifty blindfolded dentists participated (they received the injection) in a controlled clinical study comparing the standard manual syringe with *The Wand/CompuDent* system for palatal injections. Forty-eight (96%)

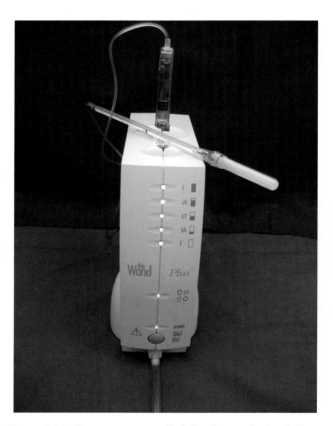

Figure 5-12. Computer-controlled local anesthetic delivery system—The Wand.

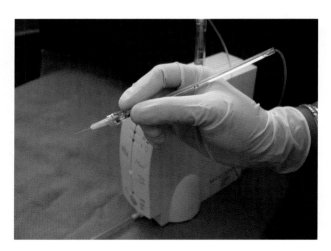

Figure 5-14. The Wand has a lightweight handpiece that provides an increase in tactile sensation and control.

preferred injections with the CCLADs. The overall pain perception was reduced twofold to threefold when compared with the standard manual syringe.

Nicholson and associates conducted a randomized clinical study using two operators administering four different types of dental injections comparing the CCLADs with the standard syringe.[13] Mean injection discomfort ratings were found to be consistently lower when using CCLADs compared with the manual syringe. Two-thirds of the patients preferred future dental injections to be performed with a CCLAD system. The investigators in the study increasingly preferred to perform all injections with CCLAD technology.

Loomer and Perry presented data from a single blind crossover study comparing CCLADs with traditional syringe delivery of local anesthetic for quadrant scaling and root planing. Twenty subjects received the new palatal injection, the AMSA injection (described in Chapter 13). Scores for the AMSA computer-controlled injection revealed highly significant difference in favor of the computer-controlled device ($p < 0.0001$).[14]

Fukayama and associates conducted a controlled clinical study evaluating pain perception of a CCLAD device. Seventeen of the 20 subjects reported a slight or no-pain rating on a visual analogue scale (VAS) for palatal injections administered with CCLADs. They concluded, "The new system provides comfortable anesthesia for patients and can be a good alternative for conventional manual syringe injection."[15]

At present, two CCLADs are available in the North American market: *The Wand/CompuDent* system and the *Comfort Control Syringe*. Another system, the *QuickSleeper*, is marketed in Europe. Similar devices, such as the *Anaeject*, are marketed in Japan (Fig. 5-15).

The Wand/CompuDent. *The Wand/CompuDent* system* utilizes a single-use disposable "safety" handpiece (Fig. 5-16). A conventional medical Luer-Lok needle (not a traditional dental needle) is attached to the handle. Luer-Lok needles are available in lengths and gauges similar to conventional dental needles. The handle (the "Wand") attaches to a cartridge holder via a 60-inch microtube, the inner diameter of which is 0.013 inch and can hold a volume of less than 0.2 ml of fluid. The cartridge holder accepts any standard 1.8 ml dental anesthetic cartridge.

The Wand handpiece provides increased tactile control and ergonomics.[11,18] In two clinical trials operators were able to achieve a more comfortable needle puncture for patients when using The Wand handpiece compared with the traditional syringe.[15,17] This was attributed to the lightweight ergonomically designed handpiece allowing for enhanced tactile sensation.

The Wand handpiece is also less threatening to the patient compared with other injection devices. Kudo and associates compared 10 different injection delivery systems.[19] *The Wand/CompuDent* system was rated the least anxiety-producing injection instrument based on the visual appearance. This may also explain why Gibson and associates found disruptive behavior in pediatric patients to be significantly reduced when using this same equipment.[12]

The penlike grasp has the additional advantage of allowing the operator to rotate the handpiece during penetration and insertion. Hochman and Friedman demonstrated that rotation of the handpiece and needle minimizes both needle deflection and the force necessary for tissue penetration during needle insertions.[20,21]

---

*The Wand/CompuDent: www.milesci.com, 1-800-862-1125.

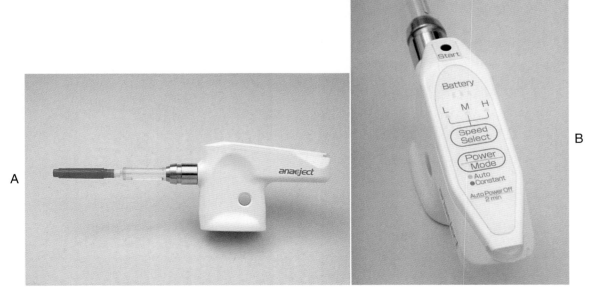

Figure 5-15. A and **B,** Anaeject computer-controlled local anesthetic delivery system.

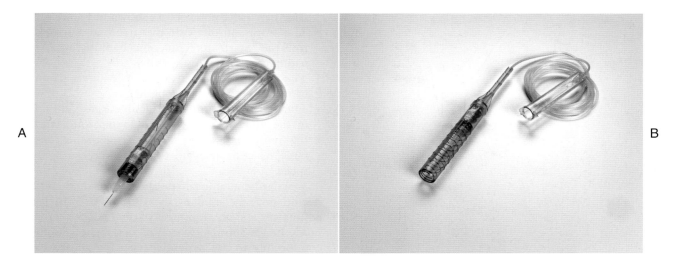

Figure 5-16. The Wand single-use disposable "safety" handpiece. **A,** Needle "open." **B,** Needle "safe."

Greater accuracy can be obtained for injections such as the inferior alveolar block injection where deeper tissue penetration is necessary.

The Wand/CompuDent system administers local anesthetic at two specific rates of delivery. The slow rate is 0.5 ml/min and the fast rate is 1.8 ml/min. An aspiration test can be activated at anytime by simply releasing the pressure on the foot-rheostat starting a 4.5-second aspiration cycle.

The Wand/CompuDent system delivers a controlled rate of flow and controls the pressure developing within the tissues as the local anesthetic is introduced. When injecting into denser tissues (with low elasticity) such as on the palate or in the PDL space using a standard manual syringe, the operator encounters significant resistance. More pressure must be applied to the plunger to overcome this resistance for the local anesthetic to be deposited into the tissue. This results in the production of extremely high pressures within nonresilient tissues, leading to pain or tissue damage. The traditional syringe possesses a mechanical design that does not allow pressure and flow rate to be precisely controlled. Pressures generated with a traditional syringe have been shown to be as high as 600 psi or even more.[22] Histological studies of the PDL injection performed with a traditional syringe demonstrated severe tissue damage from the high pressures produced with these delivery instruments.[23–25]

The Wand/CompuDent system permits both a precise rate of flow and a controlled pressure to be maintained irrespective of the type of tissue into which the local anesthetic is being deposited. Therefore even tissues with low elasticity receive a constant pressure and rate of flow, resulting in a more favorable (e.g., comfortable, less tissue damage) outcome. This has been demonstrated in a recent histological study reporting findings of minimal inflammatory changes when performing a PDL injection.[26] The controlled rate of fluid administration also explains the reduced pain perception noted by most patients during dental injections into tissues that typically elicit a high pain response (e.g., the hard palate, attached gingival, and periodontal ligament).[11]

Many doctors have found that as a result of these unique characteristics of CCLADs, most traditional dental injection techniques can be performed with greater predictability and with less discomfort. CCLAD technology has led to the development of two newly described nerve block techniques that recently have been reported in the dental literature. The anterior middle superior alveolar (AMSA)[27] injection and palatal approach-anterior superior alveolar (P-ASA)[28] injection have been described by Friedman and Hochman using the CCLADs. Both injections can be performed with a traditional syringe; however, the infusion characteristics and improved tactile control of a CCLAD system allows for more effective and comfortable drug administration. Both injections are described in Chapter 13. The advantages and disadvantages of *The Wand/CompuDent* system are listed in Box 5-9.

BOX 5-9

Advantages and Disadvantages of *The Wand/CompuDent* System

ADVANTAGES	DISADVANTAGES
Precise control of flow rate and pressure produces a more comfortable injection even in tissues with low elasticity (e.g., palate, attached gingiva, periodontal ligament)	Requires additional armamentarium Cost
Increased tactile "feel" and ergonomics from the lightweight Wand handpiece	
Nonthreatening (Wand)	
Automatic aspiration	
Rotational insertion technique minimizes needle deflection	

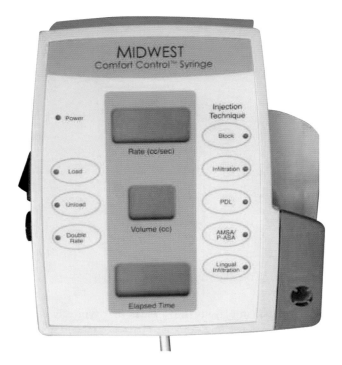

Figure 5-17. Computer-controlled local anesthetic delivery system—Comfort Control Syringe.

Comfort Control Syringe. Introduced several years after The Wand, the Comfort Control Syringe (CCS) system attempts to improve on the CCLAD concept. The CCS system is an electronic, preprogrammed delivery device that provides the operator with the control needed to make the patient's local anesthetic injection experience as pleasant as possible (Fig. 5-17). As with other CCLADs, this is achieved by depositing the local anesthetic more slowly and consistently than is possible manually. The CCS has a two-stage delivery system; the injection begins at an extremely slow rate to prevent the pain associated with quick delivery. After 10 seconds, the CCS automatically increases speed to the preprogrammed injection rate for the technique selected. There are five preprogrammed injection rates for specific injections.

The handpiece controls are shown in Figure 5-18.
- The front button with the arrow and square controls the "Start/Stop" functions by initiating or terminating the selected program.
- The middle button activates the "Aspiration" function by slightly retracting the plunger.
- The rear button initiates "Double Rate" and operates in the same manner as the Double Rate button on the unit. It doubles the preprogrammed injection rate. Selecting it again resumes the preprogrammed speed.

Standard dental local anesthetic cartridges and dental needles may be used in the CCS. Box 5-10 lists the advantages and disadvantages of the CCS.

CCLADs allow local anesthetics to be administered comfortably to the patient in virtually all areas of the oral cavity. This is of greatest importance in the palate, where the level of patient discomfort can be significant. The nasopalatine nerve block may be administered atraumatically in most patients. It is reasonable to conclude that any injection technique that has even a remote possibility of being uncomfortable to the patient can be delivered much more comfortably using a CCLAD device.

CARE AND HANDLING OF SYRINGES

Properly maintained, metal and plastic reusable syringes are designed to provide long-term service. Following is a summary of manufacturers' recommendations concerning care of these syringes:

1. After each use, the syringe should be thoroughly washed and rinsed so as to be free of any local anesthetic solution, saliva, or other foreign matter. The syringe should be autoclaved in the same manner as other surgical instruments.
2. After every five autoclavings, the syringe should be dismantled and all threaded joints and the area where the piston contacts the thumb ring and guide bearing should be lightly lubricated.

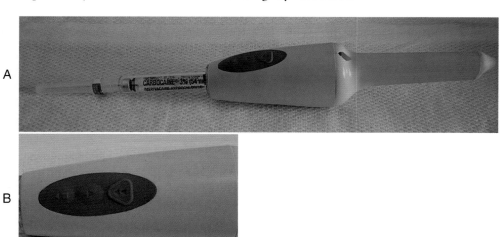

Figure 5-18. The handpiece of the Comfort Control Syringe.

BOX 5-10

Advantages and Disadvantages of the Comfort Control Syringe

ADVANTAGES	DISADVANTAGES
Familiar "syringe" type of delivery system	Requires additional armamentarium
Easy to see exactly how much local anesthetic solution has been dispensed, just like on a manual syringe	More bulky than other computer-controlled or manual local anesthesia delivery devices
Inexpensive disposables (~50¢/use)	More bulky than other computer-controlled local anesthetic delivery (CCLAD) systems or manual local anesthesia delivery devices
All controls literally at your fingertips	
Less costly than other CCLADs	
Allows selection of various rates of delivery matched to the injection technique utilized	Vibration may bother some users
	Cost

3. The harpoon should be cleaned with a brush after each use.
4. Although the harpoon is designed for long-term use, prolonged use will result in decreased sharpness and failure to remain embedded within the stopper of the cartridge. Replacement pistons and harpoons are readily available at low cost.

PROBLEMS

Leakage during Injection

When a syringe is reloaded with a second local anesthetic cartridge and a needle is already in place, care must be taken to ensure that the needle penetrates the center of the rubber diaphragm. An off-center perforation produces an ovoid puncture of the diaphragm that allows leakage of the anesthetic solution around the outside of the metal needle and into the patient's mouth (Fig. 5-19). (For further information, see Chapter 7.)

Broken Cartridge

A badly worn syringe may damage the cartridge, leading to breakage. This also can result from a bent harpoon. A needle that is bent at its proximal end (Fig. 5-20) may not perforate the diaphragm on the cartridge. Positive pressure on the thumb ring increases pressure within the cartridge, which may cause the cartridge to break.

Bent Harpoon

The harpoon must be sharp and straight (Fig. 5-21). A bent harpoon produces an off-center puncture of the rubber plunger, causing the plunger to rotate as it moves down the glass cartridge. This occasionally results in cartridge breakage.

Disengagement of the Harpoon from the Plunger during Aspiration

Disengagement occurs if the harpoon is dull or the administrator applies too much pressure to the thumb ring during aspiration. If this occurs the harpoon should be cleaned and sharpened or replaced with a new sharp harpoon. Disengagement is most likely to occur when a 30-gauge dental needle is being used because there is significant resistance produced within the needle lumen as aspiration is attempted. A very gentle backward motion of the plunger is all that is necessary for successful aspiration. Forceful action is not necessary. (See the discussion in Chapter 11.)

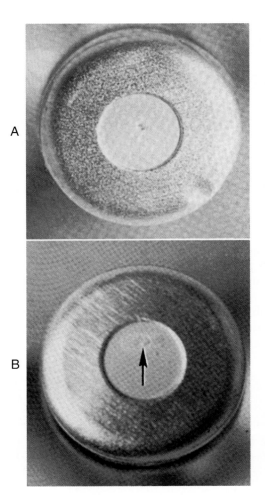

Figure 5-19. A, Centric perforation of the diaphragm by a needle prevents leakage during injection. **B,** Off-center perforation (*arrow*) permits leakage of anesthetic solution into the patient's mouth.

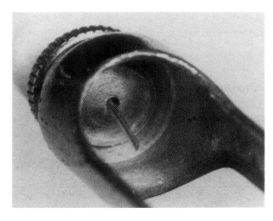

Figure 5-20. A needle bent at the proximal end may not perforate the cartridge diaphragm. Pressure on the thumb ring can lead to cartridge breakage.

Surface Deposits

An accumulation of debris, saliva, and disinfectant solution interferes with syringe function and appearance. Deposits, which can resemble rust, may be removed with a thorough scrubbing. Ultrasonic cleaning will not harm syringes.

RECOMMENDATIONS

There is no conclusive evidence that any manufacturer's syringe is superior. Therefore the ultimate decision in selection of a syringe must be left to the discretion of the buyer. It is recommended, however, that before purchasing any syringe, the buyer place a full dental cartridge into it and pick up the syringe as if to use it. It should be noted whether the fingers (thumb to other fingers) are stretched maximally because to aspirate with a harpoon-type syringe, one must be able to pull the thumb ring back several millimeters. If one is not able to do so, reliable aspiration is not possible. Although all syringes available today are of roughly the same dimensions, some variation does exist. Some manufacturers market syringes with smaller thumb rings or shorter pistons. These modifications make aspiration easier to accomplish for persons with smaller hands.

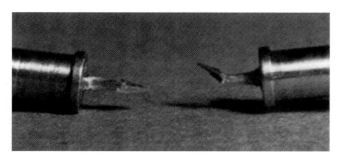

Figure 5-21. Notice the bent harpoon of the syringe on the right.

Following are additional recommendations:
1. A safety syringe, minimizing the risk of accidental needle-stick injury, is strongly recommended for use during all local anesthetic injections.
2. A self-aspirating syringe is recommended for practitioners with small hands.
3. Any syringe system used must be capable of aspiration. Nonaspirating syringes should *never* be used for local anesthetic injections.
4. All reusable syringes must be capable of being sterilized.
5. Nonreusable syringes must be disposed of properly.

REFERENCES

1. Council on Dental Materials and Devices: New American National Standards Institute/American Dental Association specification no. 34 for dental aspirating syringes, *J Am Dent Assoc* 97:236-238, 1978.
2. Council on Dental Materials, Instruments, and Equipment: Addendum to American National Standards Institute/American Dental Association specification no. 34 for dental aspirating syringes, *J Am Dent Assoc* 104:69-70, 1982.
3. Bartlett SZ: Clinical observations on the effects of injections of local anesthetic preceded by aspiration, *Oral Surg* 33:520, 1972.
4. Malamed SF: *Handbook of local anesthesia*, St Louis, 1980, Mosby.
5. Meechan JG, Blair GS, McCabe JF: Local anaesthesia in dental practice: II. A laboratory investigation of a self-aspirating system, *Br Dent J* 159:109-113, 1985.
6. Meechan JG: A comparison of three different automatic aspirating dental cartridge syringes, *J Dent* 16:40-43, 1988.
7. Peterson JK: Efficacy of a self-aspirating syringe, *Int J Oral Maxillfac Surg* 16:241-244, 1987.
8. Figge FHJ, Scherer RP: Anatomical studies on jet penetration of human skin for subcutaneous medication without the use of needles, *Anat Rec* 97:335, 1947 (abstract).
9. Margetis PM, Quarantillo EP, Lindberg RB: Jet injection local anesthesia in dentistry: a report of 66 cases, *US Armed Forces Med J* 9:625-634, 1958.
10. Hoffmann-Axthelm W: *History of dentistry*, Chicago, 1981, Quintessence, p 339.
11. Hochman MN, Chiarello D, Hochman CB, Lopatkin R, Pergola S: Computerized local anesthesia delivery vs. traditional syringe technique, *NY State Dent J* 63:24-29, 1997.
12. Gibson RS, Allen K, Hutfless S, Beiraghi S: The Wand vs. traditional injection: a comparison of pain related behaviors, *Pediatric Dent* 22:458-462, 2000.
13. Nicholson JW, Berry TG, Summitt JB, Yuan CH, Witten TM: Pain perception and utility: a comparison of the syringe and computerized local injection techniques, *Gen Dent* 167-172, 2001.
14. Perry DA, Loomer PM: Maximizing Pain Control. The AMSA Injection can provide anesthesia with few injections and less pain, *Dimensions Dent Hyg* 1:28-33, 2003.
15. Fukayama H, Yoshikawa F, Kohase H, Umino M, Suzuki N: Efficacy of anterior and middle superior alveolar (AMSA) anesthesia using a new injection system: the Wand, *Quint Int* 34:737-541, 2003.
16. Tan PY, Vukasin P, Chin ID, et al: The Wand local anesthetic delivery system, *Dis Colon Rectum* 44:686-689, 2001.

17. Landsman A, DeFronzo D, Hedman J, McDonald J: A new system for decreasing the level of injection pain associated with local anesthesia of a toe, *Am Acad Podiat Med* 2001; (abstract).

18. Friedman MJ, Hochman MN: 21st century computerized injection for local pain control, *Compend Contin Educ Dent* 18:995-1003, 1997.

19. Kudo M, Ohke H, Katagiri K, et al: The shape of local anesthetic injection syringes with less discomfort and anxiety. Evaluation of discomfort and anxiety caused by various types of local anesthetic injection syringes in high level trait-anxiety people, *J Jpn Dent Soc Anesthesiol* 29:173-178, 2001.

20. Hochman MN, Friedman MJ: In vitro study of needle deflection: a linear insertion technique versus a bi-directional rotation insertion technique, *Quint Int* 31:737-743, 2000.

21. Hochman MN, Friedman MJ: An in vitro study of needle force penetration comparing a standard linear insertion to the new bidirectional rotation insertion technique, *Quint Int* 32:789-796, 2001.

22. Pashley EL, Nelson R, Pashley DH: Pressures created by dental injections, *J Dent Res* 60:1742-1748, 1981.

23. Fuhs QM, Walker WA, Gouigh RW, Schindler WB, Hartman KS: The periodontal ligament injection: histological effects on the periodontium in dogs, *J Endodont* 9:411-415, 1983.

24. Galili D, Kaufman E, Garfunkel AA, Michaeli Y: Intraligamentary anesthesia: a histological study, *Int J Oral Surg* 12:511-516, 1984.

25. Albers DD, Ellinger RF: Histologic effects of high-pressure intraligamental injections on the periodontal ligament, *Quint Int* 19:361-363, 1988.

26. Froum SJ, Tarnow D, Caiazzo A, Hochman MN: Histologic response to intraligament injections using a computerized local anesthetic delivery system. A pilot study in Mini-Swine, *J Periodont* 71:1453-1459, 2000.

27. Friedman MJ, Hochman MN: The AMSA injection: a new concept for local anesthesia of maxillary teeth using a computer-controlled injection system, *Quint Int* 29:297-303, 1998.

28. Friedman MJ, Hochman MN: P-ASA block injection: a new palatal technique to anesthetize maxillary anterior teeth, *J Esthet Dent* 11:23-71, 1999.

The Needle

TYPES

The needle permits the local anesthetic solution to travel from the dental cartridge into the tissues surrounding the needle tip. Most needles used in dentistry are stainless steel and are disposable. Other needles are constructed of platinum or an iridium-platinum or ruthenium-platinum alloy. The stainless steel needle is highly recommended. Needles currently available for dental practices are presterilized and disposable.

Reusable needles should not be used for injections.

Because the needle represents the most dangerous component of the armamentarium, the one most likely to produce injury to patient or doctor, "safety needles" are being developed.[1] Although these needles are not yet widely used in dentistry, it is probable that within the next decade their use will become commonplace.

PARTS

The needle is composed of a single piece of tubular metal around which is placed plastic or a metal syringe adaptor and the needle hub (Fig. 6-1).

All needles have the following components in common: the bevel, the shaft, the hub, and the cartridge-penetrating end (Fig. 6-2).

The *bevel* defines the point or tip of the needle. Bevels are described by manufacturers as long, medium, and short. Several authors have confirmed that the greater the angle of the bevel with the long axis of the needle, the greater will be the degree of deflection as the needle passes through hydrocolloid (or the soft tissues of the

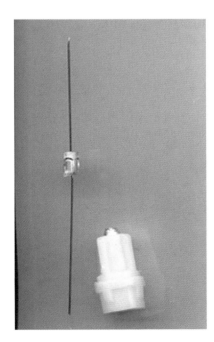

Figure 6-1. Metal disposable needle, dissembled.

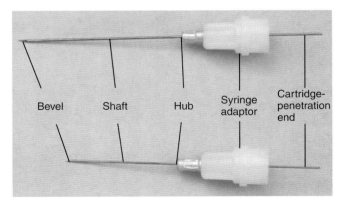

Figure 6-2. Components of dental local anesthetic needle. Long needle *(top)*; short needle *(bottom)*.

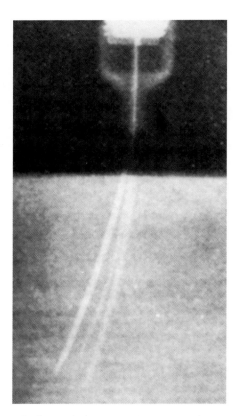

Figure 6-3. Radiograph demonstrating varying degrees of needle deflection with different gauges (left to right, 30, 27, and 25). (From Robison SE, et al: Comparative study of deflection characteristics and fragility of 25-, 27- and 30-gauge short dental needles, *J Am Dent Assoc* 109:920-924, 1984.)

mouth) (Fig. 6-3).[2-4] A needle whose point is centered on the long axis (e.g., the Huber point and the Truject needle; Fig. 6-4) will deflect less than a beveled-point needle whose point is eccentric (Fig. 6-5; Table 6-1).

Several manufacturers of dental needles have placed indicators on the plastic or metal hub to help orient the doctor to the position of the bevel.

The *shaft* of the needle is one long piece of tubular metal running from the tip of the needle, through the hub, and continuing to the piece that penetrates the cartridge (see Fig. 6-1). Two factors to be considered about this component of the needle are the diameter of its lumen (e.g., the needle gauge) and the length of the shaft from point to hub.

The *hub* is a plastic or metal piece through which the needle attaches to the syringe. The interior surface of the

plastic syringe adaptor of the needle is not prethreaded; therefore to attach a plastic-hubbed needle to a syringe, the needle must be pushed toward the syringe while it is being attached. Metallic-hubbed needles are prethreaded.

The *cartridge-penetrating end* of the dental needle extends through the needle adaptor and perforates the diaphragm of the local anesthetic cartridge. Its tip rests within the cartridge.

When needles are selected for use in various injection techniques, the two factors that must be considered are the *gauge* and the *length*.

GAUGE

Gauge refers to the diameter of the lumen of the needle: the smaller the number, the greater the diameter of the lumen. A 30-gauge needle has a smaller internal diameter than a 25-gauge needle. In the United States, needles are color-coded by gauge (Fig. 6-6).

There is a growing trend toward the use of smaller-diameter (higher number gauge) needles, based on the assumption that they are less traumatic to the patient than needles with larger diameters (Table 6-2). This assumption is unwarranted.[5] Hamburg[6] demonstrated in 1972 that patients cannot differentiate among 23-, 25-, 27-, and 30-gauge needles. A clinical experiment proves this point:
1. Several needles—25-, 27-, and 30-gauge—should be selected.
2. The buccal mucosa over the maxillary anterior teeth should be dried.
3. No topical anesthetic should be used.
4. The mucosa should be taut.
5. The mucosa should be gently penetrated (about 2 to 3 mm) with each needle without revealing to the patient which needle is being used. A different site should be selected for each penetration.
6. The patient should be questioned about the needles: Which was felt the most? Which the least?

In hundreds of clinical demonstrations, no patient could correctly determine the gauge of each needle. The usual response has been that he or she could not discern any difference.

Larger-gauge needles (e.g., 25-gauge) have distinct advantages over smaller ones (Box 6-1): *Less deflection* occurs as the needle passes through tissues (see Table 6-1 and Fig. 6-3). This leads to *greater accuracy* in needle

Figure 6-4. The tip of a nondeflecting needle is located in the center of the shaft, thereby minimizing deflection as the needle penetrates soft tissues.

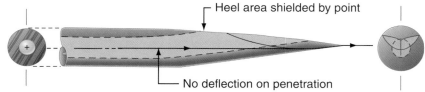

Heel area shielded by point

No deflection on penetration

Inside diameter 0.008 inch; same as 27-gauge
Outside diameter 0.014 inch

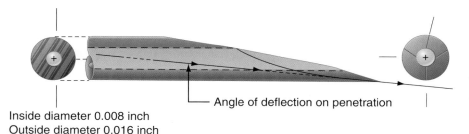

Inside diameter 0.008 inch
Outside diameter 0.016 inch
27-gauge needle with standard point

Figure 6-5. Conventional dental needle. The needle tip lies at the lower edge of the needle shaft, thereby producing deflection as the needle passes through soft tissue.

insertion and, hopefully, to increased success rates, especially for techniques in which the depth of soft tissue being penetrated is significant (e.g., the inferior alveolar, Gow-Gates mandibular, Akinosi-Vazirani mandibular, and ASA [infraorbital] nerve blocks). Needle breakage, although not common with disposable needles, is much less likely to occur with a larger needle. Numerous authors[7-10] have stated that aspiration of blood is easier and more reliable through a larger lumen. Foldes and McNall[7] reported the following findings based on an unpublished study by Monheim:

1. One hundred percent positive aspirations were achieved from blood vessels with 25-gauge needles.
2. Eighty-seven percent positive aspirations were achieved from blood vessels with 27-gauge needles.
3. Two percent positive aspirations were achieved from blood vessels with 30-gauge needles.

Trapp and Davies,[11] however, reported that in vivo human blood may be aspirated through 23-, 25-, 27-, and 30-gauge needles without a clinically significant difference in resistance to flow.

Despite this ambiguity concerning ability to aspirate blood through various-gauge needles, the use of larger needles (e.g., 25-gauge) is recommended for any injection technique used in a highly vascular area or when needle deflection through soft tissue would be a factor. Although blood may be aspirated through all 23- through 30-gauge needles, more pressure is necessary to aspirate when smaller-gauge needles are used, increasing the likelihood that the harpoon will become dislodged from the rubber plunger during aspiration.

Industry standards for needle gauge have been in place for years (Table 6-3), yet Wittrock and Fischer[12] showed in 1968 that variations in internal diameter do exist, and 35 years later such differences are still encountered. Larger-gauge needles (e.g., 25-gauge) should be used when there is a greater risk of positive aspiration, as during an inferior alveolar, posterior superior alveolar, or mental or incisive nerve block.

The most commonly used (e.g., most purchased) needles in dentistry are the 27-gauge long, and the 30-gauge short.[13] The 25-gauge, however, is the preferred needle for all injections presenting a high risk of positive aspiration. The 27-gauge can be used for all other injection techniques, provided the aspiration percentage is low and tissue penetration depth is not great (increased deflection). The 30-gauge needle is not specifically recommended for any injection, although it may be used in instances of local infiltration, as when obtaining hemostasis during periodontal therapy.

TABLE 6-1
Deflection of Needles Inserted in Hydrocolloid Tubes to Their Hubs

Needle Type	Length (mm, Tip to Hub)	Maximum Tip Deflection (mm, ± SD)
25-Gauge long (conventional)	35	7.1 ± 0.81*
27-Gauge long (conventional)	36	8.4 ± 1.2*
27-Gauge short (conventional)	26	4.6 ± 0.97†
28-Gauge long (nondeflecting)	31	1.1 ± 0.82
28-Gauge short (nondeflecting)	22	0.8 ± 0.91

Data modified from Jeske AH, Boshart BF: Deflection of conventional versus non-deflecting dental needles in vitro, *Anesth Prog* 32:62-64, 1985.
*A statistically significant difference from the nondeflecting long needle ($p < 0.01$); n = 10 needles in each group.
†A statistically significant difference from the nondeflecting short needle ($p < 0.01$); n = 10 needles in each group.

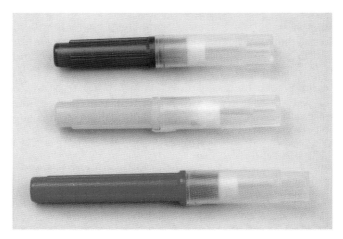

Figure 6-6. Color-coding by needle gauge: 25-gauge, red; 27-gauge, yellow; 30-gauge, blue.

TABLE **6-2**
Needle Gauges Used in Practice

Gauge	Inferior Alveolar Nerve Block (%)	Maxillary Infiltration (%)
23	1.1	0.0
25	66.9	19.1
27	32.0	60.1
30	0.0	20.8

TABLE **6-3**
Specifications for Needle Gauges

Gauge	Outer Diameter [mm]	Inner Diameter [mm]
7	4.57	3.81
8	4.19	3.43
10	3.40	2.69
11	3.05	2.39
12	2.77	2.16
13	2.41	1.80
14	2.11	1.60
15	1.83	1.32
16	1.65	1.19
17	1.50	1.04
18	1.27	0.84
19	1.07	0.69
20	0.91	0.58
21	0.81	0.51
22	0.71	0.41
23	0.64	0.33
25	0.51	0.25
26	0.46	0.25
27	0.41	0.20
30	0.31	0.15

Dental needle gauges highlighted.

Deflection becomes important when a needle must penetrate a greater thickness of soft tissue. On the standard dental needle (see Fig. 6-5), the tip of the point is located eccentrically. As the needle penetrates soft tissue, the point of the needle is deflected by the tissue through which it passes. The greater the angle of the bevel, the greater is the degree of needle deflection. Every decade or so a needle is introduced on which the tip of the point is located in the center of the lumen, thereby minimizing deflection as the needle passes through soft tissue (see Fig. 6-4). Jeske and Boshart[2] demonstrated the effectiveness of this "non-deflecting" needle (see Table 6-1). However, it needs to be shown clinically that a lesser degree of needle deflection occurring as the needle passes through soft tissues actually results in an increased rate of successful anesthesia compared with that observed with standard needles. Over years of use, dentists become accustomed to the deflecting needles they use and, over time, modify their injection techniques to accommodate this deflection. Change to a nondeflecting needle might initially lead to lower success rates.

Minimizing Needle Deflection: Rotational Insertion Technique

A new approach to reducing needle deflection has been described. The technique of rotational insertion (described as bi-rotational insertion technique [BRIT]), a technique in which the operator rotates the handpiece or needle in a back-and-forth rotational movement while advancing the needle through tissues, is similar to techniques used for acupuncture or endodontic instrumentation. Hochman and Friedman demonstrated that needle deflection could be virtually eliminated by using a rotational insertion technique during needle movement.[14] An in vitro study of 60 needle insertions was performed into a tissuelike medium with three different needle gauges comparing

rotational insertion to the traditional linear nonrotating insertion technique. The study demonstrated that deflectional bending of a needle could be minimized or eliminated, regardless of the length or gauge of a needle, as long as the insertion was performed using the rotational insertion technique.

Deflection of a needle is a consequence of the resultant forces acting on the needle bevel during tissue penetration and advancement. An eccentric pointed beveled needle generates several different forces that act on it during insertion when a nonrotating linear insertion technique is used. A linear insertion technique is the conventional technique used with the traditional dental syringe that is typically held with a palm-thumb grasp (Fig. 6-7). During this type of insertion a force perpendicular to the forward directional movement (vector) acts on the surface of the

BOX 6-1

Advantages of Larger-Gauge Needles Over Smaller-Gauge Needles

1. Less deflection, as needle advances through tissues
2. Greater accuracy in injection
3. Less chance of needle breakage
4. Easier aspiration
5. No perceptual difference in patient comfort

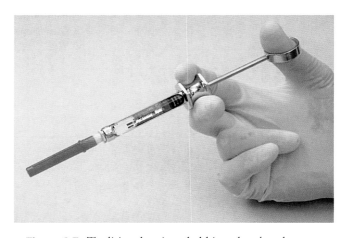

Figure 6-7. Traditional syringe held in palm-thumb grasp.

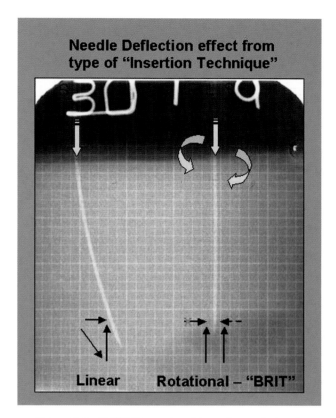

Figure 6-8. BRIT (birotational insertion technique).

eccentrically beveled needles to travel in a straight path. The traditional handheld syringe requires a palm-thumb grasp (see Fig. 6-7) that does not permit such a technique. The CCLAD device *The Wand/CompuDent* (discussed in Chapter 5) employs a lightweight handpiece that is held with a "penlike" or "dart" grasp that is easily rotated.

A subsequent study by the same authors demonstrated that the BRIT has the added benefit of reducing the force necessary for needle penetration and advancement through tissues.[15] This is explained as follows. With rotational insertion, all resultant forces are directed toward the forward path of insertion since the deflecting or bending forces have been eliminated from the rotational insertion technique, as described in the preceding. This thereby allows forward movement of the needle to occur more efficiently and with less effort (e.g., less force). In addition, rotation of the beveled needle allows the sharp cutting edge to contact the full circumference of the tissue surface, contributing to the reduction of force that is necessary during penetration and advancement. This is not unlike the rotational effect that a surgical drill bit has as it is boring through tissue or bone.

The BRIT, or birotational insertion technique, is simple and easy and has been demonstrated to improve injection techniques because the deflection of a standard needle during insertion is minimized.[16]

LENGTH

Dental needles are available in two lengths: long and short. Ultrashort needles are also available with 30-gauge needles. Despite the claim for uniformity of length by manufacturers, significant differences are found (Table 6-4).

The *average* length of a short needle is 20 mm (measured hub to tip) and 32 mm for the long dental needle (Fig. 6-9).

Needles should not be inserted into tissues to their hubs unless it is absolutely necessary for the success of the injection.

One of reasons for this precaution is needle breakage, which, although rare, does occur. The weakest (most rigid part, receiving the greatest stress) portion of the needle is at the hub, which is where needle breakage

beveled needle, causing the needle to bend or deflect in a direction opposite to which the bevel faces (e.g., if the bevel faces "up" the advancing movement causes a beveled needle to deflect "downward"). The longer the needle length, the more exaggerated bending or deflection becomes as a result of the greater distance traveled along the deflecting path. The smaller the diameter of the needle, the more exaggerated the bending or deflecting because a smaller-gauge needle is less capable of resisting the deflection or bending force on the surface of the beveled needle tip.

When the BRIT is used during needle insertion the perpendicular force that causes deflection is eliminated or "neutralized" from the constant changing of bevel orientation as it is rotated (Fig. 6-8).[14] This allows

TABLE 6-4							
Needle Lengths							
Manufacturer	**25-Gauge Long**	**25-Gauge Short**	**27-Gauge Long**	**27-Gauge Short**	**30-Gauge Long**	**30-Gauge Short**	**30-Gauge Ultrashort**
Industry standard	32	20	32	20			
Manufacturer A	30		30	21	25	21	
Manufacturer B	32 ± 1.5	22 ± 1.5	32 ± 1.5	22 ± 1.5		21 ± 1.5	12 ± 1.0
Manufacturer C			32	21	25	21	
Manufacturer D	35		35	25		25	10
Manufacturer E	32			21		19	

All measurements obtained directly from needle manufacturers.

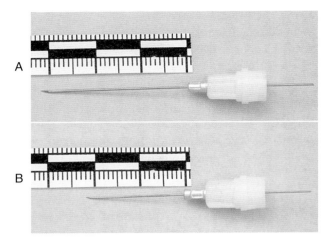

Figure 6-9. A, Long dental needle length approximately 32 mm. **B,** Short dental needle length approximately 20 mm.

happens. When a needle that is inserted into the soft tissues to its hub breaks, the elastic properties of the tissues permit them to rebound and cover (bury) the needle entirely. Retrieval usually is difficult (as discussed in Chapter 17). If even a small portion (5 mm or more) of the broken needle shaft remains visible within the oral cavity, it can be retrieved with a hemostat or pickup forceps.

A long needle is preferred for all injection techniques where the penetration of significant thicknesses of soft tissue (e.g., the inferior alveolar, Gow-Gates mandibular, Akinosi mandibular, infraorbital, and maxillary nerve blocks) is required. Short needles may be used for any injection in any patient who does not require the penetration of significant depths of soft tissue (e.g., close to or beyond 20 mm).

CARE AND HANDLING

Needles available to the dental profession today are presterilized and disposable. With proper care and handling, they should not be the cause of significant difficulties.

1. Needles must *never* be used on more than one patient.
2. Needles should be changed after several (three or four) tissue penetrations in the same patient.
   a. After three or four insertions, stainless steel disposable needles become dulled. Tissue penetration becomes more traumatic with each insertion, producing pain on insertion and soreness when sensation returns after the procedure.
3. Needles should be covered with a protective sheath when not being used to prevent accidental needle stick with a contaminated needle. (See the discussion in Chapter 9.)
4. Attention should always be paid to the position of the uncovered needle tip, whether inside or outside the patient's mouth. This minimizes the risk of potential injury to the patient and the administrator.

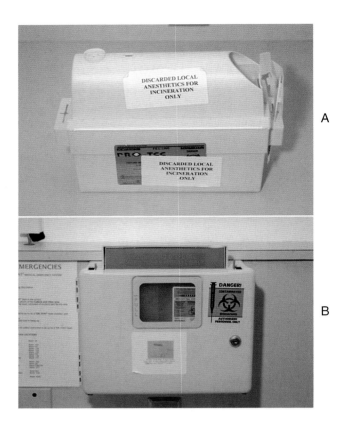

Figure 6-10. A, Container for disposal of discarded local anesthetic cartridges. **B,** "Sharps" container for disposing of contaminated needles.

5. Needles must be properly disposed of after use to prevent possible injury or reuse by unauthorized individuals. Needles can be destroyed in any of the following ways:
   a. Contaminated needles (as well as all other items contaminated with blood or saliva, such as cartridges) should be disposed of in special "contaminated" or "sharps" containers (Fig. 6-10).
   b. Proper use of a self-sheathing ("safe" needle) needle or syringe unit (as discussed in Chapter 5) minimizes risk of accidental needle stick.
   c. When needles are to be reused for subsequent injections (a unique feature of dentistry versus medicine, where second injections are rarely administered), recapping is accomplished using the "scoop" technique or a needle holder (Fig. 6-11).
   d. Contaminated needles should *never* be discarded into open trash containers.

In summary, only one local anesthetic needle is necessary in the dental office, the *25-gauge long*, which can be used for all the anesthetic techniques discussed in this book. It provides a rigidity, which is necessary in the periodontal ligament (PDL) and intraseptal injections, that is not available with higher-gauge (smaller-diameter) needles; it deflects to a lesser degree than smaller needles and seemingly provides easier and more reliable aspiration. Because there is no increase in patient discomfort with the 25-gauge

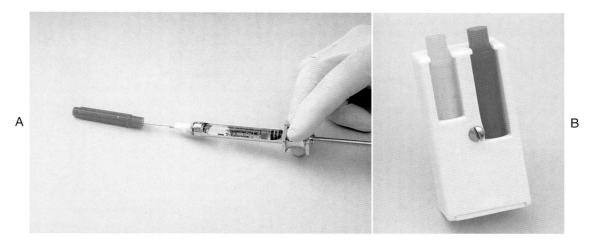

Figure 6-11. **A,** "Scoop" technique for recapping contaminated local anesthetic needle. **B,** Plastic needle cap holder.

long needle, its value is increased still further. In reality, however, it is practical to have a second needle available: The 25- or 27-gauge short needle is used for injection techniques in which the thickness of soft tissue to be penetrated is less than 20 mm and where the risk of positive aspiration is minimal, as well as in areas of the oral cavity where stabilization of a long needle might prove difficult (e.g., maxillary anterior teeth and the palate).

PROBLEMS

Pain on Insertion

The use of a dull needle can lead to pain on initial penetration of the mucosa. This pain may be prevented by using sharp, new, disposable needles and applying a topical

anesthetic at the penetration site. The needle should be changed after three or four penetrations of mucosa if reinsertion is necessary.

Breakage

Bending weakens needles, making them more likely to break on subsequent contact with hard tissues, such as bone. Needles should not be bent if they are to be inserted into soft tissue to a depth of more than 5 mm. *There is no injection technique used in dentistry (in which the needle enters into soft tissue) that mandates that the needle be bent for the injection to be successful.* Most often needles are bent by doctors administering an inferior alveolar nerve block (IANB), a posterior superior alveolar (PSA) nerve block, an intrapulpal injection, an injection into the PDL, and the intraosseous injection. The two nerve blocks mentioned can be easily administered successfully with a

Figure 6-12. Retained broken needle after inferior alveolar nerve block *(arrow).*

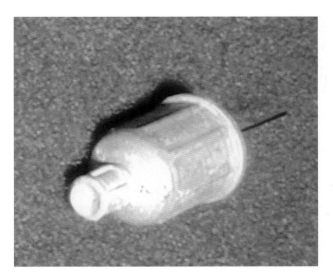

Figure 6-13. Remainder of retained local anesthetic needle shown in Figure 6-12.

straight (unbent) needle (see Chapters 13 and 14). The PDL and intrapulpal injections usually can be administered without bending the needle; however, occasions arise, such as at the distal root of a mandibular second molar (PDL), root canals in posterior teeth (intrapulpal), or injection into bone distal to a second molar (intraosseous), in which the injection site is not accessible with a straight needle. Bending of the needle is essential to success in these cases. Because the needle does not enter into soft tissue more than 2 to 4 mm (PDL), or at all (intrapulpal), there is little danger of the needle becoming nonretrievable in the unlikely event that it breaks (Figs. 6-12 and 6-13).

No attempt should be made to change the direction of a needle when it is embedded in tissue. If the direction of a needle must be changed, the needle should first be withdrawn almost completely from the tissue and then its direction altered. No attempts to force a needle against resistance should be made (needles are not designed to penetrate bone). Smaller (30- and 27-gauge) needles are more likely to break than larger (25-gauge) needles.

This author has been involved in 33 cases of broken needles that went into litigation (over a period of 30 years), and is aware of an additional 27 broken needle cases reported to manufacturers of the needles. In 59 of the 60 broken needle situations the needle involved was a 30-gauge short or ultrashort. A 27-gauge short needle was involved in the only other case.

Recommended needles for specific injection techniques are presented in the recommendations section that follows.

Pain on Withdrawal

Pain on withdrawal of the needle from tissue can be produced by "fishhook" barbs on the tip. Fishhook barbs may be produced during the manufacturing process, but it is much more likely that they develop when the needle tip forcefully contacts a hard surface, such as bone. A needle should never be forced against resistance. If in doubt about the presence of barbs, change the needle between insertions.

Injury to the Patient or Administrator

Penetration of, with injury resulting to, areas of the body with the needle can occur unintentionally. A major cause is carelessness and inattention by the administrator, although sudden unexpected movement by the patient is also a frequent cause. The needle should remain capped until it is to be used and should be made safe (sheathed or recapped) immediately after withdrawal from the mouth.

RECOMMENDATIONS

1. Sterile disposable needles should be used.
2. If multiple injections are to be administered, needles should be changed after three or four insertions in a single patient.

TABLE 6-5
Recommended Needles for Injection Techniques

Technique	Needle Gauge	Needle Length
Supraperiosteal (infiltration)	27	Short
Posterior superior alveolar nerve block	27*	Short*
Middle superior alveolar nerve block	27	Short
Anterior-middle superior alveolar nerve block (AMSA)	27	Short
Palatal approach (ASA)	30[†]	Ultrashort
Buccal (long) nerve block	27[‡]	Short[‡]
Infiltration for hemostasis	27	Short
Periodontal ligament injection (PDL or ILI)	27	Short
Intraseptal injection	27	Short
Intraosseous injection	27	Short
Intrapulpal injection	27	Short
Anterior superior alveolar nerve block ("infraorbital")	25	Long
Maxillary (V_2) nerve block	25	Long
Inferior alveolar ("mandibular") nerve block	25	Long
Gow-Gates mandibular nerve block	25	Long
Vazirani-Akinosi mandibular nerve block	25	Long

*In earlier editions of this book, the 25-gauge long needle was recommended. As a means of minimizing the risk of hematoma after the posterior superior alveolar injection, a short needle is now recommended. If available, a 25-gauge short needle should be used; where this is not available, the 27-gauge short needle is recommended. (See Chapter 13 for additional discussion.)
[†]The authors of the P-ASA paper recommend use of 30-gauge ultrashort needle.[17,18]
[‡]In most clinical situations the 25-gauge long needle, used for the IANB, is used for the buccal nerve block, which is administered immediately after the IANB.

3. Needles must *never* be used on more than one patient.
4. Needles should not be inserted into tissue to their hub unless it is absolutely necessary for success of the injection.
5. A needle's direction should not be changed while it is still in tissue.
6. A needle should never be forced against resistance.
7. Needles should remain capped until used and made safe immediately when withdrawn.
8. Needles should be discarded and destroyed after use to prevent injury or reuse by unauthorized persons.
9. The injection techniques in Table 6-5 are listed with their recommended needles (for the average-size adult).

REFERENCES

1. Cuny EJ, Fredekind R, Budenz AW: Safety needles. New requirements of the Occupational Safety and Health Administration bloodborne pathogens rule, *J Calif Dent Assoc* 27:525-530, 1999.
2. Aldous JA: Needle deflection: a factor in the administration of local anesthetics, *J Am Dent Assoc* 77:602-604, 1977.
3. Jeske AH, Boshart BF: Deflection of conventional versus non-deflecting dental needles in vitro, *Anesth Prog* 32:62-64, 1985.
4. Robison SF, Mayhew RB, Cowan RD, Hawley RJ: Comparative study of deflection characteristics and fragility of 25-, 27-, and 30-gauge short dental needles, *J Am Dent Assoc* 109:920-924, 1984.
5. Jeske AH, Blanton PL: Misconceptions involving dental local anesthesia. Part 2: Pharmacology, *Tex Dent J* 119:310-314, 2002.
6. Hamburg HL: Preliminary study of patient reaction to needle gauge, *NY State Dent J* 38:425-426, 1972.
7. Foldes FF, McNall PG: Toxicity of local anesthetics in man, *Dent Clin North Am* 5:257-258, 1961.
8. Harris S: Aspirations before injection of dental local anesthetics, *J Oral Surg* 25:299-303, 1957.
9. Kramer H, Mitton V: Dental emergencies, *Dent Clin North Am* 17:443-460, 1973.
10. McClure DB: Local anesthesia for the preschool child, *J Dent Child* 35:441-448, 1968.
11. Trapp LD, Davies RO: Aspiration as a function of hypodermic needle internal diameter in the in-vivo human upper limb, *Anesth Prog* 27:49-51, 1980.
12. Wittrock JW, Fischer WE: The aspiration of blood through small-gauge needles, *J Am Dent Assoc* 76:79-81, 1968.
13. Personal communications, Septodont Inc., Newark, Del., April 2003.
14. Hochman MN, Friedman MJ: In vitro study of needle deflection: A linear insertion technique versus a bi-directional rotation insertion technique, *Quint Int* 31:737-743, 2000.
15. Hochman MN, Friedman MJ: An in vitro study of needle force penetration comparing a standard linear insertion to the new bidirectional rotation insertion technique, *Quint Int* 32:789-796, 2001.
16. Aboushala A, Kugel G, Efthimiadis N, Korchak M: Efficacy of a computer-controlled injection system of local anesthesia in vivo. IADR Abstract. 2000; Abst#2775.1.
17. Friedman MJ, Hochman MN: P-ASA block injection: a new palatal technique to anesthetize maxillary anterior teeth, *J Esthet Dent* 11:23-71, 1999.
18. Hochman MN, Friedman MJ: Using AMSA and P-ASA nerve blocks for esthetic restorative dentistry, *Gen Dent* 49:506-511, 2001.

The Cartridge

CHAPTER 7

The dental cartridge is a glass cylinder containing the local anesthetic drug, among other ingredients. The glass cylinder itself can hold 2 ml of solution; however, as prepared today in the United States the dental cartridge contains 1.8 ml of local anesthetic solution. Local anesthetic products manufactured by Septodont list their minimum volume as 1.7 ml (although in actuality they contain 1.8 ml of local anesthetic solution). In other countries, notably the United Kingdom and Australia, the prefilled dental cartridge contains 2.2 ml of local anesthetic solution.

The dental cartridge is, by common usage, referred to as a "carpule" by dental professionals. The term *carpule* is actually a registered trade name for the dental cartridge prepared by Cook-Waite Laboratories, who introduced it into dentistry in 1920.

In recent years local anesthetic manufacturers in some countries (but not as of yet in the United States) have introduced a local anesthetic cartridge composed of plastic.[1] Plastic cartridges have several negative features, primarily leakage of solution in injection techniques, requiring considerable force to be applied to the plunger of the syringe (e.g., PDL, nasopalatine),[1] and the plunger not "gliding" down the plastic cartridge as smoothly as it does down the glass cartridge, leading to sudden spurts of local anesthetic being administered, which can produce pain in the patient.

COMPONENTS

The prefilled 1.8-ml dental cartridge consists of four parts (Fig. 7-1):
1. Cylindrical glass tube
2. Stopper (plunger, bung)
3. Aluminum cap
4. Diaphragm

The *stopper* (plunger) is located at the end of the cartridge that receives the harpoon of the aspirating syringe. The harpoon is embedded into the silicone (non–latex-containing) rubber plunger with gentle finger pressure applied to the thumb ring of the syringe. The plunger occupies a little less than 0.2 ml of the volume of the entire cartridge. Until recently, the stopper was sealed with paraffin (wax) to produce an airtight seal against the glass walls of the cartridge. Glycerin was added in channels around the stopper as a lubricant, permitting it to traverse

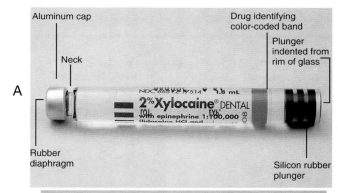

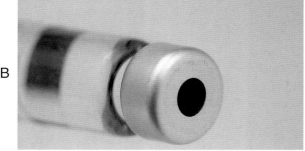

Figure 7-1. A and **B**, Components of the glass dental local anesthetic cartridge.

the glass cylinder more easily. Today most local anesthetic manufacturers treat the stopper with silicone, eliminating both the paraffin and glycerin. "Sticky stoppers" (stoppers that do not move smoothly down the glass cartridge) are infrequent today. In recent years there has been a move toward use of a uniform black rubber stopper in all local anesthetic drug combinations. Virtually gone are the color-coded red, green, and blue stoppers that aided in identification of the drug. Where black stoppers are used, a color-coding band, required by the American Dental Association (ADA) as of June 2003 for products to receive the ADA Seal of Approval, is found around the glass cartridge (Table 7-1).

In an intact dental cartridge (Fig. 7-2), the stopper is slightly indented from the lip of the glass cylinder. Cartridges whose plungers are flush with or extruded beyond the glass of the cylinder should not be used. This problem is discussed later in this chapter. (See "Problems.")

An *aluminum cap* is located at the opposite end of the cartridge from the rubber plunger. It fits snugly around the neck of the glass cartridge, holding the thin diaphragm in position. It is silver colored on all cartridges.

The *diaphragm* is a semipermeable membrane, usually latex rubber, through which the needle penetrates into the cartridge. When properly prepared, the perforation of the needle is centrally located and round, forming a tight seal around the needle. Improper preparation of the needle and cartridge can produce an eccentric puncture with ovoid holes leading to leakage of the anesthetic solution during injection. The permeability of the diaphragm allows any solution in which the dental cartridge may be stored to diffuse into the cartridge, contaminating the local anesthetic solution.

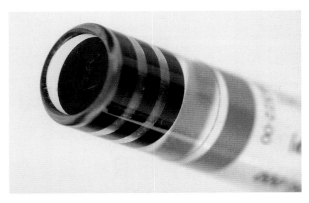

Figure 7-2. Silicone rubber plunger is slightly indented from rim of glass.

Persons with latex allergy may be at increased risk when administered a local anesthetic through a glass cartridge.[2] However, a recent literature review by Shojaei and Haas stated that although the possibility of an allergic reaction precipitated by latex in the dental local anesthetic cartridge does exist, "there are no reports of studies or cases in which a documented allergy was due to the latex component of cartridges for dental anesthesia."[3]

A thin Mylar plastic label is applied to all cartridges (Fig. 7-3). It protects the patient and administrator in the event the glass cracks and also provides specifications about the enclosed drug. In addition, some manufacturers include a volume indicator on their label, making it easier for the administrator to deposit precise volumes of anesthetic (Fig. 7-4).

CARTRIDGE CONTENTS

The composition of the solution found in the dental cartridge varies depending on whether or not a vasopressor is included (Table 7-2).

The *local anesthetic drug* is the raison d'être for the entire dental cartridge. It interrupts the propagated nerve impulse, preventing it from reaching the brain. The drug contained within the cartridge is listed by its percent

TABLE 7-1
Color-Coding of Local Anesthetic Cartridges, as per American Dental Association Council on Scientific Affairs

Local Anesthetic Solution	Color of Cartridge Band
Articaine HCl 4% with epinephrine 1:100,000	Gold
Bupivacaine 0.5% with epinephrine 1:200,000	Blue
Lidocaine HCl 2%	Light blue
Lidocaine HCl 2% with epinephrine 1:50,000	Green
Lidocaine HCl 2% with epinephrine 1:100,000	Red
Mepivacaine HCl 3%	Tan
Mepivacaine HCl 2% with levonordefrin 1:20,000	Brown
Prilocaine HCl 4%	Black
Prilocaine HCl 4% with epinephrine 1:200,000	Yellow

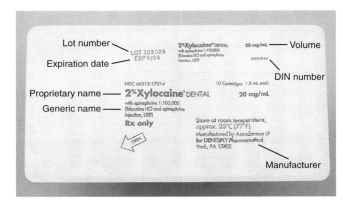

Figure 7-3. Mylar plastic label.

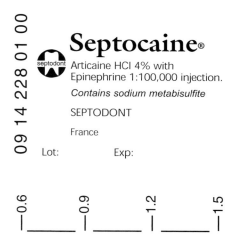

09 14 228 01 00

Septocaine®
Articaine HCl 4% with
Epinephrine 1:100,000 injection.
Contains sodium metabisulfite

SEPTODONT

France

Lot: Exp:

0.6   0.9   1.2   1.5

Figure 7-4. Label with volume indicator. (Courtesy Septodont, New Castle, Del.)

concentration. The number of milligrams of the agent can be calculated by multiplying the percent concentration (e.g., 2% = 20 mg/ml) by 1.8 (US) or 2.2 (UK) (number of milliliters in the cartridge). Thus a 1.8 ml cartridge of a 2% solution contains 36 mg (Table 7-3). The local anesthetic drug is stable and is capable of being autoclaved, heated, or boiled without breaking down. However, other components of the cartridge are more labile (e.g., vasopressor drug and cartridge seals) and are easily destroyed.

A *vasopressor drug* is included in most anesthetic cartridges to increase safety and the duration and depth of action of the local anesthetic. The pH of dental cartridges containing vasopressors is lower (more acidic) than that of cartridges not containing vasopressors (pH of 3.3 to 4.0 versus 5.5 to 6.0). Because of this pH difference, plain local anesthetics have a somewhat more rapid onset of clinical action and are more comfortable (less "burning" on injection).[4-6]

Cartridges containing vasopressors also contain an *antioxidant*, most often sodium (meta) bisulfite. It prevents the oxidation of the vasopressor by oxygen, which might

be trapped in the cartridge during manufacture or diffuse through the semipermeable diaphragm after filling. Sodium bisulfite reacts with oxygen before the oxygen is able to destroy the vasopressor. Sodium bisulfite is oxidized to sodium bisulfate, which has an even lower pH. The clinical relevance of this lies in the fact that increased burning (discomfort) is experienced by the patient on injection of an "older" cartridge of anesthetic with vasopressor than with a fresher cartridge. Allergy to bisulfites also must be considered in the medical evaluation of all patients before local anesthetic administration[7,8] (see Chapter 10).

Sodium chloride is added to the cartridge to make the solution isotonic with the tissues of the body. In the past, isolated instances have been reported in which local anesthetic solutions containing too much sodium chloride (hypertonic solutions) produced tissue edema or paresthesia, sometimes lasting for several months, after drug administration.[9] This is no longer a problem.

Distilled water is used as the diluent to provide the volume of solution in the cartridge.

A significant change in cartridge composition in the United States and most other countries was the removal of methylparaben, a bacteriostatic agent. A ruling by the United States Food and Drug Administration (FDA) mandated the removal of methylparaben from dental local anesthetic cartridges manufactured after January 1, 1984. Methylparaben possesses bacteriostatic, fungistatic, and antioxidant properties. It and related compounds (ethylparaben, propylparaben, and butylparaben) are commonly used as preservatives in ointments, creams, lotions, and dentifrices. In addition, paraben preservatives are found in all multiple-dose vials of drugs. Methylparaben is commonly used in a 0.1% concentration (1 mg/ml). Its removal from local anesthetic cartridges was predicated on two facts. First, dental local anesthetic cartridges are single-use items meant to be discarded and not reused. Therefore inclusion of a bacteriostatic agent is unwarranted. Second, repeated exposure to paraben has led to

TABLE 7-2
Composition of Local Anesthetic Solution

Component	Function	"Plain" Local Anesthetic Solution	Vasopressor-containing Local Anesthetic Solution
Local anesthetic drug (e.g., lidocaine HCl)	Blockade of nerve conduction	●	●
Sodium chloride	Isotonicity of the solution	●	●
Sterile water	Volume	●	●
Vasopressor (e.g., epinephrine, levonordefrin)	↑ Depth and ↑ duration of anesthesia; ↓ absorption of local anesthetic and vasopressor		●
Sodium (meta) bisulfite	Antioxidant		●
Methylparaben*	Bacteriostatic agent		

*Methylparaben is no longer included in single-use dental cartridges of local anesthetic; however, it is found in ALL multidose vials of injectable drugs.

TABLE **7-3**
Calculation of Milligrams per Cartridge

Percent Solution	=	Milligrams (mg) per Milliliter (ml)	×	Volume of Cartridge	=	Milligrams per Cartridge
0.5	=	5	×	1.8	=	9
1.0	=	10	×	1.8	=	18
2.0	=	20	×	1.8	=	36
3.0	=	30	×	1.8	=	54
4.0	=	40	×	1.8	=	72

reports of increased allergic reactions in some persons.[10,11] Responses have been limited to localized edema, pruritus, and urticaria. Fortunately, to date there has not been a systemic allergic reaction to a paraben. Removal of methylparaben has further decreased an already minimal risk of allergy to local anesthetic drugs.

CARE AND HANDLING

Local anesthetics are marketed either in vacuum-sealed tin containers of 50 cartridges or in blister packs. Although no manufacturer makes any claim of sterility about the exterior surface of the cartridge, bacterial cultures taken immediately on opening a container usually fail to produce any growth. Therefore it seems obvious that extraordinary measures related to cartridge sterilization are unwarranted. Indeed, the glass dental cartridge should not be autoclaved. The seals on the cartridge cannot withstand the extreme temperatures of autoclaving, and

the heat-labile vasopressors are destroyed in the process. Plastic cartridges cannot be autoclaved.

More commonly today, local anesthetics are marketed in cardboard boxes of approximately 50 cartridges. Within the box are 5 sealed units of 10 cartridges each (Fig. 7-5), called *blister packs*. Kept in this container until use, cartridges remain clean and uncontaminated.

Local anesthetic cartridges should be stored in their original container, preferably at room temperature (e.g., 21°C to 22°C [70°F to 72°F]) and in a dark place. There is no need to "prepare" a cartridge before use. The doctor or assistant should insert it into the syringe. However, many doctors feel compelled to somehow "sterilize" the cartridge. When this urge strikes, the doctor should apply an alcohol wipe moistened with undiluted 91% isopropyl alcohol or 70% ethyl alcohol to the rubber diaphragm (Fig. 7-6).

If a clear plastic cartridge dispenser is used, 1 day's supply of cartridges should be placed with the aluminum cap and diaphragm facing downward. Several (two or

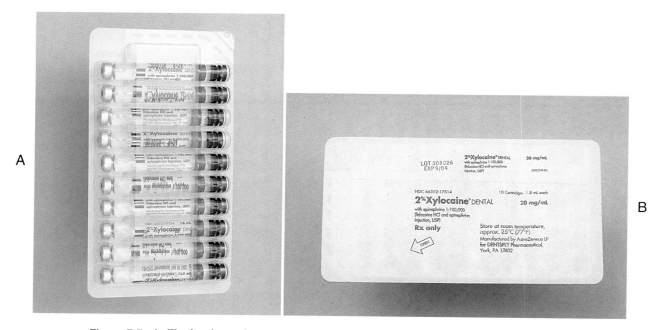

Figure 7-5. A, Ten local anesthetic cartridges are contained in a sealed "blister pack." **B,** Back of blister pack contains information about drug.

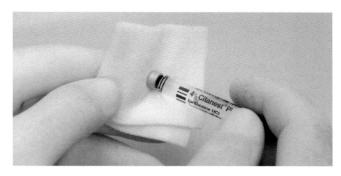

Figure 7-6. Preparing local anesthetic cartridge for use by wiping rubber diaphragm with alcohol.

three) sterile dry 2 × 2-inch gauze wipes are placed in the center of the dispenser and moistened with (not immersed in) either 91% isopropyl alcohol or 70% ethyl alcohol. There should be no liquid alcohol present around the cartridges. Before loading the syringe, the aluminum cap and rubber diaphragm are rubbed against the moistened gauze.

Cartridges should not be permitted to soak in either alcohol or other sterilizing solutions because the semipermeable diaphragm permits diffusion of these solutions into the dental cartridge, contaminating it. Therefore it is recommended that cartridges be kept in their original container until they are to be used.

Cartridge warmers are not necessary. Indeed, occasionally they may produce problems. Overheating the local anesthetic solution can lead to discomfort for the patient and the more rapid destruction of a heat-labile vasopressor (producing a shorter duration of anesthesia). It has been demonstrated that after the warmed glass cartridge is removed from the cartridge warmer and placed in a metal syringe and the solution forced through a fine metal needle, its temperature has decreased almost to room temperature.[4,12]

Cartridge warmers, designed to maintain anesthetic solutions at "body temperature," are not needed and cannot be recommended. Local anesthetics in cartridges maintained at room temperature (20°C to 22°C) do not cause the patient any discomfort on injection into tissues, nor do patients complain of the solution being too cold.[13] On the other hand, warmed local anesthetic solutions at 27°C (80°F) or above have a much greater incidence of being described as too hot or burning on injection.[12]

Local anesthetic cartridges should not be left exposed to direct sunlight because some contents may undergo accelerated deterioration. The primary clinical effect of this will be destruction of the vasopressor, with a corresponding decrease in the duration of clinical action of the anesthetic solution.

Included in every package of local anesthetic is an important document: the *drug package insert*. It contains valuable information about the product such as dosages, warnings, precautions, and care and handling. All persons

Figure 7-7. A, All local anesthetic containers have a product identification package insert, which should be read. **B,** Important information is contained in all package inserts.

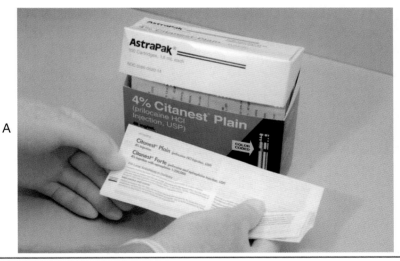

A

B

WARNINGS

DENTAL PRACTITIONERS WHO EMPLOY LOCAL ANESTHETICS IN THEIR OFFICES SHOULD BE WELL VERSED IN DIAGNOSIS AND MANAGEMENT OF EMERGENCIES WHICH MIGHT ARISE FROM THEIR USE. RESUSCITATIVE EQUIPMENT, OXYGEN, AND OTHER RESUSCITATIVE DRUGS SHOULD BE AVAILABLE FOR IMMEDIATE USE.

Reactions resulting in fatality have occurred on rare occasions with the use of local anesthetics, even in the absence of a history of hypersensitivity.

involved in the handling or administration of local anesthetics should review this document periodically (Fig. 7-7).

PROBLEMS

Occasionally problems develop with dental cartridges. Although most are minor, producing slight inconvenience to the drug administrator, others are more significant and might prove harmful to the patient:

1. Bubble in the cartridge
2. Extruded stopper
3. Burning on injection
4. Sticky stopper
5. Corroded cap
6. "Rust" on the cap
7. Leakage during injection
8. Broken cartridge

Bubble in the Cartridge

A small bubble of approximately 1 to 2 mm diameter (described as "BB"-sized) frequently is found in the dental cartridge. It is composed of nitrogen gas, which was bubbled into the local anesthetic solution during its

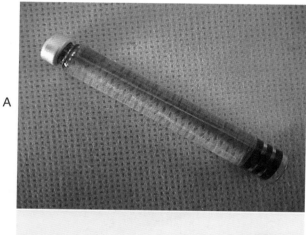

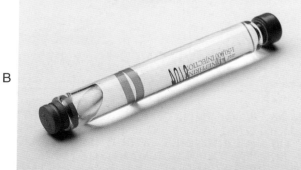

Figure 7-8. A, Normal cartridge with no bubble or a small BB-sized bubble. Notice that the rubber stopper is indented from the glass rim. **B,** Local anesthetic cartridge with an extruded stopper and large bubble caused by freezing.

manufacture to prevent oxygen from being trapped in the cartridge and potentially destroying the vasopressor. The nitrogen bubble may not always be visible in a normal cartridge (Fig. 7-8, *A*).

A larger bubble, which may be present with a plunger that is extruded beyond the rim of the cartridge, is the result of the freezing of the anesthetic solution (Fig. 7-8, *B*). Such cartridges should not be used because sterility of the solution cannot be assured. Instead, the cartridges should be returned to their manufacturer for replacement.

Extruded Stopper

The stopper can become extruded when a cartridge is frozen and the liquid inside expands. In this case the solution can no longer be considered sterile and should not be used for injection. Frozen cartridges can be identified by the presence of a large (>2 mm) air bubble by the extruded stopper.

An extruded stopper with no bubble is indicative of prolonged storage in a chemical disinfecting solution and diffusion of the solution into the cartridge. Shannon and Wescott demonstrated that alcohol enters a cartridge through the diaphragm in measurable amounts within 1 day if the diaphragm is immersed in alcohol.[14] Local anesthetic solutions containing alcohol produce an uncomfortable burning on injection. Alcohol in sufficiently high concentration is a neurolytic agent and can produce long-term paresthesia. The greatest concentration of alcohol reported to date in a dental cartridge has been 8%, which is not likely to produce significant long-term injury.[15]

Antirust tablets should not be used in disinfectant solutions. The sodium nitrate (or similar agent) that they contain is capable of releasing metal ions, which have been related to an increased incidence of edema after local anesthetic administration.[16]

It should be remembered that small quantities of sterilizing solution can diffuse into a dental cartridge without any visible movement of the plunger. Care always must be taken in storage of local anesthetic cartridges.

Burning on Injection

A burning sensation on injection of anesthetic solution may be the result of one of the following:

1. Normal response to the pH of the drug
2. Cartridge containing sterilizing solution
3. Overheated cartridge
4. Cartridge containing a vasopressor

During the few seconds immediately after deposition of a local anesthetic solution the patient may complain of a slight sensation of burning. This normal reaction is caused by the pH of the local anesthetic solution; it lasts a second or two, until the anesthetic takes effect, and is noted mainly by sensitive patients.

A more intense burning on injection is usually the result of the diffusion of disinfecting solution into the dental cartridge and its subsequent injection into the oral mucous membranes. Although burning is most often a mere annoyance, the inclusion of disinfecting agents such as alcohol in dental cartridges can lead to more serious sequelae, such as postinjection paresthesia and tissue edema.[14,15]

Overheating of the solution in a cartridge warmer also may produce burning on injection. The (Christmas tree) bulb-type cartridge warmer is most often at fault in this regard. Unless local anesthetic cartridges are unusually cold, there is little justification for use of a cartridge warmer. Local anesthetic solutions injected at room temperature are well tolerated by tissues and patients.

Use of a vasopressor-containing local anesthetic solution also may be responsible for the sensation of burning on injection. The addition of a vasopressor and an antioxidant (sodium bisulfite) lowers the pH of the solution to between 3.3 and 4, significantly more acidic than solutions not containing a vasopressor (pH about 5.5).[4,5,16] Patients are more likely to feel the burning sensation with these solutions. A further decrease in the pH of the local anesthetic solution results when the sodium bisulfite is oxidized to sodium bisulfate. This response can be minimized by carefully checking the expiration date of all cartridges before use. Conversely, increasing the pH of the anesthetic solution has the effect of making local anesthetic administration more comfortable for the patient.[17]

Sticky Stopper

The "sticky stopper" has become rare today, with the inclusion of silicone as a lubricant and the removal of paraffin as a sealant in the cartridge. Where paraffin is still used, difficulty in advancing the stopper may occur on colder days as the paraffin hardens. Using cartridges at room temperature minimizes this problem; using silicone-coated stoppers eliminates it. Plastic cartridges appear to suffer from this problem to a greater degree than glass cartridges.

Corroded Cap

The aluminum cap on a local anesthetic cartridge can be corroded if immersed in disinfecting solutions that contain quaternary ammonium salts, such as benzalkonium chloride (e.g., "cold" sterilizing solution). These salts are electrolytically incompatible with aluminum. Aluminum-sealed cartridges should be disinfected in either 91% isopropyl alcohol or 70% ethyl alcohol. Cartridges with corroded caps must not be used. Corrosion (Fig. 7-9) may be easily distinguished from rust, which appears as a red deposit on an intact aluminum cap.

Rust on the Cap

Rust found on a cartridge indicates that at least one cartridge in the tin container has broken or leaked. The

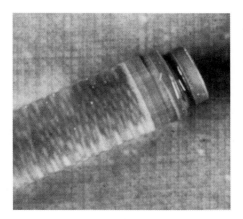

Figure 7-9. Damaged (corroded) metal cap.

"tin" container (actually steel dipped in molten tin) rusts, and the deposit comes off on the cartridges. Cartridges containing rust should not be used. If any cartridge contains rust or a crack (Fig. 7-10), all cartridges in the container must be carefully checked before use. With the introduction of nonmetal packaging, rust is rarely seen.

Leakage during Injection

Leakage of local anesthetic solution into the patient's mouth during injection occurs if the cartridge and needle are prepared improperly and the needle puncture of the diaphragm is ovoid and eccentric. Properly placed on the syringe after the cartridge is inserted, the needle produces a centric perforation of the diaphragm that tightly seals itself around the needle. When pressure is applied to the plunger during injection, all of the solution is directed into the lumen of the needle. If the cartridge is placed in a breech-loading syringe *after* the needle, an eccentric ovoid perforation may occur and, with pressure on the plunger, some solution is directed into the lumen

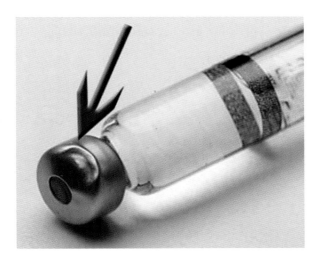

Figure 7-10. Local anesthetic cartridge with damaged cap. The glass around the neck of the cartridge should be examined carefully for cracks.

of the needle while some may leak out of the cartridge between the needle and the diaphragm and run into the patient's mouth (see Fig. 5-19). When the safety syringe is used, it is necessary to insert the cartridge after the needle has been attached; however, because the cartridge slides directly into the syringe, not from the side, leakage during injection is rarely a problem. Verbal and written communications from doctors using plastic cartridges indicate that the occurrence of leakage appears to be considerably greater with them.

The plastic dental cartridge does not withstand the application of injection pressure and the traditional glass cartridge. Meechan and associates applied pressures equal to that achieved during the periodontal ligament (PDL) injection to both glass and plastic local anesthetic cartridges.[1] Leakage of anesthetic occurred in 1.4% of glass cartridges, whereas leakage was noted in 75.1% of plastic cartridges.

Broken Cartridge

The most common cause of cartridge breakage is the use of a cartridge that has been cracked or chipped during shipping. Dented metal containers or damaged boxes should be returned to the supplier immediately for exchange. If a broken cartridge is found in a container, all remaining cartridges must be examined for hairline cracks or chips. Two areas that must be examined carefully are the thin neck of the cartridge where it joins the cap (Fig. 7-10) and the glass surrounding the plunger (Fig. 7-11). Subjecting a cracked cartridge to the pressure of injection often causes the cartridge to shatter or "explode." If this occurs inside the patient's mouth, serious sequelae may result from the ingestion of glass. It is essential to suction the patient's mouth thoroughly and consult with a physician or emergency department about follow-up therapy before discharging the patient. The addition of a thin Mylar plastic label to the glass cartridge minimizes such injury. Additionally, if the aluminium "cap" on the cartridge is damaged, the cartridge should not be used because the underlying glass also may have been damaged (Fig. 7-10).

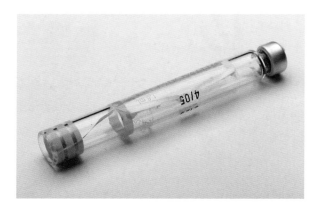

Figure 7-11. Cracked glass on dental cartridge.

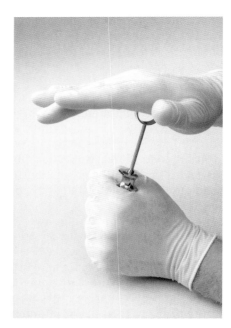

Figure 7-12. If force is necessary to embed the harpoon in the rubber plunger, the glass face of the syringe should be covered with the hand.

Plastic cartridges do not fracture when subjected to PDL injection pressures.[1] Excessive force used to engage the aspirating harpoon in the stopper has resulted in numerous cases of shattered cartridges. Although they have not broken in the patient's mouth, there has been injury to dental personnel. Hitting the thumb ring of the syringe in an attempt to engage the harpoon in the rubber stopper should be avoided. If this technique is essential to embed the harpoon in the rubber plunger (as it is with the plastic safety syringe), one hand should be used to cover the entire exposed glass face of the cartridge (Fig. 7-12). Proper preparation of the armamentarium (Chapter 9) minimizes this problem.

Breakage also can occur as a result of attempting to use a cartridge with an extruded plunger. Extruded plungers can be forced back into the cartridge only with difficulty, if at all. Cartridges with extruded plungers should not be used.

Syringes with bent harpoons may cause cartridges to break (see Fig. 5-21). Bent needles that are no longer patent create a pressure buildup within the cartridge during attempted injection (see Fig. 5-20). *No* attempt should be made to force local anesthetic solution from a dental cartridge against significant resistance.

RECOMMENDATIONS

1. Dental cartridges must never be used on more than one patient.
2. Cartridges should be stored at room temperature.
3. It is not necessary to warm cartridges before use.

4. Cartridges should not be used beyond their expiration date.

5. Cartridges should be checked carefully for cracks, chips, and the integrity of the stopper and cap before use.

REFERENCES

1. Meechan JG, McCabe JF, Carrick TE: Plastic dental anaesthetic cartridges: a laboratory investigation, *Br Dent J* 169: 254-256, 1990.

2. Sussman GL, Beezhold DH: Allergy to latex rubber, *Ann Intern Med* 122:143-146, 1995.

3. Shojaei AR, Haas DA: Local anesthetic cartridges and latex allergy: a literature review, *J Can Dent Assoc* 68: 10622-10626, 2002.

4. Jeske AH, Blanton PL: Misconceptions involving dental local anesthesia. Part 2: Pharmacology, *Tex Dent J* 119: 4310-4314, 2002.

5. Wahl MJ, Schmitt MM, Overton DA, Gordon MK: Injection of bupivacaine with epinephrine vs. prilocaine plain, *J Am Dent Assoc* 133:111652-111656, 2002.

6. Wahl MJ, Overton DA, Howell J, et al: Pain on injection of prilocaine plain vs. lidocaine with epinephrine: a prospective double-blind study, *J Am Dent Assoc* 132: 101396-101401, 2001.

7. Seng GF, Gay BJ: Dangers of sulfites in dental local anesthetic solutions: warning and recommendations, *J Am Dent Assoc* 113:769-770, 1986.

8. Perusse R, Goulet JP, Turcotte JY: Contraindications to vasoconstrictors in dentistry: Part II. Hyperthyroidism, diabetes, sulfite sensitivity, cortico-dependent asthma, and pheochromocytoma, *Oral Surg* 74:5687-5691, 1992.

9. Nickel AA: Paresthesia resulting from local anesthetics, *J Oral Maxillofac Surg* 42:52-79, 1984.

10. Wurbach G, Schubert H, Pillipp I: Contact allergy to benzyl alcohol and benzyl paraben, *Contact Dermatitis* 28:3187-3188, 1993.

11. Klein CE, Gall H: Type IV allergy to amide-type anesthetics, *Contact Dermatitis* 25:145-148, 1991.

12. Volk RJ, Gargiulo AV: Local anesthetic cartridge warmer-first in, first out, *Ill Dent J* 53:292-294, 1984.

13. Rogers KB, Fielding AF, Markiewicz SW: The effect of warming local anesthetic solutions prior to injection, *Gen Dent* 37:6496-6499, 1989.

14. Shannon IL, Wescott WB: Alcohol contamination of local anesthetic cartridges, *J Acad Gen Dent* 22:20-21, 1974.

15. Oakley J: Personal communications, 1985.

16. Moorthy AP, Moorthy SP, O'Neil R: A study of pH of dental local anesthetic solutions, *Br Dent J* 157: 11394-11395, 1984.

17. Crose VW: Pain reduction in local anesthetic administration through pH buffering, *J Ind Dent Assoc* 70: 224-225, 1991.

Additional Armamentarium

CHAPTER

8

In previous chapters the three major components of local anesthetic armamentarium—syringe, needle, and cartridge—have been discussed. There are other important items in the local anesthetic armamentarium, however, including the following:

1. Topical antiseptic
2. Topical anesthetic
3. Applicator sticks
4. Cotton gauze (2 × 2 inches)
5. Hemostat

TOPICAL ANTISEPTIC

A topical antiseptic may be used to prepare the tissues at the site of injection before the initial needle penetration. Its function is to produce a transient decrease in the bacterial population at the injection site, thereby minimizing any risk of postinjection infection.

The topical antiseptic, on an applicator stick, is placed at the site of injection for 15 to 30 seconds. There is no need to place a large quantity on the applicator stick; it should be sufficient just to moisten the cotton portion of the swab.

Available agents include Betadine (povidone-iodine) and Merthiolate (thimerosal). Topical antiseptics containing alcohol (e.g., *tincture* of iodine or *tincture* of Merthiolate) should not be used because the alcohol produces tissue irritation. In addition, allergy to iodine-containing compounds is common.[1] Before any iodine-containing topical antiseptic is applied to tissues, care should be taken to determine if adverse reactions to iodine have previously developed.

In a survey of local anesthetic techniques in dental practice,[2] 7.9% of the dentists mentioned that they always used topical antiseptics before injection, 22.4% sometimes used them, and 69.7% never used them.

Postinjection infections can and do occur, and the regular use of a topical antiseptic can virtually eliminate them. If a topical antiseptic is not available, a sterile gauze wipe may serve to prepare the tissues adequately before injection.

The application of a topical antiseptic is considered an optional step in tissue preparation before intraoral injection.

TOPICAL ANESTHETIC

Topical anesthetic preparations are discussed in depth in Chapter 4. Their use before initial needle penetration of the mucous membrane is strongly recommended. With proper application the *initial* penetration of mucous membrane usually can be made anywhere in the oral cavity without the patient being aware of it.

For effectiveness, it is recommended that a minimal quantity of topical anesthetic be applied to the end of the applicator stick and placed directly at the site of penetration for approximately 1 minute. Gill and Orr have demonstrated that when topical anesthetics are applied according to the manufacturer's instructions (approximately 10 to 15 seconds), their effectiveness is no greater than that of a placebo, especially for palatal injections.[3] Stern and Giddon showed that application of the topical anesthetic to mucous membrane for 2 to 3 minutes leads to profound soft-tissue analgesia.[4]

A variety of topical anesthetic agents are available for use today. Most contain the ester local anesthetic benzocaine. The likelihood of occurrence of allergic reactions to esters is significantly greater than that to amide topical anesthetics; however, because benzocaine is not absorbed systemically, allergic reactions usually are localized to the site of application. Of the amides, only lidocaine possesses topical anesthetic activity in clinically acceptable concentrations.

The risk of overdose with amide topical anesthetics is greater than that with the esters and increases with the area of application of the topical anesthetic. Topical forms of lidocaine are available as ointments, gels, pastes, and sprays.

EMLA (eutectic mixture of local anesthetics) is a combination of lidocaine and prilocaine in a topical cream formulation, designed to provide surface anesthesia of intact skin. Its primary indications are for use before venipuncture and in pediatric surgical procedures, such as circumcision.[5,6] EMLA has been used effectively intraorally; however, it is not designed for intraoral administration, so it contains no flavoring agent and is bitter tasting.[7,8]

Unmetered sprays of topical anesthetics are potentially dangerous and are not recommended for routine use. Because topical anesthetics require greater concentration to penetrate mucous membranes, and because topical anesthetics are absorbed rapidly into the cardiovascular system, only small measured doses should be administered. Topical anesthetic sprays that deliver a continuous stream of topical anesthetic until being deactivated are capable of delivering overly high doses of the topical anesthetic. If absorbed into the cardiovascular system, the topical anesthetic may induce high local anesthetic blood levels, increasing the risk of an overdose reaction. Metered sprays that deliver a fixed dose with each administration, regardless of the length of time the nozzle is depressed, are preferred for topical formulations that are absorbed systemically. An example of this form of topical anesthetic spray is Xylocaine, which delivers 10 mg per administration.

Yet another potential problem with topical anesthetic sprays is difficulty keeping the spray nozzle sterile. This is a very important consideration when selecting the form of topical anesthetic to be used. Most topical anesthetic sprays today come with disposable applicator nozzles (Fig. 8-1).

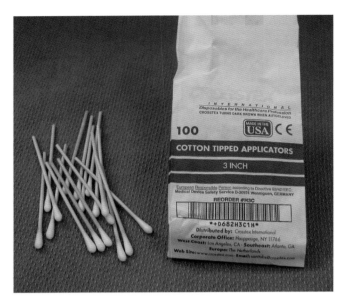

Figure 8-2. Cotton-tipped applicator sticks.

It should be remembered that some topical anesthetic formulations contain preservatives, such as methylparaben, that may be significant in instances of allergy to local anesthetics.

APPLICATOR STICKS

Applicators should be available as part of the local anesthetic armamentarium. They are wooden sticks with a cotton swab at one end, and they can be used to apply topical antiseptic and anesthetic solutions to mucous membranes (Fig. 8-2) and compress tissue during palatal injections.

COTTON GAUZE

Cotton gauze is included in the local anesthetic armamentarium for wiping the area of injection before the administration of a local anesthetic and drying the mucous membrane to aid retraction for increased visibility.

Many dentists select gauze in lieu of topical antiseptic solution for cleansing the soft tissue at the site of needle penetration. The gauze effectively dries the injection site and removes any gross debris from the area (Fig. 8-3). It is *not* as effective as the topical antiseptic but is an acceptable substitute.

Retraction of lips and cheeks for improved access and visibility to the injection site is important during all intraoral injections. Quite often this task becomes unnecessarily difficult if these tissues are moist, and it is made even more vexing wearing gloves. A dry cotton gauze makes the tissues easier to grasp and retract.

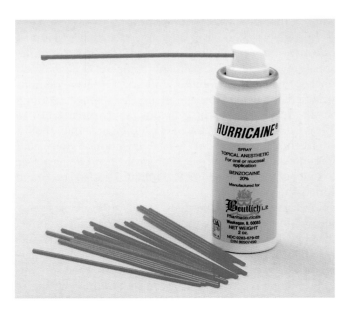

Figure 8-1. Disposable nozzle for topical anesthetic spray.

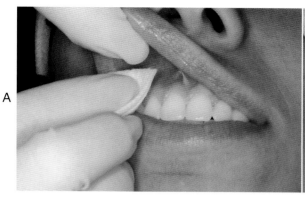
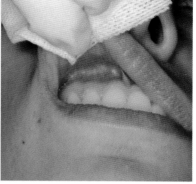

Figure 8-3. Sterile gauze is used to wipe mucous membrane, **A,** at site of needle penetration and, **B,** to aid in tissue retraction if necessary.

A variety of sizes of cotton gauze are available, but the most practical and the most commonly used is the 2 × 2 inch size.

HEMOSTAT

Although not considered an essential element of the local anesthetic armamentarium, a hemostat or pickup forceps should be readily available at all times in the dental office. Its primary function in local anesthesia is the removal of a needle from the soft tissues of the mouth in the unlikely event that the needle breaks off within tissues (Fig. 8-4).

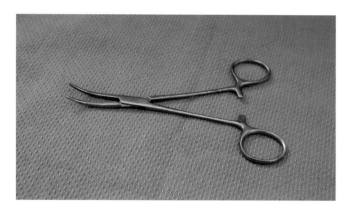

Figure 8-4. Hemostat.

REFERENCES

1. Bennasr S, Magnier S, Hassan M, Jacqz-Aigrain E: Anaphylactic shock and low osmolarity contrast medium, *Arch Pediatr* 1:155-157, 1994.
2. Malamed SF: *Handbook of local anesthesia*, ed 1, St Louis, 1980, Mosby.
3. Gill CJ, Orr DL II: A double blind crossover comparison of topical anesthetics, *J Am Dent Assoc* 98:213-214, 1979.
4. Stern I, Giddon DB: Topical anesthesia for periodontal procedures, *Anesth Prog* 22:105-108, 1975.
5. Fetzer SJ: Reducing venipuncture and intravenous insertion pain with eutectic mixture of local anesthetic: a meta-analysis, *Nurs Res* 51:119-124, 2002.
6. Taddio A: Pain management for neonatal circumcision, *Paediatric Drugs* 3:101-111, 2001.
7. Bernardi M, Secco F, Benech A: Anesthetic efficacy of a eutectic mixture of lidocaine and prilocaine (EMLA) on the oral mucosa: prospective double-blind study with a placebo, *Minerva Stomatal* 48(1-2):39-43, 1999.
8. Munshi AK, Hegde AM, Latha R: Use of EMLA: is it an injection free alternative? *J Clin Pediatr Dent* 25:215-219, 2001.

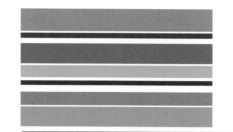

Preparation of the Armamentarium

CHAPTER
9

Proper care and handling of the local anesthetic armamentarium can prevent or at least minimize the development of complications associated with the needle, syringe, and cartridge, many of which have been discussed in the preceding chapters. Other complications and minor annoyances may be prevented through proper preparation of the armamentarium.

BREECH-LOADING, METALLIC OR PLASTIC, CARTRIDGE-TYPE SYRINGE

1. Remove the sterilized syringe from its container (Fig. 9-1).
2. Retract the piston fully before attempting to load the cartridge (Fig. 9-2).

3. Insert the cartridge, while the piston is fully retracted, into the syringe. Insert the rubber stopper end of the cartridge first (Fig. 9-3).
4. Engage the harpoon. Holding the syringe as if injecting, *gently* push the piston forward until the harpoon is firmly engaged in the plunger (Fig. 9-4). Excessive force is not necessary. Do *not* hit the piston in an effort to engage the harpoon (Fig. 9-5). This frequently leads to cracked or shattered glass cartridges.
5. Attach the needle to the syringe. Remove the white or clear protective plastic cap from the syringe end of the needle and screw the needle onto the syringe (Fig. 9-6). Metal-hubbed needles have threading, but plastic-hubbed needles do not, and the needle must be constantly pushed toward the metal hub of the syringe while being turned.

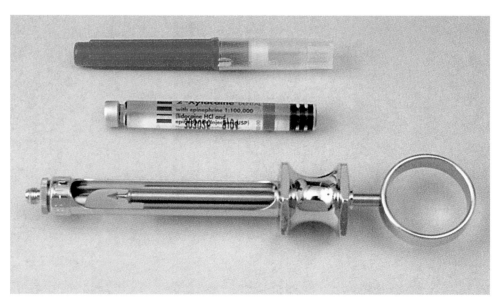

Figure 9-1. Local anesthetic armamentarium *(from top)*: needle, cartridge, syringe.

Figure 9-2. Retract the piston.

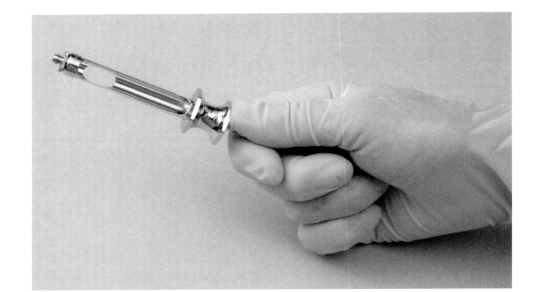

Figure 9-3. Insert the cartridge.

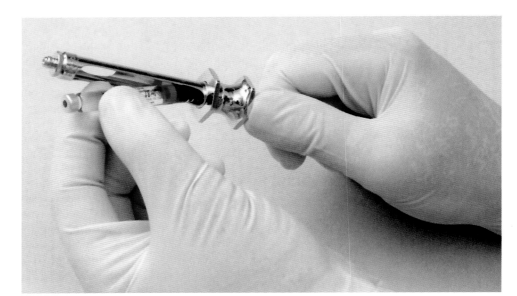

Figure 9-4. Engage the harpoon in plunger with *gentle* finger pressure.

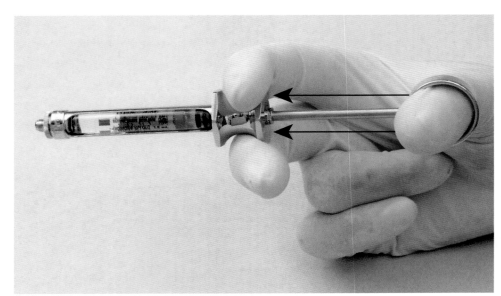

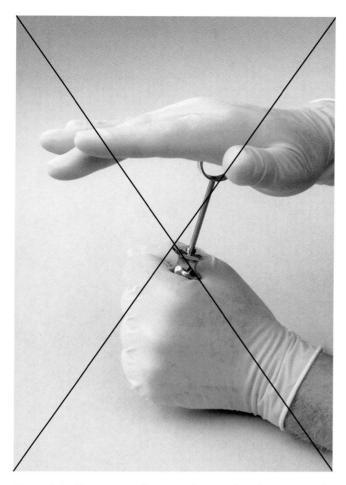

Figure 9-5. Do *not* exert force on plunger; the glass may crack.

6. Carefully remove the colored plastic protective cap from the opposite end of the needle and *expel a few drops of solution* to test for proper flow.
7. The syringe is now ready for use.

Note: It is common practice in dentistry to attach the needle to the syringe *before* placing the cartridge. This requires hitting the piston hard to engage the harpoon, a process that can lead to broken cartridges or leakage of anesthetic solution into the patient's mouth during the injection. The recommended sequence, described in the preceding, virtually eliminates this possibility and always should be used.

Recapping the Needle

After removal of the syringe from the patient's mouth, the needle should be recapped immediately. Recapping is *the* time when health professionals are most likely to be injured (stuck) with a needle, and probably the most dangerous time to be stuck because the needle is now contaminated with blood, saliva, and debris. Although a variety of techniques and devices for recapping have been suggested, the technique recommended by most state safety and health agencies is termed the "scoop" technique (Fig. 9-7), in which the uncapped needle is slid into the needle sheath lying on the instrument tray or table. Until a better method is designed, the scoop technique should be used for needle recapping.

Safety needles and syringes are in development; however, some systems currently available for dental use leave much to be desired.

Various needle cap holders are available, either commercially made or self-made (from acrylic) (Fig. 9-8) that hold the cap stationary while the needle is being inserted into it, making the recapping somewhat easier to accomplish.

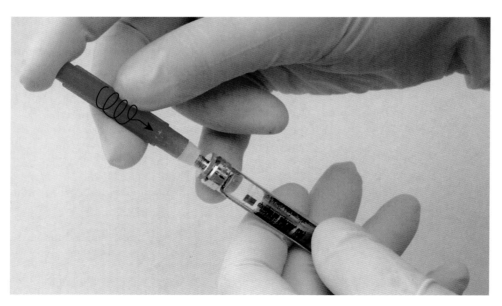

Figure 9-6. A plastic hubbed needle must be screwed onto the syringe while simultaneously being pushed into the metal needle adaptor of the syringe *(arrow)*.

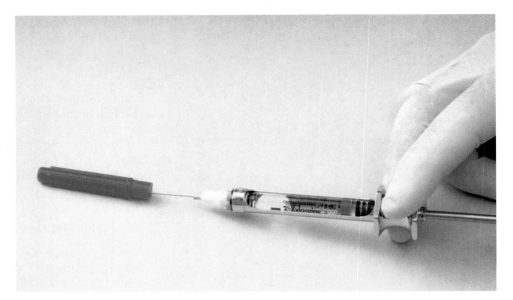

Figure 9-7. "Scoop" technique for recapping needle after use.

Unloading the Breech-loading, Metallic or Plastic, Cartridge-type Syringe

After administration of the local anesthetic, the following sequence is suggested for removing the used cartridge:

1. Retract the piston and pull the cartridge away from the needle with your thumb and forefinger as you retract the piston (Fig. 9-9), until the harpoon disengages from the plunger.
2. Remove the cartridge from the syringe by inverting the syringe, permitting the cartridge to fall free (Fig. 9-10).
3. *Discard the used needle.* All needles must be discarded after use to prevent injury or intentional misuse by unauthorized persons. Carefully unscrew the now-recapped needle, being careful not to accidentally

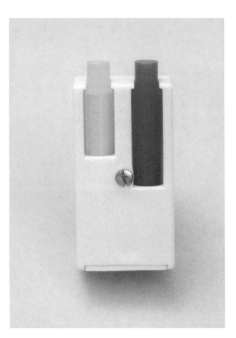

Figure 9-8. Plastic needle cap holder.

discard the metal needle adaptor (Fig. 9-11). The use of a sharps container is recommended (Fig. 9-12) for needle disposal.

SELF-ASPIRATING SYRINGE*

1. Insert the cartridge (as in the preceding instructions).
2. Attach the needle.
3. The syringe is now ready for use.

Because of the absence of a harpoon, loading and unloading the self-aspirating syringe are simple procedures.

ULTRASAFE ASPIRATING SYRINGE†

Loading the Safety Syringe

1. Insert the anesthetic cartridge into the body assembly (Fig. 9-13), making certain that the needle pierces the rubber diaphragm on the cartridge.
2. Grasp the octagonal plug on the body assembly between the thumb and index finger. *Align the legs with the notches and snap the two sections (body and plunger) together* (Fig. 9-14). A very distinct snapping sound is heard when the two sections are forced together.
3. Grasp the body assembly below its collar between the thumb and the index finger. Point the needle end of the syringe down (Fig. 9-15).
4. *Engage the harpoon into the stopper of the cartridge* by striking the flat top of the plunger with the palm of the hand (Fig. 9-16).

---

*From Dentsply, *www.dentsply.com*. This is a portion of the instructions that Dentsply encloses with its syringes.
†From Safety Syringes, Arcadia, CA. *www.safetysyringes.com*. This is a portion of the instructions that Safety Syringes encloses with its syringes.

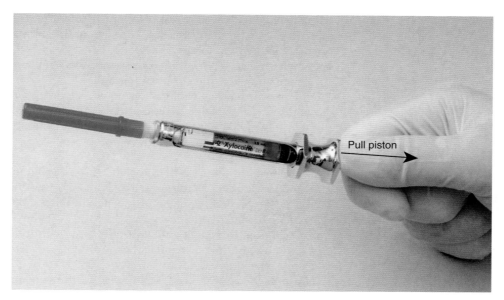

Figure 9-9. Retract the piston.

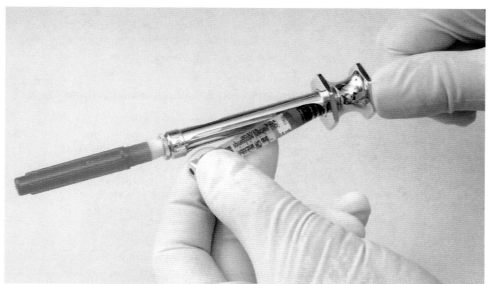

Figure 9-10. Remove the used cartridge.

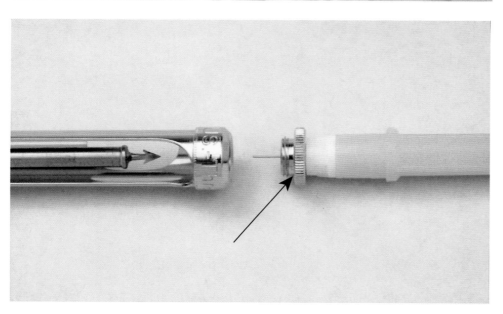

Figure 9-11. When discarding needle, check to be sure that the metal needle adaptor from the syringe is not inadvertently discarded too (*arrow*).

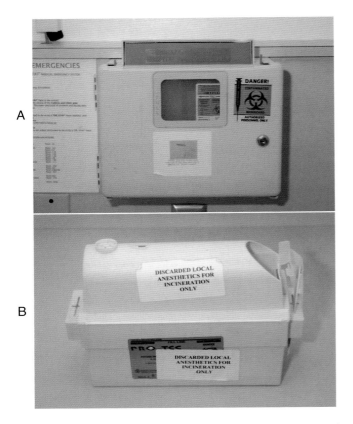

Figure 9-12. A, A sharps container is required for storage of discarded contaminated needles. **B,** A separate sealed container is recommended for discarded local anesthetic cartridges.

5. Express several drops of anesthetic solution to ensure proper preparation of the syringe.
6. The syringe is now ready for use (Fig. 9-17).

Unloading the UltraSafe Aspirating Syringe

The syringe is designed for single use. After the last injection, the entire device should be discarded into a sharps container as soon as possible. The UltraSafe aspirating syringe may be reloaded with an additional cartridge as follows:

1. *Release the harpoon from the rubber stopper* by pulling back the plunger to its original position.
2. Holding the body assembly in one hand, use the other hand to grasp the plug with the thumb and the index finger. Twist the plug counter counterclockwise until the plug releases from the body assembly.
3. *Remove the cartridge.*
4. a. Holding the guard near the collar, use the thumb and index finger to release the lock by pinching the walls of the body assembly forward until the needle clears the guard opening.
   b. Load the cartridge and push forward with the thumb until the body and cartridge are fully loaded into their original positions.
5. Grasp the octagonal plug, align the legs with the body notches, and push forward firmly until the sections snap together.
6. Reengage the harpoon by striking the flat top of the plunger with the palm of the hand. The syringe is ready for the next injection.

Making the UltraSafe Aspirating Syringe "Safe"

One-handed Guarding Technique

1. After completion of the injection, gently move the index and middle fingers against the front collar of the guard (Fig. 9-18).
2. Pull back on the needle (pulling back the plunger) until it is retracted into the guard and the guard legs lock into the body notches (Fig. 9-19).

Two-handed Guarding Technique

Use of the two-handed guarding technique is suggested when the entire cartridge has not been administered or if the administrator has small or petite glove-size hands.

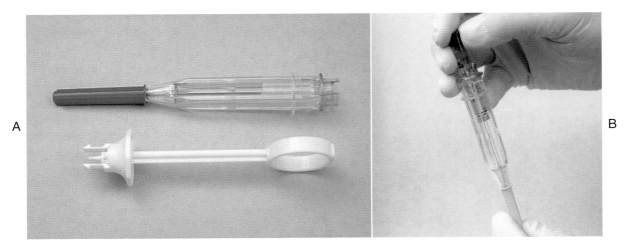

Figure 9-13. A, Safety syringe components. **B,** Insert local anesthetic cartridge into the syringe.

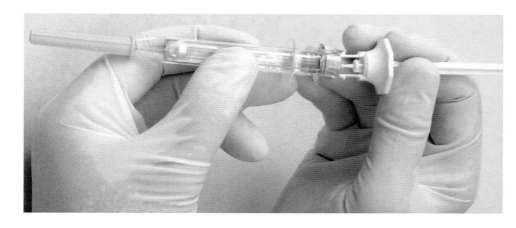

Figure 9-14. Snap the two sections together.

1. Grasp the guard near its collar with the free hand (Fig. 9-20).
2. Pull the body back until the needle is retracted into the guard and the guard legs lock into the body notches (Fig. 9-21).

The needle is now safe. The entire assembly unit can be discarded in the sharps container.

The manufacturer of the UltraSafe aspirating syringe recommends several safety precautions:
1. Keep hands behind the needle at all times during use and disposal.
2. Do not attempt to override or defeat the locking safety mechanism.
3. Use the syringe only once.

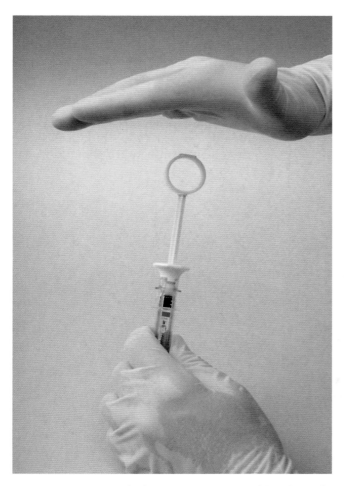

Figure 9-15. Prepare for harpoon insertion. Hold with needle facing down.

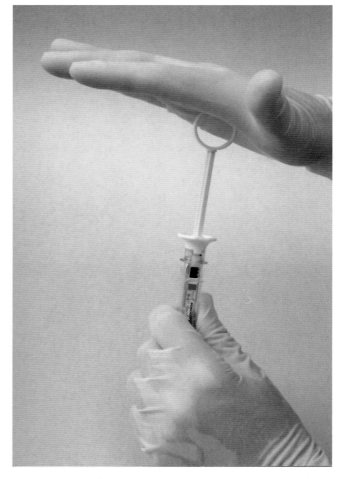

Figure 9-16. Strike the thumb ring with the palm of the hand to embed the harpoon into the plunger of the cartridge.

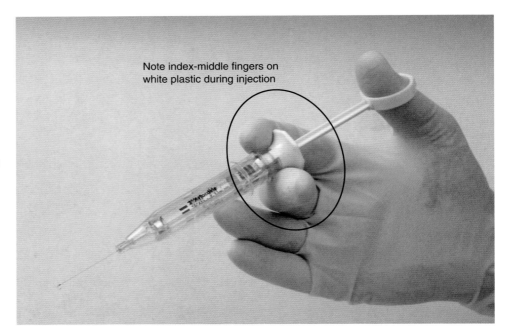

Note index-middle fingers on white plastic during injection

Figure 9-17. The safety syringe is ready for use.

4. For aspiration, use standard operating procedures for the administration of an anesthetic.

ULTRA SAFETY PLUS XL*

Loading the ULTRA Safety Plus XL System

1. Tear back paper seal and remove the sterile ULTRA Safety Plus XL unit from the blister pack. Grip the

*From Septodont, Inc. New Castle, Del. *www.septodontinc.com*. This is a portion of the instructions that Septodont encloses with its syringes.

barrel firmly and fully insert the anesthetic cartridge into the open end of the syringe (Fig. 9-22).

2. Grip the ULTRA Safety Plus XL plunger handle; push the finger holder to the end until it stops and covers the silicone o-ring. Support the finger holder from behind with your thumb, then "pushing forward," *roll* the "bull-nose" of the handle in behind the cartridge. Be sure the base of the unit is fully attached to the handle (Fig. 9-23).

3. Slide the sheath protecting the needle backward toward the handle until it *clicks* onto the handle. Make sure there is no gap between the transparent

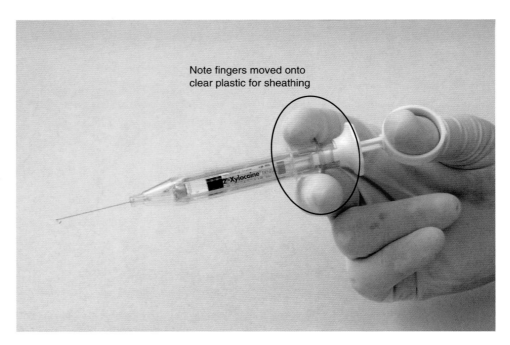

Note fingers moved onto clear plastic for sheathing

Figure 9-18. One-handed guarding technique: place fingers on front of the guard.

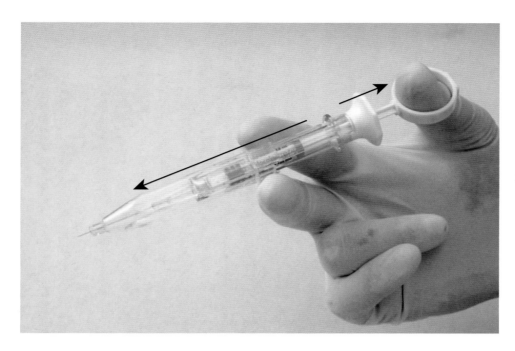

Figure 9-19. One-handed guarding technique: pull back until a "click" is heard.

sheath and the black handle. (The click is made as the sheath hits the handle and *locks* the unit together [Fig. 9-24]).

How the Instrument Locks Onto the Handle

Inside at the end of the cartridge barrel are ridges that, when the protective sheath is "clicked" into place, are crimped behind the "bull-nose" of the handle in the gutter provided.

4. All movements now are away from the needle. Remove the needle cap and discard it. The system is now ready to use (Fig. 9-25).

Passive Aspiration

As you press forward on the plunger, a small cylinder inside the hub moves the cartridge diaphragm further into the cartridge, building a negative pressure. Your release of the forward pressure on the plunger will aspirate the system. You can utilize this system multiple times during an injection.

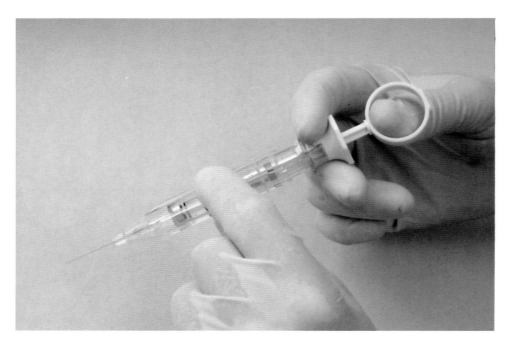

Figure 9-20. Two-handed guarding technique: grasp guard near its collar with free hand.

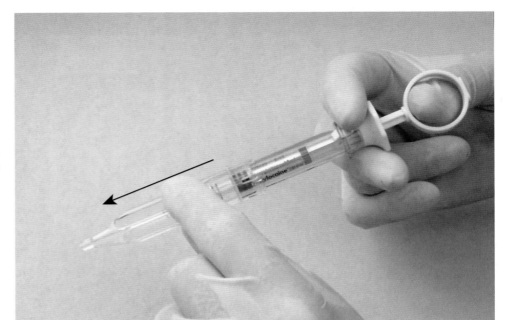

Figure 9-21. Two-handed guarding technique: pull pack the needle until locked *(arrow)*.

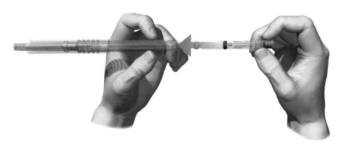

Figure 9-22. Insert the anesthetic cartridge into the open end of the injection unit. (Courtesy Septodont, New Castle, Del.)

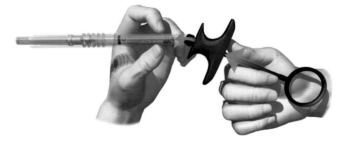

Figure 9-23. With the T-bar pushed all the way forward, snap the injection unit onto the syringe handle. (Courtesy Septodont, New Castle, Del.)

Figure 9-24. Pull back on the protective sheath until it is flush with the syringe handle and it clicks; the capped needle is now visible. (Courtesy Septodont, New Castle, Del.)

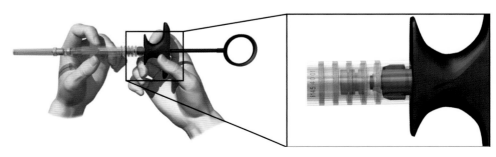

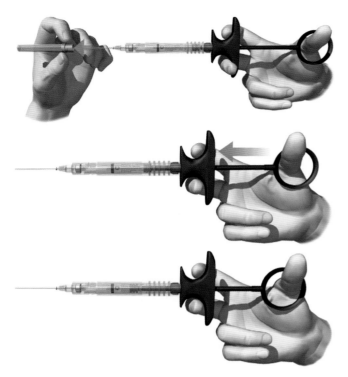

Figure 9-25. Remove and discard the needle cap, exposing the sterile needle. (Courtesy Septodont, New Castle, Del.)

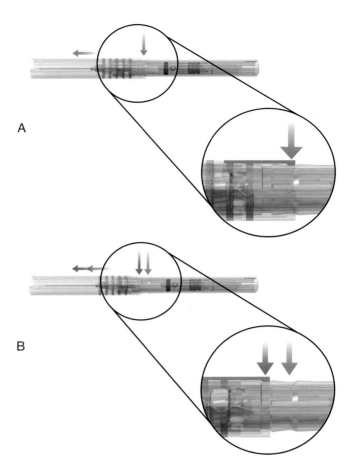

A

B

Figure 9-26. After the initial injection, slide the protective sheath toward the needle until it reaches the holding position, **A.** Slide the protective sheath toward the locking position, **B,** which is the second notch at the end of the barrel. (Courtesy Septodont, New Castle, Del.)

> NOTE: Failure to retract the sheath fully until you hear the *click,* which locks the instrument securely, may result in the system disassembling during use; leave no gap between the transparent sheath and the black handle.

Active Aspiration

The clear, silicone o-ring on the end of the plunger handle creates a tight vacuum within the cartridge and allows multiple aspirations of the stopper during routine injection. A small portion of solution must be injected to fully utilize this method.

> REMINDER: Please use the finger grips to prevent wet, gloved fingers from slipping when the outer protective sheath is activated.

How To Use

5. **When using only one cartridge.** During multiple injection procedures using one cartridge, you may safely retain the syringe for further use by moving the sheath toward the needle until it reaches the holding position (Fig. 9-26, *A*). When the procedure is complete, slide the protective sheath toward the locking position (Fig. 9-26, *B*) until it clicks (the second notch at the end of the barrel). This has now permanently locked the needle safely in the protective sheath.

6. When you have finished with the ULTRA Safety Plus XL and have locked it into position, you will need to separate the plunger handle. Hold the barrel with one hand and with the other hand, place a finger in the ring of the plunger handle and pull backward until the plunger is fully retracted.

Once you have fully retracted the plunger, pull off the handle in one movement. When the handle has been removed, the unit can be disposed of safely into your sharps container; the handle is ready to be autoclaved (Fig. 9-27).

Should you need to insert a second cartridge, follow Steps 7-8:

7. **Inserting a second cartridge.** During procedures that require more than one cartridge, retract the protective sheath to the holding position (see Fig. 9-26, *A*). To reload a second cartridge after you have finished with the first one, take hold of the ULTRA Safety Plus XL handle; with the other hand, grip the protective sheath and slide it toward the holding position.

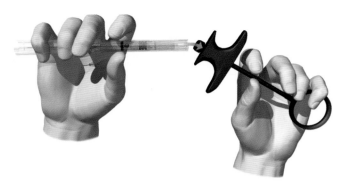

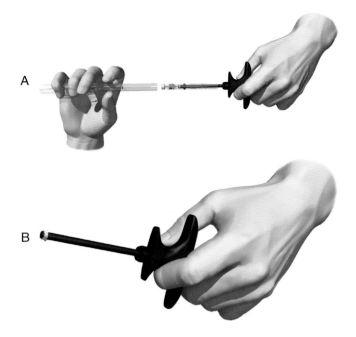

Figure 9-27. While holding the middle of the plastic barrel in one hand, use the other hand to pull back on the T-bar only, not the plunger. The injection unit is now separated from the syringe holder; the empty cartridge is removed. (Courtesy Septodont, New Castle, Del.)

Hold the barrel with one hand; with the other hand, place a finger in the ring of the plunger handle and pull backward until the plunger is fully retracted (Fig. 9-28).

When you have fully retracted the plunger, pull off the handle in one movement.

> NOTE: Should the system be inadvertently fully locked in position (see Fig. 9-26, *B*), do not attempt to unlock it. Discard the unit (Step 8) and use a new ULTRA Safety Plus XL unit.

8. You are now ready to take out the empty cartridge. Take hold of the plunger handle and pull the finger grip handle back toward the ring, exposing the silicone o-ring. Insert the tip of the plunger into the empty cartridge, which is inside the ULTRA Safety Plus XL barrel. Pull out the cartridge attached to the plunger by the silicone o-ring, remove the cartridge from the plunger, and dispose of it safely in your sharps container (Fig. 9-29). You are now ready to insert a fresh new cartridge and proceed from Step 1.

Figure 9-29. Hold the T-bar and pull the thumb ring all the way back so that the plunger is completely backed out of the anesthetic cartridge. Simply "snap" off the entire injection unit with the anesthetic cartridge still inside. (Courtesy Septodont, New Castle, Del.)

PLACING AN ADDITIONAL CARTRIDGE IN A (TRADITIONAL) SYRINGE

On occasion it is necessary to deposit an additional cartridge of local anesthetic solution. To do so, the following sequence is suggested with the metallic or plastic breech-loading syringe.

1. Recap the needle using the scoop (or other appropriate) technique and remove it from the syringe.
2. Retract the piston (which disengages the harpoon from the rubber stopper).
3. Remove the used cartridge.

Figure 9-28. While holding the plastic barrel in one hand, place a finger in the ring of the plunger handle and pull backward until the plunger is fully retracted. Then pull the handle away in one movement. (Courtesy Septodont, New Castle, Del.)

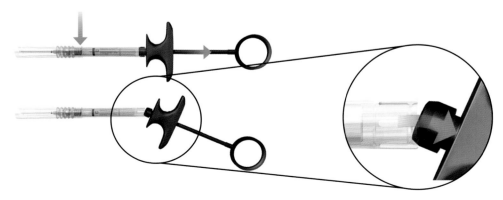

4. Insert the new cartridge.
5. Embed the harpoon.
6. Reattach the needle.

The estimated time necessary to complete this procedure is 10 to 15 seconds.

In light of the fact that most doctors do not remove the needle when reloading a syringe, the following is offered as an alternative procedure for reloading a local anesthetic syringe:

1. Recap the needle using the scoop (or other appropriate) technique.
2. Retract the piston (which disengages the harpoon from the rubber stopper).

3. Remove the used cartridge.
4. Fully retract the piston; insert the new local anesthetic cartridge.
   a. Ensure that the piston is fully retracted so that the cartridge is placed into the syringe without bending the needle stylus.
5. Embed the harpoon into the stopper of the cartridge.
   a. This requires the administrator to strike a hard, sharp blow with the hand on the thumb ring of the syringe.
6. Ensure proper placement and lack of glass breakage by expressing a small volume of anesthetic solution before administering the next injection.

IN THIS PART

PART THREE

Techniques of Regional Anesthesia in Dentistry

The anatomy of the head, neck, and oral cavity is presented as a prelude to detailed descriptions of the techniques of regional anesthesia. Techniques that are commonly used in dentistry are presented. Although many of the techniques described in these chapters also may be carried out successfully with an extraoral, rather than intraoral, approach, the author has limited descriptions to intraoral techniques, primarily because of the extremely limited use of extraoral nerve blocks in contemporary dental practice. The interested reader is referred to textbooks that describe extraoral techniques at some length.[1,2] In the second edition of this book, the *Vazirani-Akinosi closed-mouth mandibular block* and *periodontal ligament injection* were introduced, both of which have received favorable clinical acceptance since the publication of the first edition in 1980. In this fifth edition, the rediscovered "intraosseous" technique is described in depth, and two new techniques, the anterior middle superior alveolar nerve block (AMSA) and the palatal approach to the anterior superior alveolar nerve block (P-ASA), are described.[3-5]

There are usually several variations of each injection technique. Subtle differences are noted when techniques are taught to students by different persons. The reader must always keep in mind that there is never only one "correct" technique. The goals in the administration of local anesthesia are to provide clinically adequate pain control without unnecessarily increasing risk or provoking any immediate or delayed complications in the patient.[1,2] Any technique meeting these two criteria is acceptable. The techniques presented in this section are those that this author finds most acceptable. In several situations alternative approaches to the technique are also described.

A subject that is all too often neglected—the requirements for pain control and local anesthesia within the dental specialties—is discussed after describing these injection techniques. These vary somewhat, from endodontics to pediatric dentistry to periodontics to prosthodontics to oral and maxillofacial surgery, and require special attention (Chapter 16). The administration of local anesthetics to the geriatric patient, a significant and growing segment of the population, is also reviewed.

The beginning of this section, Chapters 10 and 11, addresses two important subjects relating to all injections: the physical and psychological evaluation of the patient before injection and basic injection technique (e.g., the preparation of the patient and tissues for administration of any local anesthetic, and the procedure for an atraumatic [painless] injection).

REFERENCES

1. Mulroy MF: *Regional anesthesia: an illustrated procedural guide*, ed 3, Philadelphia, 2002, Lippincott Williams & Wilkins.
2. Mulroy MF: *Peripheral nerve blocks.* In Longnecker DE, Tinker JH, Morgan GE Jr, editors: *Principles and practice of anesthesiology*, ed 2, St Louis, 1998, Mosby.
3. Friedman MJ, Hochman MN: The AMSA injection: a new concept for local anesthesia of maxillary teeth using a computer-controlled injection system. *Quint Int* 31:79-80, 2000.
4. Friedman MJ, Hochman MN: The AMSA injection: a new concept for local anesthesia of maxillary teeth using a computer-controlled injection system. *Quint Int* 29:297-303, 1998.
5. Friedman MJ, Hochman MN: P-ASA block injection: a new palatal technique to anesthetize maxillary anterior teeth. *J Esthet Dent* 11:63-71, 1999.

Physical and Psychological Evaluation

CHAPTER

10

Before starting any dental therapy, the doctor or hygienist must determine whether the patient can tolerate, both physically and psychologically, the planned dental procedures in relative safety. If this is not the case, the specific treatment modifications necessary to decrease the risk presented by the patient must be determined. This is especially important whenever drugs are to be administered during treatment and includes all drugs, such as analgesics, anxiolytics, inhalation sedation (N_2O-O_2), sedative-hypnotics, and local anesthetics. Before administering local anesthetics, the administrator must determine the relative risk presented by the patient. This is important because local anesthetics, like all drugs, exert actions on many parts of the body (see Chapter 2). Local anesthetics' actions include depressant effects on excitable membranes (e.g., the central nervous system [CNS] and the cardiovascular system [CVS]). Because local anesthetics undergo biotransformation, primarily in the liver (amides) or blood (esters), the functional status of these systems should be determined before drug administration. Because a percentage of all local anesthetics is excreted in an active (unmetabolized) form in the kidneys, they should also be evaluated. Other questions should be asked: *Has the patient ever received a local anesthetic for either medical or dental care?* If so, *Were any adverse reactions observed?*

Most undesirable reactions to local anesthetics are produced not by the drugs themselves but as a response to the act of drug administration.[1] These reactions are usually psychogenic and have the potential to be life threatening. The two most commonly occurring psychogenic reactions are vasodepressor syncope and hyperventilation. Other psychogenically induced reactions noted as a response to local anesthetic administration include tonic–clonic convulsions, bronchospasm, and angina pectoris.

However, local anesthetics are not absolutely innocuous drugs, nor is the act of local anesthetic administration entirely benign. The doctor must seek to uncover as much information as possible concerning the patient's physical and mental status before the administration of a local anesthetic. Fortunately the means to do so exist in the form of the patient's completed medical history questionnaire, the dialogue history, and the physical examination of the patient. Adequate use of these safeguards can lead to an accurate determination of a patient's physical status and prevent up to 90% of all life-threatening medical emergencies in dental practice.[2]

• • •

A brief review of the procedure of physical evaluation recommended for all dental patients follows, with emphasis on patients who are to receive local anesthesia.

• • •

MEDICAL HISTORY QUESTIONNAIRE

As a general standard of care,* dentists have their patients complete a medical history questionnaire at the initial office visit. This history should be updated regularly (e.g., every 6 months or whenever the patient has been absent from the office for an extended time). Although many such questionnaires are available, two basic types exist from which most others are derived: the short- and long-form medical histories. Both provide a knowledgeable practitioner with adequate information from which to determine a patient's physical status. A short-form medical history questionnaire is shown in Fig. 10-1.

---

*Standard of care: what a reasonably prudent doctor would do, or would not do, in a given situation.

MEDICAL HISTORY

CIRCLE

1. Are you having pain or discomfort at this time? . . . . .YES   NO
2. Do you feel very nervous about having dentistry treatment? . . . . .YES   NO
3. Have you ever had a bad experience in the dentistry office? . . . . .YES   NO
4. Have you been a patient in the hospital during the past two years? . . . . .YES   NO
5. Have you been under the care of a medical doctor during the past two years? . . . . .YES   NO
6. Have you taken any medicine or drugs during the past two years? . . . . .YES   NO
7. Are you allergic to (i.e., itching, rash, swelling of hands, feet or eyes) or made sick by
    penicillin, aspirin, codeine, or any drugs or medication? . . . . .YES   NO
8. Have you ever had any excessive bleeding requiring special treatment? . . . . .YES   NO
9. Circle any of the following which you have had or have at present:

Heart failure	Emphysema	AIDS
Heart Disease or Attack	Cough	Hepatitis A (infectious)
Angina Pectoris	Tuberculosis (TB)	Hepatitis B (serum)
High Blood Pressure	Asthma	Liver Disease
Heart Murmur	Hay Fever	Yellow Jaundice
Rheumatic Fever	Sinus Trouble	Blood Transfusion
Congenital Heart Lesions	Allergies or Hives	Drug Addiction
Scarlet Fever	Diabetes	Hemophilia
Artificial Heart Valve	Thyroid Disease	Venereal Disease (Syphilis, Gonorrhea)
Heart Pacemaker	X-ray or Cobalt Treatment	Cold Sores
Heart Surgery	Chemotherapy (Cancer, Leukemia)	Genital Herpes
Artificial Joint	Arthritis	Epilepsy or Seizures
Anemia	Rheumatism	Fainting or Dizzy Spells
Stroke	Cortisone Medicine	Nervousness
Kidney Trouble	Glaucoma	Psychiatric Treatment
Ulcers	Pain in Jaw Joints	Sickle Cell Disease
		Bruise Easily

10. When you walk up stairs or take a walk, do you ever have to stop because of pain in your chest,
    or shortness of breath, or because you are very tired? . . . . .YES   NO
11. Do your ankles swell during the day? . . . . .YES   NO
12. Do you use more than 2 pillows to sleep? . . . . .YES   NO
13. Have you lost or gained more than 10 pounds in the past year? . . . . .YES   NO
14. Do you ever wake up from sleep short of breath? . . . . .YES   NO
15. Are you on a special diet? . . . . .YES   NO
16. Has your medical doctor ever said you have a cancer or tumor? . . . . .YES   NO
17. Do you have any disease, condition, or problem not listed?
18. WOMEN: Are you pregnant now? . . . . .YES   NO
              Are you practicing birth control? . . . . .YES   NO
              Do you anticipate becoming pregnant? . . . . .YES   NO

To the best of my knowledge, all of the preceding answers are true and correct. If I ever have any change in my health, or if my medicines change, I will inform the doctor of dentistry at the next appointment without fail.

_____   _____   _____
Date   *Faculty Signature*   *Signature of Patient, Parent or Guardian*

MEDICAL HISTORY / PHYSICAL EVALUATION DATE

Date   *Addition*   *Student/Faculty Signatures*

_____   _____   _____   _____

_____   _____   _____   _____

_____   _____   _____   _____

Figure 10-1. University of Southern California School of Dentistry medical history questionnaire.

A long-form medical history questionnaire is especially valuable in teaching institutions and in those situations in which a doctor manages many patients with significant medical disorders. In addition, the long form is valuable for the doctor lacking extensive experience in physical evaluation. The in-depth questions found on this form elicit more information from a patient than those on most short-form histories. The short form is more frequently used by doctors experienced in physical evaluation.

The following questions in the medical history questionnaire should be carefully evaluated for any patient who is to receive a local anesthetic.

Question 1: Are you having pain or discomfort at this time?

Comment: The requirement for immediate treatment is gathered from this question. Also the doctor can determine whether any additional steps (e.g., sedation, oral analgesics) may be necessary to aid in achieving pain control. It is frequently more difficult to achieve adequate analgesia when chronic pain or inflammation is present.

Question 2: Do you feel very nervous about having dental treatment?

Question 3: Have you ever had a bad experience in the dental office?

Comment: These represent critical questions that are often not found on the medical history questionnaire. The patient's psychological outlook toward dentistry should be assessed before the start of treatment. A positive response to either question requires the evaluator to pursue a detailed dialogue history and to consider the possible use of psychosedation during treatment. Many patients state that they have had bad experiences related to injections or "shots" in the dental office. These situations should be pursued so that the same problem does not recur.

Question 4: Have you been a patient in the hospital during the past 2 years?

Question 5: Have you been under the care of a medical doctor during the past 2 years?

Comment: These questions seek information about any health problems for which the patient required medical intervention and that might be of significance to the planned dental therapy. Question 9 provides somewhat more detail in this area.

Question 6: Have you taken any medicine or drugs during the past 2 years?

Comment: Although few, interactions with local anesthetics or vasopressors can occur when certain drugs are taken by patients for medical disorders. These include potential drug–drug interactions between the following:

- Summation interactions with local anesthetics (use of multiple local anesthetics)
- Local anesthetics with opioid sedation
- Vasoconstrictor and nonselective β-adrenoreceptor antagonist
- Vasoconstrictor with general anesthetic
- Vasoconstrictor and cocaine
- Vasoconstrictor with tricyclic antidepressants

Potential interactions are discussed later in this chapter. In light of the plethora of *nonprescription drugs* and *herbal remedies* being taken by people, it is prudent to include them, along with *prescription drugs*, in our questioning.

Question 7: Are you allergic to (e.g., experience itching, rash, or swelling of hands, feet, or eyes) or made sick by penicillin, aspirin, codeine, or any medications?

Comment: Determine the name of the drug(s) involved and the nature of the adverse reaction that developed. Evaluation of alleged allergy to local anesthetics ("Doctor, I'm allergic to Novocain") is described in depth in Chapter 18. The incidence of true, documented, and reproducible allergy to the amide local anesthetics is virtually nil.[3,4] However, reports of alleged allergy to local anesthetics are common.[5,6] Thorough investigation of the alleged allergy is essential if the patient is not to be consigned the label of "allergic to all -caine drugs," thereby precluding dental (and surgical) care in a normal manner. Either avoidance of dental care or the receipt of dental care under general anesthesia is the alternative in these cases.

Reports of allergy to "epinephrine" or "adrenaline" also must be evaluated carefully. Most often such reports prove to be simply an exaggerated physiological response by the patient to either the injected epinephrine or, more commonly, to endogenous catecholamine release in response to the act of administering the local anesthetic (the "adrenal squeeze" as a colleague called it recently).

Question 8: Have you ever had excessive bleeding that required special treatment?

Comment: Before inserting a needle into the vascular soft tissues of the oral cavity, it should be determined if the patient is at risk for excessive bleeding. In the presence of coagulopathies or other bleeding disorders, injection techniques with a greater incidence of positive aspiration should be avoided in favor of supraperiosteal, periodontal ligament (PDL), intraosseous (IO), or other techniques less likely to produce bleeding. Techniques that might be avoided when bleeding disorders are present include the maxillary nerve block (high tuberosity approach), posterior superior alveolar nerve block, inferior alveolar nerve block, mental or incisive nerve block, and probably both the Gow-Gates and Vazirani-Akinosi mandibular nerve blocks. Although both the Gow-Gates and Vazirani-Akinosi nerve blocks have relatively low positive aspiration rates, bleeding occurring after their administration is likely to be deep in the tissues and therefore might be more difficult to manage. Modifications in therapy should be listed on the patient's chart (Fig. 10-2).

Question 9: Have you ever had any of the following conditions or treatments?

Heart failure

Comment: The degree of heart failure must be assessed. Ambulatory patients with congestive heart failure (CHF) may be considered as ASA II, III, or IV risks. CHF patients who demonstrate disability (undue fatigue, shortness of breath) at rest (ASA IV) or who are unable to complete normal functions without disability (ASA III) likely demonstrate some degree of decreased liver perfusion, leading to an increase in the half-life of amide local anesthetics.[7] Also, in more significant heart failure a greater percentage of cardiac stroke volume is delivered to the cerebral circulation (14% to 15% normal, up to 30% in more severe heart failure), increasing the risk of an overdose reaction to the local anesthetic.[7] ASA III and IV heart failure patients are less tolerant of stress, having a decreased functional reserve. Anxiety must be dealt with, not ignored. Psychosedation is appropriate (inhalation sedation preferred). Placement of the patient into the "ideal" position

Figure 10-2. Possible treatment modifications are listed on the patient's chart.

for receipt of local anesthetics (supine) and dental treatment may not prove possible because of the presence of orthopnea. Compromise in patient positioning may be necessary.

Heart disease or heart attack

Comment: Recent (<6 months) or repeated myocardial infarction (MI) increases risk to patients during dental care or the administration of local anesthetics. Patients ought not receive elective dental care within 6 months of an MI (ASA IV) because reinfarction is more likely to occur during this time.[8,9] After this period of recuperation, most status post-MI patients are treatable (ASA III) with appropriate therapy modification. The administration of local anesthetics containing vasopressors in cardiac risk patients is a never-ending question and is discussed more fully in Chapter 20. Suffice it to say here that all ASA I and some ASA II and III patients may safely receive the concentrations of vasoconstrictor contained in local anesthetic cartridges. For the more severely cardiovascular compromised ASA III patient, the dose of vasoconstrictor should be limited. The ASA IV cardiovascular risk patient is not a candidate for vasopressors or elective dental care.

Angina pectoris

Comment: Angina pectoris is defined as a transient chest pain produced by myocardial ischemia, relieved by rest or the administration of a vasodilator. Stable angina pectoris (angina of exertion) represents an ASA III risk. Any factor, such as anxiety or inadequate pain control, that increases myocardial oxygen requirements may provoke an anginal episode. The judicious use of vasopressors in local anesthetics is not contraindicated in stable angina. Unstable angina (preinfarction angina) represents an ASA IV risk.[10]

High blood pressure

Comment: The United States National Heart, Lung and Blood Institute recently revised definitions of high blood pressure for adult Americans (Table 10-1).[11] Patients with mild to moderate elevations in systolic or diastolic pressure are acceptable risks for dental care, including use of local anesthetics with vasopressors. Hypertensive

patients should have their blood pressure monitored at each appointment and be managed according to the most recent reading. It must be remembered that patient noncompliance with antihypertensive drug regimens is epidemic. Patients should be reminded to take these potentially life-saving medications as prescribed by their physician.

Heart murmur, rheumatic fever, congenital heart lesions, or scarlet fever

Comment: Patients with clinical manifestations of heart disease (e.g., valvular defects or murmurs) must undergo a more in-depth evaluation (dialogue history and physical evaluation) to determine whether any degree of disability or stress intolerance exists and whether antibiotic prophylaxis is necessary before dental care, including local anesthetic administration. Patients with mitral valve prolapse are included in this evaluation. Current prophylactic regimens from the American Heart Association are presented in Boxes 10-1, 10-2, and 10-3.[12]

The administration of local anesthetics does not, in and of itself, require antibiotic prophylaxis. The one exception to this is the PDL injection.[13] However, because it is highly unlikely that a local anesthetic would be administered without dental treatment being carried out subsequently, the nature of the dental treatment would likely dictate whether or not antibiotic prophylaxis is required.

Artificial heart valve

Comment: The presence of a prosthetic heart valve indicates the need for antibiotic prophylaxis before any dental care. Specific regimens may be individualized, and consultation with the patient's primary care physician is required before initiating any form of dental care.[12]

Heart pacemaker

Comment: Significant rhythm disturbances of the heart may necessitate the insertion of a pacemaker. Most current pacemakers are of the demand type (functioning only when needed), and these patients usually do not require antibiotic prophylaxis. Local anesthetics with vasoconstrictors may be administered safely to these patients.

TABLE **10-1**

Classification and Management of Blood Pressure for Adults

BP Classification	SBP* mmHg	DBP* mmHg	Lifestyle Modification	Initial Drug Therapy Without Compelling Indications	With Compelling Indications
Normal	<120	and <80	Encourage		
Prehypertension	120–139	or 80–89	Yes	No antihypertensive drug indicated.	Drug(s) for compelling indications.[‡]
Stage 1 Hypertension	140–159	or 90–99	Yes	Thiazide-type diuretics for most. May consider ACEI, ARB, BB, CCB, or combination	Drug(s) for the compelling indications.[‡] Other antihypertensive drugs (diuretics, ACEI, ARB, BB, CCB) as needed.
Stage 2 Hypertension	≥160	or ≥100	Yes	Two-drug combination for most[†] (usually thiazide-type diuretic and ACEI or ARB or BB or CCB).	

(Data from National Heart, Lung, and Blood Institute, Bethesda, Md, 2003.)
*Treatment determined by highest BP category.
[†]Initial combined therapy should be used cautiously in those at risk for orthostatic hypotension.
[†]Treat patients with chronic kidney disease or diabetes to BP goal of <130/80 mmHg.
ACEI = angiotensin converting enzyme inhibitor; ARB = angiotensin receptor blocker; BB = β-blocker; CCB = calcium channel blocker; DBP = diastolic blood pressure; SBP = systolic blood pressure.

Implanted cardioverter/defibrillator (ICD)

Comment: Many persons with significant atrial and ventricular cardiac dysrhythmias have received implanted cardioverter or defibrillators. These devices, computers, can sense the onset of potentially life-threatening irregularities in the heart's rhythm and deliver either a synchronized shock (cardioversion) or a shock to defibrillate the heart. The size of a deck of playing cards, the ICD is implanted under the skin on the left side of the chest. Leads are placed into the heart to monitor its rhythm and deliver a shock, if needed. Because this device is not located within the heart, there is no need for antibiotic prophylaxis. However, given the nature of this cardiac condition, a consultation with the patient's cardiologist is suggested before the start of dental treatment.

Heart operation

Comment: The nature of the surgical procedure (e.g., valve replacement, insertion of a pacemaker, coronary artery bypass), the degree of any current disability, and whether there is a need for antibiotic prophylaxis should be determined. In most cases patients with these conditions, with proper treatment modification, may safely receive dental care, including local anesthetics with vasoconstrictors, with little or no increase in risk. Physician consultation may be required.

Anemia

Comment: The presence of methemoglobinemia, either congenital or idiopathic, represents a *relative*

contraindication to the administration of prilocaine.[14,15] Methemoglobinemia is discussed in detail on p. 155.

Other forms of anemia, iron deficiency and sickle cell, do not impact the administration of local anesthetics with or without vasopressors.

Stroke

Comment: Patients with a history of cerebrovascular accident (CVA, "brain attack") or transient ischemic attack (TIA) require treatment modification to decrease risk. Blood pressure should be monitored routinely and treatment modified accordingly. Use of minimal effective doses of local anesthetics with vasoconstrictors is indicated. Intravascular administration of vasopressors should be scrupulously avoided in these patients. Most status post-CVA patients are considered ASA II or III risks 6 months or more after the acute incident.

Kidney trouble

Comment: A small percentage of injected local anesthetic is excreted unmetabolized in the urine. Patients who are functionally anephric (have kidney failure) could theoretically attain high levels of local anesthetic in their blood, thereby increasing their risk of local anesthetic overdose. In actual clinical situations, usual doses of local anesthetics do not pose any increased risk in these patients.

Hay fever, sinus trouble, or allergies or hives

Comment: A positive response to any of these items, which might indicate the presence of allergy, requires that a more complete dialogue history be performed to

BOX 10-1

Cardiac Conditions Associated with Endocarditis

ENDOCARDITIS PROPHYLAXIS RECOMMENDED
High-risk category
Prosthetic cardiac valves, including bioprosthetic and homograft valves
Previous bacterial endocarditis
Complex cyanotic congenital heart disease (e.g., single ventricle states, transposition of the great arteries, tetralogy of Fallot)
Surgically constructed systemic pulmonary shunts or conduits
Moderate-risk category
Most other congenital cardiac malformations (other than above and below)
Acquired valvar dysfunction (e.g., rheumatic heart disease)
Hypertrophic cardiomyopathy
Mitral valve prolapse with valvular regurgitation or thickened leaflets

ENDOCARDITIS PROPHYLAXIS NOT RECOMMENDED
Negligible-risk category (no greater risk than the general population)
Isolated secundum atrial septal defect
Surgical repair of atrial septal defect, ventricular septal defect, or patent ductus arteriosus (without residua beyond 6 months)
Previous coronary artery bypass graft surgery
Mitral valve prolapse without valvular regurgitation
Physiological, functional, or innocent heart murmurs
Previous Kawasaki disease without valvular dysfunction
Previous rheumatic fever without valvular dysfunction
Cardiac pacemakers (intravascular and epicardial) and implanted defibrillators

(From Dajani AS, Taubert K, Wilson W: Prevention of bacterial endocarditis: recommendations by the American Heart Association. *JAMA*, 277(22):1794-1801, 1997.)

BOX 10-2

Dental Procedures and Endocarditis Prophylaxis

ENDOCARDITIS PROPHYLAXIS RECOMMENDED*
Dental extractions
Periodontal procedures including surgery, scaling and root planing, probing, and recall maintenance
Dental implant placement and reimplantation of avulsed teeth
Endodontic (root canal) instrumentation or surgery only beyond the apex
Subgingival placement of antibiotic fibers or strips
Initial placement of orthodontic bands but not brackets
Intraligamentary local anesthetic injections
Prophylactic cleaning of teeth or implants where bleeding is anticipated

ENDOCARDITIS PROPHYLAXIS NOT RECOMMENDED
Restorative dentistry[†] (operative and prosthodontic) with or without retraction cord[‡]
Local anesthetic injections (nonintraligamentary)
Intracanal endodontic treatment; after placement and build-up
Placement of rubber dams
Postoperative suture removal
Placement of removable prosthodontic or orthodontic appliances
Taking of oral impressions
Fluoride treatments
Taking of oral radiographs
Orthodontic appliance adjustment
Shedding of primary teeth

(From Dajani AS, Taubert K, Wilson W: Prevention of bacterial endocarditis: Recommendations by the American Heart Association. *JAMA* 277(22):1794-1801, June 11, 1997.)
*Prophylaxis is recommended for patients with high- and moderate-risk cardiac conditions.
[†]This includes restoration of decayed teeth (filling cavities) and replacement of missing teeth.
[‡]Clinical judgment may indicate antibiotic use in selected circumstances that may create significant bleeding.

BOX 10-3

Prophylactic Regimens for Dental, Oral, Respiratory Tract, or Esophageal Procedures

SITUATION	AGENT	REGIMEN*
Standard general prophylaxis	Amoxicillin	Adults: 2.0 g; children: 50 mg/kg orally 1 hour before procedure
Unable to take oral medications	Ampicillin	Adults: 2.0 g IM or IV; children: 50 mg/kg IM or IV within 30 minutes before procedure
Allergic to penicillin	Clindamycin OR	Adults: 600 mg; children: 20 mg/kg orally 1 hour before procedure
	Cephalexin[†] or Cefadroxil[†] OR	Adults: 2.0 g; children: 50 mg/kg orally 1 hour before procedure
	Azithromycin or Clarithromycin	Adults: 500 mg; children: 15 mg/kg orally 1 hour before procedure
Allergic to penicillin and unable to take oral medications	Clindamycin OR	Adults: 600 mg; children: 20 mg/kg intravenously within 30 minutes before procedure
	Cefazolin[†]	Adults: 1.0 g; children: 25 mg/kg IM or IV within 30 minutes before procedure

(From Dajani AS, Taubert K, Wilson W: Prevention of bacterial endocarditis: Recommendations by the American Heart Association. *JAMA*, Vol 277(22):1794-1801, 1997.)
*Total children's dose should not exceed adult dose.
[†]Cephalosporins should not be used in individuals with immediate-type hypersensitivity reaction (urticaria, angioedema, or anaphylaxis) to penicillins.

elucidate the precise nature of the problem (described further in Chapter 18).

Thyroid disease

Comment: Patients who are clinically hyperthyroid (e.g., sensitive to heat; sweat easily; and have experienced tachycardia, palpitation, weight loss, increased body temperature, tremor of extremities, and increased nervousness) are sensitive to catecholamines and may demonstrate an exaggerated response to vasopressors included in local anesthetic solutions. Although unlikely to be significant (even though they do "bother" the patient), such reactions can be prevented or minimized through the use of minimum concentrations of epinephrine and other vasopressors. Patients with surgically corrected or medication-controlled hyperthyroid or hypothyroid conditions are termed *euthyroid* and respond in a normal manner to catecholamines.

Pain in jaw joints

Comment: The patient may be unable to open his or her mouth adequately, thus rendering certain injection techniques impossible to employ (e.g., the Gow-Gates and inferior alveolar nerve blocks). If dental care must be completed, alternate techniques should be considered (e.g., the Vazirani-Akinosi closed-mouth mandibular block or extraoral nerve blocks).

Acquired immunodeficiency syndrome (AIDS), hepatitis A (infectious), hepatitis B (serum), liver disease, jaundice, drug addiction, hemophilia

Comment: The unifying bonds among these conditions are an increased risk of infection (AIDS, hepatitis A and B) via blood or saliva and an increased risk of liver dysfunction (hepatitis A and B, liver disease, jaundice, drug addiction, and hemophilia). Thorough evaluation of the disorder is needed so the degree of risk to the administrator and to the patient can be ascertained before starting treatment. With significant (ASA IV) liver dysfunction (only rarely encountered in ambulatory patients), the half-life of the amide local anesthetics may be significantly prolonged, thereby increasing the risk of overdose.

Epilepsy or seizures

Comment: Stress may provoke a seizure even in patients with well-controlled epilepsy. Appropriate stress reduction procedures should be employed to minimize the risk of a seizure developing during treatment. Hypoglycemia and hyperventilation are two other causes of seizures in the dental environment. Severe local anesthetic overdose reactions manifest themselves clinically as generalized tonic–clonic convulsions. However, the administration of local anesthetics is not contraindicated in seizure-prone patients. (Indeed, carefully administered intravenous local anesthetics may be used as anticonvulsants in a patient during grand mal seizures.)[16]

Fainting, dizzy spells, and nervousness

Comment: These may indicate the presence of abnormal anxiety, fear, seizures, or possible orthostatic (postural) hypotension. The nature of the problem should be determined before starting dental care. Psychosedation or other treatment modifications may be required when a psychogenic etiology is present.

Psychiatric treatment

Comment: Patients under psychiatric care usually can receive a local anesthetic with no increased risk. Patients may be taking psychotropic drugs that alter their behavior patterns. Two types of drugs are frequently prescribed: tricyclic antidepressants (TCAs) and monoamine oxidase inhibitors (MAOIs). These pose a minimal risk to the administration of vasopressor-containing local anesthetics, provided the catecholamine dose is kept minimal (as was also noted for cardiovascular risk patients). See the discussion later in this chapter.

In the recent past MAOIs were considered to be relative contraindications to the administration of vasopressors. Recent information has demonstrated that this is *not* the case.[17,18]

Bruise easily

Comment: Any potential bleeding disorder must be evaluated before administering a local anesthetic, especially with a technique in which the risk of blood vessel penetration is increased, such as with the inferior alveolar nerve block, posterior superior alveolar nerve block, and mental or incisive nerve block.

Questions 10 through 16 provide the patient an opportunity to volunteer the presence of clinical signs and symptoms of diseases or syndromes that may not as yet have been diagnosed by a physician. Questions 10 through 14 pertain to clinical symptoms of various cardiovascular disorders (as well as disorders of other systems). The reader should consult *Medical Emergencies in the Dental Office*[19] for an in-depth discussion of the significance of each of these questions.

Question 17: Do you have any disease, condition, or problem not listed?

Comment: This question allows the patient to mention any disease process not noted in Question 9. Two disorders are worthy of additional discussion: *malignant hyperthermia* (MH; hyperpyrexia) and *atypical plasma cholinesterase*. MH represents a *relative contraindication* to dental care. Previously MH was considered to represent an absolute contraindication to the administration of amide local anesthetics.[20] At present it is thought that MH does *not* represent a contraindication to the administration of any local anesthetic.[21–23] MH is considered a relative contraindication because a medical consultation should be obtained before starting any dental care on patients with MH.

Atypical plasma cholinesterase also represents a *relative contraindication*, but only to the administration of ester local anesthetics.

Idiopathic or *congenital methemoglobinemia* also might be mentioned here, although its presence is most likely elicited in response to Question 9. These three entities are evaluated more fully later in this chapter.

Question 18: Women: Are you pregnant now? Are you practicing birth control? Do you anticipate becoming pregnant?

TABLE 10-2

Food and Drug Administration Pregnancy Categories

Pregnancy Category	Definition
A	[Generally considered safe] Controlled studies show no risk in first trimester; no evidence of second or third trimester risk; risk of fetal harm remote
B	[Caution advised] Animal studies show no risk or adverse fetal effects but controlled human first trimester studies not available/do not confirm; no evidence of second or third trimester risk; fetal harm possible but unlikely; see package insert for drug-specific recommendations
C	[Weigh risk and benefit] Animal studies show adverse fetal effect(s) but no controlled human studies OR no animal or human studies; weigh possible fetal risk versus maternal benefit; see package insert for drug-specific recommendations
C/D/D	[Weigh risk and benefit] Category C in first trimester but positive evidence of human fetal risk in second and third trimester; maternal benefit may outweigh fetal risk in serious or life-threatening situations; see package insert for drug-specific recommendations
D	[Weigh risk and benefit] Positive evidence of human fetal risk; maternal benefit may outweigh fetal risk in serious or life-threatening situations; see package insert for drug-specific recommendations
X	[Contraindicated] Positive evidence of serious fetal abnormalities in animals, humans, or both; fetal risks clearly outweigh maternal benefit

---

Comment: Pregnancy represents a *relative contraindication* to elective dental care, especially during the first trimester (thus the need for the latter two questions). Consultation with the patient's physician before commencing any treatment is indicated, especially if there are any problems with this or prior pregnancies. Local anesthetics and vasopressors are not teratogens and may be administered to pregnant patients during any trimester. However, it is prudent to be conservative in administering any drugs to pregnant women. Tables 10-2, 10-3, and 10-4 present the United States Food and Drug Administration's drug classification ratings for pregnancy and lactation.

Patients are asked to read the statement after Question 18 and to sign (in ink) the questionnaire, attesting that the answers provided are true and correct to the best of their knowledge. The doctor or hygienist reviewing the questionnaire should countersign the form.

• • •

The medical history questionnaire should be updated on a regular basis (e.g., every 6 months or whenever a patient has been away from the office for an extended period of time) and any changes or additions noted on the form (see the bottom of Fig. 10-1) or in the patient's dental record. The patient should be asked two questions: "Has there been any change in your health since your last visit?" and, "Are you now taking any drugs or medications?" The answers should be noted in the record (e.g., date, medical history update—no change).

DIALOGUE HISTORY

After the patient completes the medical history questionnaire, the doctor must review it for any medical disorders of possible significance. If disorders are present, the doctor next discusses these with the patient to obtain as much information as possible concerning the severity of the problem and its potential impact on the planned dental care. This questioning of the patient is called the *dialogue history*, and it constitutes an essential part of the physical evaluation process. The doctor must use all available knowledge of the disease entity to accurately assess the degree of risk represented by the patient. Dialogue history related to the administration of local anesthetic in patients with alleged allergy is presented in Chapter 18.

PHYSICAL EXAMINATION

The doctor should next conduct a physical examination of the patient. Although the scope of such an examination

---

TABLE 10-3

Food and Drug Administration Lactation Categories

Lactation Category	Definition
S	Safe for nursing infant; medication usually compatible with breast-feeding
S?	Safety in nursing infants unknown; inadequate literature available
S*	Potential for significant effects on nursing infants; medication should be given with caution
NS	Not safe for nursing infants; medication contraindicated or requires cessation of breast-feeding

TABLE 10-4

Food and Drug Administration Drug Classification Ratings for Pregnancy and Lactation

Drug	Pregnancy Category	Lactation Category
Articaine	C	Unknown-exercise caution
Bupivacaine	C	S?
Lidocaine	B	S
Mepivacaine	C	S?
Prilocaine	B	Unknown-exercise caution
Epinephrine	C	NS

is not limited and can include heart and lung auscultation and laboratory and function tests, if desired, the following *minimum* physical examination is recommended for dental patients. It includes visual inspection and the recording of vital signs.

Visual Inspection

Visual examination can provide the doctor with valuable information concerning the patient's medical status. Observation of a patient's posture, body movements, speech patterns, and skin can assist in a diagnosis of possibly significant disorders that may have previously gone undetected. The interested reader is referred to textbooks that deal with physical examination in greater depth.[19,24]

Vital Signs

There are six vital signs: blood pressure, heart rate and rhythm (pulse), respiratory rate, temperature, height, and weight. Vital signs should be recorded on the patient's dental chart (Fig. 10-3). For a minimum examination, it is recommended that the blood pressure and heart rate and rhythm be monitored for all patients seeking dental care. Table 10-5 presents guidelines for dental management of adult patients according to their blood pressure. Adherence to these guidelines minimizes the development of acute complications of high blood pressure, such as CVA. A patient with a systolic pressure in excess of 200 mmHg or a diastolic in excess of 115 (ASA IV) is

at significant risk and ought not to undergo invasive elective dental care until the blood pressure elevation has been brought under control. The act of administering local anesthetics can only further elevate the blood pressure of an already anxious patient.

The heart rate, or pulse, can be measured at any readily accessible artery. The brachial or radial artery is the most frequently used for routine assessment. Three factors should be evaluated when monitoring the pulse: the heart *rate* (recorded as beats per minute), the heart *rhythm* (regular or irregular), and the *quality* of the pulse (thready, bounding, or weak). The normal resting adult heart rate ranges from 60 to 110 beats per minute. It is suggested that any adult patient with a heart rate below 60 or above 110 undergo further evaluation. Anxiety is the most frequent cause of an elevated heart rate in the dental environment. The rhythm of the heart is equally, if not more, important. A normal pulse maintains a relatively regular rhythm. The occasional premature ventricular contraction (PVC) is not uncommon, and results from smoking, fatigue, stress, various drugs and medications (e.g., epinephrine), and the ingestion of alcohol. A PVC is noted as a "missed beat" when a peripheral pulse is taken. If PVCs occur at a rate of five or more per minute with no obvious cause, medical consultation must be considered. Unusually frequent PVCs in a high-risk cardiovascular patient (ASA III or IV) indicate myocardial irritability (ischemia) and may presage more serious ventricular dysrhythmias (tachycardia and fibrillation).[25] The administration of epinephrine-containing local anesthetics is relatively contraindicated in patients with cardiac dysrhythmias unresponsive to medical therapy. Dysrhythmias frequently are induced by an ischemic or irritable myocardium. Epinephrine and other catecholamines may provoke further irritability, leading to potentially more serious, possibly lethal dysrhythmias.

Determination of Medical Risk

Having completed all components of the physical evaluation and a thorough intraoral dental examination, the doctor must then gather this information and answer the following questions:

1. Is the patient capable, both physiologically and psychologically, of tolerating in relative safety the stresses involved in the proposed treatment?

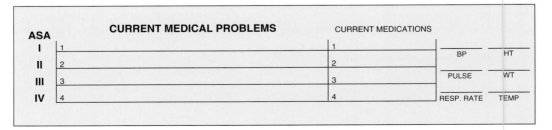

Figure 10-3. Baseline vital signs are recorded on the patient's chart.

TABLE 10-5
Adult Blood Pressure Guidelines

Blood Pressure (mm Hg)			ASA	
Systolic		Diastolic	Classification	Dental Treatment Considerations
<140	and	<90	I	Routine dental management Recheck in 6 months
140 to 159	and /or	90 to 94	II	Recheck blood pressure before dental treatment for three consecutive appointments; if all exceed these guidelines, seek medical consultation
160 to 179	and/or	95 to 104	IIIa	Recheck blood pressure in 5 minutes Routine dental therapy Consider stress reduction protocol
180 to 199	and/or	105 to 114	IIIb	Recheck blood pressure in 5 minutes If still elevated, seek medical consultation before dental treatment If all other medical history factors are within normal limits (WNL), routine dental therapy Seriously consider stress reduction protocol
>200	and/or	>115	IV	Recheck blood pressure in 5 minutes Immediate medical consultation if still elevated No dental care, elective or emergent, until blood pressure is decreased (Noninvasive) Emergency care with drugs: analgesics, antibiotics Refer to hospital for invasive dental care

2. Does the patient represent a greater risk (of morbidity or mortality) than normal during this treatment?
3. If the patient does represent an increased risk, what modifications are necessary in the planned treatment to minimize this risk?
4. Is the risk too great for the patient to be managed safely as an outpatient in the medical or dental office?

The U.S.C. School of Dentistry developed a physical evaluation system, based on the American Society of Anesthesiologists (ASA) Physical Status Classification System that enables the doctor to readily evaluate a patient's risk status before starting treatment. This system, defined in Table 10-6, is described in considerable detail in other monographs.[26–28] Components of the stress reduction protocol (SRP) for medically compromised ASA categories II, III, and IV are presented in Box 10-4.[29,30]

Careful consideration of the pretreatment evaluation enables the doctor to accurately determine a potential patient's ability to withstand the stresses associated with dental care. If there is any doubt concerning a patient's ability to tolerate these stresses, medical consultation should be obtained, leading to possible modifications in the planned dental treatment. Contraindications, both relative and absolute, to the use of local anesthetic solutions are summarized in Chapter 4.

• • •

Potential drug–drug interactions involving either local anesthetics or vasopressors, and three *relative*

TABLE 10-6
University of Southern California Physical Evaluation System

American Society of Anesthesiologists Physical Status Classification and Definition		Dental Therapy Modifications
I	Normal, healthy patient	None (stress reduction protocol [SRP], as indicated)
II	Patient with mild to moderate systemic disease	Possible SRP and other modifications as indicated
III	Patient with severe systemic disease that limits activity but is not incapacitating	Possible strict modifications; SRP and medical consultations are priorities
IV	Patient with severe systemic disease that limits activity and is a constant threat to life	Elective care contraindicated. Noninvasive emergency care in office; hospitalize for invasive emergency care; medical consultation urged
V	Moribund patient not expected to survive 24 hours with or without the operation	Hospitalized; dental care limited to palliative treatment only
VI	Clinically dead patient being maintained for harvesting of organs	

BOX 10-4

Stress Reduction Protocol

1. Sedation: evening before, and morning of, appointment
2. Sedation: intraoperative
3. Effective pain control
4. Morning appointment
5. Time factor: Do not exceed patient's tolerance
6. Hot, humid weather
7. Postoperative prescriptions, prn
8. Postoperative telephone call:
   ASA III, IV
   Postparenteral sedation, general anesthesia
   Prolonged, or traumatic, procedure

contraindications to the administration of local anesthetics—malignant hyperthermia or malignant hyperpyrexia, atypical plasma cholinesterase, and idiopathic or congenital methemoglobinemia—are detailed in the following discussion. A fourth—allergy (an *absolute contraindication*)—is discussed in Chapter 18.

The importance of each potential interaction is listed in its Significance Rating designed by Moore and associates.[31] The rating system is defined in Box 10-5.

BOX 10-5

Significance Ratings for Dental Drug Interactions

RATING	DEFINITION
1	Major reactions that are established, probable, or suspected
2	Moderate reactions that are established, probable, or suspected
3	Minor reactions that are established, probable, or suspected
4	Major or minor reactions that are possible
5	Minor reactions that are possible; all reactions that are unlikely

SEVERITY RATING

Major	Potentially life threatening or capable of causing permanent damage
Moderate	Could cause deterioration of patient's clinical status; additional treatment or hospitalization might be necessary
Minor	Mild effects that are bothersome or unnoticed; should not significantly affect therapeutic outcome

DOCUMENTATION RATING

Established	Proved to occur in well-controlled studies
Probable	Very likely, but not proved clinically
Suspected	Could occur; some good data exist, but more study is needed
Possible	Could occur; data are very limited
Unlikely	Doubtful; there is no consistent and reliable evidence of an altered clinical effect

DRUG–DRUG INTERACTIONS

Amide Local Anesthetics with Inhibitors of Metabolism (e.g., Cimetidine and Lidocaine) (Significance Rating = 5)

The H_2-receptor blocker *cimetidine* modifies the biotransformation of lidocaine by competing with it for binding to hepatic oxidative enzymes. Other H_2-receptor blockers, such as ranitidine and famotidine, do not inhibit lidocaine biotransformation.[32,33] The net result of this interaction with cimetidine is an increase in the half-life of the circulating local anesthetic. With typical dental practice usage of local anesthetics, this interaction is of little clinical significance. The interaction between amide local anesthetics and cimetidine might be of greater clinical significance in the presence of a history of CHF (ASA III or greater), where the percentage of cardiac output delivered to the liver falls while the percentage of cardiac output delivered to the brain increases.[34] With greater blood levels of lidocaine secondary to cimetidine, and an increased percentage in blood being delivered to the brain, the risk of local anesthetic overdose is increased somewhat. The inhibition of local anesthetic metabolism has little effect on peak plasma levels of the local anesthetic when given as a single injection.[35] This combination of factors—cimetidine and ASA III + CHF—represents a *relative contraindication* to the use of amide local anesthetics. Minimal doses of amide local anesthetics should be administered.

Summation Interactions with Local Anesthetics (Significance Rating = 1)

Combinations of local anesthetics may be administered together without unnecessary increase in risk of a toxic reaction (overdose) developing. Toxicity of local anesthetics is additive when they are administered in combination. To minimize this risk, the total dose of all local anesthetics administered should not exceed the maximum recommended dose (MRD) of the drugs used.

Sulfonamides and Esters (Significance Rating = 5)

Ester local anesthetics, such as procaine and tetracaine, may inhibit the bacteriostatic action of the sulfonamides. With the uncommon use of sulfonamides today, along with the extremely rare administration of ester local anesthetics in dentistry, this potential drug interaction is unlikely to be noted. As a rule, ester local anesthetics should not be administered to patients receiving sulfonamides.

Local Anesthetics with Opioid Sedation (Significance Rating = 1)

Sedation with opioid analgesics may increase the risk of developing local anesthetic overdose. This is of primary concern in children. Therefore the dosage of local anesthetic should be minimized.

Local Anesthetic-induced Methemoglobinemia (Significance Rating = 4)

Methemoglobin usually results when prilocaine is administered in excessive dosages.[15] Local anesthetic-induced methemoglobinemia is discussed later in this chapter.

Vasoconstrictor and Tricyclic Antidepressant (e.g., Levonordefrin and Amitriptyline) (Significance Rating = 1)

Tricyclic antidepressants (TCAs) are commonly prescribed in the management of major depression. TCAs may enhance the cardiovascular actions of exogenously administered vasopressors. This enhancement of activity is approximately fivefold to tenfold with levonordefrin and norepinephrine, but is only twofold with epinephrine and phenylephrine.[36] This interaction has been reported to have resulted in a series of hypertensive crises, one of which led to the death of a patient (after a small dose of norepinephrine).[37] *The administration of norepinephrine and levonordefrin should be avoided in patients receiving TCAs.* Patients receiving epinephrine-containing local anesthetics should be administered the smallest effective dose. Yagiela and associates recommend limiting the epinephrine dose to patients receiving TCAs in a dental appointment to 0.05 mg or 5.4 ml of a 1:100,000 epinephrine concentration.[38] Commonly prescribed TCAs are listed in Box 10-6.

Vasoconstrictors and Nonselective β-adrenoceptor Antagonist (β-blocker) (e.g., Propranolol and Epinephrine) (Significance Rating = 1)

The administration of vasopressors in patients being treated with nonselective β-blockers increases the likelihood of a serious elevation of the blood pressure accompanied by a reflex bradycardia. Several cases have been reported in the medical literature and appear to be dose

---

BOX 10-6

Antidepressant Medications

TRICYCLIC ANTIDEPRESSANTS	MONOAMINE OXIDASE INHIBITORS
Amitriptyline (Elavil)	Isocarboxazid (Marplan)
Nortriptyline (Aventyl, Pamelor)	Phenelzine (Nardil)
Imipramine (Tofranil)	Tranylcypromine (Parnate)
Doxepin (Sinequan)	Trimipramine (Surmontil)
Amoxapine (Asendin)	
Desipramine (Norpramin)	
Protriptyline (Vivactil)	
Clomipramine (Anafranil)	

BOX 10-7

β-adrenoceptor Antagonists (β-blockers)

NONSELECTIVE (β₁ AND β₂ ADRENORECEPTORS)	CARDIOSELECTIVE (β₁ ADRENORECEPTORS)
Penbutolol (Levatol)	Atenolol (Tenormin)
Carteolol (Cartrol)	Betaxolol (Kerlone)
Pindolol (Visken)	Metoprolol (Lopressor)
Timolol (Blocadren)	Acebutolol (Sectral)
Sotalol (Betapace)	Esmolol (Brevibloc)
Nadolol (Corgard)	Bisoprolol (Zebeta)
Propranolol (Inderal, Betachron)	

---

related.[39,40] Reactions have occurred with epinephrine doses ranging from 0.04 to 0.32 mg, the equivalent of the administration of from 4 to 32 ml of local anesthetic with a 1:100,000 epinephrine concentration.[41] Box 10-7 lists both nonselective and cardioselective β-blockers.

Monitoring preoperative vital signs—specifically the blood pressure and heart rate and rhythm—is strongly recommended for all patients, but is especially recommended in patients receiving β-blockers. Rerecording these vital signs at 5 to 10 minutes after the administration of a vasopressor-containing local anesthetic is strongly suggested.

Vasoconstrictor with General Anesthetic (e.g., Halothane and Epinephrine) (Significance Rating = 1)

There is an increased possibility of cardiac dysrhythmias when patients receiving certain halogenated general anesthetic gases are administered epinephrine.[42,43] Discussion with the anesthesiologist before local anesthetic administration during general anesthesia is suggested.

Vasoconstrictor with Cocaine (Significance Rating = 1)

Cocaine is a local anesthetic drug that also possesses significant stimulatory properties on the CNS and CVS. Cocaine stimulates norepinephrine release and inhibits its reuptake in adrenergic nerve terminals, thus producing a state of catecholamine hypersensitivity.[44,45] Tachycardia and hypertension frequently are observed with cocaine administration, both of which increase cardiac output and myocardial oxygen requirements.[46] When this results in myocardial ischemia, potentially lethal dysrhythmias, anginal pain, myocardial infarction, or cardiac arrest may ensue.[47-49] The risk of such problems is elevated in dentistry when a local anesthetic containing a vasopressor is accidentally administered intravascularly in a patient with already high cocaine blood levels. After intranasal application of cocaine, peak blood levels develop within 30 minutes and usually disappear after 4 to 6 hours.[50] *Whenever possible, local anesthetics containing vasopressors should not be administered to patients who have used cocaine on the day of their dental appointment.*[51] Unfortunately, it is the rare abuser of cocaine who will volunteer this vital information to the dentist. The use of epinephrine-impregnated gingival retraction cord, although not recommended for use in any dental patient, is absolutely contraindicated in the cocaine abuser.

The administration of local anesthetics to cocaine abusers also can increase the risk of local anesthetic overdose. If there is any suspicion about a patient having used cocaine recently, the patient should be questioned directly. *If cocaine has been used within 24 hours of the dental appointment, or it is suspected that cocaine has been used within 24 hours, the planned dental treatment should be postponed.*[52,53]

Vasoconstrictor with Antipsychotic or Other α-Adrenoceptor Blocker (Significance Rating = 4)

Hypotension as a result of antipsychotic overdose may be intensified. Vasoconstrictor should be used with caution.[54]

Vasoconstrictor with Adrenergic Neuronal Blocker (Significance Rating = 4)

Sympathomimetic effects may be enhanced. The vasoconstrictor should be used cautiously.[55] Phenothiazines are psychotropic drugs usually prescribed for the management of serious psychotic disorders. The most commonly observed side effect of phenothiazines involving the cardiovascular system is *postural hypotension.* The phenothiazines suppress the vasoconstricting actions of epinephrine, permitting its milder vasodilating actions to work unopposed. This response is not likely to develop when local anesthetics are administered extravascularly; however, accidental intravascular administration of a vasopressor-containing local anesthetic could lead to hypotension in patients receiving phenothiazines.[53]

Local anesthetics containing vasopressors are not contraindicated in patients receiving phenothiazines; however, it is recommended that *the smallest volume of vasopressor-containing local anesthetic that is compatible with clinically adequate pain control be administered.*

Vasoconstrictor with Thyroid Hormone (e.g., Epinephrine and Thyroxine) (Significance Rating = 4)

Summation of effects is possible when thyroid hormones are taken in excess. Vasoconstrictor should be used with caution when clinical signs and symptoms indicating hyperthyroidism are present.[56,57]

Vasoconstrictor and Monoamine Oxidase Inhibitors (Significance Rating = 5)

Monoamine oxidase inhibitors (MAOIs) are prescribed in the management of major depression, certain phobic-anxiety states, and obsessive-compulsive disorders

(Box 10-6).[53] They are capable of potentiating the actions of vasopressors used in dental local anesthetics by inhibiting their biodegradation by the enzyme monoamine oxidase (MAO) at the presynaptic neuron level.[44]

Historically the administration of local anesthetics containing vasopressors has been absolutely contraindicated for patients receiving MAOIs because of the increased risk of hypertensive crisis. However, Yagiela and others demonstrated that such an interaction among epinephrine, levonordefrin, norepinephrine, and MAO did not occur.[38,53] Such a response, hypertensive crisis, did develop with phenylephrine, a vasopressor not used at present in dental local anesthetic solutions.

Therefore it seems appropriate to state that, "there seems to be no restriction, from a theoretical basis, to use local anesthetic with vasoconstrictor other than phenylephrine in patients currently treated with MAOIs."[53]

For a thorough review of potentially significant drug interactions occurring in dentistry, the reader is referred to the excellent series of papers that appeared in 1999 in the *Journal of the American Dental Association.*[18,31,35,58,59]

• • •

Most known drug–drug interactions involving local anesthetics or vasopressors occur with CNS and CVS depressants. Whenever a potential drug–drug interaction exists, doses of local anesthetics should be decreased. There is no formula for the correct degree of reduction. Prudence dictates, however, that the smallest dose of local anesthetic or vasopressor that is clinically effective be used.

Knowledge of all drugs and medications, including prescription and nonprescription drugs, as well as herbal remedies, being taken by a patient better enables the doctor to evaluate the patient's overall physical and psychological well-being. Drug references such as *Mosby's Drug Consult, Compendium of Pharmaceuticals and Specialities* (CPS) (Canada),* or *ePocrates.com*† are valuable resources in determining drug information, including the potential for drug–drug interactions. Current medications should be listed in the dental record.

MALIGNANT HYPERTHERMIA

Malignant hyperthermia (MH; malignant hyperpyrexia) is one of the most intense and life-threatening complications associated with the administration of general anesthesia. It occurs rarely: a 1:15,000 incidence among children receiving general anesthesia and a 1:50,000 incidence in adults.[60] The syndrome is transmitted genetically by an autosomally dominant gene. Reduced penetrance and variable expressivity in siblings of families inheriting the syndrome are also characteristic of its genetic transmission. MH is seen more frequently in males than

---

*Compendium of Pharmaceuticals and Specialities *www.pharmacists.ca.*
†*www.epocrates.com.*

females, a finding that increases with increasing age. To date, the youngest reported case of MH was in a boy aged 2 months and the oldest in a 78-year-old man.

The reports of MH in North America appear to be clustered in three regions: Toronto (in Canada) and Wisconsin and Nebraska (in the United States). Most persons with MH are functionally normal, the presence of MH becoming known only when the individual is exposed to triggering agents or through specific testing.

For many years it was thought that MH could be triggered when susceptible patients were exposed to amide local anesthetics.[61] Indeed, in both the first and second editions of this textbook, MH was considered an absolute contraindication to amide local anesthetics. However, more recent findings[62-64] and publications by the Malignant Hyperthermia Association of the United States (MHAUS)[23] have demonstrated that amide local anesthetics are not likely to trigger such episodes; thus MH has been recategorized as a *relative contraindication* in the third and subsequent editions.

Mechanism

It is felt that the mechanism underlying MH is a defect in the distribution of myoplasmic calcium (Ca^{++}). The primary event in an acute episode is a rise in Ca^{++} concentration in the myoplasm, which serves to explain the observed muscular rigidity, metabolic acidosis, and elevated body temperature.

Elevation of Ca^{++} levels occurs in normal muscles and MH-susceptible (MHS) muscles. Increased Ca^{++} concentration acts on the contractile proteins troponin and tropomyosin. Tropomyosin molecules are repositioned as a result of Ca^{++} binding to troponin so the myosin heads can contact the actin molecules. Muscle fibrils shorten and the muscle contracts. When the myoplasmic Ca^{++} level decreases to its initial concentration, muscle relaxation occurs. The strength of muscle contraction is a function of the concentration of free Ca^{++} in the cytoplasm. Kalow and associates[66] first demonstrated the increased contractility of MHS muscle using exposure to caffeine. Subsequent studies have shown spontaneous contractures of MHS muscle with exposure to halothane and succinylcholine.[67,68] Halothane increases myoplasmic Ca^{++} concentration by a direct action on the cell membrane. Succinylcholine increases Ca^{++} levels through muscle fasciculation.

Why do Ca^{++} concentrations remain elevated in MHS patients? The reason might be a continuous release of Ca^{++} or a defect in the mechanism of Ca^{++} reuptake. Nelson and Denborough[69] demonstrated that halothane produces a continuous release of Ca^{++} into the myoplasm of MHS muscle. Cheah and Cheah[70] reported a Ca^{++} efflux rate from mitochondria of MH-sensitive pigs in anaerobic circumstances twice that of stress-resistant animals: a rate that is further enhanced with exposure to halothane.

Lactic acidosis occurring in MH results from the activation of phosphorylase by Ca^{++} so that glycogen is broken down into lactic acid. Phosphorylase activation helps to supply the fructose-1,6-diphosphate for adenosine triphosphate (ATP) production by glycolysis. Heat is generated during the continuous synthesis and utilization of ATP during glycolysis in both muscle and the liver (increased metabolism), which is a possible explanation for the elevated temperature seen in MH patients.

Clinical Signs and Symptoms

The MH syndrome is characterized by tachycardia, fever (increased body core temperature), tachypnea, cardiac dysrhythmias, muscle rigidity, cyanosis, and death, which occurs when the patient is exposed to a triggering agent, usually a drug used to induce or maintain general anesthesia. Most episodes of MH have occurred on the patient's first exposure to general anesthesia; however, some have developed after a prior uneventful exposure to these same drugs.

The initial clinical sign of MH is frequently an unexplained tachycardia, produced by the hypermetabolic state that is starting to manifest itself. Tachypnea and cyanosis also develop in response to the increased production of carbon dioxide and the body's increased demand for oxygen. Muscle rigidity frequently develops, particularly in the masseter, and may occur after the administration of a muscle relaxant drug such as succinylcholine.

Increased body temperature does not occur immediately in all cases of MH. Pyrexia usually follows muscle rigidity and is a result, not a cause, of the reaction. Increases in body temperature may occur gradually over many hours or may rise abruptly within 10 to 15 minutes. Core temperatures of greater than 110°F (43°C) have been monitored. The mortality associated with MH was 80% but has been reduced to 10% since 1985 through the combination of increased awareness and early recognition and treatment.[71] A syndrome with a mortality of even 10% despite vigorous treatment remains one that all health professionals should respect and seek to prevent.

Etiology

All reported cases of MH (associated with drug administration) have developed during the administration of general anesthesia.[72] There appears to be no association with the type of surgical procedure being performed. Several cases of MH have been reported among anesthetized patients receiving dental care, including one case in a dental office.[73,74]

Anesthetic agents that have been associated with cases of MH are as follows (several of these drugs, such as lidocaine and mepivacaine, have been associated with MH only anecdotally): succinylcholine (77% of all cases), halothane (60%), enflurane, isoflurane, desflurane, and sevoflurane.

Two drugs have been associated with a preponderance of MH cases: succinylcholine, a skeletal muscle relaxant

(77% of all cases), and halothane (60%).[75] Of significance to dentistry is the fact that the two most commonly used (amide) local anesthetics, lidocaine and mepivacaine, had been administered along with other potential trigger agents in cases in which MH developed. Initially it was considered that a history of documented MH or a high risk of MH should be considered an absolute contraindication to the administration of all amide local anesthetics. However, *more recent evidence indicates that MH is not a likely occurrence with amide local anesthetics as used in dentistry and as such should only be considered a relative contraindication.* The MHAUS published a policy statement on the use of local anesthetics:[65] "Based on limited clinical and laboratory evidence, all local anesthetic drugs appear to be safe for MH susceptible individuals." This statement followed several reports in the literature, including one by Adragna,[76] which stated, "After an extensive search of the literature, I have been unable to find any reports of any malignant hyperthermic crisis caused solely by the use of amide local anesthetics without epinephrine. . . . In fact, lidocaine has been used successfully to treat the arrhythmias of a severe MH reaction and, in fact, lidocaine has been used routinely as a local anesthetic without problems on MHS patients in at least one institution. . . . The question I am posing is clear. Is there any evidence that amide local anesthetics are contraindicated in MHS patients, or is our habit of avoiding them just a habit?" Because the MH syndrome has yet to be reported in a situation in which local anesthetic was the sole drug administered, it is reasonable for the dentist to manage the dental needs of such patients using either amide or ester local anesthetics. Prior consultation with the patient's physician is strongly suggested.

Adriani and Sundin reported that in susceptible patients MH may be precipitated by factors other than the drugs just listed.[77] These include emotional factors (excitement and stress) and physical factors (mild infection, muscle injury, vigorous exercise, and elevated environmental temperatures). It appears then that the dental office could be a site where the susceptible patient, exposed to excessive stresses such as pain and fear, might exhibit symptoms of MH.

Recognition of the High-risk Malignant Hyperthermia Patient

There are no questions on medical history questionnaires currently used in dental practice that specifically address MH. The only one on the health history questionnaire that might elicit this information is Question 17: *Do you have any disease, condition, or problem not listed?* The patient with MH or a family member at risk has to volunteer this information to the doctor at an early visit.

Family members are usually evaluated for their risk after the occurrence of MH. Initial evaluation involves determination of the blood levels of creatinine phosphokinase (CPK).[78] Elevated CPK levels are seen when muscle damage has occurred. With an elevated CPK, a second phase of evaluation is required, involving the histological examination of a biopsy specimen taken from the quadriceps muscle (with the patient under a type of anesthesia known to be safe) and testing of the specimen for an increased contracture response to when exposed to halothane and caffeine.

Dental Management of the Malignant Hyperthermia Patient

On disclosure of the presence of MH, or when there is a high risk of its occurrence, it is recommended that the dentist contact the patient's primary care physician to discuss treatment options.

Dental management on an outpatient basis is possible in most cases, but with higher-risk patients it might be prudent to conduct such treatment within the confines of a hospital, where immediate emergency care is available should the MH syndrome be triggered. "Normal" doses of amide local anesthetics may be used with little increase in risk.[65] Ester local anesthetics may also be used for nerve block or infiltration anesthesia. Esters include chloroprocaine and procaine/propoxycaine. Vasoconstrictors may be included with either the esters or the amides to provide longer periods of pain control or hemostasis.

General anesthesia may be used when it is absolutely necessary, although with great care and preparation. Agents that may be administered safely to MHS patients include the following:[79]

1. Amide and ester local anesthetics with or without vasoconstrictors
2. Barbiturates
3. Benzodiazepines
4. Etomidate
5. Ketamine
6. Narcotics
7. Nitrous oxide
8. Opioids
9. Propofol

Safe muscle relaxants:[78]

1. Atracurium
2. Doxacurium
3. Mivacurium
4. Pancuronium
5. Pipecuronium
6. Rocuronium
7. Vecuronium

Unfortunately, risk is still present even with this list of "safe" drugs because triggering agents may have been administered to the patient uneventfully on prior occasions but may subsequently produce the syndrome. As always, the potential risk of drug administration must be carefully weighed against the benefits to be gained.

The development and use of dantrolene sodium (Dantrium), a long-acting hydantoin-type muscle relaxant (it is the only direct-acting skeletal muscle relaxant), has greatly benefited both the prevention and treatment of MH. Dantrolene effectively blocks the release of Ca^{++} from the sarcoplasmic reticulum. It became available in oral form in 1972 and as an injectable in 1978 and has been used extensively in the treatment of MH. MHAUS does not recommend prophylactic administration of dantrolene before dental treatment.[79]

Management of Acute Episodes

Current MHAUS guidelines for emergency treatment of patients with MH follow:[79]

Immediate consultation with MHAUS may be obtained (in the United States) by calling 1-800-MH-HYPER or 1-800-644-9737.

1. Discontinue triggering agents.
2. Hyperventilate with 100% oxygen at three to four times normal minute volume.
3. Give dantrolene sodium IV 2.5 mg/kg, repeated as necessary based on ongoing signs of MH.
   a. 36 vials of dantrolene sodium should be on hand (20 mg/vial).
   b. Add 60 ml of sterile water without bacteriostatic agent to each vial of dantrolene to reconstitute the drug.
   c. Shake vigorously to reconstitute (until clear).
   d. Use IV spike transfer pins to reconstitute.
   e. Once mixed, protect from direct light.
   f. 2.5 mg/kg body weight should be given initially and repeated every 5 to 10 minutes.
   g. Continue administration until signs of MH abate.
   h. Use reconstituted drug within 6 hours.
4. Give bicarbonate 1 to 2 mEq/kg in absence of blood gas analysis.
5. In case of hyperthermia administer:
   a. Cold IV fluids
   b. External ice packs to groin and axilla
   c. Lavage of stomach with cold solutions
6. Dysrhythmias usually respond to management of acidosis and hyperkalemia. Antidysrhythmic drugs, excluding calcium-channel blockers, may be used for refractory or life-threatening dysrhythmias.
7. After a fulminant MH episode, the patient should be placed in an intensive care unit for at least 24 hours after all signs have returned to normal.
8. Monitor CPK, calcium, and potassium concentrations until such time as they return to baseline levels.
9. Initiate electrocardiograph monitoring and continue it during the postoperative period.
10. Monitor body temperature closely, because hypothermia may result from overvigorous treatment of MH. Core temperatures of 106°F (41°C to 42°C) are compatible with survival and normal brain function if recognized and treated promptly.
11. Ensure adequate output of urine (>2 ml/kg per hour).
12. Convert from intravenous to oral dantrolene when the condition permits. It is currently recommended that 4 mg/kg per day in divided doses be given orally for 48 hours after operation.

Summary

As these guidelines for treatment indicate, MH is a life-threatening event. The drugs, equipment, techniques, and facilities required for its management are available only in a well-equipped medical center. Therefore prevention is the key to successful dental management of the MH-susceptible patient. Immediate medical consultation with the patient's primary care physician, the anesthesiology department of a local medical center, or MHAUS is important. When the patient is well prepared and well monitored, prophylaxis with dantrolene sodium and the use of "safe" drugs can lead to a successful dental experience.

ATYPICAL PLASMA CHOLINESTERASE

Choline–ester substrates, such as the depolarizing muscle relaxant succinylcholine and the ester local anesthetics, are hydrolyzed in the blood by the enzyme plasma cholinesterase, which is produced in the liver. Hydrolysis of these chemicals is usually quite rapid, their blood levels decreasing rapidly, thereby terminating the drug's action (succinylcholine) or minimizing the risk of overdose (ester local anesthetics).

Approximately 1 out of every 2820 persons possesses an atypical form of plasma cholinesterase, transmitted as an inherited autosomal recessive trait.[80] Although a number of genetic variations of atypical plasma cholinesterase are identifiable, not all produce clinically significant signs and symptoms.

Determination

In most cases the presence of atypical plasma cholinesterase is determined through the patient's response to succinylcholine, a depolarizing skeletal muscle relaxant. Succinylcholine is commonly administered during the induction of general anesthesia to facilitate intubation of the trachea. Apnea is produced for a brief time with spontaneous ventilation returning as the succinylcholine is hydrolyzed by plasma cholinesterase. When atypical plasma cholinesterase is present, the apneic period is prolonged from minutes to many hours. Patient management simply involves the maintenance of controlled ventilation until effective spontaneous respiratory efforts return. After recovery the patient and family members are tested for a serum cholinesterase survey. The dibucaine number is determined from a sample of blood. Normal patients have dibucaine numbers between 66 and 86. Atypical plasma cholinesterase patients exhibiting prolonged response to succinylcholine have dibucaine numbers as low as 20, with other genetic variants exhibiting intermediate values. Patients with low dibucaine numbers are more likely to exhibit prolonged succinylcholine-induced apnea.[81]

Significance in Dentistry

The presence of atypical plasma cholinesterase should alert the doctor to the increased risk of prolonged apnea in patients receiving succinylcholine during general anesthesia. Also, and of greater significance in the typical ambulatory dental patient not receiving general anesthesia or succinylcholine, is the increased risk of developing elevated blood levels of the ester local anesthetics. Signs and symptoms of local anesthetic overdose are more apt to be noted in these patients, even after "normal" dosages.

Atypical plasma cholinesterase represents a *relative contraindication* to the administration of the ester local anesthetics. Whenever possible, amide local anesthetics should be administered. Because they undergo biotransformation in the liver, amide anesthetics do not present the increased risk of overly high blood levels in these patients. Ester anesthetics may be administered, if deemed necessary by the doctor, but their doses should be minimized.

METHEMOGLOBINEMIA

Methemoglobinemia is a condition in which a cyanosis-like state develops in the absence of cardiac or respiratory abnormalities. When the condition is severe, the blood appears chocolate brown, and clinical signs and symptoms, including respiratory depression and syncope, may be noted. Death, although unlikely, can result. Methemoglobinemia may occur through inborn errors of metabolism or may be acquired through the administration of drugs or chemicals that are able to increase the formation of methemoglobin. The injectable local anesthetic prilocaine can produce methemoglobinemia in patients with subclinical methemoglobinemia when administered in large doses.[82,83]

Administration of prilocaine to patients with congenital methemoglobinemia or other clinical syndromes in which the oxygen-carrying capacity of blood is reduced should be avoided because of the increased risk of producing clinically significant methemoglobinemia. The topical anesthetic benzocaine also can induce methemoglobinemia, but only when administered in very large doses.[84,85]

Etiology

Iron is normally present in the reduced or ferrous state (Fe^{++}) in the hemoglobin molecule. Each hemoglobin molecule contains four ferrous atoms, each loosely bound to a molecule of oxygen. In the ferrous state, hemoglobin can carry oxygen that is available to the tissues. Because hemoglobin in the erythrocyte is inherently unstable, it is continuously being oxidized to the ferric form (Fe^{+++}), in which state the oxygen molecule is more firmly attached and cannot be released to the tissues. This form of hemoglobin is called *methemoglobin*. To permit an adequate oxygen-carrying capacity in the blood, an enzyme system is present that continually reduces the ferric form to the ferrous form. In usual clinical situations approximately 97% to 99% of hemoglobin is found in the more functional ferrous state, and 1% to 3% is found in the ferric state. This enzyme system is known commonly as methemoglobin reductase (erythrocyte nucleotide diaphorase), and it acts to reconvert the iron from the ferric to the ferrous state at a rate of 0.5 g/dl per hour, thus maintaining a level of less than 1% methemoglobin (0.15 g/dl) in the blood at any given time. As blood levels of methemoglobin increase, clinical signs and symptoms of cyanosis and respiratory distress may become noticeable. In most instances they are not observed until a methemoglobin blood level of 1.5 to 3.0 g/dl (10% to 20% methemoglobin) is reached.[86]

Acquired Methemoglobinemia

Although prilocaine can produce elevated methemoglobin levels, other chemicals and substances can also do this, including acetanilid, aniline derivatives (e.g., crayons, ink, shoe polish, and dermatologicals), benzene derivatives, cyanides, methylene blue in large doses, nitrates (antianginals), para-aminosalicylic acid, and sulfonamides.[15] Sarangi and Kumar reported the case of a fatality that occurred because of a chemically induced methemoglobinemia from writing ink.[87] Daly and associates reported the case of a child born with 16% (2.3 g/dl) methemoglobin that supposedly resulted because the mother, while still pregnant, had stood with wet bare feet on a bath mat colored with aniline dye.[88] In these situations the nitrates in the pen and dye were absorbed and converted to nitrites, which oxidized the ferrous atoms to ferric atoms and thus produced methemoglobinemia.

The production of methemoglobin by prilocaine is dose related. Toluene is present in the prilocaine molecule, which as the drug is biotransformed becomes *o*-toluidine, a compound capable of oxidizing ferrous iron to ferric iron and of blocking the methemoglobin reductase pathways. Peak blood levels of methemoglobin develop approximately 3 to 4 hours after drug administration and persist for 12 to 14 hours.

Clinical Signs and Symptoms and Management

The signs and symptoms of methemoglobinemia usually appear 3 to 4 hours after administration of large doses of prilocaine in healthy patients, or of smaller doses in patients with the congenital disorder. Most dental patients will have left the office by this time, thus provoking a worried telephone call to the doctor. Although the signs and symptoms vary with blood levels of methemoglobin, typically the patient appears lethargic and in respiratory distress; mucous membranes and nail beds will be cyanotic; the skin pale gray (ashen). Diagnosis of methemoglobinemia is made on the presentation of cyanosis unresponsive to oxygen administration and a distinctive brown color of arterial blood.[86] Administration of 100% oxygen does not lead to significant improvement (ferric atoms cannot surrender oxygen to tissues). Venous blood (gingival puncture) may appear chocolate brown and will not turn redder when exposed to oxygen. Definitive treatment of this situation requires the slow IV administration of 1% methylene blue (1.5 mg/kg or 0.7 mg/lb). This dose may be repeated every 4 hours if cyanosis persists or returns. Methylene blue acts as an electron acceptor in the transfer of electrons to methemoglobin, thus hastening conversion of ferric to ferrous atoms. However, methylene blue, if administered to excess, can itself cause methemoglobinemia.

Another treatment, although not as rapid-acting as methylene blue and therefore not as popular, is the IV or IM administration of ascorbic acid (100 to 200 mg/day). Ascorbic acid accelerates the metabolic pathways that produce ferrous atoms.

Methemoglobinemia should not develop in a healthy ambulatory dental patient, provided doses of local anesthetic remain within recommended limits. The presence of congenital methemoglobinemia remains a *relative contraindication* to the administration of prilocaine. Although prilocaine may be administered if absolutely necessary, its dose must be minimized. Whenever possible, alternate local anesthetics should be used.

The maximum recommended dose of prilocaine is listed by the manufacturer as 8.0 mg/kg [2.7 mg/lb]. Methemoglobinemia is unlikely to develop at doses below this level.

REFERENCES

1. Daublander M, Muller R, Lipp MD: The incidence of complications associated with local anesthesia in dentistry, *Anesth Prog* 44:132-141, 1997.
2. McCarthy FM: *Essentials of safe dentistry for the medically compromised patient*, Philadelphia, 1989, WB Saunders.
3. Sindel LJ, deShazo RD: Accidents resulting from local anesthetics. True or false allergy? *Clin Rev Allergy* 9:379-395, 1991.
4. Haas DA: An update on local anesthetics in dentistry, *J Can Dent Assoc* 68:446-551, 2002.
5. Jackson D, Chen AH, Bennett CR: Identifying true lidocaine allergy, *J Am Dent Assoc* 125:1362-1366, 1994.
6. Shojaei AR, Haas DA: Local anesthetic cartridges and latex allergy: a literature review, *J Can Dent Assoc* 68:622-626, 2002.
7. Thompson P, Melmon K, Richardson J, et al: Lidocaine pharmacokinetics in advanced heart failure, liver disease, and renal failure in humans, *Ann Intern Med* 78:499, 1973.
8. Tarhan S, Giuliani ER: General anesthesia and myocardial infarction, *Am Heart J* 87:137, 1974.
9. Weinblatt E, Shapiro S, Frank CW, et al: Prognosis of men after first myocardial infarction: mortality and first recurrence in relation to selected parameters, *Am J Public Health* 58:1329, 1968.
10. Gottlieb SO, Flaherty JT: Medical therapy of unstable angina pectoris, *Cardiol Clin* 9:19-98, 1991.
11. National High Blood Pressure Education Program: The Seventh Report of the Joint National Committee on Prevention, Detection, Evaluation, and Treatment of High Blood Pressure (JNC-7). U.S. Department of Health and Human Services. National Heart, Lung, and Blood Institute. Bethesda, Md, 2003.
12. Dajani AS, Taubert KA, Wilson W, et al: Prevention of bacterial endocarditis. Recommendations by the American Heart Association, *JAMA* 277:1794-1801, 1997.
13. Quilici DL: Contraindications in the use of the periodontal ligament injection, *Compendium* 11:26-100, 1990.
14. Bardoczky GI, Wathieu M, Dhollander A: Prilocaine-induced methemoglobinemia evidenced by pulse oximetry, *Acta Anaesthesiol Scand* 34:162-164, 1990.
15. Wilburn-Goo D, Lloyd LM: When patients become cyanotic: acquired methemoglobinemia, *J Am Dent Assoc* 130:26-31, 1999.
16. DeToledo JC: Lidocaine and seizures, *Therap Drug Monit* 22:320-322, 2000.
17. Naftalin LW, Yagiela JA: Vasoconstrictors: indications and precautions, *Dent Clin N Amer* 46:433-446, 2002.
18. Yagiela JA: Adverse drug interactions in dental practice: interactions associated with vasoconstrictors. Part V of a series, *J Am Dent Assoc* 130:501-709, 1999.
19. Malamed SF: *Medical emergencies in the dental office*, ed 5, St Louis, 1999, Mosby.
20. Strazis KP, Fox AW: Malignant hyperthermia: a review of published cases, *Anesth Analg* 77:297-304, 1993.
21. Minasian A, Yagiela JA: The use of amide local anesthetics in patients susceptible to malignant hyperthermia, *Oral Surg, Oral Med, Oral Pathol* 66:405-415, 1988.
22. Monaghan A, Hindle I: Malignant hyperthermia in oral surgery: case report and literature review, *Br J Oral Maxillofac Surg* 32:190-193, 1994.
23. Malignant Hyperthermia Association of the United States. *www.mhaus.org.*
24. Bates B, Bickley LS, Hoekelman RA, eds: *A guide to physical examination and history taking*, ed 6, Philadelphia, 1995, JB Lippincott.
25. Buxton AE, Kirk MM, Michaud GF: Current approaches to evaluation and management of patients with ventricular arrhythmias, *Med Health* 84:28-62, 2001.
26. American Society of Anesthesiologists: new classification of physical status, *Anesthesiology* 24:111, 1963.
27. Wong CA: Preoperative patient preparation, *J Post Anesth Nurs* 5:49-156, 1990.
28. Malamed SF: *Sedation: a guide to patient management*, ed 4, St Louis, 2003, Mosby.
29. McCarthy FM, Malamed SF: Physical evaluation system to determine medical risk and indicated dental therapy modifications, *J Am Dent Assoc* 99:181-184, 1979.
30. McCarthy FM: Recognition, assessment and safe management of the medically compromised patient in dentistry, *Anesth Prog* 37:217-222, 1990.

31. Moore PA, Gage TW, Hersh EV, et al: Adverse drug interactions in dental practice. Professional and educational implications, *J Am Dent Assoc* 130:17-54, 1999.

32. Kishikawa K, Namiki A, Miyashita K, et al: Effects of famotidine and cimetidine on plasma levels of epidurally administered lignocaine, *Anaesthesia* 45:719-721, 1990.

33. Wood M: Pharmacokinetic drug interactions in anaesthetic practice, *Clin Pharmacokinet* 21:85-307, 1991.

34. Wu FL, Razzaghi A, Souney PE: Seizure after lidocaine for bronchoscopy: case report and review of the use of lidocaine in airway anesthesia, *Pharmacotherapy* 13:12-78, 1993.

35. Moore PA: Adverse drug interactions in dental practice: interactions associated with local anesthetics, sedatives and anxiolytics. Part IV of a series, *J Am Dent Assoc* 130: 441-554, 1999.

36. Jastak JT, Yagiela JA: Vasoconstrictors and local anesthesia: a review and rational use, *J Am Dent Assoc* 107:623-630, 1983.

37. Boakes AJ, Laurence DR, Lovel KW, et al: Adverse reactions to local anesthetic vasoconstrictor preparations: a study of the cardiovascular responses to xylestesin and host-cain with noradrenalin, *Br Dent J* 133:137-140, 1972.

38. Yagiela JA, Duffin SR, Hunt LM: Drug interactions and vasoconstrictors used in local anesthetic solutions, *Oral Surg* 59:565-571, 1985.

39. Hansbrough JF, Near A: Propanolol-epinephrine antagonism with hypertension and stroke, *Ann Intern Med* 92:717, 1980 (letter).

40. Kram J, Bourne HR, Melmon KL, et al: Propanolol, *Ann Intern Med* 80:282, 1974 (letter).

41. Foster CA, Aston SJ: Propanolol-epinephrine interaction: a potential disaster, *Reconstr Surg* 72:74-78, 1983.

42. Ghoneim MM: Drug interactions in anaesthesia. A review, *Can Anaesthet Soc J* 18:353-375, 1971.

43. Reichle FM, Conzen PF: Halogenated inhalational anaesthetics. Best practice and research, *Clin Anaesthesiol* 17:19-46, 2003.

44. Hardman JG, Limbird LE, eds: *Goodman and Gilman's the pharmacological basis of therapeutics*, ed 10, New York, 2001, McGraw-Hill.

45. Hoffman BB, Lefkowitz RJ, Taylor P: *Neurotransmission: the autonomic and somatic motor nervous systems*. In *Goodman and Gilman's the pharmacological basis of therapeutics*, ed 9, New York, 1996, McGraw-Hill.

46. Benzaquen BS, Cohen V, Eisenberg MJ: Effects of cocaine on the coronary arteries, *Am Heart J* 142:302-410, 2001.

47. Gradman AH: Cardiac effects of cocaine: a review, *Biol Med* 61:137-141, 1988.

48. Vasica G, Tennant CC: Cocaine use and cardiovascular complications, *Med J Austral* 177:260-262, 2002.

49. Hahn IH, Hoffman RS: Cocaine use and acute myocardial infarction, *Emerg Med Clin North Am* 19:493-510, 2001.

50. Myerburg RJ: Sudden cardiac death in persons with normal (or near normal) hearts, *Am J Cardiol* 79(6A):3-9, 1997.

51. Van Dyke D, Barash PG, Jatlow P, Byck R: Cocaine: plasma concentrations after intranasal application in man, *Science* 191:859-861, 1976.

52. Friedlander AH, Gorelick DA: Dental management of the cocaine addict, *Oral Surg* 65:45-48, 1988.

53. Perusse R, Goulet J-P, Turcotte J-Y: Contraindications to vasoconstrictors in dentistry. Part III. Pharmacologic interactions, *Oral Surg, Oral Med, Oral Pathol* 74:592-697, 1992.

54. Debruyne FM: Alpha blockers: are all created equal? *Urology* 56(5 suppl 1):20-22, 2000.

55. Emmelin N, Engstrom J: Supersensitivity of salivary glands following treatment with bretylium or guanethidine, *Br J Pharmacol Chemother* 16:15-319, 1961.

56. McDevitt DG, Riddel JG, Hadden DR, et al: Catecholamine sensitivity in hyperthyroidism and hypothyroidism, *Br J Clin Pharmacol* 6:97-301, 1978.

57. Johnson AB, Webber J, Mansell P, et al: Cardiovascular and metabolic responses to adrenaline infusion in patients with short-term hypothyroidism, *Clin Endocrinol* 43:647-751, 1995.

58. Hersh EV: Adverse drug interactions in dental practice: interactions involving antibiotics, Part II of a series, *J Am Dent Assoc* 130:236-251, 1999.

59. Haas DA: Adverse drug interactions in dental practice: interactions associated with analgesics, Part III of a series, *J Am Dent Assoc* 130:397-407, 1999.

60. Rosenberg H, Fletcher JE: An update on the malignant hyperthermia syndrome, *Ann Acad Med Singapore* 23(suppl 6): 84-97, 1994.

61. Carson JM, Van Sickels JE: Preoperative determination of susceptibility to malignant hyperthermia, *J Oral Maxillofac Surg* 40:432-435, 1982.

62. Gielen M, Viering W: 3-in-1 lumbar plexus block for muscle biopsy in malignant hyperthermia patients: amide local anaesthetics may be used safely, *Acta Anaesthesiol Scand* 30:581-583, 1986.

63. Paasuke RT, Brownell AKW: Amine local anaesthetics and malignant hyperthermia, *Can Anaesth Soc J* 33:126-129, 1986 (editorial).

64. Ording H: Incidence of malignant hyperthermia in Denmark, *Anesth Analg* 64:700-704, 1985.

65. Malignant Hyperthermia Association of the United States: MHAUS Professional Advisory Council adopts new policy statement on local anesthetics, *Communicator* 3:4, 1985.

66. Kalow W, Britt BA, Terreau ME, et al: Metabolic error of muscle metabolism after recovery from malignant hyperthermia, *Lancet* 2:895-898, 1970.

67. Donnelly AJ: Malignant hyperthermia: epidemiology, pathophysiology, treatment, *AORN J* 59:393-395, 398-400, 403-405, 1994.

68. Mastaglia FL: Adverse effects of drugs on muscles, *Drugs* 24:304-321, 1982.

69. Nelson TE, Denborough MA: Studies on normal human skeletal muscle in relation to the pH and pathopharmacology of malignant hyperpyrexia, *Clin Exp Pharmacol Physiol* 4:315-322, 1977.

70. Cheah KS, Cheah AM: Mitochondrial calcium transport and calcium-activated phospholipase in porcine malignant hyperthermia, *Biochim Biophys Acta* 634:70-84, 1981.

71. Kolb ME, Horne ML, Martz R: Dantrolene in human malignant hyperthermia, *Anesthesiology* 56:254-262, 1982.

72. Jurkat-Rott K, McCarthy T, Lehmann-Horn F: Genetics and pathogenesis of malignant hyperthermia, *Muscle Nerve* 23:1-17, 2000.

73. Steelman R, Holmes D: Outpatient dental treatment of pediatric patients with malignant hyperthermia: report of three cases, *ASDC J Dent Child* 59:12-65, 1992.

74. Amato R, Giordano A, Patrignani F, et al: Malignant hyperthermia in the course of general anesthesia in oral surgery: a case report, *J Int Assoc Dent Child* 12:15-28, 1981.

75. The European Malignant Hyperpyrexia Group: A protocol for the investigation of malignant hyperpyrexia (MH) susceptibility, *Br J Anaesthe* 56:1267-1269, 1984.

76. Adragna MG: Medical protocol by habit: avoidance of amide local anesthetics in malignant hyperthermia susceptible patients, *Anesthesiology* 62:99-100, 1985 (letter).

77. Adriani J, Sundin R: Malignant hyperthermia in dental patients, *J Am Dent Assoc* 108:180-184, 1984.

78. Kaus SJ, Rockoff MA: Malignant hyperthermia, *Pediatr Clin North Am* 41:121-237, 1994.

79. MHAUS: Malignant hyperthermia: a concern in dentistry and oral and maxillofacial surgery. On-line brochure: *www.mhaus.org*

80. Williams FM: Clinical significance of esterases in man, *Clin Pharmacokinet* 10:392-403, 1985.

81. Abernethy MH, George PM, Herron JL, et al: Plasma cholinesterase phenotyping with use of visible-region spectrophotometry, *Clin Chem* 32(1 pt 1):194-197, 1986.

82. Prilocaine-induced methemoglobinemia-Wisconsin, 1993, *MMWR Morb Mortal Wkly Rep* 43:555-657, 1994.

83. Bellamy MC, Hopkins PM, Hallsall PJ, Ellis FR: A study into the incidence of methaemoglobinaemia after "three-in-one" block with prilocaine, *Anaesthesia* 47:1084-1085, 1992.

84. Guertler AT, Pearce WA: A prospective evaluation of benzocaine-associated methemoglobinemia in human beings, *Ann Emerg Med* 24:426-630, 1994.

85. Rodriguez LF, Smolik LM, Zbehlik AJ: Benzocaine-induced methemoglobinemia: a report of a severe reaction and review of the literature, *Ann Pharmacother* 28:543-649, 1994.

86. Eilers MA, Garrison TE: *General management principles.* In Marx J, Hockberger R, Walls R: *Rosen's emergency medicine: concepts and clinical practice*, ed 5, St Louis, 2002, Mosby.

87. Sarangi MP, Kumar B: Poisoning with writing ink, *Indian Pediatr* 31:756-857, 1994.

88. Daly DJ, Davenport J, Newland MC: Methemoglobinemia following the use of prilocaine, *Br J Anaesth* 36:737-739, 1964.

Basic Injection Technique

CHAPTER 11

Nothing that is done by a dentist for a patient is of greater importance than the administration of a drug that prevents pain during dental treatment. Yet the very act of administering a local anesthetic frequently induces great anxiety or is associated with pain in the recipient. Patients frequently mention that they would prefer anything to the injection or "shot" (to use the patients' term for the local anesthetic injection). Not only can the injection of local anesthetics produce fear and pain, it also may be a factor in the occurrence of emergency medical situations. In a review of medical emergencies developing in Japanese dental offices, Matsuura determined that 54.9% of the emergency situations arose either during the administration of the local anesthetic or in the 5 minutes immediately after its administration.[1] Most of these emergency situations were directly related to the increased stress associated with the receipt of the anesthetic (the injection) and not to the drug being used. Moreover, in a survey on the occurrence of medical emergencies in dental practices in North America, 4309 dentists responded that a total of more than 30,000 emergency situations had developed in their offices over the previous 10 years.[2] Ninety-five percent of respondents stated that they had experienced a medical emergency in their office in this time period. More than half of the emergencies, 15,407, were vasodepressor syncope (common faint), the majority of which occurred during or immediately after the administration of the local anesthetic.

Local anesthetics can and should be administered in a nonpainful, or atraumatic, manner. Most dental students' first injections were given to classmate "patients" who then gave the same injection to the student who had just injected them. Most likely these students went out of their way to make *their* injection as painless as possible. At the University of Southern California School of Dentistry, these first injections are usually absolutely atraumatic. Students are routinely surprised by this, some having experienced the more usual (painful) injection at some time in the past when they were "real" dental patients. Why should there be a difference in dental injections and degree of pain between the injections administered by the inexperienced beginning student and those given by the more experienced practitioner? All too often, local anesthetic administration becomes increasingly traumatic to the patient the longer a dentist has been out of school. Can this discouraging situation be corrected?

Local anesthetic administration should not be painful. Every one of the local anesthetic techniques presented in the following chapters may be done atraumatically, including the administration of local anesthetics on the palate (normally the most sensitive area in the oral cavity). Several skills and attitudes are required of the drug administrator, the most important of which is probably *empathy*. If the administrator truly believes that local anesthetic injections do not have to be painful, then through a conscious or subconscious effort it is possible to make minor changes in technique that will lead to making formerly traumatic procedures less painful for the patient.

There are two components to an atraumatic injection: a technical and a communicative aspect.*

◆ **STEP 1: Use a sterilized sharp needle.** Stainless steel disposable needles currently used in dentistry are sharp and rarely produce any pain on insertion or withdrawal.

---

*The atraumatic injection technique was developed over many years by Dr. Nathan Friedman and the Department of Human Behavior at the University of Southern California School of Dentistry. These principles are incorporated into this section.

However, because these needles are machine manufactured, occasionally (exceedingly rare) a fishhook-type barb may appear on the tip. This results in an atraumatic insertion of the needle that is followed by painful withdrawal as the tip tears the unanesthetized tissue. This may be avoided by use of sterile 2 × 2 inch gauze. Place the needle tip against the gauze and draw the needle backward. If the gauze is snagged, a barb is present and the needle should be discarded. (*This procedure is optional and may be omitted if fear of needle contamination is great.*)

Disposable needles are sharp on first insertion. However, with each succeeding penetration their sharpness diminishes. By the third or fourth penetration the operator can sense increased tissue resistance to needle penetration. Clinically this is evidenced by increased pain on penetration and increased postanesthetic tissue discomfort. Therefore it is recommended that stainless steel disposable needles be changed after every three or four tissue penetrations.

The increasing use of disposable safety syringes precludes reuse of the needle, minimizing the problem of dulling needles.

The gauge of the needle should be determined solely by the injection to be administered. Pain caused by needle penetration in the absence of adequate topical anesthesia can be eliminated in dentistry through the use of needles not larger than 25 gauge. Studies have demonstrated that patients cannot differentiate among 25-, 27-, and 30-gauge needles inserted into mucous membranes, even without the benefit of topical anesthesia.[3] Twenty-three-gauge and larger needles are associated with increased pain on initial insertion.

◆   **STEP 2: Check the flow of local anesthetic solution.** After properly loading the cartridge into the syringe, and with the aspirator tip (harpoon) embedded into the silicone rubber stopper (if appropriate), a few drops of local anesthetic should be expelled from the cartridge. This ensures a free flow of solution when it is deposited at the target area. The stoppers on the anesthetic cartridge are made of a silicone rubber to ensure ease of administration. Only a few drops of the solution should be expelled from the needle to determine if a free flow of solution exists.

◆   **STEP 3: Determine whether or not to warm the anesthetic cartridge or syringe.** There is no reason for a local anesthetic cartridge to be warmed before its injection into soft tissues, if the cartridge is stored at room temperature (approximately 72°F, 22°C). The patient will not perceive local anesthetic solution stored at room temperature as too cold or too hot when it is injected.

Most complaints concerning overly warm local anesthetic cartridges come from those stored in cartridge warmers heated by a (Christmas tree-type) light bulb. Temperatures within these cartridges frequently become excessive, leading to patient discomfort and adverse effects on the contents of the cartridge[4] (see Chapter 7).

Cartridges stored in refrigerators or other cool areas should be brought to room temperature before use.

Some persons advocate a slight warming of the *metal syringe* before its use. The rationale is that a cold metal object is psychologically more disturbing to the patient than is the same object at room temperature. It is recommended that both the local anesthetic cartridge and the metal syringe be as close to room temperature as possible, preferably without the use of any mechanical devices to achieve these temperatures. Holding the loaded metal syringe in the palm of one's hand for half a minute before injection warms the metal. Plastic syringes do not pose this problem.

◆   **STEP 4: Position the patient.** Any patient receiving local anesthetic injections should be in a physiologically sound position before and during the injection.

Vasodepressor syncope (common faint), the most commonly seen medical emergency in dentistry, most often occurs before, during, and, on occasion, immediately after local anesthetic administration. The primary pathophysiological component of this situation is cerebral ischemia secondary to an inability of the heart to supply the brain with an adequate volume of oxygenated blood. When a patient is seated in an upright position, the effect of gravity is such that the blood pressure in cerebral arteries is decreased by 2 mmHg for each inch above the level of the heart.

In the presence of anxiety, blood flow is increasingly directed toward the skeletal muscles at the expense of other organ systems such as the gastrointestinal tract (the "fight-or-flight" response). In the absence of muscular movement ("I can take it like a man!"), the increased volume of blood in skeletal muscles remains there, decreasing venous return to the heart and decreasing the volume of blood available to be pumped by the heart (uphill) to the brain. Decreased cerebral blood flow is evidenced by the appearance of signs and symptoms of vasodepressor syncope (e.g., light-headedness, dizziness, tachycardia, and palpitation). If this situation continues, cerebral blood flow declines still further and consciousness is lost.

To prevent this occurrence, it is recommended that during local anesthetic administration the patient be placed in a supine position (head and heart parallel to the floor) with the feet elevated slightly (Fig. 11-1). Although this position may vary according to the dentist's preference, the patient's medical status, and the specific injection technique, all techniques of regional block anesthesia can be carried out successfully with the patient in this position.

◆   **STEP 5: Dry the tissue.** A 2 × 2 inch gauze should be used to dry the tissue in and around the site of needle penetration and to remove any gross debris (Fig. 11-2). In addition, if the lip must be retracted to obtain adequate visibility during the injection, it too should be dried to make retraction easier (Fig. 11-3).

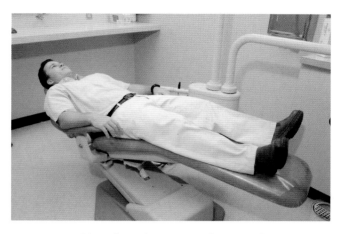

Figure 11-1. Physiological position of patient for receipt of local anesthetic injection.

◆ **STEP 6: Apply topical antiseptic (optional).** After the tissues are dried, a suitable topical antiseptic should be applied at the site of injection. This further decreases the risk of introducing septic materials into the soft tissues, producing either inflammation or infection. Antiseptics include Betadine (povidone-iodine) and Merthiolate (thimerosal). Alcohol-containing antiseptics can cause burning of the soft tissue and should be avoided. (*This step is optional*; however, the preceding step [no. 5] of drying the tissue must *not* be eliminated.)

◆ **STEP 7A: Apply topical anesthetic.** A topical anesthetic is applied after the topical antiseptic. As with the topical antiseptic, it should be applied only at the site of needle penetration. All too often excessive amounts of topical anesthetic are used on large areas of soft tissues, producing undesirably wide areas of anesthesia (e.g., the soft palate and pharynx), an unpleasant taste, and, perhaps even more importantly, with some topical anesthetics (such as lidocaine), a rapid absorption into the cardiovascular system (CVS), leading to higher local anesthetic blood levels and an increased risk of overdose. Only a small quantity of topical anesthetic should be placed on

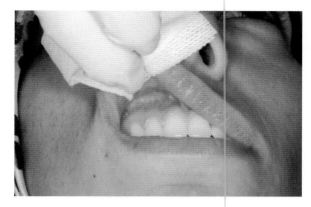

Figure 11-3. Sterilized gauze also may be used as an aid in tissue retraction.

the cotton applicator stick and applied directly at the injection site (Fig. 11-4).

Topical anesthetics produce anesthesia of the outermost 2 or 3 mm of mucous membrane; this tissue is quite sensitive. Ideally the topical anesthetic should remain in contact with the tissue for 2 minutes to ensure effectiveness.[5,6] A minimum application of 1 minute is recommended.

◆ **STEP 7B: Communicate with the patient.** During the application of the topical anesthetic it is desirable for the operator to speak to the patient about the reasons for its use. Tell the patient, "I'm applying a topical anesthetic to the tissue so that the remainder of the procedure will be much more comfortable." This statement places a positive idea in the patient's mind concerning the upcoming injection.

Note that the words *injection*, *shot*, *pain*, or *hurt* are not used. These words have a negative connotation; they tend to increase a patient's fears. Their use should be avoided if at all possible. More positive (e.g., less threatening) words can be substituted in their place. "Administer the local anesthetic" is used in place of "give an injection" or "give a shot." The latter is a particularly poor choice of words and must be avoided. A statement such as, "This

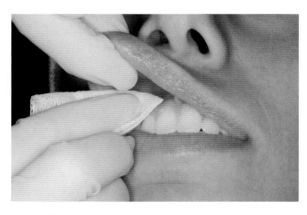

Figure 11-2. Sterilized gauze is used to gently wipe tissue at site of needle penetration.

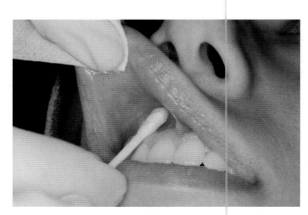

Figure 11-4. A small quantity of topical anesthetic is placed at the site of needle penetration and kept in place for at least 1 minute.

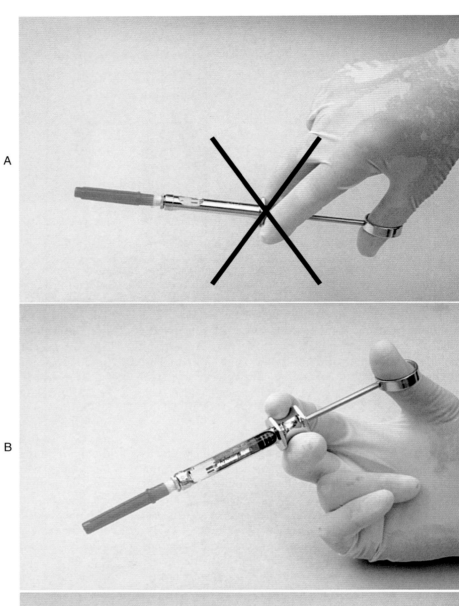

A

Figure 11-5. Hand positions for injections. **A,** Palm down: poor control over the syringe; *not recommended*. **B,** Palm up: better control over the syringe because it is supported by the wrist; *recommended*. **C,** Palm up and finger support: greatest stabilization; *highly recommended*.

B

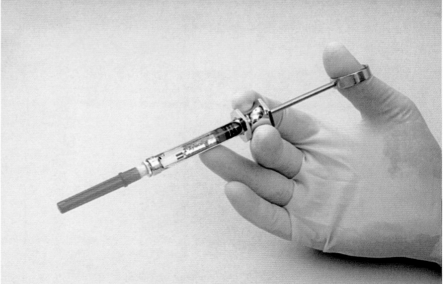

C

will not hurt" also should be avoided. Patients hear only the word *hurt*, ignoring the rest of the statement. The same is true for the word *pain*. An alternative to this is the word *discomfort*. Although their meanings are similar, *discomfort* is much less threatening and produces less fear.

◆ **STEP 8: Establish a firm hand rest.** After the topical anesthetic swab is removed from the tissue, the prepared local anesthetic syringe should be picked up (see Chapter 9). It is essential to maintain complete control over it at all times. To do so requires a steady hand so that tissue penetration may be accomplished readily, accurately, and without inadvertent nicking of tissues. A firm hand rest is necessary. The types of hand rest vary according to the practitioner's likes, dislikes, and physical abilities. Persons with long fingers can use finger rests on the patient's face for many injections; those with shorter fingers may need elbow rests. Figures 11-5 to 11-7 illustrate a variety of hand and finger rests that can be used to stabilize syringes.

Any finger or hand rest that permits the anesthetic syringe to be stabilized without increasing risk to a patient

is acceptable. Two techniques to be avoided are using no syringe stabilization of any kind,[1] and placing the arm holding the syringe directly on the patient's arm or shoulder[2] (Fig. 11-8). In the first situation it is highly unlikely that a needle can be adequately stabilized without the use of some form of rest. The operator has less control over the syringe, thereby increasing the possibility of inadvertent needle movement and injury. Resting on a patient's arm or shoulder is also dangerous and can lead to patient or administrator needle-stick injury. If the patient inadvertently moves during the injection, damage can occur as the needle tip moves around within the mouth. Apprehensive patients, especially children, frequently move their arms during local anesthetic administration.

◆ **STEP 9: Make the tissue taut.** The tissues at the site of needle penetration should be stretched before insertion of the needle (Fig. 11-9). This can be accomplished in all areas of the mouth except the palate (where the tissues are naturally quite taut). Stretching of the tissues permits the sharp stainless steel needle to *cut* through the

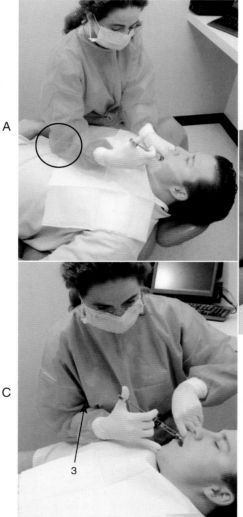
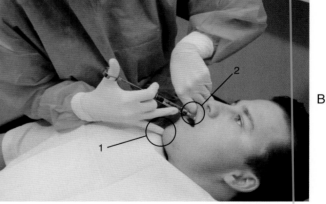

Figure 11-6. A, Use of the patient's chest for stabilization of syringe during a right inferior alveolar nerve block *(circle)*. *Never use the patient's arm to stabilize a syringe.* **B,** Use of the *chin (1)* as a finger rest, with the syringe barrel stabilized by the patient's lip *(2)*. **C,** When necessary, stabilization may be increased by drawing the administrator's arm in against his or her chest *(3)*.

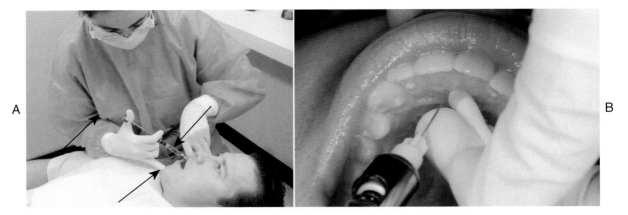

Figure 11-7. A, Syringe stabilization for a right posterior superior alveolar nerve block: syringe barrel on the patient's lip, one finger resting on the chin and one on the syringe barrel *(arrows)*, upper arm kept close to the administrator's chest to maximize stability. **B,** Syringe stabilization for a nasopalatine nerve block: index finger used to stabilize the needle, syringe barrel resting in the corner of the patient's mouth.

mucous membrane with a minimum of resistance. Loose tissues, on the other hand, are pushed and torn by the needle as it is inserted, producing more discomfort on injection and more postoperative soreness.

Techniques of distraction also are effective in this regard. Some dentists advocate jiggling the lip as the needle is inserted; others recommend leaving the needle tip stationary and pulling the soft tissues over the needle tip (Fig. 11-10). Although there is nothing inherently wrong with these distraction techniques, there generally is no need for either. Because the operator should maintain sight of the needle tip at all times, needles should not be inserted blindly into tissues, as is necessitated by many of the distraction techniques.

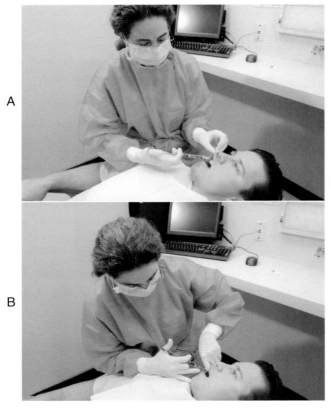

Figure 11-8. A, Incorrect position: no hand or finger rest for stabilization of syringe. **B,** Incorrect position: administrator resting elbow on patient's arm.

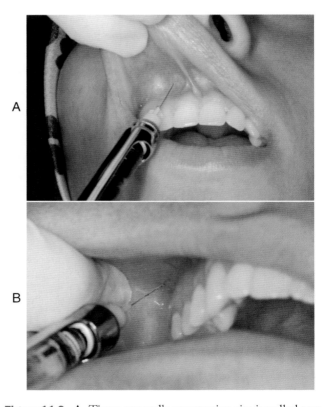

Figure 11-9. A, Tissue at needle penetration site is pulled taut, aiding both visibility and atraumatic needle insertion. **B,** Taut tissue provides excellent visibility of the penetration site for a posterior superior alveolar nerve block.

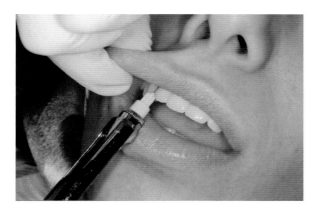

Figure 11-10. When soft tissues are pulled over the needle, visualization of the injection site is impaired.

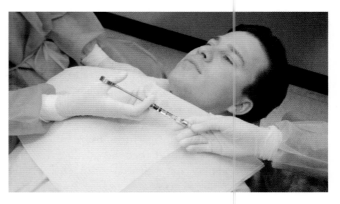

Figure 11-12. Passing syringe from assistant to administrator below the patient's line of sight.

Proper application of topical anesthetic, taut tissues, and a firm hand rest can produce an unnoticed initial penetration of tissues virtually 100% of the time.

◆ **STEP 10: Keep the syringe out of the patient's line of sight.** With the tissue prepared and the patient positioned, the assistant should pass the syringe to the administrator behind the patient's head or across and in front of the patient but below the patient's line of sight. A right-handed practitioner administrating a right-side injection can sit facing the patient (Fig. 11-11) or, if administering a left-side injection, facing in the same direction as the patient (Fig. 11-12). In all cases it is better if the syringe is not visible to the patient. Proper positioning for left-handed operators is a mirror image of that for right-handed ones. (Specific recommendations for administrator positioning during local anesthetic injections are discussed in Chapters 13 and 14.)

◆ **STEP 11A: Insert the needle into the mucosa.** With the needle bevel properly oriented (see specific injection technique for bevel orientation; however, as a general rule *the bevel of the needle should be oriented toward bone*),

insert the needle *gently* into the tissue at the injection site (where the topical anesthetic was placed) to the depth of the bevel. With a firm hand rest and adequate tissue preparation, this potentially traumatic procedure is accomplished without the patient ever being aware of it.

◆ **STEP 11B: Watch and communicate with the patient.** During Step 11a, the patient should be watched and communicated with; the patient's face should be observed for evidence of discomfort during needle penetration. Signs such as furrowing of the brow or forehead and blinking of the eyes may indicate discomfort (Fig. 11-13). More frequently, no change will be noticed in the patient's facial expression at this time (indicating a painless, or atraumatic, needle insertion).

The practitioner should communicate with the patient as Step 11a is carried out. The patient should be told in a positive manner, "I don't expect you to feel this," as the needle penetrates the tissues. The words, "This will not hurt," should not be said; this is a negative statement, and the patient hears only the word *hurt*.

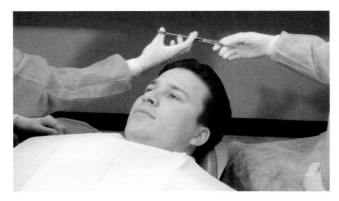

Figure 11-11. Passing syringe from assistant to administrator behind the patient, out of his or her line of sight.

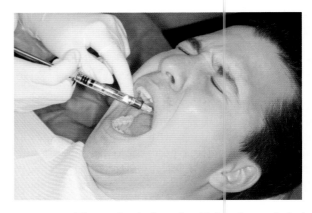

Figure 11-13. The patient's face should be observed during administration of the local anesthetic, and any squinting of the eyes or furrowing of the brows, indicating discomfort, should be noted.

◆ **STEP 12:** Inject several drops of local anesthetic solution (optional).

◆ **STEP 13:** Slowly advance the needle toward the target. Steps 12 and 13 are carried out together. The soft tissue in front of the needle may be anesthetized with a few drops of local anesthetic solution. After waiting 2 or 3 seconds for anesthesia to develop, the needle should be advanced into this area and a little more anesthesia deposited. The needle should then be advanced again. These procedures may be repeated until the needle reaches the desired target area.

In most patients the injection of local anesthetic during insertion of the needle toward the target area is entirely unnecessary. Pain is rarely encountered between the surface mucosa and the mucoperiosteum. If patients are asked what they feel as a needle is being advanced through soft tissue (as in an inferior alveolar or posterior superior alveolar nerve block), the usual reply is that they are aware that something is there but that it does not hurt.

On the other hand, patients who are apprehensive about injections of local anesthetics are more likely to react to any sensation as though it were painful. These patients are said to have a lowered pain reaction threshold. These patients should be told, "To make you more comfortable I will deposit a little anesthetic as I advance (the needle) toward the target." Minimal amounts of the local anesthetic should be injected as the process continues. In an injection such as the inferior alveolar nerve block, for which the average depth of needle insertion is 20 to 25 mm, not more than one eighth of a cartridge of local anesthetic should be deposited as the soft tissues are penetrated. Aspiration does not need to be performed at this stage because of the small amount of anesthetic solution that is being continually deposited over a changing injection site. If a vessel were to be penetrated during this procedure, only a drop or two (<1 mg) of anesthetic would be deposited intravascularly. As the needle is advanced further, it leaves the vessel. However, aspiration always must be carried out before depositing any significant volume of solution (Steps 15 and 16).

◆ **STEP 14:** Deposit several drops of local anesthetic before touching the periosteum. In techniques of regional block anesthesia in which the needle touches or comes close to the periosteum, several drops of solution should be deposited just before contact. The periosteum is richly innervated, and contact with the needle tip produces pain. Anesthetizing the periosteum permits atraumatic contact. Regional block injection techniques that require this are the inferior alveolar, Gow-Gates mandibular, and infraorbital nerve blocks.

Knowledge of when to deposit the local anesthetic comes with experience. The depth of penetration of soft tissue at any injection site varies from patient to patient; therefore the periosteum may be contacted inadvertently.

However, a keen tactile sense is developed with repetition, enabling the needle to be used gently as a probe. This enables the administrator to detect subtle changes in tissue density as the needle approaches bone. With experience and development of this tactile sense, a small volume of local anesthetic solution may be deposited just before gently contacting the periosteum.

◆ **STEP 15:** Aspirate. Aspiration always must be carried out before deposing a volume of local anesthetic at any site. Aspiration dramatically minimizes the possibility of an intravascular injection. The goal of aspiration is to determine whether the needle tip lies within a blood vessel. To aspirate, one must create a negative pressure within the dental cartridge. The self-aspirating syringe does this whenever the operator stops applying positive pressure to the thumb ring (plunger). With the more commonly used harpoon-type syringe the administrator must make a conscious effort to create this negative pressure within the cartridge.

Adequate aspiration necessitates that the tip of the needle remain unmoved, neither pushed further into nor pulled out of the tissues during aspiration. Adequate stabilization is mandatory. Beginners have a tendency to pull the syringe out of the tissues while attempting to aspirate.

The thumb ring should be pulled back gently. Movement of only 1 or 2 mm is needed. This produces a negative pressure within the cartridge that then translates to the tip of the needle. Whatever is lying in the soft tissues around the needle tip (e.g., blood, tissue, or air) will be drawn back into the anesthetic cartridge. By observing the needle end lying within the cartridge for signs of blood return, the administrator can determine if a positive aspiration has occurred. *Any sign of blood is a positive aspiration*, and local anesthetic solution should not be deposited at that site (Fig. 11-14). No return at all, or an air bubble, indicates a negative aspiration. Aspiration should be performed at least twice before administering local anesthetic, with the orientation of the bevel changed (rotate barrel of syringe about 45 degrees for second aspiration test) to ensure that the bevel of the needle is not located inside a blood vessel but abutting against the wall of the vessel, providing a false-negative aspiration. Several additional aspiration tests are suggested during the administration of the anesthetic drug. This serves two functions: to slow down the rate of anesthetic administration,[1] and preclude the deposition of large volumes of anesthetic into the cardiovascular system.[2]

The major factor determining whether aspiration can be reliably performed is the needle gauge. Larger-gauge needles (e.g., 25) are recommended more than smaller-gauge needles (e.g., 27 and 30) whenever a greater risk of positive aspiration exists.

◆ **STEP 16A:** Slowly deposit the local anesthetic solution. With the needle in position at the target area and

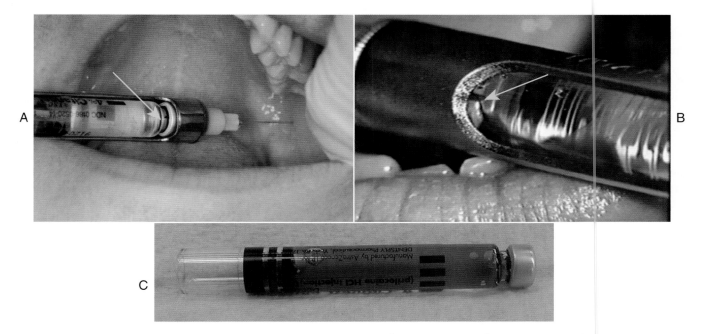

Figure 11-14. **A,** Negative aspiration. With the needle in position at the injection site, the administrator pulls the thumb ring of the harpoon aspirator syringe 1 or 2 mm. The needle tip should *not* move. Check the cartridge at the site where the needle penetrates the diaphragm *(arrow)* for a bubble or blood. **B,** Positive aspiration. A slight reddish discoloration at the diaphragm end of the cartridge *(arrow)* on aspiration usually indicates venous penetration. Reposition the needle, reaspirate, and if negative, deposit the solution. **C,** Positive aspiration. Bright red blood rapidly filling the cartridge usually indicates arterial penetration. Remove the syringe from the mouth, change the cartridge, and repeat the procedure.

aspirations completed and *negative,* the administrator should begin pressing gently on the plunger to start administering the predetermined (for the technique) volume of anesthetic. Slow injection is vital for two reasons: of utmost significance is the safety factor (discussed in greater detail in Chapter 18);[1] slow injection also prevents the solution from tearing the tissue into which it is deposited.[2] Rapid injection results in immediate discomfort (for a few seconds) followed by a prolonged soreness when the action of the local anesthetic is terminated.

Slow injection is defined as the deposition of 1 ml of local anesthetic solution in not less than 60 seconds. Therefore a full 1.8-ml cartridge requires approximately 2 minutes. Through slow deposition the solution is able to diffuse along normal tissue planes without producing postoperative discomfort.

Most local anesthetic administrators tend to administer these drugs too rapidly. In a survey completed several years previously,[7] 84% of more than 200 respondents stated that the average time spent to deposit 1.8 ml of local anesthetic solution was less than 20 seconds.

In actual clinical practice, it therefore seems highly improbable to expect doctors to change their rate of injection from less than 20 seconds to a safe and comfortable 2 minutes per cartridge. *A more realistic time span in a*

clinical situation is 60 seconds for a full 1.8-ml cartridge. This rate of deposition of solution does not produce tissue damage either during or after anesthesia and, in the event of accidental intravascular injection, does not produce a serious reaction. There are few injection techniques that require the administration of 1.8 ml for success.

For many years the author has used one particular method for slowing the rate of injection. After two negative aspirations, he deposits a volume of solution (approximately one fourth of the total to be deposited) and then aspirates again. If the aspiration is negative, he deposits another fourth of the solution, reaspirates, and continues this process until the total volume of solution for the given injection is deposited. This enables him to do two positive things during injection: to reaffirm through multiple negative aspirations that the solution is in fact being deposited extravascularly,[1] and to stop the injection for aspiration, which automatically slows the rate of deposit and thereby minimizes patient discomfort.[2] In the first situation, if positive aspiration occurs after deposition of one fourth of a cartridge, only 9 mg of a 2% solution, or 13.5 mg of a 3% solution, or 18 mg of a 4% solution will have been deposited intravascularly—doses unlikely to provoke any adverse reaction. The needle tip should be repositioned, negative aspiration (×2) achieved, and the injection continued. The incidence of adverse reactions caused by intravascular injection is greatly minimized in this manner.

◆ **STEP 16B: Communicate with the patient.** The patient should be communicated with during deposition of the local anesthetic. Most patients are accustomed to receiving their local anesthetic injections rapidly. Statements such as, *"I'm depositing the solution (or I'm doing this) slowly so it will be more comfortable for you, but you're not receiving any more than is usual"* go far to allay a patient's apprehension at this time. The second part of the statement is important, because patients might not realize that there is a fixed volume of anesthetic solution in the syringe. A reminder that they are not receiving any more than is usual is a comfort to the patient.

◆ **STEP 17: Slowly withdraw the syringe.** After completion of the injection, the syringe should be slowly withdrawn from the soft tissues and the needle made safe by drawing its protective sheath over it (safety syringe) or by capping it immediately with its plastic sheath via the scoop technique.

Recent concerns about the possibility of needle-stick injuries and the spread of infection caused by inadvertent sticking with contaminated needles have led to the formulation of guidelines for the recapping of needles.[8] It has been demonstrated that the time health professionals are most apt to be injured with needles is when recapping after the administration of an injection.[9,10] At this time the needle is contaminated with blood, tissue, and (after intraoral injection) saliva. A number of devices have been marketed to aid the health professional in recapping the needle safely. Needle guards, placed over the needle cap *before* injection, prevent fingers from being stuck during recapping. Although no guidelines are yet in effect, the following are most often mentioned for preventing

accidental needle stick: *Needles should not be reused.*[1] After their use, needles should immediately be discarded into a sharps container. This policy, although applicable in most nondental hospital situations in which only one injection is administered, is impractical in dentistry, where multiple injections are commonplace.[2] *The "scoop" technique* (Fig. 11-15)—in which the needle cap has been placed on the instrument tray and after injection the administrator simply slides the needle tip into the cap (without touching the cap), scooping up the needle cap—can be used for multiple injections without increased risk. The capped needle is then discarded in a sharps container.[3] An acrylic needle holder can be purchased or fabricated that holds the cap upright during injection. The needle then can be reinserted into the cap without difficulty after injection (Fig. 11-16).

◆ **STEP 18: Observe the patient.** After completion of the injection the doctor, hygienist, or assistant should remain with the patient while the anesthetic begins to take effect (and its blood level increases). Most adverse drug reactions, especially those to intraorally administered local anesthetics, develop either during the injection or within 5 to 10 minutes of completion of the injection. All too often reports are heard of situations in which a local anesthetic was administered and the doctor left the patient alone for a few minutes only to return to find the patient in convulsions or unconscious. Matsuura reported that 54.9% of all medical emergencies arising in Japanese dental offices developed either during the injection of local anesthetics or in the 5 minutes immediately after their administration.[1] *Patients should never be left unattended after administration of a local anesthetic.*

◆ **STEP 19: Record the injection on the patient's chart.** An entry must be made of the local anesthetic drug used, vasoconstrictor used (if any), dose (in milligrams) of the

Figure 11-15. "Scoop" technique for recapping needle after use.

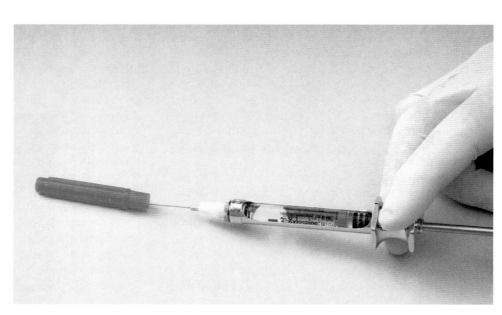

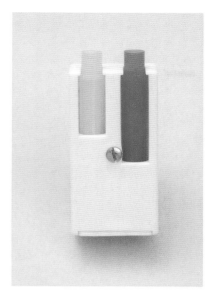

Figure 11-16. Plastic needle cap holder.

Atraumatic Injection Technique
1. Use a sterilized sharp needle.
2. Check the flow of local anesthetic solution.
3. Determine whether to warm the anesthetic cartridge or syringe.
4. Position the patient.
5. Dry the tissue.
6. Apply topical antiseptic (optional).
7a. Apply topical anesthetic.
7b. Communicate with the patient.
8. Establish a firm hand rest.
9. Make the tissue taut.
10. Keep the syringe out of the patient's line of sight.
11a. Insert the needle into the mucosa.
11b. Watch and communicate with the patient.
12. Inject several drops of local anesthetic solution (optional).
13. Slowly advance the needle toward the target.
14. Deposit several drops of local anesthetic before touching the periosteum.
15. Aspirate.
16a. Slowly deposit the local anesthetic solution.
16b. Communicate with the patient.
17. Slowly withdraw the syringe. Cap the needle and discard.
18. Observe the patient after the injection.
19. Record the injection on the patient's chart.

solution(s) used, the needle(s) used, the injection(s) given, and the patient's reaction.[1-6] For example, on the patient's dental progress notes the following might be inscribed: *R-IANB, 25-long, 2% lido + 1:100,000 epi, 36 mg. Tolerated procedure well.*

* * *

The administrator of local anesthetics who adheres to these steps develops a reputation among patients as a "painless doctor." It is not possible to guarantee that every injection will be absolutely atraumatic, because the reactions of both patients and doctors are far too variable. However, even when they feel some discomfort, patients invariably state that the injection was better than any other they had previously experienced. This should be the goal sought with every local anesthetic injection.

REFERENCES

1. Matsuura H: Analysis of systemic complications and deaths during dental treatment in Japan, *Anesth Prog* 36:219-228, 1989.
2. Malamed SF: Managing medical emergencies, *J Am Dent Assoc* 124:50-53, 1993.
3. Mollen AJ, Ficara AJ, Provant DR: Needles—25 gauge versus 27 gauge—can patients really tell? *Gen Dent* 29:417-418, 1981.
4. Rogers KB, Fielding AF, Markiewicz SW: The effect of warming local anesthetic solutions before injection, *Gen Dent* 37:496-499, 1989.
5. Gill CJ, Orr DL: A double blind crossover comparison of topical anesthetics, *J Am Dent Assoc* 98:213, 1979.
6. Jeske AH, Blanton PL: Misconceptions involving dental local anesthesia. Part 2: Pharmacology, *Tex Dent J* 119:310-314, 2002.
7. Malamed SF: Results of a survey of 209 dentists. *Handbook of local anesthesia*, ed 4, St Louis, 1997, Mosby.
8. Goldwater PN, Law R, Nixon AD, et al: Impact of a recapping device on venipuncture-related needlestick injury, *Infect Control Hosp Epidemiol* 10:11-25, 1989.
9. McCormick RD, Maki DG: Epidemiology of needle-stick injuries in hospital personnel, *Am J Med* 70:928-932, 1981.
10. Berry AJ, Greene ES: The risk of needlestick injuries and needlestick-transmitted diseases in the practice of anesthesiology, *Anesthesiology* 77:1007-1021, 1992.

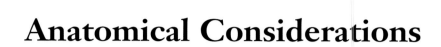

Anatomical Considerations

CHAPTER
12

TRIGEMINAL NERVE

An understanding of the management of pain in dentistry requires thorough knowledge of the fifth cranial nerve (Fig. 12-1). The right and left trigeminal nerves provide, among other functions, the overwhelming majority of sensory innervation from the teeth, bone, and soft tissues of the oral cavity. The trigeminal nerve is also the largest cranial nerve. It is composed of a small motor root and a considerably larger (tripartite) sensory root. The motor root supplies the muscles of mastication and other muscles in the region. The three branches of the sensory root supply the skin of the entire face and the mucous membrane of the cranial viscera and oral cavity, except for the pharynx and base of the tongue. Table 12-1 summarizes the functions of the trigeminal and the 11 other cranial nerves.

Motor Root

The motor root of the trigeminal nerve arises separately from the sensory root, originating in the motor nucleus within the pons and medulla oblongata (Fig. 12-2). Its fibers, forming a small nerve root, travel anteriorly along with, but entirely separate from, the larger sensory root to the region of the semilunar (or gasserian) ganglion. At the semilunar ganglion the motor root passes in a lateral and inferior direction under the ganglion toward the foramen ovale, through which it leaves the middle cranial fossa along with the third division of the sensory root, the mandibular nerve (Figs. 12-3 and 12-4). Just after leaving the skull, the motor root unites with the sensory root of the mandibular division to form a single nerve trunk.

Motor fibers of the trigeminal nerve supply the following muscles:
1. Masticatory
   a. Masseter
   b. Temporalis
   c. Pterygoideus medialis
   d. Pterygoideus lateralis
2. Mylohyoid
3. Anterior belly of the digastric
4. Tensor tympani
5. Tensor veli palatini

Sensory Root

Sensory root fibers of the trigeminal nerve comprise the central processes of ganglion cells located in the trigeminal (semilunar or gasserian) ganglion. There are two ganglia, one innervating each side of the face. They are located in Meckel's cavity, on the anterior surface of the petrous portion of the temporal bone (see Fig. 12-3). The ganglia are flat and crescent shaped and measure approximately 1.0×2.0 cm; their convexities face anteriorly and downward. Sensory root fibers enter the concave portion of each crescent, and the three sensory divisions of the trigeminal nerve exit from the convexity:
1. The *ophthalmic division* (V_1) travels anteriorly in the lateral wall of the cavernous sinus to the medial part of the superior orbital fissure, through which it exits the skull into the orbit.
2. The *maxillary division* (V_2) travels anteriorly and downward to exit the cranium through the foramen rotundum into the upper portion of the pterygopalatine fossa.
3. The *mandibular division* (V_3) travels almost directly downward to exit the skull, along with the motor root, through the foramen ovale. These two roots then intermingle, forming one nerve trunk that enters the infratemporal fossa.

On exiting the cranium through their respective foramina, the three divisions of the trigeminal nerve divide into a multitude of sensory branches.

• • •

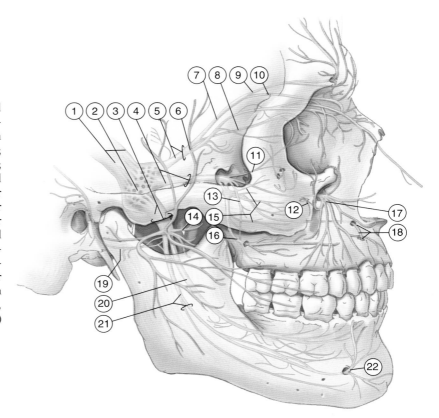

Figure 12-1. Distribution of the trigeminal nerve. *1,* The branches are as follows: *2,* gasserian ganglion; *3,* mandibular nerve and foramen ovale; *4,* maxillary nerve and foramen rotundum; *5,* ophthalmic nerve and superior orbital fissure; *6,* nasociliary nerve; *7,* frontal nerve; *8,* lacrimal nerve; *9,* supraorbital nerve; *10,* supratrochlear nerve; *11,* zygomatic nerve; *12,* anterior superior alveolar branches; *13,* posterior superior alveolar branches; *14,* buccal nerve; *15,* posterior nasal branches; *16,* greater palatine nerve; *17,* infraorbital nerve; *18,* nasopalatine nerve; *19,* auriculotemporal nerve; *20,* lingual nerve; *21,* inferior alveolar nerve; *22,* mental nerve. (Redrawn from Haglund J, Evers H: *Local anaesthesia in dentistry,* ed 2, Södertälje, Sweden, 1975, Astra Läkemedel.)

Each of the three divisions of the trigeminal nerve is described, but more attention is devoted to the maxillary and mandibular divisions because of their greater importance in pain control in dentistry. Figure 12-5 illustrates the sensory distribution of the trigeminal nerve.

Ophthalmic Division (V_1). The ophthalmic division is the first branch of the trigeminal nerve. It is exclusively sensory and is the smallest of the three divisions. It leaves the cranium and enters the orbit through the superior orbital fissure (Fig. 12-6). The nerve trunk is approximately 2.5 cm long. It supplies the eyeball, conjunctiva, lacrimal gland, parts of the mucous membrane of the nose and paranasal sinuses, and the skin of the forehead, eyelids, and nose. When the ophthalmic nerve (V_1) is paralyzed, the ocular conjunctiva becomes insensitive to touch.

Just before the ophthalmic nerve passes through the superior orbital fissure, it divides into its three main branches: the nasociliary, frontal, and lacrimal nerves.

Nasociliary nerve. The nasociliary nerve travels along the medial border of the orbital roof, giving off branches to the nasal cavity and ending in the skin at the root of the nose. It then branches into the *anterior ethmoidal* and *external nasal nerves.* The *internal nasal nerve* (from the anterior ethmoidal) supplies the mucous membrane of the anterior part of the nasal septum and the lateral wall of the nasal cavity. The *ciliary ganglion* contains sensory

fibers that travel to the eyeball via the *short ciliary nerves.* There are two or three *long ciliary nerves* supplying the iris and cornea. The *infratrochlear nerve* supplies the skin of the lacrimal sac and the lacrimal caruncle, the *posterior ethmoidal nerve* supplies the ethmoidal and sphenoidal sinuses, and the *external nasal nerve* supplies the skin over the apex (tip) and the ala of the nose.

TABLE **12-1**
Cranial Nerves

Number	Name	Type
I	Olfactory	Sensory
II	Optic	Sensory
III	Oculomotor	Motor
IV	Trochlear	Motor
V	Trigeminal	Mixed
V_1: sensory		
V_2: sensory		
V_3: sensory, motor		
VI	Abducens	Motor
VII	Facial	Motor
VIII	Auditory	Sensory
IX	Glossopharyngeal	Mixed
X	Vagus	Mixed
XI	Accessory	Motor
XII	Hypoglossal	Motor

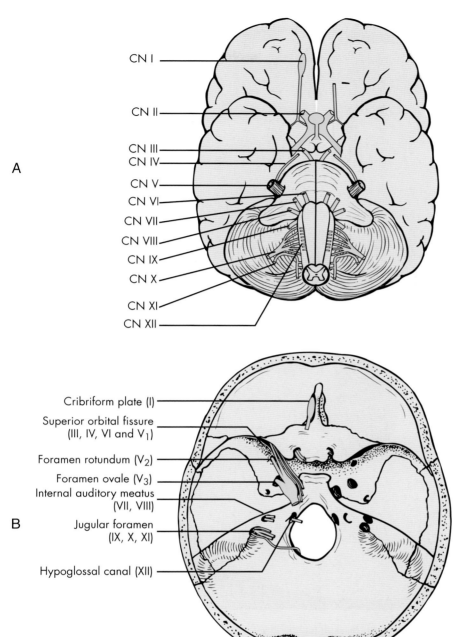

CN I
CN II
CN III
CN IV
CN V
CN VI
CN VII
CN VIII
CN IX
CN X
CN XI
CN XII

A

Cribriform plate (I)
Superior orbital fissure
(III, IV, VI and V₁)
Foramen rotundum (V₂)
Foramen ovale (V₃)
Internal auditory meatus
(VII, VIII)
Jugular foramen
(IX, X, XI)
Hypoglossal canal (XII)

B

Figure 12-2. A, Inferior view showing cranial nerves arising from brain. **B,** Internal aspect of base of skull showing foramina through which cranial nerves exit skull. *CN*, Cranial nerve. (Data from Liebgott B: *The anatomical basis of dentistry*, ed 2, St Louis, 2001, Mosby.)

Frontal nerve. The frontal nerve travels anteriorly in the orbit, dividing into two branches: the *supratrochlear* and *supraorbital*. The frontal is the largest branch of the ophthalmic division. The supratrochlear nerve supplies the conjunctiva and skin of the medial aspect of the upper eyelid and the skin over the lower and mesial aspects of the forehead. The supraorbital nerve is sensory to the upper eyelid, the scalp as far back as the parietal bone, and the lambdoidal suture.

Lacrimal nerve. The lacrimal nerve is the smallest branch of the ophthalmic division. It supplies the lateral part of the upper eyelid and a small adjacent area of skin.

Maxillary Division (V₂). The maxillary division of the trigeminal nerve arises from the middle of the trigeminal ganglion. Intermediate in size between the ophthalmic and mandibular divisions, it is purely sensory in function.

Origins. The maxillary nerve passes horizontally forward, leaving the cranium through the foramen rotundum (see Fig. 12-3). The foramen rotundum is located in the greater wing of the sphenoid bone. Once outside the cranium, the maxillary nerve crosses the uppermost part of the pterygopalatine fossa, between the pterygoid plates of the sphenoid bone and the palatine bone. As it crosses the pterygopalatine fossa, it gives off branches to the

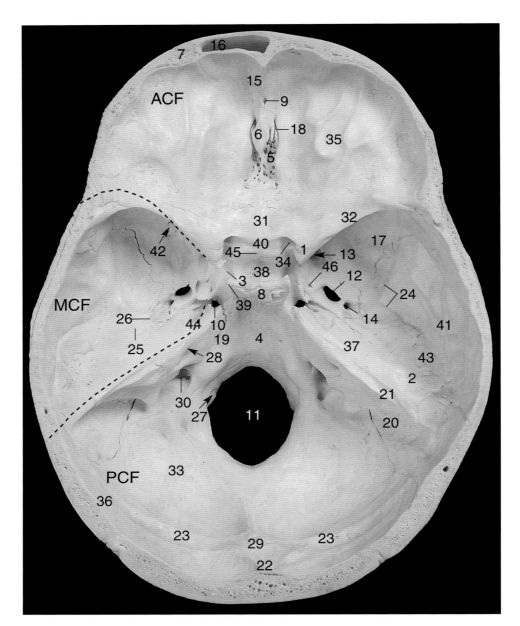

Figure 12-3. Internal surface of the base of the skull (cranial fossa). *ACF,* Anterior cranial fossa; *MCF,* middle cranial fossa; *PCF,* posterior cranial fossa. *1,* Anterior clinoid process; *2,* arcuate eminence; *3,* carotid groove; *4,* clivus; *5,* cribriform plate of ethmoid bone; *6,* crista galli; *7,* diploë; *8,* dorsum sellae; *9,* foramen caecum; *10,* foramen lacerum; *11,* foramen magnum; *12,* foramen ovale; *13,* foramen rotundum; *14,* foramen spinosum; *15,* frontal crest; *16,* frontal sinus; *17,* greater wing of sphenoid bone; *18,* groove for anterior ethmoidal nerve and vessels; *19,* groove for inferior petrosal sinus; *20,* groove for sigmoid sinus; *21,* groove for superior petrosal sinus; *22,* groove for superior sagittal sinus; *23,* groove for transverse sinus; *24,* grooves for middle meningeal vessels; *25,* hiatus and groove for greater petrosal nerve; *26,* hiatus and groove for lesser petrosal nerve; *27,* hypoglossal canal; *28,* internal acoustic meatus; *29,* internal occipital protuberance; *30,* jugular foramen; *31,* jugum of sphenoid bone; *32,* lesser wing of sphenoid bone; *33,* occipital bone; *34,* optic canal; *35,* orbital part of frontal bone; *36,* parietal bone (posteroinferior angle only); *37,* petrous part of temporal bone; *38,* pituitary fossa (sella turcica); *39,* posterior clinoid process; *40,* prechiasmatic groove; *41,* squamous part of temporal bone; *42,* superior orbital fissure; *43,* tegmen tympani; *44,* trigeminal impression; *45,* tuberculum sellae; *46,* venous foramen. (Data from Abrahams PH, Marks SC Jr, Hutchings RT: *McMinn's color atlas of human anatomy,* ed 5, St Louis, 2003, Mosby.)

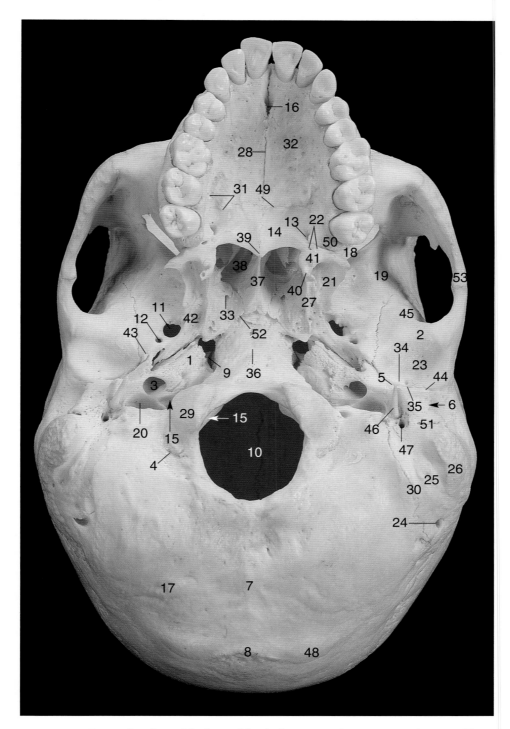

Figure 12-4. External surface of the base of the skull. *1*, Apex of petrous part of temporal bone; *2*, articular tubercle; *3*, carotid canal; *4*, condylar canal (posterior); *5*, edge of tegmen tympani; *6*, external acoustic meatus; *7*, external occipital crest; *8*, external occipital protuberance; *9*, foramen lacerum; *10*, foramen magnum; *11*, foramen ovale; *12*, foramen spinosum; *13*, greater palatine foramen; *14*, horizontal plate of palatine bone; *15*, hypoglossal (anterior condylar) canal; *16*, incisive fossa; *17*, inferior nuchal line; *18*, inferior orbital fissure; *19*, infratemporal crest of greater wing of sphenoid bone; *20*, jugular foramen; *21*, lateral pterygoid plate; *22*, lesser palatine foramina; *23*, mandibular fossa; *24*, mastoid foramen; *25*, mastoid notch; *26*, mastoid process; *27*, medial pterygoid plate; *28*, median palatine (intermaxillary) suture; *29*, occipital condyle; *30*, occipital groove; *31*, palatine grooves and spines; *32*, palatine process of maxilla; *33*, palatinovaginal canal; *34*, petrosquamous fissure; *35*, petrotympanic

Continued.

Figure 12-4, cont'd.   fissure; *36,* pharyngeal tubercle; *37,* posterior border of vomer; *38,* posterior nasal aperture (choana); *39,* posterior nasal spine; *40,* pterygoid hamulus; *41,* pyramidal process of palatine bone; *42,* scaphoid fossa; *43,* spine of sphenoid bone; *44,* squamotympanic fissure; *45,* squamous part of temporal bone; *46,* styloid process; *47,* stylomastoid foramen; *48,* superior nuchal line; *49,* transverse palatine (palatomaxillary) suture; *50,* tuberosity of maxilla; *51,* tympanic part of temporal bone; *52,* vomerovaginal canal; *53,* zygomatic arch. (Data from Abrahams PH, Marks SC Jr, Hutchings RT: *McMinn's color atlas of human anatomy,* ed 5, St Louis, 2003, Mosby.)

---

sphenopalatine ganglion, the posterior superior alveolar nerve, and the zygomatic branches. It then angles laterally in a groove on the posterior surface of the maxilla, entering the orbit through the inferior orbital fissure. Within the orbit it occupies the infraorbital groove and becomes the infraorbital nerve, which courses anteriorly into the infraorbital canal.

The maxillary division emerges on the anterior surface of the face through the infraorbital foramen, where it divides into its terminal branches, supplying the skin of the face, nose, lower eyelid, and upper lip (Fig. 12-7). The following is a breakdown of maxillary division innervation:

1. Skin:
   a. Middle portion of the face
   b. Lower eyelid
   c. Side of the nose
   d. Upper lip
2. Mucous membrane:
   a. Nasopharynx
   b. Maxillary sinus
   c. Soft palate
   d. Tonsil
   e. Hard palate
3. Maxillary teeth and periodontal tissues

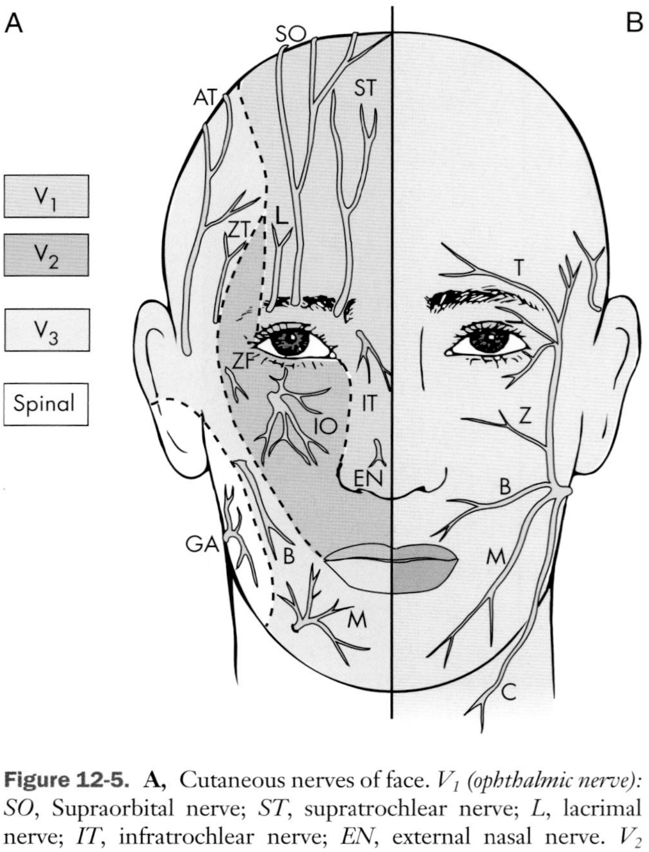

Figure 12-5. A, Cutaneous nerves of face. *V₁ (ophthalmic nerve): SO,* Supraorbital nerve; *ST,* supratrochlear nerve; *L,* lacrimal nerve; *IT,* infratrochlear nerve; *EN,* external nasal nerve. *V₂ (maxillary nerve): IO,* Infraorbital nerve; *ZT,* zygomatico temporal nerve; *ZF,* zygomaticofacial nerve. *V₃ (mandibular nerve): AT,* Auriculotemporal nerve; *B,* buccal nerve; *M,* mental nerve. *Spinal nerve: GA,* Great auricular nerve. **B,** Motor nerves to muscles of facial expression. *Facial branches of CN VII: T,* Temporal branches; *Z,* zygomatic branches; *B,* buccal branches; *M,* mandibular branches; *C,* cervical branches. (Data from Liebgott B: *The anatomical basis of dentistry,* ed 2, St Louis, 2001, Mosby.)

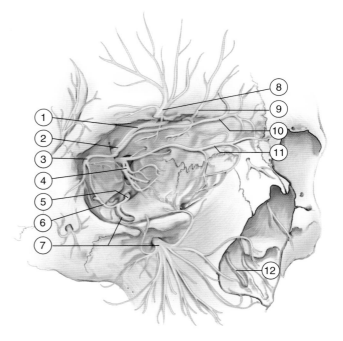

Figure 12-6. Distribution of the ophthalmic division (V₁). *1,* Supraorbital nerve; *2,* frontal nerve; *3,* lacrimal nerve; *4,* nasociliary nerve; *5,* maxillary nerve; *6,* zygomatic nerve; *7,* infraorbital nerve; *8,* lateral branch of the frontal nerve; *9,* medial branch of the frontal nerve; *10,* supratrochlear nerve; *11,* infratrochlear nerve; *12,* nasopalatine nerve. (Data from Haglund J, Evers H: *Local anaesthesia in dentistry,* ed 2, Södertälje, Sweden, 1975, Astra Läkemedel.)

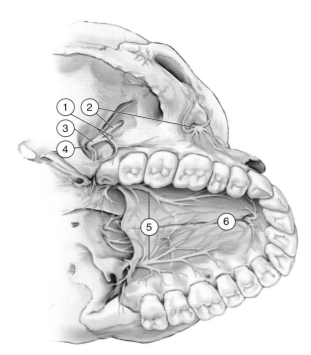

Figure 12-7. Distribution of the maxillary division (V₂). *1*, Posterior superior alveolar branches; *2*, infraorbital nerve; *3*, maxillary nerve; *4*, foramen rotundum; *5*, greater palatine nerve; *6*, nasopalatine nerve. (Data from Haglund J, Evers H: *Local anaesthesia in dentistry*, ed 2, Södertälje, Sweden, 1975, Astra Läkemedel.)

Branches. The maxillary division gives off branches in four regions: within the cranium, in the pterygopalatine fossa, in the infraorbital canal, and on the face.

Branch within the cranium. Immediately after separating from the trigeminal ganglion, the maxillary division gives off a small branch, the *middle meningeal nerve,* which travels with the middle meningeal artery to provide sensory innervation to the dura mater.

Branches in the pterygopalatine fossa. After exiting the cranium through the foramen rotundum, the maxillary division crosses the pterygopalatine fossa. In this fossa several branches are given off (Fig. 12-8): the zygomatic nerve, the pterygopalatine nerves, and the posterior superior alveolar nerve.

The *zygomatic nerve* comes off the maxillary division in the pterygopalatine fossa and travels anteriorly, entering the orbit through the inferior orbital fissure, where it divides into the zygomaticotemporal and zygomaticofacial nerves: the *zygomaticotemporal* supplying sensory innervation to the skin on the side of the forehead, and the *zygomaticofacial* supplying the skin on the prominence of the cheek. Just before leaving the orbit, the zygomatic nerve sends a branch that communicates with the lacrimal nerve of the ophthalmic division. This branch carries secretory fibers from the sphenopalatine ganglion to the lacrimal gland.

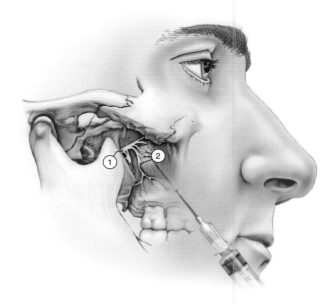

Figure 12-8. Branches of V₂ in the pterygopalatine fossa. *1,* Maxillary nerve; *2,* posterior superior alveolar branches. (Data from Haglund J, Evers H: *Local anaesthesia in dentistry,* ed 2, Södertälje, Sweden, 1975, Astra Läkemedel.)

The *pterygopalatine nerves* are two short trunks that unite in the pterygopalatine ganglion and are then redistributed into several branches. They also serve as a communication between the pterygopalatine ganglion and the maxillary nerve (V₂). Postganglionic secretomotor fibers from the pterygopalatine ganglion pass through these nerves and back along V₂ to the zygomatic nerve, through which they are routed to the lacrimal nerve and lacrimal gland.

Branches of the pterygopalatine nerves include those that supply four areas: the orbit, nose, palate, and pharynx.

1. The orbital branches supply the periosteum of the orbit.
2. The nasal branches supply the mucous membranes of the superior and middle conchae, the lining of the posterior ethmoidal sinuses, and the posterior portion of the nasal septum. One branch is significant in dentistry, the *nasopalatine nerve,* which passes across the roof of the nasal cavity downward and forward, where it lies between the mucous membrane and the periosteum of the nasal septum. The nasopalatine nerve continues downward, reaching the floor of the nasal cavity and giving branches to the anterior part of the nasal septum and the floor of the nose. It then enters the incisive canal, through which it passes into the oral cavity via the incisive foramen, located in the midline of the palate about 1 cm posterior to the maxillary central incisors. The right and left nasopalatine nerves emerge together through this foramen and provide sensation to the palatal mucosa in the region of the premaxilla (canines through central incisors) (Fig. 12-9).

A

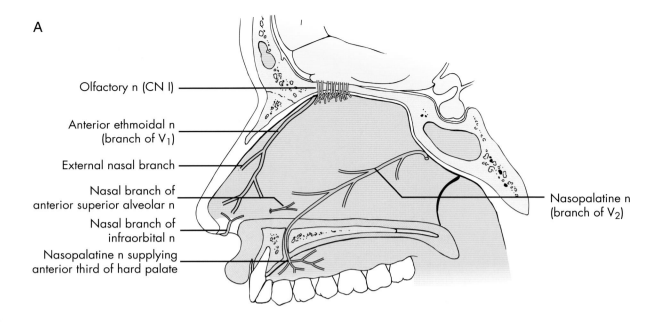

Olfactory n (CN I)

Anterior ethmoidal n (branch of V₁)

External nasal branch

Nasal branch of anterior superior alveolar n

Nasal branch of infraorbital n

Nasopalatine n supplying anterior third of hard palate

Nasopalatine n (branch of V₂)

B

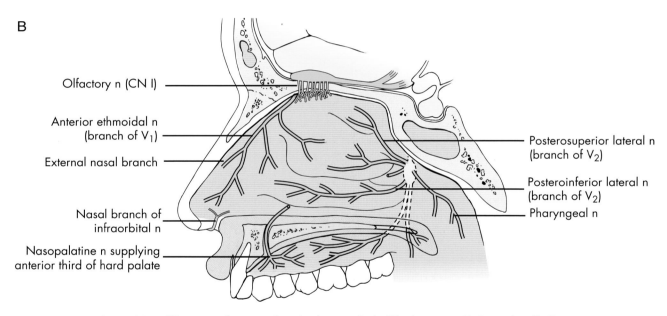

Olfactory n (CN I)

Anterior ethmoidal n (branch of V₁)

External nasal branch

Nasal branch of infraorbital n

Nasopalatine n supplying anterior third of hard palate

Posterosuperior lateral n (branch of V₂)

Posteroinferior lateral n (branch of V₂)

Pharyngeal n

Figure 12-9.   Nerve supply to nasal cavity (*n*, nerve). **A,** Nasal septum. **B,** Lateral wall. (Data from Liebgott B: *The anatomical basis of dentistry*, ed 2, St Louis, 2001, Mosby.)

3. The palatine branches are the greater (or anterior) palatine nerve and the lesser (middle and posterior) palatine nerves (Fig. 12-10). The *greater (or anterior) palatine nerve* descends through the pterygopalatine canal, emerging on the hard palate through the greater palatine foramen (which is usually located about 1 cm toward the palatal midline, just distal to the second molar). Sicher and DuBrul have stated that the greater palatine foramen may be located 3 to 4 mm in front of the posterior border of the hard palate.[1] The nerve courses anteriorly between the mucoperiosteum and the osseous hard palate, supplying sensory innervation to the palatal soft tissues and bone as far anterior as the first premolar, where it communicates with terminal fibers of the nasopalatine nerve (see Fig. 12-10). It also provides sensory innervation to some parts of the soft palate. The *middle palatine nerve* emerges from the lesser palatine foramen, along with the *posterior palatine nerve.* The middle palatine nerve provides sensory innervation to the mucous membrane of the soft palate; the tonsillar region is innervated, in part, by the posterior palatine nerve.

ARTERIES   **NERVES**

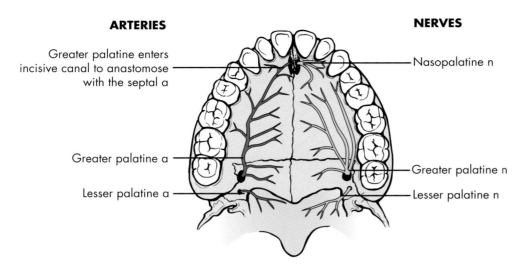

Greater palatine enters incisive canal to anastomose with the septal a

Greater palatine a

Lesser palatine a

Nasopalatine n

Greater palatine n

Lesser palatine n

Figure 12-10. Blood and sensory nerve supply to hard and soft palate. (*a*, artery; *n*, nerve) (Data from Liebgott B: *The anatomical basis of dentistry*, ed 2, St Louis, 2001, Mosby.)

4. The pharyngeal branch is a small nerve that leaves the posterior part of the pterygopalatine ganglion, passes through the pharyngeal canal, and is distributed to the mucous membrane of the nasal part of the pharynx, posterior to the auditory (eustachian) tube.

The *posterior superior alveolar (PSA) nerve* descends from the main trunk of the maxillary division in the pterygopalatine fossa just before the maxillary division enters the infraorbital canal (see Fig. 12-7). Commonly there are two PSA branches, but on occasion a single trunk arises. Passing downward through the pterygopalatine fossa, they reach the inferior temporal (posterior) surface of the maxilla. When two trunks are present, one remains external to the bone, continuing downward on the posterior surface of the maxilla to provide sensory innervation to the buccal gingiva in the maxillary molar region and adjacent facial mucosal surfaces, whereas the other branch enters into the maxilla (along with a branch of the internal maxillary artery) through the PSA canal to travel down the posterior or posterolateral wall of the maxillary sinus and provide sensory innervation to the mucous membrane of the sinus. Continuing downward, this second branch of the PSA nerve provides sensory innervation to the alveoli, periodontal ligaments, and pulpal tissues of the maxillary third, second, and first molars (with the exception [in 28% of patients] of the mesiobuccal root of the first molar).

Branches in the infraorbital canal. Within the infraorbital canal, the maxillary division (V_2) gives off two branches of significance in dentistry, the middle superior and anterior superior alveolar nerves. While in the infraorbital groove and canal, the maxillary division is known as the infraorbital nerve.

The *middle superior alveolar (MSA) nerve* branches off the main nerve trunk (V_2) within the infraorbital canal to form a part of the superior dental plexus,[1] composed of the posterior, middle, and anterior superior alveolar nerves. The site of origin of the MSA nerve varies, from

the posterior portion of the infraorbital canal to the anterior portion, near the infraorbital foramen. The MSA nerve provides sensory innervation to the two maxillary premolars and, perhaps, to the mesiobuccal root of the first molar and the periodontal tissues, buccal soft tissue, and bone in the premolar region. Traditionally it has been stated that the MSA nerve is absent in 30%[2] to 54%[3] of individuals. In a more recent dissection study, Loetscher and Walton[4] found the MSA nerve to be present in 72% of the specimens examined. In its absence its usual innervations are provided by either the PSA or the ASA nerves; most frequently the latter.[1]

The *anterior superior alveolar (ASA) nerve*, a relatively large branch, is given off the infraorbital nerve (V_2) approximately 6 to 10 mm before the latter's exit from the infraorbital foramen. Descending *within* the anterior wall of the maxillary sinus, it provides pulpal innervation to the central and lateral incisors and the canine, and sensory innervation to the periodontal tissues, buccal bone, and mucous membranes of these teeth (Fig. 12-11).

The ASA nerve communicates with the MSA nerve and gives off a small nasal branch that innervates the anterior part of the nasal cavity, along with branches of the pterygopalatine nerves. In persons without an MSA nerve, the ASA nerve frequently provides sensory innervation to the premolars and occasionally the mesiobuccal root of the first molar.

The actual innervation of individual roots of all teeth, bone, and periodontal structures in both the maxilla and mandible derives from terminal branches of larger nerves in the region. These nerve networks are termed the *dental plexus.*

The superior dental plexus is composed of smaller nerve fibers from the three superior alveolar nerves (and in the mandible, from the inferior alveolar nerve). Three types of nerves emerge from these plexuses: dental nerves, interdental branches, and interradicular branches. Each is accompanied along its pathway by a corresponding artery.

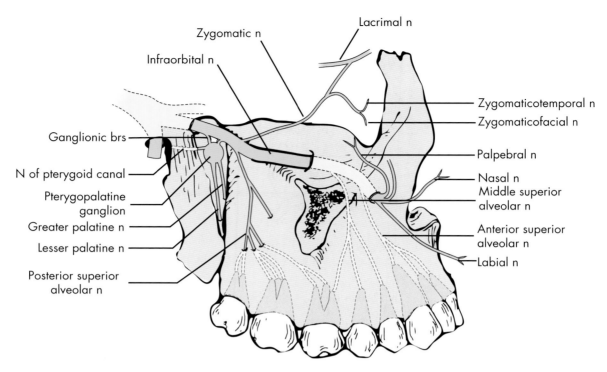

Figure 12-11. Maxillary nerve and its branches (*brs*, branches; *n*, nerve). (Data from Liebgott B: *The anatomical basis of dentistry*, ed 2, St Louis, 2001, Mosby.)

The *dental nerves* are those that enter a tooth through the apical foramen, dividing into many small branches within the pulp. Pulpal innervation of all teeth is derived from dental nerves. Although in most instances one easily identifiable nerve is responsible, in some cases (usually the maxillary first molar) more than one nerve is responsible.

The *interdental branches* (also termed *perforating branches*) travel through the entire height of the interradicular septum, providing sensory innervation to the periodontal ligaments of adjacent teeth through the alveolar bone. They emerge at the height of the crest of the interalveolar septum and enter the gingiva to innervate the interdental papillae and buccal gingiva.

The *interradicular branches* traverse the entire height of the interradicular or interalveolar septum, providing sensory innervation to the periodontal ligaments of adjacent roots. They terminate in the periodontal ligament (PDL) at the root furcations.

Branches on the face. The infraorbital nerve emerges through the infraorbital foramen onto the face to divide into its terminal branches: the inferior palpebral, external nasal, and superior labial. The *inferior palpebral branches* supply the skin of the lower eyelid with sensory innervation, the *external nasal branches* provide sensory innervation to the skin on the lateral aspect of the nose, and the *superior labial branches* afford sensory innervation to the skin and mucous membranes of the upper lip.

Although anesthesia of these nerves is not necessary for adequate pain control during dental treatment, they are frequently blocked in the process of carrying out other anesthetic procedures.

Summary. The following is a summary of the branches of the maxillary division (italicized nerves denote those of special significance in dental pain control):
1. Branches within the cranium
   a. Middle meningeal nerve
2. Branches within the pterygopalatine fossa
   a. Zygomatic nerve
      Zygomaticotemporal nerve
      Zygomaticofacial nerve
   b. Pterygopalatine nerves
      Orbital branches
      Nasal branches
         Nasopalatine nerve
      Palatine branches
      Greater (anterior) palatine nerve
         Lesser (middle and posterior) palatine nerves
         Pharyngeal branch
   c. *Posterior superior alveolar nerve*
3. Branches within the infraorbital canal
   a. *Middle superior alveolar nerve*
   b. *Anterior superior alveolar nerve* (Fig. 12-12)
4. Branches on the face
   a. Inferior palpebral branches
   b. External nasal branches
   c. Superior labial branches

Mandibular Division (V_3). The mandibular division is the largest branch of the trigeminal nerve. It is a mixed nerve with two roots: a large sensory root and a smaller motor root (the latter representing the entire motor component of the trigeminal nerve). The sensory root of the mandibular division originates at the inferior angle of the trigeminal ganglion, whereas the motor root arises in motor cells located in the pons and medulla oblongata. The two roots emerge from the cranium separately through the foramen ovale, the motor root lying medial to the sensory. They unite just outside the skull and form the main trunk of the third division. This trunk remains undivided for only 2 to 3 mm before it splits into a small anterior and large posterior division (Figs. 12-13 and 12-14).

The areas innervated by V_3 are included in the following outline:

1. Sensory root
   a. Skin:
      Temporal region
      Auricula
      External auditory meatus
      Cheek
      Lower lip
      Lower part of the face (chin region)
   b. Mucous membrane:
      Cheek
      Tongue (anterior two thirds)
      Mastoid cells
   c. Mandibular teeth and periodontal tissues
   d. Bone of the mandible
   e. Temporomandibular joint
   f. Parotid gland

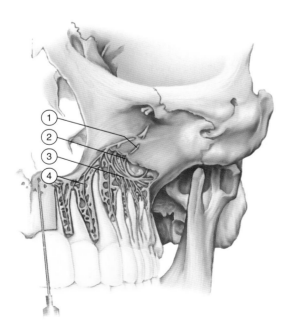

Figure 12-12. Anterior superior alveolar (ASA) nerve (bone over the nerves removed). *1,* Branches of the ASA nerve; *2,* superior dental plexus; *3,* dental branches; *4,* interdental and interradicular branches. (Data from Haglund J, Evers H: *Local anaesthesia in dentistry,* ed 2, Södertälje, Sweden, 1975, Astra Läkemedel.)

2. Motor root
   a. Masticatory muscles
      Masseter
      Temporalis
      Pterygoideus medialis
      Pterygoideus lateralis
   b. Mylohyoid
   c. Anterior belly of the digastric
   d. Tensor tympani
   e. Tensor veli palatini

Branches. The third division of the trigeminal nerve gives off branches in three areas: from the undivided nerve, and the anterior and posterior divisions.

Branches from the undivided nerve. On leaving the foramen ovale, the main undivided nerve trunk gives off two branches during its 2- to 3-mm course. These are the nervus spinosus (meningeal branch of the mandibular nerve) and the medial pterygoid nerve. The *nervus spinosus* reenters the cranium through the foramen spinosum along with the middle meningeal artery to supply the dura mater and mastoid air cells. The *medial pterygoid nerve* is a motor nerve to the medial (internal) pterygoid muscle. It gives off small branches that are motor to the tensor veli palatini and tensor tympani.

Branches from the anterior division. Branches from the anterior division of V_3 provide motor innervation to the muscles of mastication and sensory innervation to the mucous membrane of the cheek and buccal mucous membrane of the mandibular molars.

The anterior division is significantly smaller than the posterior. It runs forward under the lateral (external) pterygoid muscle for a short distance and then reaches the external surface of that muscle by either passing between its two heads or, less frequently, winding over its upper border. From this point it is known as the *buccal nerve.* Although under the lateral pterygoid muscle, the buccal nerve gives off several branches: the *deep temporal nerves* (to the temporal muscle) and the *masseter* and *lateral pterygoid nerves* (providing motor innervation to the respective muscles).

The buccal nerve, also known as the *buccinator nerve* and the *long buccal nerve,* usually passes between the two heads of the lateral pterygoid to reach the external surface of that muscle. It then follows the inferior part of the temporal muscle and emerges under the anterior border of the masseter muscle, continuing in an anterolateral direction. At the level of the occlusal plane of the mandibular third or second molar, it crosses in front of the anterior border of the ramus and enters the cheek through the buccinator muscle. Sensory fibers are distributed to the skin of the cheek. Other fibers pass into the retromolar triangle, providing sensory innervation to the buccal gingiva of the mandibular molars and the mucobuccal fold in that region. The buccal nerve does *not* innervate the buccinator muscle; the facial nerve does.

Nor does it provide sensory innervation to the lower lip or corner of the mouth. This is significant because some doctors do not administer the "long" buccal injection after inferior alveolar nerve block until the lower lip has become numb. Their thinking is that the long buccal nerve block will provide anesthesia of the lower lip and therefore might lead them to believe that their inferior alveolar nerve block has been successful, when in fact it has been missed. Such concern is unwarranted. *The long buccal nerve block should be administered immediately after inferior alveolar nerve block.*

Anesthesia of the buccal nerve is important for dental procedures requiring soft-tissue manipulation on the buccal surface of the mandibular molars.

Branches of the posterior division. The posterior division of V_3 is primarily sensory with a small motor component. It descends for a short distance downward and medially to the lateral pterygoid muscle, at which point it branches into the auriculotemporal, lingual, and inferior alveolar nerves.

The *auriculotemporal nerve* is not profoundly significant in dentistry. It traverses the upper part of the parotid gland and then crosses the posterior portion of the zygomatic arch. It gives off a number of branches, all of which

are sensory. These include a communication with the facial nerve, providing sensory fibers to the skin over the areas of innervation of the following motor branches of the facial nerve: the zygomatic, buccal, and mandibular; a communication with the otic ganglion, providing sensory, secretory, and vasomotor fibers to the parotid gland; the anterior auricular branches, supplying the skin over the helix and tragus of the ear; branches to the external auditory meatus, innervating the skin over the meatus and the tympanic membrane; articular branches to the posterior portion of the temporomandibular joint; and the superficial temporal branches, supplying the skin over the temporal region.[1-6]

The *lingual nerve* is the second branch of the posterior division of V_3. It passes downward medial to the lateral pterygoid muscle and, as it descends, lies between the ramus and the medial pterygoid muscle in the pterygomandibular space. It runs anterior and medial to the inferior alveolar nerve, whose path it parallels. It then continues downward and forward, deep to the pterygomandibular raphe and below the attachment of the superior constrictor of the pharynx, to reach the side of the base of the tongue slightly below and behind the mandibular third molar (Figs. 12-13 and 12-14). Here it lies just below the mucous membrane in the lateral

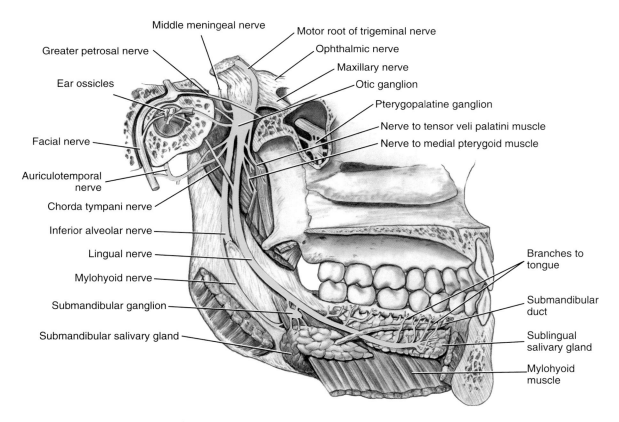

Figure 12-13. Medial view of the mandible showing the motor and sensory branches of the mandibular nerve. (Data from Fehrenbach MJ, Herring SW: *Illustrated anatomy of the head and neck*, ed 2, Philadelphia, 2002, WB Saunders.)

lingual sulcus, where it is so superficial in some persons that it may be seen just below the mucous membrane. It then proceeds anteriorly across the muscles of the tongue, looping downward and medial to the submandibular (Wharton's) duct to the deep surface of the sublingual gland, where it breaks up into its terminal branches.

The lingual nerve is the sensory tract to the anterior two thirds of the tongue. It provides both general sensation and gustation (taste) for this region. It is the nerve that supplies fibers for general sensation, whereas the chorda tympani (a branch of the facial nerve) supplies fibers for taste. In addition, the lingual nerve provides sensory innervation to the mucous membranes of the floor of the mouth and the gingiva on the lingual of the mandible.

The *inferior alveolar nerve* is the largest branch of the mandibular division (Fig. 12-14). It descends medial to the lateral pterygoid muscle and lateroposterior to the lingual nerve, to the region between the spheno-mandibular ligament and the medial surface of the mandibular ramus, where it enters the mandibular canal at the level of the mandibular foramen. Throughout its path it is accompanied by the inferior alveolar artery (a branch of the internal maxillary artery) and the inferior alveolar vein. The artery lies just anterior to the nerve. The nerve, artery, and vein travel anteriorly in the mandibular canal as far forward as the mental foramen, where the nerve divides into terminal branches: the incisive nerve and the mental nerve.

Bifid (from the Latin meaning "cleft into two parts") inferior alveolar nerves and mandibular canals have been observed radiographically and categorized by Langlais and associates.[5] In 6000 panoramic radiographs studied, bifid mandibular canals were evident in 0.95%. The bifid mandibular canal is clinically significant in that it increases the difficulty of achieving adequate anesthesia in the mandible with conventional techniques. This is especially so in the Type 4 variation (Fig. 12-15), in which two separate mandibular foramina are present on each side of the mouth.

The *mylohyoid nerve* branches from the inferior alveolar nerve before the latter's entry into the mandibular canal (see Figs. 12-13 and 12-14). It runs downward and forward in the mylohyoid groove on the medial surface of the ramus and along the body of the mandible to reach the mylohyoid muscle. The mylohyoid is a mixed nerve, being motor to the mylohyoid muscle and the anterior belly of the digastric. It is thought to contain sensory fibers that supply the skin on the inferior and anterior surfaces of the mental protuberance. It also may provide sensory innervation to the mandibular incisors. There is evidence that the mylohyoid also may be involved in supplying pulpal innervation to portions of the mandibular molars in some persons, usually the mesial root of the mandibular first molar.[6]

Once the inferior alveolar nerve enters the mandibular canal, it travels anteriorly along with the inferior alveolar

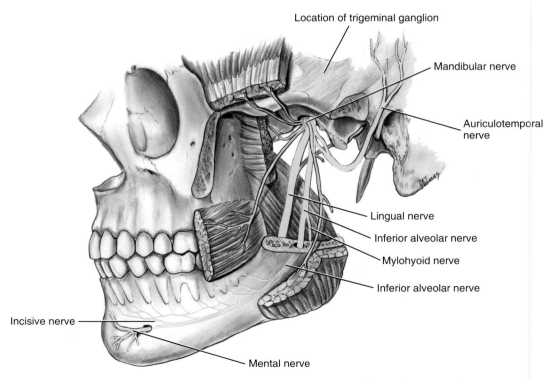

Figure 12-14. The pathway of the posterior trunk of the mandibular division of the trigeminal nerve. (Data from Fehrenbach MJ, Herring SW: *Illustrated anatomy of the head and neck*, ed 2, Philadelphia, 2002, WB Saunders.)

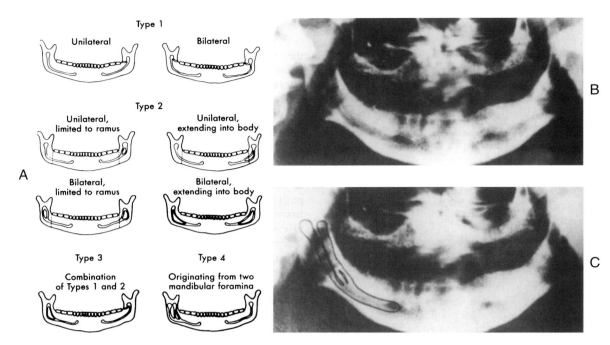

Figure 12-15. A, Variations of bifid mandibular canals. **B** and **C,** Radiographs of a Type 4 bifid mandibular canal (**B,** on the patient's right; **C,** outlined). (Data from Langlais RP, Broadus R, Glass BJ: Bifid mandibular canals in panoramic radiographs, *J Am Dent Assoc* 110:923-926, 1985.)

artery and vein. The *dental plexus* serves the mandibular posterior teeth, entering through their apices and providing pulpal innervation. Other fibers supply sensory innervation to the buccal periodontal tissues of these same teeth.

The inferior alveolar nerve divides into its two terminal branches, the incisive nerve and the mental nerve at the mental foramen (see Fig. 12-14). The *incisive nerve* remains within the mandibular canal and forms a nerve plexus that innervates the pulpal tissues of the mandibular first premolar, canine, and incisors via the dental branches. The *mental nerve* exits the canal through the mental foramen and divides into three branches that innervate the skin of the chin and the skin and mucous membrane of the lower lip.

Summary. The following outline summarizes the branches of the mandibular division (italicized nerves denote those especially significant in dental pain control):
1. Undivided nerve
   a. Nervus spinosus
   b. Nerve to the medial pterygoid muscle
2. Divided nerve
   a. Anterior division
      Nerve to the lateral pterygoid muscle
      Nerve to the masseter muscle
      Nerve to the temporal muscle
      Buccal nerve

   b. *Posterior division*
      Auriculotemporal nerve
      Lingual nerve
      Mylohyoid nerve
      Inferior alveolar nerve: dental branches
      Incisive branch: dental branches
      Mental nerve

OSTEOLOGY: MAXILLA

In addition to the neuroanatomy of pain control in dentistry, one should be aware of the relationship of these nerves to the osseous and soft tissues through which they course.

The maxilla (more properly, the right and left maxillae) is the largest bone of the face, excluding the mandible. Its anterior (or facial) surface (Fig. 12-16) is directed both forward and laterally. At its inferior borders are a series of eminences that correspond to the roots of the maxillary teeth. The most prominent usually is found over the canine tooth, often referred to as the *canine eminence.* Superior to the canine fossa (located just distal to the canine eminence) is the infraorbital foramen, through which blood vessels and terminal branches of the infraorbital nerve emerge. Bone in the region of the maxillary teeth is quite commonly of the more porous cancellous variety, leading to a significantly greater incidence of clinically adequate anesthesia than in areas where more dense cortical bone

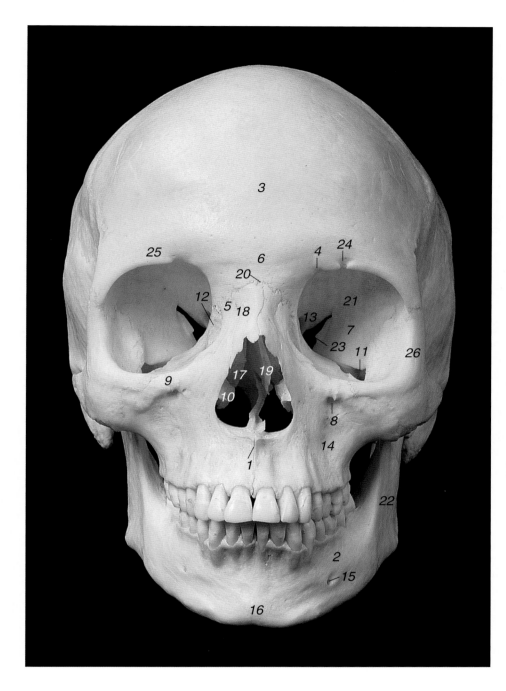

Figure 12-16. Anterior view of the skull. *1*, Anterior nasal spine; *2*, body of mandible; *3*, frontal bone; *4*, frontal notch; *5*, frontal process of maxilla; *6*, glabella; *7*, greater wing of sphenoid bone; *8*, infraorbital foramen; *9*, infraorbital margin; *10*, inferior nasal concha; *11*, inferior orbital fissure; *12*, lacrimal bone; *13*, lesser wing of sphenoid bone; *14*, maxilla; *15*, mental foramen; *16*, mental protuberance; *17*, middle nasal concha; *18*, nasal bone; *19*, nasal septum; *20*, nasion; *21*, orbit (orbital cavity); *22*, ramus of mandible; *23*, superior orbital fissure; *24*, supraorbital foramen; *25*, supraorbital margin; *26*, zygomatic bone. (Data from Abrahams PH, Marks SC Jr, Hutchings RT: *McMinn's color atlas of human anatomy*, ed 5, St Louis, 2003, Mosby.)

is present, such as in the mandible. In many areas, bone over the apices of the maxillary teeth either is tissue-paper thin or shows evidence of dehiscence.

The inferior temporal surface of the maxilla is directed backward and laterally (Fig. 12-17). Its posterior surface is pierced by several alveolar canals that transmit the posterior superior alveolar nerves and blood vessels. The maxillary tuberosity, a rounded eminence, is found on the inferior posterior surface. On the superior surface is a groove, directed laterally and slightly superiorly, through which the maxillary nerve passes. This groove is continuous with the infraorbital groove.

The palatal processes of the maxilla are thick horizontal projections that form a large portion of the floor of

the nose and roof of the mouth. The bone here is considerably thicker anteriorly than posteriorly. Its inferior (or palatal) surface constitutes the anterior three fourths of the hard palate (Fig. 12-18). Many foramina (passages for nutrient blood vessels) perforate it. Along its lateral border, at the junction with the alveolar process, is a groove through which the anterior palatine nerve passes from the greater palatine foramen. In the midline in the anterior region is the funnel-shaped opening of the incisive foramen. Four canals are located in this opening: two for the descending palatine arteries and two for the nasopalatine nerves. In many skulls, especially those of younger persons, a fine suture line extends laterally from the incisive foramen to the border of the palatine process

Figure 12-17. Infratemporal aspect of the maxilla. *1*, Articular tubercle; *2*, external acoustic meatus; *3*, horizontal plate of palatine bone; *4*, inferior orbital fissure; *5*, infratemporal crest; *6*, infratemporal (posterior) surface of maxilla; *7*, infratemporal surface of greater wing of sphenoid bone; *8*, lateral pterygoid plate; *9*, mandibular fossa; *10*, mastoid notch; *11*, mastoid process; *12*, medial pterygoid plate; *13*, occipital condyle; *14*, occipital groove; *15*, pterygoid hamulus; *16*, pterygomaxillary fissure and pterygopalatine fossa; *17*, pyramidal process of palatine bone; *18*, spine of sphenoid bone; *19*, styloid process and sheath; *20*, third molar tooth; *21*, tuberosity of maxilla; *22*, vomer; *23*, zygomatic arch. (Data from Abrahams PH, Marks SC Jr, Hutchings RT: *McMinn's color atlas of human anatomy*, ed 5, St Louis, 2003, Mosby.)

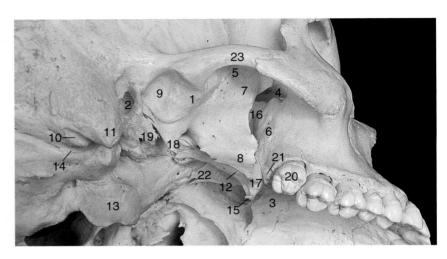

by the canine teeth. The small area anterior to this suture is termed the *premaxilla*.

The horizontal plate of the palatine bone forms the posterior fourth of the hard palate. Its anterior border articulates with the palatine process of the maxilla, and its posterior border serves as the attachment for the soft palate. Foramina are present on its surface, representing the lower end of the pterygopalatine canal, through which descending palatine blood vessels and the anterior palatine nerve run.

OSTEOLOGY: MANDIBLE

The mandible is the largest and strongest bone of the face. It consists of a curved horizontal portion (the body) and two perpendicular portions (the rami). The buccal cortical plate of the mandible most often is sufficiently dense so as to preclude effective infiltration anesthesia in its vicinity.[7]

The external (lateral) surface of the *body* of the mandible is marked in the midline by a faint ridge, an

indication of the symphysis of the two pieces of bone from which the mandible is created (Fig. 12-19, *A* and *C*). The bone forming the buccal alveolar processes in the anterior region (incisors) is usually less dense than that over the posterior teeth, permitting infiltration (supraperiosteal) anesthesia to be employed with some expectation of success (in adults usually in the area of the lateral incisor only). In the region of the second premolar on each side, midway between the upper and lower borders of the body, lies the mental foramen. Phillips and associates, in an evaluation of 75 dry, adult human mandibles, determined that the usual position of the mental foramen is below the crown of the second premolar.[8] The mental nerve, artery, and vein exit the mandibular canal here. Bone along this external surface of the mandible is commonly quite thick cortical bone.

The lingual border of the body of the mandible is concave from side to side (Fig. 12-19, *B* and *D*). Extending upward and backward is the mylohyoid line, giving origin to the mylohyoid muscle. Bone along the lingual of the mandible is usually quite thick; however, in approximately 68% of mandibles there are lingual

Figure 12-18. Inferior view of the hard palate. (Data from Fehrenbach MJ, Herring SW: *Illustrated anatomy of the head and neck*, ed 2, Philadelphia, 2002, WB Saunders.)

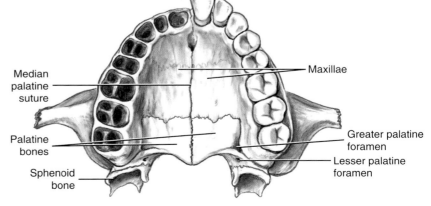

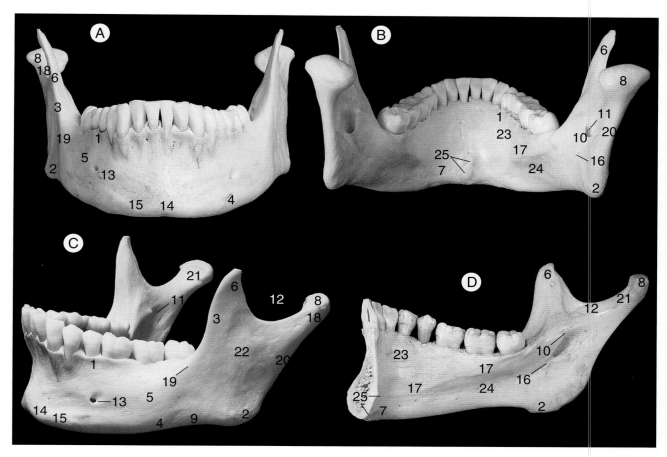

Figure 12-19. The mandible from the front **(A),** from behind and above **(B),** from the left and front **(C),** and internal view from the left **(D).** *1,* Alveolar part; *2,* angle; *3,* anterior border of ramus; *4,* base; *5,* body; *6,* coronoid process; *7,* digastric fossa; *8,* head; *9,* inferior border of ramus; *10,* lingula; *11,* mandibular foramen; *12,* mandibular notch; *13,* mental foramen; *14,* mental protuberance; *15,* mental tubercle; *16,* mylohyoid groove; *17,* mylohyoid line; *18,* neck; *19,* oblique line; *20,* posterior border of ramus; *21,* pterygoid fovea; *22,* ramus; *23,* sublingual fossa; *24,* submandibular fossa; *25,* superior and inferior mental spines (genial tubercles). (Data from Abrahams PH, Marks SC Jr, Hutchings RT: *McMinn's color atlas of human anatomy,* ed 5, St Louis, 2003, Mosby.)

foramina located in the posterior (molar) region.[9] The function of these foramina is as yet unclear, but some may contain sensory fibers from the mylohyoid nerve that innervate portions of mandibular molars.[2]

The lateral surface of each *ramus* is flat, composed of dense cortical bone and providing attachment for the masseter muscle along most of its surface (see Fig. 12-19, *C*). The medial surface (see Fig. 12-19, *D*) contains the mandibular foramen, located roughly halfway between the superior and inferior borders and two thirds to three fourths the distance from the anterior border of the ramus to its posterior border.[10] Other studies of the anteroposterior location of the mandibular foramen have provided differing locations. Hayward and associates[11] found the foramen most often in the third quadrant from the anterior part of the ramus, Monheim[12] found it at the midpoint of the ramus, whereas Hetson and associates[13]

located it at 55% distal to the anterior ramus (a range of 44.4% to 65.5%). The mandibular canal extends obliquely downward and anteriorly within the ramus. It then courses horizontally forward in the body, distributing small dental branches to the mandibular teeth posterior to the mental foramen. The mandibular foramen is the entrance through which the inferior alveolar nerve, artery, and vein enter the mandibular canal. The height of this foramen varies greatly, ranging from 1 to 19 mm or more above the level of the occlusal plane.[11] A prominent ridge, the lingula mandibulae, lies on the anterior margin of the foramen. The lingula serves as an attachment for the sphenomandibular ligament. At the lower end of the mandibular foramen the mylohyoid groove begins, coursing obliquely downward and anteriorly. In this groove lie the mylohyoid nerve and vessels.

Bone along the lingual surface of the mandible usually is dense (see Fig. 12-19, *D*). On rare occasions bone over the lingual aspect of the third molar roots is less dense, permitting a greater chance of supraperiosteal anesthesia.

The superior border of the ramus has two processes: the coronoid anteriorly and condylar posteriorly. Between these two processes is a deep concavity, the mandibular (sigmoid) notch. The coronoid process is thinner than the condylar. Its anterior border is concave, the coronoid notch. The coronoid notch represents a landmark for determining the height of needle penetration in the inferior alveolar nerve block technique. The condylar process is thicker than the coronoid. The condylar head, the thickened articular portion of the condyle, sits atop the constricted neck of the condyle. The condylar neck is flattened front to back. The attachment for the external pterygoid muscle is on its anterior surface.

When cut horizontally at the level of the mandibular foramen, the ramus of the mandible can be seen to be thicker in its anterior region than it is posteriorly. This is of clinical importance during the inferior alveolar nerve block. The thickness of soft tissues between needle penetration and the osseous tissues of the ramus at the level of the mandibular foramen averages about 20 to 25 mm. Because of the increased thickness of bone in the anterior third of the ramus, the thickness of soft tissue is decreased accordingly (approximately 10 mm). Knowing the depth of penetration of soft tissue before contacting osseous tissues can aid the administrator in determining correct positioning of the needle tip.

REFERENCES

1. DuBrul EL: *Sicher's oral anatomy,* ed 7, St Louis, 1980, Mosby.
2. Heasman PA: Clinical anatomy of the superior alveolar nerves, *Br J Oral Maxillofac Surg* 22:439-447, 1984.
3. McDaniel WL: Variations in nerve distributions of the maxillary teeth, *J Dent Res* 35:916-921, 1956.
4. Loetscher CA, Walton RE: Patterns of innervation of the maxillary first molar: a dissection study, *Oral Surg* 65: 86-90, 1988.
5. Langlais RP, Broadus R, Glass BJ: Bifid mandibular canals in panoramic radiographs, *J Am Dent Assoc* 110:923-926, 1985.
6. Frommer J, Mele FA, Monroe CW: The possible role of the mylohyoid nerve in mandibular posterior tooth sensation, *J Am Dent Assoc* 85:113-117, 1972.
7. Blanton PL, Jeske AH: The key to profound local anesthesia: neuroanatomy, *J Amer Dent Assoc* 134:753-760, 2003.
8. Phillips JL, Weller N, Kulild JC: The mental foramen: Part III. Size and position on panoramic radiographs, *J Endodont* 18:383-386, 1992.
9. Shiller WR, Wiswell OB: Lingual foramina of the mandible, *Anat Rec* 119:387-390, 1954.
10. Bremer G: Measurements of special significance in connection with anesthesia of the inferior alveolar nerve, *Oral Surg* 5:966-988, 1952.
11. Hayward J, Richardson ER, Malhotra SK: The mandibular foramen: its anteroposterior position, *Oral Surg* 44:837-843, 1977.
12. Monheim LM: Local anesthesia and pain control in dental practice, ed 4, St Louis, 1969, Mosby.
13. Hetson G, Share J, Frommer J, et al: Statistical evaluation of the position of the mandibular ramus, *Oral Surg* 65: 32-34, 1988.

Techniques of Maxillary Anesthesia

CHAPTER 13

There are several general methods of obtaining pain control with local anesthetics. The site of deposition of the drug relative to the area of operative intervention determines the type of injection administered. Three major types of local anesthetic injection can be differentiated: local infiltration, field block, and nerve block.

◆ **Local infiltration**

Small terminal nerve endings in the area of the dental treatment are flooded with local anesthetic solution. Incision (or treatment) is then made into the same area in which the local anesthetic has been deposited (Fig. 13-1). An example of local infiltration is the administration of a local anesthetic into an interproximal papilla before root planing.

◆ **Field block**

Local anesthetic solution is deposited near the larger terminal nerve branches so the anesthetized area will be circumscribed, preventing the passage of impulses from the tooth to the central nervous system (CNS). Incision (or treatment) is then made into an area away from the site of injection of the anesthetic (Fig. 13-2). Maxillary injections administered above the apex of the tooth to be treated are properly termed *field blocks* (although common usage identifies them as *infiltration* or *supraperiosteal*).

◆ **Nerve block**

Local anesthetic is deposited close to a main nerve trunk, usually at a distance from the site of operative intervention (Fig. 13-3). Posterior superior alveolar, inferior alveolar, and nasopalatine injections are examples of nerve blocks.

◆ **Discussion**

Technically, the injection commonly referred to in dentistry as a *local infiltration* is a field block, because anesthetic solution is deposited at or above the apex of the tooth to be treated. Terminal nerve branches to the

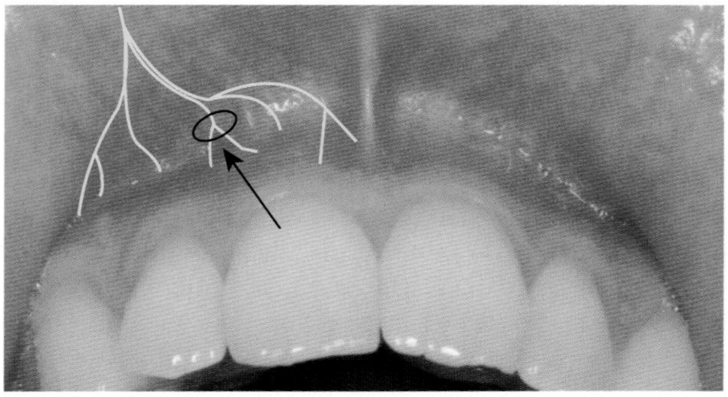

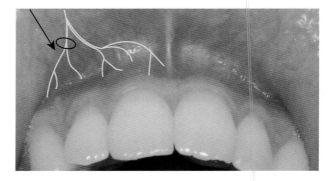

Figure 13-1. Local infiltration. The area of treatment is flooded with local anesthetic. An incision is made into the same area *(arrow)*.

Figure 13-2. Field block. Local anesthetic is deposited near the larger terminal nerve endings *(arrow)*. An incision is made away from the site of injection.

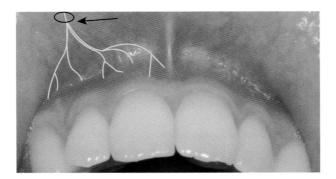

Figure 13-3. Nerve block. Local anesthetic is deposited close to the main nerve trunk, located at a distance from the site of incision *(arrow)*.

pulpal and soft tissues distal to the injection site are anesthetized.

Field block and nerve block may be distinguished by the extent of anesthesia achieved. In general, field blocks are more circumscribed, involving the tissues in and around one or two teeth, whereas nerve blocks affect a larger area (e.g., that observed after inferior alveolar or infraorbital nerve block).

The type of injection administered for a given treatment is determined by the extent of the operative area. For management of small, isolated areas, infiltration anesthesia may suffice. When two or three teeth are being restored, field block is indicated, whereas for pain control in quadrant dentistry, regional block anesthesia is recommended.

MAXILLARY INJECTION TECHNIQUES

A number of injection techniques are available to aid in providing clinically adequate anesthesia of the teeth and soft and hard tissues in the maxilla. Selection of the specific technique to be used is determined, in large part, by the nature of the treatment to be provided. The following techniques are available:

1. Supraperiosteal (infiltration), recommended for limited treatment protocols
2. Periodontal ligament (PDL, intraligamentary) injection, recommended as an adjunct to other techniques or for limited treatment protocols
3. Intraseptal injection, recommended primarily for periodontal surgical techniques
4. Intracrestal injection, recommended for single teeth (primarily mandibular molars) when other techniques have failed
5. Intraosseous (IO) injection, recommended for single teeth (primarily mandibular molars) when other techniques have failed
6. Posterior superior alveolar (PSA) nerve block, recommended for management of several molar teeth in one quadrant

7. Middle superior alveolar (MSA) nerve block, recommended for management of premolars in one quadrant
8. Anterior superior alveolar (ASA, infraorbital) nerve block, recommended for management of anterior teeth in one quadrant
9. Maxillary (second division) nerve block, recommended for extensive buccal, palatal, and pulpal management in one quadrant
10. Greater (anterior) palatine nerve block, recommended for palatal soft- and osseous-tissue treatment distal to the canine in one quadrant
11. Nasopalatine nerve block, recommended for palatal soft- and osseous-tissue management from canine to canine bilaterally
12. Anterior middle superior alveolar (AMSA) nerve block, recommended for extensive management of anterior teeth, palatal and buccal soft and hard tissues
13. Palatal approach-anterior superior alveolar (P-ASA) nerve block, recommended for treatment of maxillary anterior teeth, their palatal and facial soft, and hard tissues

The supraperiosteal, periodontal ligament, intraseptal, and intraosseous injections are appropriate for administration in either the maxilla or mandible. Because of the great success of the supraperiosteal injection in the maxillary arch, it is discussed in this chapter. The periodontal ligament, intraseptal, intracrestal, and intraosseous injections are supplemental injections that are of somewhat greater importance in the mandible and are described in Chapter 15.

TEETH AND BUCCAL SOFT AND HARD TISSUES

Supraperiosteal Injection

The supraperiosteal injection, more commonly (but incorrectly) called *local infiltration*, is the most frequently used technique for obtaining pulpal anesthesia in maxillary teeth. Although it is a simple procedure to accomplish successfully, there are several valid reasons for using other techniques (e.g., regional nerve blocks) whenever more than two or three teeth are involved in treatment.

Multiple supraperiosteal injections necessitate numerous needle penetrations of the tissue, each with the potential to produce pain, either during the procedure or after the anesthetic effect has resolved. In addition, and perhaps even more important, using supraperiosteal injections for pulpal anesthesia on multiple teeth leads to the administration of a larger volume of local anesthetic solution, with an attendant increase (though usually minor) in the risk of systemic and local complications.

The supraperiosteal injection is indicated whenever dental procedures are confined to a relatively circumscribed area in either the maxilla or mandible.

Other Common Names. Local infiltration, paraperiosteal injection

Nerves Anesthetized. Large terminal branches of the dental plexus

Areas Anesthetized. The entire region innervated by the large terminal branches of this plexus: pulp and root area of the tooth, buccal periosteum, connective tissue, mucous membrane (Fig. 13-4).

Indications
1. Pulpal anesthesia of the maxillary teeth when treatment is limited to one or two teeth
2. Soft-tissue anesthesia when indicated for surgical procedures in a circumscribed area

Contraindications
1. Infection or acute inflammation in the area of injection.
2. Dense bone covering the apices of teeth (can be determined only by trial and error; most likely over the permanent maxillary first molar in children, its apex lies beneath the zygomatic bone, which is relatively dense). The apex of an adult's central incisor may also be located beneath denser bone (e.g., of the nose), thereby increasing the failure rate (although not significantly).

Advantages
1. High success rate (>95%)
2. Technically easy injection
3. Usually entirely atraumatic

Disadvantages. Not recommended for large areas, because of the need for multiple needle insertions and the necessity to administer larger total volumes of local anesthetic

Positive Aspiration. Negligible, but possible (<1%)

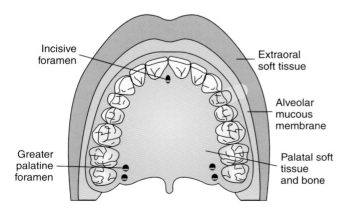

Incisive foramen

Greater palatine foramen

Extraoral soft tissue

Alveolar mucous membrane

Palatal soft tissue and bone

Figure 13-4. Supraperiosteal injection in the anterior region of the maxilla. Notice the placement of the needle and the area anesthetized.

Alternatives. PDL, IO, regional nerve block

Technique
1. A 25- or 27-gauge short needle is recommended
2. Area of insertion: height of the mucobuccal fold above the apex of the tooth being anesthetized
3. Target area: apical region of the tooth to be anesthetized
4. Landmarks
   a. Mucobuccal fold
   b. Crown of the tooth
   c. Root contour of the tooth
5. Orientation of the bevel:* toward bone
6. Procedure
   a. Prepare tissue at the injection site.
      (1) Clean with sterile dry gauze.
      (2) Apply topical antiseptic (optional).
      (3) Apply topical anesthetic for minimum of 1 minute.
   b. Orient needle so bevel faces bone.
   c. Lift the lip, pulling the tissue taut.
   d. Hold the syringe parallel with the long axis of the tooth (Fig. 13-5).
   e. Insert the needle into the height of the mucobuccal fold over the target tooth.
   f. Advance the needle until its bevel is at or above the apical region of the tooth (Table 13-1). In most instances the depth of penetration is only a few millimeters. Because the needle is in soft tissue (not touching bone), there should be no resistance to its advancement, nor should there be any patient discomfort with this injection.
   g. Aspirate ×2.
      (1) If negative, deposit approximately 0.6 ml (one third of a cartridge) slowly over 20 seconds. (Do not permit the tissues to balloon.)
   h. Slowly withdraw the syringe.
   i. Make the needle safe.
   j. Wait 3 to 5 minutes before commencing the dental procedure.

Signs and Symptoms
1. Subjective: feeling of numbness in the area of administration
2. Objective: absence of pain during treatment

---

*Bevel orientations are specified for all injection techniques in Chapters 13 and 14. The orientation of the needle bevel is *not* a significant factor in the success or failure of an injection technique, and these recommendations need not be rigidly adhered to; yet there will be a fuller expectation of successful anesthesia if they are followed, provided all other technical and anatomical principles are maintained. In general, whenever possible, the bevel of the needle is to be facing toward bone; then, in the unlikely event that the needle comes into contact with bone, the bevel will slide over the periosteum, provoking minor discomfort, but not tearing the periosteum. If the bevel faces away from bone, the sharp point of the needle would contact the periosteum, tearing it and leading to a more painful (subperiosteal) injection. Postinjection discomfort is considerably greater with subperiosteal than with supraperiosteal injections.

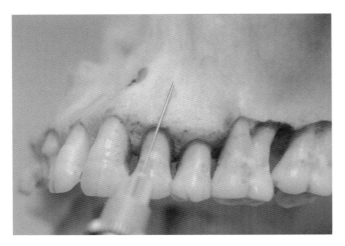

Figure 13-5. The syringe should be held parallel with the long axis of the tooth and inserted at the height of the mucobuccal fold over the tooth.

Safety Features
1. Minimal risk of intravascular administration
2. Slowness of injection, aspiration

Precautions. This injection should not be used for larger areas. A greater number of tissue penetrations increases the possibility of pain both during and after the injection, and the larger volume of solution administered increases the possibility of local anesthetic overdose and postinjection pain.

Failures of Anesthesia
1. Needle tip lies below the apex (along the root) of the tooth (see Table 13-1). Depositing anesthetic solution below the apex of a maxillary tooth results in excellent soft-tissue anesthesia but poor or absent pulpal anesthesia.
2. Needle tip lies too far from the bone (solution deposited in the buccal soft tissues). To correct: Redirect the needle closer to the periosteum.

Complications. Pain on needle insertion with the needle tip against periosteum. To correct: Withdraw the needle and reinsert it farther from the periosteum.

Posterior Superior Alveolar Nerve Block

The posterior superior alveolar (PSA) nerve block is a commonly used dental nerve block. Although it is a highly successful technique (>95%), there are several issues to weigh when considering its use. These include the extent of anesthesia produced and the potential for hematoma formation.

When used to achieve pulpal anesthesia, the PSA nerve block is effective for the maxillary third, second, and first molars in 77% to 100% of patients.[1] However, the mesiobuccal root of the maxillary first molar is not consistently innervated by the PSA nerve. In a dissection study by Loetscher and associates[2] the middle superior alveolar nerve provided sensory innervation to the mesiobuccal root of the maxillary first molar in 28% of the specimens examined. Therefore a second injection, usually supraperiosteal, is indicated after the PSA nerve block when effective anesthesia of the first molar does not develop. Loetscher and associates[2] concluded by stating that the PSA nerve usually provides sole pulpal innervation to the maxillary first molar and that a single PSA

TABLE 13-1
Average Tooth Length

	Length of Crown (mm) +	Length of Root (mm) =	Length of Tooth
MAXILLARY			
Central incisors	11.6	12.4	24.0
Lateral incisors	9.0 to 10.2	12.3 to 13.5	22.5
Canines	10.9	16.1	27.0
First premolars	8.7	13.0	21.7
Second premolars	7.9	13.6	21.5
First molars	7.7	13.6	21.3
Second molars	7.7	13.4	21.1
Third molars	Extremely variable	Extremely variable	Extremely variable
MANDIBULAR			
Central incisors	9.4	12.0	21.4
Lateral incisors	9.9	13.3	23.2
Canines	11.4	14.0	25.4
First premolars	7.5 to 11.0	11.0 to 16.0	18.5 to 27.0
Second premolars	8.5	14.7	23.2
First molars	8.3	14.5	22.8
Second molars	8.1	14.7	22.8
Third molars	Extremely variable	Extremely variable	Extremely variable

nerve block usually provides clinically adequate pulpal anesthesia.

The risk of a potential complication also must be considered whenever the PSA block is used. Insertion of the needle too far distally may lead to a temporarily (10 to 14 days) unaesthetic hematoma. When the PSA is to be administered, one must always consider the patient's skull size in determining the depth of soft-tissue penetration. An "average" depth of penetration in a patient with a smaller than average-sized skull may produce a hematoma, whereas a needle inserted "just right" in a larger-skulled patient might not provide anesthesia to any teeth. As a means of decreasing the risk of hematoma formation after a PSA nerve block, the use of a "short" dental needle is recommended for all but the largest of patients. Because the average depth of soft-tissue penetration from the insertion site (the mucobuccal fold over the maxillary second molar) to the area of the PSA nerves is 16 mm, the short dental needle (~20 mm) can be successfully and safely used. Overinsertion of the needle is less likely to occur, thereby minimizing the risk of hematoma. A 25-gauge short needle is preferred, but in its absence a 27-gauge short needle may be used, as long as aspiration is performed carefully and the local anesthetic is injected slowly. One must remember to aspirate several times before and during drug deposition during the PSA nerve block to avoid inadvertent intravascular injection.

Other Common Names. Tuberosity block, zygomatic block

Nerves Anesthetized. Posterior superior alveolar and branches

Areas Anesthetized
1. Pulps of the maxillary third, second, and first molars (entire tooth = 72%; mesiobuccal root of the maxillary first molar not anesthetized = 28%)
2. Buccal periodontium and bone overlying these teeth (Fig. 13-6)

Indications
1. When treatment involves two or more maxillary molars
2. When supraperiosteal injection is contraindicated (e.g., with infection or acute inflammation)
3. When supraperiosteal injection has proved ineffective

Contraindication. When the risk of hemorrhage is too great (as with a hemophiliac), in which case a supraperiosteal or PDL injection is recommended

Advantages
1. Atraumatic; administered properly, no pain is experienced by the patient receiving the PSA because of the relatively large area of soft tissue into which the local anesthetic is deposited and the fact that bone is not contacted.

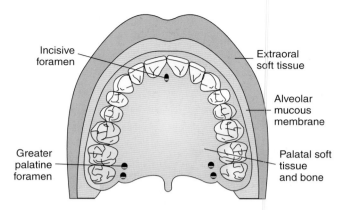

Figure 13-6. Area anesthetized by a posterior superior alveolar (PSA) nerve block. Infratemporal surface of maxilla; maxillary tuberosity.

2. High success rate (>95%)
3. Minimum number of necessary injections
   a. One injection compared with option of three infiltrations
4. Minimizes the total volume of local anesthetic solution administered
   a. Equivalent volume of anesthetic solution necessary for three supraperiosteal injections = 1.8 ml

Disadvantages
1. Risk of hematoma, which is usually diffuse; also discomfiting and embarrassing to the patient
2. Technique somewhat arbitrary: no bony landmarks during insertion
3. Second injection necessary for treatment of the first molar (mesiobuccal root) in 28% of patients

Positive Aspiration. Approximately 3.1%

Alternatives
1. Supraperiosteal or PDL injections for pulpal and root anesthesia
2. Infiltrations for the buccal periodontium and hard tissues
3. Maxillary nerve block

Technique
1. A 25-gauge short needle recommended, although the 27-gauge short is more likely to be available and is also acceptable
2. Area of insertion: height of the mucobuccal fold above the maxillary second molar
3. Target area: PSA nerve—posterior, superior, and medial to the posterior border of the maxilla (Fig. 13-7)
4. Landmarks
   a. Mucobuccal fold
   b. Maxillary tuberosity
   c. Zygomatic process of the maxilla
5. Orientation of the bevel: toward bone during the injection. If bone is accidentally touched, the sensation is less unpleasant.

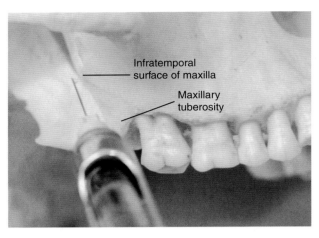

Figure 13-7. Needle at the target area for a posterior superior alveolar (PSA) nerve block.

6. Procedure
   a. Assume the correct position (Fig. 13-8).
      (1) For a left PSA nerve block, a right-handed administrator should sit at the 10 o'clock position facing the patient.
      (2) For a right PSA block, a right-handed administrator should sit at the 8 o'clock position facing the patient.
   b. Prepare the tissues at the height of the mucobuccal fold for penetration.
      1. Dry with a sterile gauze.
      2. Apply a topical antiseptic (optional).
      3. Apply topical anesthetic for a minimum of 1 minute.
   c. Orient the bevel of the needle toward bone.
   d. Partially open the patient's mouth, pulling the mandible to the side of injection.
   e. Retract the patient's cheek with your finger (for visibility).
   f. Pull the tissues at the injection site taut.
   g. Insert the needle into the height of the mucobuccal fold over the second molar (Fig. 13-9).
   h. Advance the needle slowly in an upward, inward, and backward direction (Fig. 13-10) in one movement (not three).
      (1) Upward: superiorly at a 45-degree angle to the occlusal plane
      (2) Inward: medially toward the midline at a 45-degree angle to the occlusal plane (Fig. 13-11)
      (3) Backward: posteriorly at a 45-degree angle to the long axis of the second molar
   i. Slowly advance the needle through soft tissue.
      (1) There should be no resistance and therefore no discomfort to the patient.
      (2) If resistance (bone) is felt, the angle of the needle in toward the midline is too great
         (a) Withdrawn the needle slightly (but do not remove it entirely from the tissues) and bring the syringe barrel closer to the occlusal plane.
         (b) Readvance the needle.
   j. Advance the needle to the desired depth (see Fig. 13-11).
      (1) In an adult of normal size, penetration to a depth of 16 mm places the needle tip in the immediate vicinity of the foramina through which the PSA nerves enter the posterior surface of the maxilla. When a long needle is used (average length 32 mm), it is inserted half its length into the tissue. With a short needle (average length 20 mm), approximately 4 mm should remain visible.

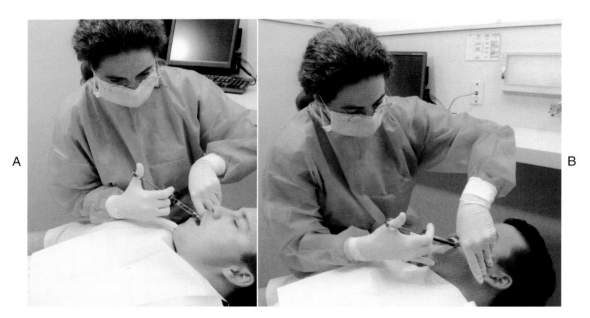

Figure 13-8. Position of the administrator for an, **A,** right and, **B,** left posterior superior alveolar (PSA) nerve block.

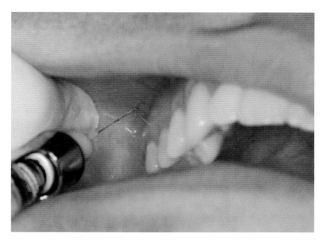

Figure 13-9. Posterior superior alveolar (PSA) nerve block. Tissue retracted at the site of penetration. Notice orientation of needle: inward, upward, backward.

(2) For smaller adults and children it is prudent to halt the advance of the needle short of its usual depth of penetration to avoid a possible hematoma caused by overpenetration. Penetrating to a depth of 10 to 14 mm places the needle tip in the target area in most small-skulled patients.
Note: The goal is to deposit local anesthetic close to the PSA nerves, located posterosuperior and medial to the maxillary tuberosity.

k. Aspirate in two planes.
   (1) Rotate the syringe barrel (needle bevel) one-fourth turn and reaspirate.

l. If both aspirations are negative:
   (1) Slowly, over 30 to 60 seconds, deposit 0.9 to 1.8 ml of anesthetic solution.
   (2) Aspirate several additional times (in one plane) during the procedure.
   (3) The PSA injection is normally atraumatic because of the large tissue space available to accommodate the anesthetic solution and the fact that bone is not touched.

m. Slowly withdraw the syringe.
n. Make the needle safe.
o. Wait 3 to 5 minutes before commencing the dental procedure.

Signs and Symptoms
1. Subjective: usually none; the patient has difficulty reaching this region to determine the extent of anesthesia
2. Objective: absence of pain during therapy

Safety Features
1. Slow injection, repeated aspirations
2. No anatomical safety features to prevent overinsertion of the needle; therefore careful observation is necessary

Precaution. The depth of needle penetration should be checked: overinsertion (too deep) increases the risk of hematoma; too shallow might still provide adequate anesthesia

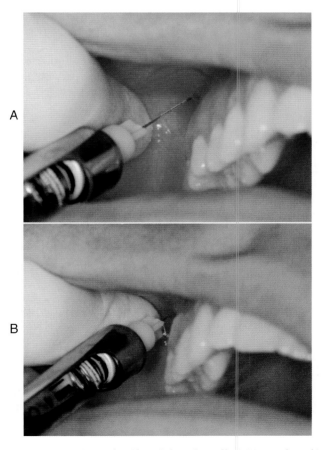

Figure 13-11. A, With a "long" dental needle (~32-mm length) in an average-sized adult, the depth of penetration is half its length. Use of "long" needle on posterior superior alveolar (PSA) nerve block increases risk of overinsertion and hematoma. **B,** PSA nerve block using a "short" dental needle (~20-mm length). Overinsertion is less likely.

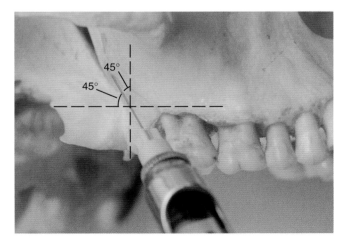

Figure 13-10. Advance the needle upward, inward, and backward.

Failures of Anesthesia

1. Needle too lateral. To correct: Redirect the needle tip medially (see complication 2).
2. Needle not high enough. To correct: Redirect the needle tip superiorly.
3. Needle too far posterior. To correct: Withdraw the needle to the proper depth.

Complications

1. Hematoma
   a. This is commonly produced by inserting the needle too far posteriorly into the pterygoid plexus of veins. In addition, the maxillary artery may be perforated. Use of a short needle (25 or 27 g) minimizes the risk of pterygoid plexus puncture.
   b. A visible intraoral hematoma develops within several minutes, usually noted in the buccal tissues of the mandibular region. (See Chapter 17.)
      (1) There is no easily accessible area to which pressure can be applied to stop the hemorrhage.
      (2) Bleeding continues until the pressure of the extravascular blood is equal to or greater than that of intravascular blood.
2. Mandibular anesthesia
   a. The mandibular division of the fifth cranial nerve (V_3) is located lateral to the PSA nerves. Deposition of local anesthetic lateral to the desired location may produce varying degrees of mandibular anesthesia. Most often, when this occurs, patients mention that their tongue and perhaps their lower lip are anesthetized.

Middle Superior Alveolar Nerve Block

The middle superior alveolar (MSA) nerve is present in only about 28% of the population, thereby limiting the clinical usefulness of this block. However, where the infraorbital nerve block fails to provide pulpal anesthesia distal to the maxillary canine, the MSA block is indicated for procedures on premolars and for the mesiobuccal root of the maxillary first molar. The success rate of the MSA nerve block is high.

Nerves Anesthetized. Middle superior alveolar and terminal branches

Areas Anesthetized

1. Pulps of the maxillary first and second premolars, mesiobuccal root of the first molar
2. Buccal periodontal tissues and bone over these same teeth (Fig. 13-12)

Indications

1. When infraorbital nerve block fails to provide pulpal anesthesia distal to the maxillary canine
2. Dental procedures involving both maxillary premolars only

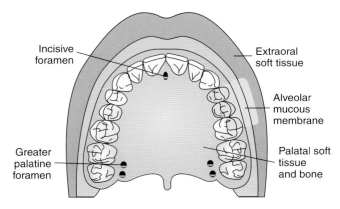

Figure 13-12. Area anesthetized by a middle superior alveolar (MSA) nerve block.

Contraindications

1. Infection or inflammation in the area of injection or needle insertion or drug deposition
2. Where the MSA nerve is absent, innervation is through the anterior superior alveolar (ASA) nerve; branches of the ASA innervating the premolars and mesiobuccal root of the first molar can be anesthetized by means of the MSA technique.

Advantages. Minimizes the number of injections and volume of solution

Disadvantages. None

Positive Aspiration. Negligible (<3%)

Alternatives

1. Local infiltration (supraperiosteal), PDL, IO injections
2. Infraorbital nerve block for the first and second premolar and mesiobuccal root of the first molar

Technique

1. A 25-gauge short or long needle is recommended, although the 27-gauge short is more likely to be available and is perfectly acceptable
2. Area of insertion: height of the mucobuccal fold above the maxillary second premolar
3. Target area: maxillary bone above the apex of the maxillary second premolar (Fig. 13-13)
4. Landmark: mucobuccal fold above the maxillary second premolar
5. Orientation of the bevel: toward bone
6. Procedure
   a. Assume the correct position (Fig. 13-14).
      (1) For a right MSA nerve block, a right-handed administrator should face the patient from the 10 o'clock position.
      (2) For a left MSA nerve block, a right-handed administrator should face the patient directly from the 8 or 9 o'clock position.

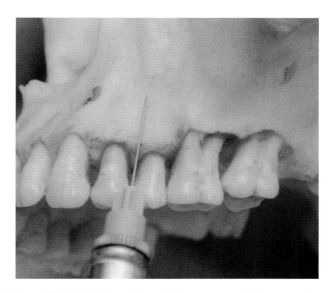

Figure 13-13. Position of needle between maxillary premolars for a middle superior alveolar (MSA) nerve block.

b. Prepare the tissues at the site of injection.
   (1) Dry with sterile gauze.
   (2) Apply topical antiseptic (optional).
   (3) Apply topical anesthetic for a minimum of 1 minute.
c. Stretch the patient's upper lip to make the tissues taut and to gain visibility.
d. Insert the needle into the height of the mucobuccal fold above the second premolar with the bevel directed toward bone.
e. Penetrate the mucous membrane and and slowly advance the needle until its tip is located well above the apex of the second premolar (Fig. 13-15).
f. Aspirate.

g. Slowly deposit 0.9 to 1.2 ml (one half to two thirds cartridge) of solution (approximately 30 to 40 seconds).
h. Withdraw the syringe and make the needle safe.
i. Wait 3 to 5 minutes before commencing dental therapy.

Signs and Symptoms
1. Subjective: upper lip numb
2. Objective: no pain during dental therapy

Safety Features. Relatively avascular area, anatomically safe

Precautions. To prevent pain, do not insert too close to the periosteum and do not inject too rapidly; the MSA should be an atraumatic injection.

Failures of Anesthesia
1. Anesthetic solution not deposited high above the apex of the second premolar
   a. To correct: Check radiographs and increase the depth of penetration.
2. Deposition of solution too far from the maxillary bone with the needle placed in tissues lateral to the height of the mucobuccal fold
   a. To correct: Reinsert at the height of the mucobuccal fold.
3. Bone of the zygomatic arch at the site of injection preventing the diffusion of anesthetic
   a. To correct: Use the supraperiosteal, infraorbital, or PSA injection in place of the MSA.

Complications (rare). A hematoma may develop at the site of injection. Apply pressure with sterile gauze over

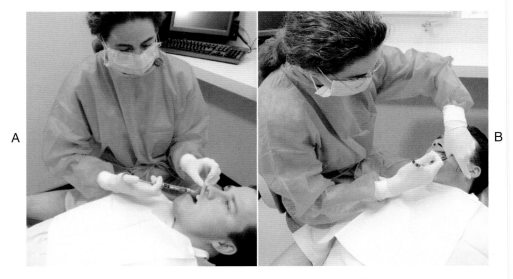

Figure 13-14. Position of the administrator for an, **A,** right and, **B,** left middle superior alveolar (MSA) nerve block.

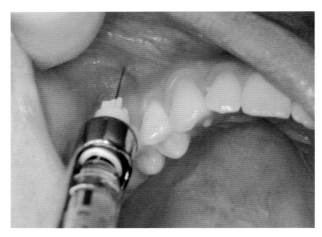

Figure 13-15. Needle penetration for a middle superior alveloar (MSA) nerve block.

the site of swelling and discoloration for a minimum of 60 seconds.

Anterior Superior Alveolar Nerve Block (Infraorbital Nerve Block)

The anterior superior alveolar (ASA) nerve block does not enjoy the popularity of the PSA block, primarily because there is a general lack of experience with this highly successful and extremely safe technique. It provides profound pulpal and buccal soft-tissue anesthesia from the maxillary central incisor through the premolars in about 72% of patients.

Used in place of supraperiosteal injections, the ASA nerve block necessitates a smaller volume of local anesthetic solution to achieve equivalent anesthesia: 0.9 to 1.2 ml versus 3.0 ml for supraperiosteal injections of the same teeth.

Generally speaking, the major factor inhibiting dentists from using the ASA nerve block is fear of injury to the patient's eye. Fortunately this fear is unfounded. Adherence to the following protocol produces a high success rate devoid of complications and adverse side effects.

Other Common Name. Infraorbital nerve block (technically, the infraorbital nerve provides anesthesia to the soft tissues of the anterior portion of the face, not to the teeth or intraoral soft and hard tissues; therefore it is inaccurate to call the ASA nerve block the *infraorbital nerve block*)

Nerves Anesthetized
1. Anterior superior alveolar
2. Middle superior alveolar
3. Infraorbital nerve
   a. Inferior palpebral
   b. Lateral nasal
   c. Superior labial

Areas Anesthetized
1. Pulps of the maxillary central incisor through the canine on the injected side
2. In about 72% of patients, pulps of the maxillary premolars and mesiobuccal root of the first molar
3. Buccal (labial) periodontium and bone of these same teeth
4. Lower eyelid, lateral aspect of the nose, upper lip (Fig. 13-16)

Indications
1. Dental procedures involving more than two maxillary teeth and their overlying buccal tissues
2. Inflammation or infection (which contraindicates supraperiosteal injection); if a cellulitis is present, the maxillary nerve block may be indicated in lieu of the infraorbital nerve block
3. When supraperiosteal injections have been ineffective because of dense cortical bone

Contraindications
1. Discrete treatment areas (one or two teeth only; supraperiosteal preferred)
2. Hemostasis of localized areas, when desirable, cannot be adequately achieved with this injection; local infiltration into the treatment area is indicated.

Advantages
1. Comparatively simple technique
2. Comparatively safe; minimizes the volume of solution used and the number of needle punctures necessary to achieve anesthesia

Disadvantages
1. Psychological
   a. Administrator: There may be an initial fear of injury to the patient's eye (experience with the technique leads to confidence).

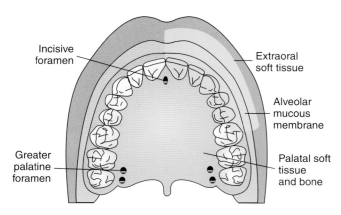

Figure 13-16. Anterior superior alveolar (ASA) nerve block, showing area anesthetized in 72% of patients.

b. Patient: An extraoral approach to the infraorbital nerve may prove disturbing; however, intraoral techniques are rarely a problem.
2. Anatomical: difficulty defining landmarks

Positive Aspiration. 0.7%

Alternatives
1. Supraperiosteal, PDL, or IO injection for each tooth
2. Infiltration for the periodontium and hard tissues
3. Maxillary nerve block

Technique
1. A 25-gauge long needle is recommended, although the 25-gauge short also may be used, especially for children and smaller adults.
2. Area of insertion: height of the mucobuccal fold directly over first premolar
   Note: The needle may be inserted into the height of the mucobuccal fold over any tooth from the second premolar anteriorly to the central incisor. The ensuing path of penetration is toward the target area, the infraorbital foramen. The first premolar usually provides the shortest route to this target area.
3. Target area: infraorbital foramen (below the infraorbital notch)
4. Landmarks
   a. Mucobuccal fold
   b. Infraorbital notch
   c. Infraorbital foramen
5. Orientation of the bevel: toward bone
6. Procedure
   a. Assume the correct position (Fig. 13-17). For a right or left ASA nerve block, a right-handed administrator should sit at the 10 o'clock position, directly facing the patient or facing in the same direction as the patient.
   b. Position the patient supine (much preferred) or semisupine with the neck extended slightly. If the patient's neck is not extended, the patient's chest may interfere with the syringe barrel.
   c. Prepare the tissues at the injection site (height of the mucobuccal fold) for penetration.
      (1) Dry with sterile gauze.
      (2) Apply topical antiseptic (optional).
      (3) Apply topical anesthetic for a minimum of 1 minute.
   d. Locate the infraorbital foramen (Fig. 13-18).
      (1) Feel the infraorbital notch.
      (2) Move your finger downward from the notch, applying gentle pressure to the tissues.
      (3) The bone immediately inferior to the notch is convex (felt as an outward bulge). This represents the lower border of the orbit and the roof of the infraorbital foramen (see Fig. 13-18, *B*).
      (4) As your finger continues inferiorly, a concavity is felt; this is the infraorbital foramen.

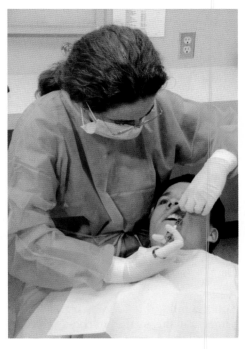

Figure 13-17. Position of the administrator for a right or left anterior superior alveolar (ASA) nerve block. The patient's head should be turned slightly to improve visibility.

      (5) Applying pressure, feel the outlines of the infraorbital foramen at this site. The patient senses a mild soreness when the foramen is palpated.
   e. Maintain your finger on the foramen or mark the skin at the site (Fig. 13-19).
   f. Retract the lip, pulling the tissues in the mucobuccal fold taut and increasing visibility. A 2 × 2 inch sterile gauze placed beneath your gloved finger aids in retraction of the lip during the ASA injection.
   g. Insert the needle into the height of the mucobuccal fold over the first premolar with the bevel facing bone (Fig. 13-20).
   h. Orient the syringe toward the infraorbital foramen.
   i. The needle should be held parallel with the long axis of the tooth as it is advanced, to avoid premature contact with bone (Fig. 13-21).
   j. Advance the needle slowly until bone is gently contacted.
      (1) The point of contact should be the upper rim of the infraorbital foramen.
      (2) The general depth of needle penetration is 16 mm for an adult of average height (equivalent to about half the length of a long needle).
      (3) The depth of penetration varies, of course. In a patient with a high (deep) mucobuccal fold or a low infraorbital foramen, less tissue penetration is necessary than in one with a shallow mucobuccal fold or high infraorbital foramen.
      (4) A preinjection approximation of the depth of penetration can be made by placing one finger

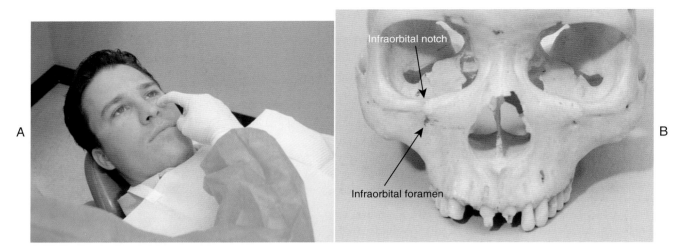

Figure 13-18. A, Palpate the infraorbital notch. **B,** Location of the infraorbital foramen in relation to the infraorbital notch.

on the infraorbital foramen and another on the injection site in the mucobuccal fold and estimating the distance between them.

k. Before injecting the anesthetic solution, check for the following:
   (1) Depth of needle penetration (adequate to reach the foramen)
   (2) Any lateral deviation of the needle from the infraorbital foramen; correct before injecting solution
   (3) Orientation of the bevel (facing bone)

l. Position the needle tip during injection with the bevel facing into the infraorbital foramen and the needle tip touching the roof of the foramen (Fig. 13-22).

m. Aspirate.

n. Slowly deposit 0.9 to 1.2 ml (over 30 to 40 seconds). Little or no swelling should be visible as the solution is deposited. If the needle tip is properly inserted at the opening of the foramen, solution is directed toward the foramen.
   (1) The administrator is able to "feel" the anesthetic solution as it is deposited beneath the finger on the foramen if the needle tip is in the correct position. At the conclusion of the injection, the foramen should no longer be palpable (because of the volume of anesthetic in this position).

   The infraorbital nerve block, providing anesthesia to the soft tissues on the anterior portion of the face and lateral aspect of the nose, is complete. To complete the anterior superior alveolar nerve block, providing anesthesia to the teeth and their supporting structures:

o. Maintain firm pressure with your finger over the injection site both during and for at least 1 minute after the injection (to increase the diffusion of local anesthetic solution into the infraorbital foramen).

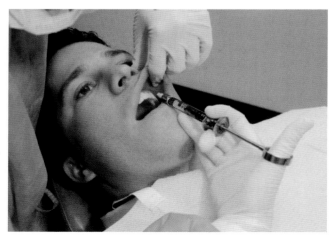

Figure 13-19. Using a finger over the foramen, lift the lip, and hold the tissues in the mucobuccal fold taut.

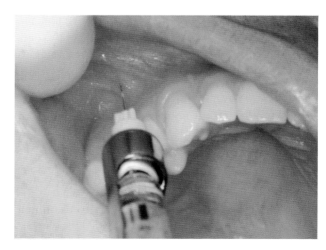

Figure 13-20. Insert the needle for anterior superior alveolar (ASA) nerve block in mucobuccal fold over maxillary first premolar.

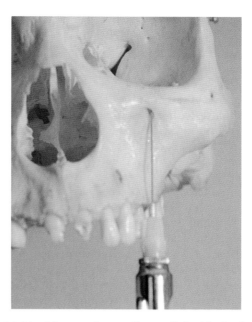

Figure 13-21. Advance the needle parallel with the long axis of the tooth to preclude prematurely contacting bone. Notice how the bone of the maxilla becomes concave between the root eminence and infraorbital foramen *(note shadow)*.

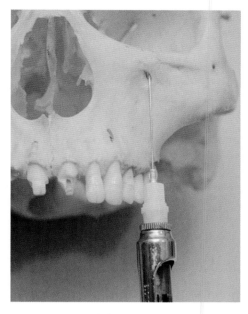

Figure 13-22. Position of the needle tip before deposition of local anesthetic at the infraorbital foramen.

p. Withdraw the syringe slowly and immediately make the needle safe.
q. Maintain direct finger pressure over the injection site for a minimum of 1 minute, preferably 2 minutes, after injection.
r. Wait 3 to 5 minutes after completion of the injection before commencing the dental procedure.

Signs and Symptoms
1. Subjective: tingling and numbness of the lower eyelid, side of the nose, and upper lip indicate anesthesia of the infraorbital nerve, not the ASA or MSA nerve (develops almost instantly as the anesthetic is being administered)
2. Subjective and objective: numbness in the teeth and soft tissues along the distribution of the ASA and MSA nerves (developing within 3 to 5 minutes if pressure is maintained over the injection site)
3. Objective: no pain during dental therapy

Safety Features
1. Needle contact with bone at the roof of the infraorbital foramen prevents inadvertent overinsertion and possible puncture of the orbit.
2. A finger positioned over the infraorbital foramen helps direct the needle toward the foramen.
   a. The needle should not be palpable. If it is felt then its path is too superficial (away from the bone). If this occurs, withdraw the needle slightly and redirect it toward the target area.
   b. In most patients it is not possible to palpate the needle through soft tissues over the foramen unless

it is too superficial. However, in some patients with less well-developed facial musculature, a properly positioned needle may be palpable.

Precautions
1. For pain on insertion of the needle and tearing of the periosteum, reinsert the needle in a more lateral (away from bone) position or deposit solution as the needle advances through soft tissue.
2. For overinsertion of the needle, estimate the depth of penetration before injection (review procedure) and exert finger pressure over the infraorbital foramen.
   a. Overinsertion is unlikely because of the rim of bone that forms the superior rim of the infraorbital foramen. The needle tip contacts this rim.

Failures of Anesthesia
1. Needle contacting bone below (inferior to) the infraorbital foramen; anesthesia of the lower eyelid, lateral side of the nose, and upper lip develop, with little or no dental anesthesia; a bolus of solution may be felt beneath the skin in the area of deposition, which lies at a distance from the infraorbital foramen (which remains palpable after the local anesthetic solution has been injected). These are, by far, the most common causes of anesthetic failure within the distribution of the ASA nerve. In essence a failed ASA is a supraperiosteal injection over the first premolar. To correct:
   a. Keep the needle in line with the infraorbital foramen during penetration. Do not direct the needle toward bone.
   b. Estimate the depth of penetration before injecting.

2. Needle deviation medial or lateral to the infraorbital foramen. To correct:
   a. Direct the needle toward the foramen immediately after inserting and before advancing it through the tissue.
   b. Recheck needle placement before aspirating and depositing the anesthetic solution.

Complications. Hematoma (rare) may develop across the lower eyelid and the tissues between it and the infraorbital foramen. To manage, apply pressure on the soft tissue over the foramen for 2 to 3 minutes. Hematoma is extremely rare because pressure is routinely applied to the injection site both during and after the ASA nerve block.

PALATAL ANESTHESIA

Anesthesia of the hard palate is necessary for dental procedures involving manipulation of palatal soft or hard tissues. For many dental patients, palatal injections prove to be a very traumatic experience. For many dentists the administration of palatal anesthesia is one of the most traumatic procedures they perform in dentistry.[3] Indeed, many dentists and dental hygienists advise their patients that they expect them to feel pain (dental professionals usually use the term *discomfort* rather than *pain* when describing uncomfortable procedures) during palatal injections! Forewarning the patient about procedural pain permits the patient to become more prepared psychologically and relieves the administrator of responsibility when the pain occurs. When the patient acknowledges the existence of pain, the administrator can console the patient with a shrug of the shoulders and a kind word, once again confirming to both the patient and the administrator that palatal injections always hurt!

However, palatal anesthesia can be achieved atraumatically. At best, patients are unaware of the needle penetration of soft tissues and deposition of the local anesthetic solution (they won't even feel it!). At worst, when the following techniques are adhered to, patients state that although they still were somewhat uncomfortable, this palatal injection was the least painful they had ever received.

With the introduction of computer-controlled local anesthetic delivery (CCLAD) systems (The Wand and Comfort Control Syringe [see Chapter 5]), delivery of atraumatic palatal injections has become even more simplified.[4,5]

The steps in the atraumatic administration of palatal anesthesia are as follows:

1. Provide adequate topical anesthesia at site of needle penetration.
2. Use pressure anesthesia at the site both before and during needle insertion and the deposition of solution.
3. Maintain control over the needle.
4. Deposit the anesthetic solution slowly.
5. Trust yourself . . . that you can complete the procedure atraumatically.

Adequate topical anesthesia at the injection site can be provided by allowing topical anesthetic to remain in contact with the soft tissues for at least 2 minutes. The palate is the one area in the mouth where the cotton swab must be held in position by the administrator the entire time.

Pressure anesthesia can be produced at the site of injection by applying considerable pressure to the tissues adjacent to the injection site with a firm object, such as the cotton applicator stick previously used to apply the topical anesthetic. Other objects, such as the handle of a mouth mirror, are used by some, but because these objects are metal or plastic they are more likely to hurt the patient. The goal is to produce anesthesia of the soft tissues through the gate control theory of pain.[6] The applicator stick should be pressed firmly enough to produce ischemia (blanching) of the normally pink tissues at the penetration site and a feeling of intense pressure (dull and tolerable, not sharp and painful) (Fig. 13-23). Pressure anesthesia should be maintained during penetration of the soft tissues with the needle and must be maintained throughout the time that the needle remains in the palatal soft tissues.

Control over the needle is probably of greater importance in palatal anesthesia than in other intraoral injections. To achieve this control, the administrator must secure a firm hand rest. Several positions are illustrated in Chapter 11. When palatal anesthesia is administered, it is also possible on occasion to stabilize the needle with both hands (Fig. 13-24). Perfection of this technique only develops with experience.

The 27-gauge short needle is recommended for palatal injection techniques because patients are unable to distinguish the "feel" between a 27- and 30-gauge needle.[7]

Slow deposition of the local anesthetic is important in all injection techniques, not only as a safety feature but also as a means of providing an atraumatic injection.

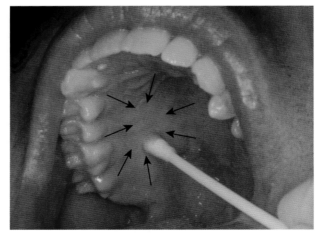

Figure 13-23. Notice ischemia *(arrows)* of palatal tissues produced by pressure from the applicator stick.

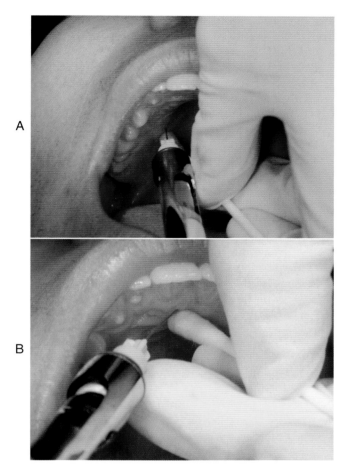

Figure 13-24. Stabilization of the needle for an, **A,** greater palatine and, **B,** nasopalatine nerve block. With both injections, the barrel of the syringe should rest against the patient's lower lip.

Because of the density of the palatal soft tissues and their firm adherence to the underlying bone, slow deposition is of even greater importance here. Rapid injection of the solution produces high tissue pressure, which tears the palatal soft tissues and leads to both pain on injection and localized soreness when the anesthetic actions are terminated. Slow injection of the local anesthetic does not produce discomfort.

Probably the most important factor in providing an atraumatic palatal injection is the belief by the administrator that it can be done painlessly; special care is then taken to minimize discomfort to the patient, and this generally results in a more atraumatic palatal injection.

• • •

Five palatal injections are described. Three—the anterior (or greater) palatine nerve block, providing anesthesia of the posterior portions of the hard palate; the nasopalatine nerve block, producing anesthesia of the anterior hard palate; and local infiltration of the hard palate—are used primarily to achieve soft tissue anesthesia and hemostasis before surgical procedures. None provides any pulpal anesthesia to the maxillary teeth. The AMSA and P-ASA

are recently introduced techniques that provide extensive areas of pulpal and palatal anesthesia.[5,8]

Greater Palatine Nerve Block

The greater palatine nerve block is useful for dental procedures involving the palatal soft tissues distal to the canine. Minimum volumes of solution (0.45 to 0.6 ml) provide profound hard- and soft-tissue anesthesia. Although potentially traumatic, the greater palatine nerve block is less so than the nasopalatine nerve block because the tissues surrounding the greater palatine foramen are better able to accommodate the volume of solution deposited.

Other Common Name. Anterior palatine nerve block

Nerve Anesthetized. Greater palatine

Areas Anesthetized. The posterior portion of the hard palate and its overlying soft tissues, anteriorly as far as the first premolar and medially to the midline (Fig. 13-25)

Indications
1. When palatal soft-tissue anesthesia is necessary for restorative therapy on more than two teeth (e.g., with subgingival restorations and insertion of matrix bands subgingivally)
2. For pain control during periodontal or oral surgical procedures involving the palatal soft and hard tissues

Contraindications
1. Inflammation or infection at the injection site
2. Smaller areas of therapy (one or two teeth)

Advantages
1. Minimizes needle penetrations and volume of solution
2. Minimizes patient discomfort

Disadvantages
1. No hemostasis except in the immediate area of injection
2. Potentially traumatic

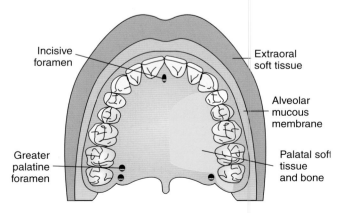

Figure 13-25. Area anesthetized by greater palatine nerve block.

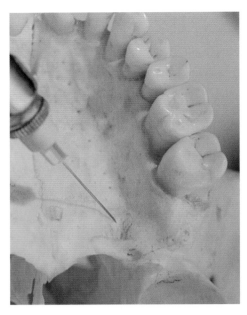

Figure 13-26. Target area for a greater palatine nerve block.

Positive Aspiration. Less than 1%

Alternatives
1. Local infiltration into specific regions
2. Maxillary nerve block

Technique
1. A 27-gauge short needle is recommended (although the 25-gauge short also may be used).
2. Area of insertion: soft tissue slightly anterior to the greater palatine foramen
3. Target area: greater (anterior) palatine nerve as it passes anteriorly between the soft tissues and bone of the hard palate (Fig. 13-26)

4. Landmarks: greater palatine foramen and junction of the maxillary alveolar process and palatine bone
5. Path of insertion: advance the syringe from the opposite side of the mouth at a right angle to the target area.
6. Orientation of the bevel: toward the palatal soft tissues. (See steps *g* and *h*, p. 205.)
7. Procedure
   a. Assume the correct position (Fig. 13-27).
      (1) For a right greater palatine nerve block, a right-handed administrator should sit facing the patient at the 7 or 8 o'clock position.
      (2) For a left greater palatine nerve block, a right-handed administrator should sit facing in the same direction as the patient at the 11 o'clock position.
   b. Request the patient, who is in a supine position (Fig. 13-28, *A*), to do the following:
      (1) Open wide.
      (2) Extend the neck.
      (3) Turn the head to the left or right (for improved visibility).
   c. Locate the greater palatine foramen (Fig. 13-28, *B* and Table 13-2).
      (1) Place a cotton swab at the junction of the maxillary alveolar process and the hard palate.
      (2) Start in the region of the maxillary first molar and palpate posteriorly by pressing firmly into the tissues with the swab.
      (3) The swab "falls" into the depression created by the greater palatine foramen (Fig. 13-29).
      (4) The foramen is most frequently located distal to the maxillary second molar, but it may be either anterior or posterior to its usual position. (See "Maxillary Nerve Block," p. 220.)

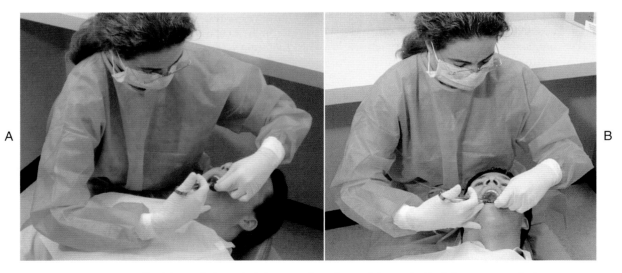

A   B

Figure 13-27. Position of the administrator for, **A,** a right and, **B,** left greater palatine nerve block.

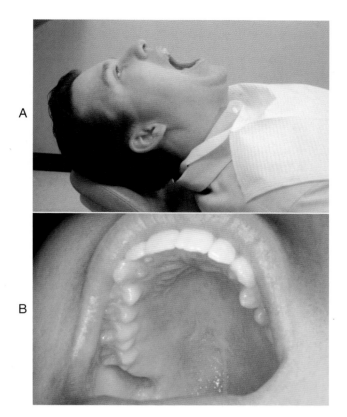

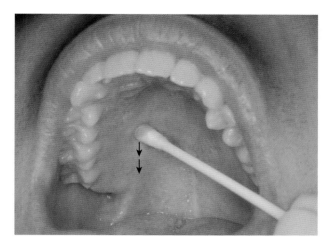

Figure 13-29. A cotton swab is pressed against the hard palate at the junction of the maxillary alveolar process and palatal bone. The swab is slowly moved distally *(arrows)* until a depression in the tissue is felt. This is the greater (anterior) palatine foramen.

Figure 13-28. A, Patient position for a greater palatine nerve block. **B,** Administrator's view of hard palate when patient is properly positioned.

    d. Prepare the tissue at the injection site, just 1 to 2 mm anterior to the greater palatine foramen.
      (1) Clean and dry with sterile gauze.
      (2) Apply topical antiseptic (optional).
      (3) Apply topical anesthetic for 2 minutes.
    e. After 2 minutes of topical anesthetic application, move the swab posteriorly so it is directly over the greater palatine foramen.
      (1) Apply considerable pressure at the area of the foramen with the swab in the left hand (if right-handed).
      (2) Note the ischemia (whitening of the soft tissues) at the injection site.

      (3) Apply pressure for a minimum of 30 seconds, and while doing this proceed to do the following:
    f. Direct the syringe into the mouth from the opposite side with the needle approaching the injection site at a right angle (Fig. 13-30).
    g. Place the bevel (not the point) of the needle gently against the previously blanched (ischemic) soft tissue at the injection site. It must be well stabilized to prevent accidental penetration of the tissues.
    h. With the bevel lying against the tissue:
      (1) Apply enough pressure to bow the needle slightly.
      (2) Deposit a small volume of anesthetic. The solution is forced against the mucous membrane, and a droplet forms (Fig. 13-31).
    i. Straighten the needle and permit the bevel to penetrate mucosa.

TABLE 13-2
Location of the Greater Palatine Foramen*

Location	No.	Percent
Anterior half second molar	0	0
Posterior half second molar	63	39.87
Anterior half third molar	80	50.63
Posterior half third molar	15	9.49

From Malamed SF, Trieger N: Intraoral maxillary nerve block: an anatomical and clinical study, *Anesth Prog* 30:44-48, 1983.
*Measurements from 158 skulls with the maxillary second and third molars present.

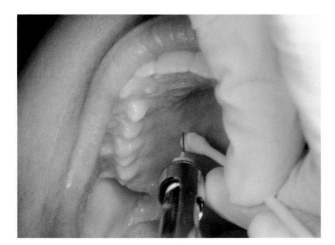

Figure 13-30. Notice the angle of needle entry into the mouth. The insertion is into ischemic tissues slightly anterior to the applicator stick. The barrel of the syringe is stabilized by the corner of the mouth and the teeth.

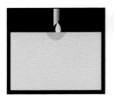
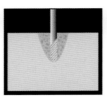
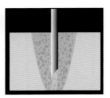

Figure 13-31. Prepuncture technique: bevel of needle placed on soft tissue; pressure exerted by cotton applicator stick. Local anesthetic solution deposited before needle enters tissues.

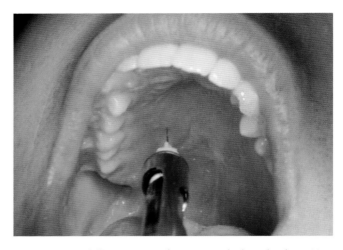

1. Continue to deposit small volumes of anesthetic throughout the procedure.
2. Ischemia spreads into the adjacent tissues as the anesthetic (usually with a vasoconstrictor) is deposited (Figs. 13-32 and 13-33).

j. Continue to apply pressure anesthesia throughout the deposition of the anesthetic solution (see Fig. 13-32). Ischemia spreads as the vasoconstrictor decreases tissue perfusion.

k. Slowly advance the needle until palatine bone is gently contacted.
  (1) The depth of penetration is usually less than 10 mm.
  (2) Continue to deposit small volumes of anesthetic. As the tissue is entered, there is increased resistance to the deposition of solution, which is entirely normal in the greater palatine nerve block.

l. Aspirate.
m. If negative, slowly deposit (30-second minimum) not more than one fourth to one third of a cartridge (0.45 to 0.6 ml).
n. Withdraw the syringe.
o. Make the needle safe.
p. Wait 2 to 3 minutes before commencing the dental procedure.

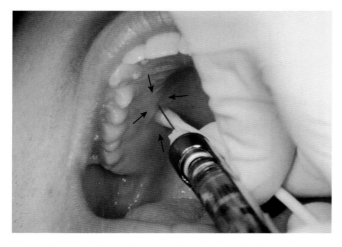

Figure 13-32. Notice the spread of ischemia *(arrows)* as the anesthetic is deposited.

Figure 13-33. The cotton swab is removed when the deposition of solution ceases.

Signs and Symptoms
1. Subjective: numbness in the posterior portion of the palate
2. Objective: no pain during dental therapy

Safety Features
1. Contact with bone
2. Aspiration

Precautions. Do not enter the greater palatine canal. Although this is not hazardous, there is no reason to enter the canal for this technique to be successful.

Failures of Anesthesia
1. The greater palatine nerve block is not a technically difficult injection to administer. Its incidence of success is well above 95%.
2. If local anesthetic is deposited too far anterior to the foramen, adequate soft-tissue anesthesia may not develop in the palatal tissues posterior to the site of injection (partial success).
3. Anesthesia on the palate in the area of the maxillary first premolar may prove inadequate because of overlapping fibers from the nasopalatine nerve (partial success).
  a. To correct: Local infiltration may be necessary as a supplement in the area of inadequate anesthesia.

Complications
1. Few of significance
2. Ischemia and necrosis of soft tissues when highly concentrated vasoconstricting solution used for hemostasis over a prolonged period
  a. Norepinephrine should never be used for hemostasis on the palatal soft tissues (not available in local anesthetics in the United States or Canada)
3. Hematoma is possible but rare because of the density and firm adherence of the palatal tissues to underlying bone

4. Some patients may be uncomfortable if their soft palate becomes anesthetized, a distinct possibility when the middle palatine nerve exits near the injection site

Nasopalatine Nerve Block

The nasopalatine nerve block is an invaluable technique for palatal pain control in that, with the administration of a minimum volume of anesthetic solution (maximally, one quarter of a cartridge), a wide area of palatal soft-tissue anesthesia is achieved, thereby minimizing the need for multiple palatal injections. Unfortunately, the nasopalatine nerve block has the distinction of being a potentially highly traumatic (e.g., painful) injection. With no other injection technique is the need for strict adherence to the protocol of atraumatic injection more important than with the nasopalatine nerve block. Two approaches to this injection are presented. Readers should become familiar with both techniques and then use the one with which they feel more comfortable (e.g., that works best in their hands).

The first approach involves only one tissue penetration, just lateral to the incisive papilla on the palatal aspect of the maxillary central incisors. The soft tissue in this area is dense, firmly adherent to underlying bone, and quite sensitive; three factors that combine to increase patient discomfort during injection. The second approach was recommended by a number of readers of earlier editions of this book. It involves two or three needle punctures but, when carried out properly, is significantly less traumatic than the more direct single-puncture technique. In it the labial soft tissues between the maxillary central incisors are anesthetized (injection #1), then the needle is directed from the labial aspect through the interproximal papilla between the centralis toward the incisive papilla to anesthetize the nasopalatine nerves (injection #2). In some instances these two injections suffice to provide acceptable nasopalatine nerve block; in others a third injection, directly into the now partially anesthetized palatal soft tissues overlying the nasopalatine nerve, is necessary. Although a single-needle puncture technique may be preferred whenever possible, the second approach can produce effective nasopalatine anesthesia with a minimum of discomfort.

Other Common Names. Incisive nerve block, sphenopalatine nerve block

Nerves Anesthetized. Nasopalatine nerves bilaterally

Areas Anesthetized. Anterior portion of the hard palate (soft and hard tissues) from the mesial of the right first premolar to the mesial of the left first premolar (Fig. 13-34)

Indications
1. When palatal soft-tissue anesthesia is necessary for restorative therapy on more than two teeth (e.g.,

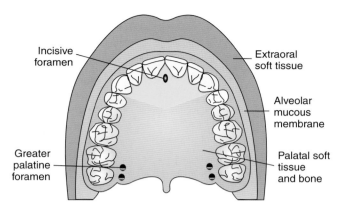

Figure 13-34. Area anesthetized by a nasopalatine nerve block.

subgingival restorations and insertion of matrix bands subgingivally)
2. For pain control during periodontal or oral surgical procedures involving palatal soft and hard tissues

Contraindications
1. Inflammation or infection at the injection site
2. Smaller area of therapy (one or two teeth)

Advantages
1. Minimizes needle penetrations and volume of solution
2. Minimal patient discomfort from multiple needle penetrations

Disadvantages
1. No hemostasis except in the immediate area of injection
2. Potentially the most traumatic intraoral injection; however, the protocol for an atraumatic injection or use of a CCLAD system can minimize or entirely eliminate discomfort

Positive Aspiration. Less than 1%

Alternatives
1. Local infiltration into specific regions
2. Maxillary nerve block

Technique (Single Needle Penetration of the Palate)
1. A 27-gauge short needle is recommended (although a 25-gauge short may be used).
2. Area of insertion: palatal mucosa just lateral to the incisive papilla (located in the midline behind the central incisors); the tissue here is more sensitive than other palatal mucosa
3. Target area: incisive foramen, beneath the incisive papilla (Fig. 13-35)
4. Landmarks: central incisors and incisive papilla
5. Path of insertion: approach the injection site at a 45-degree angle toward the incisive papilla
6. Orientation of the bevel: toward the palatal soft tissues (review procedure for the basic palatal injection)

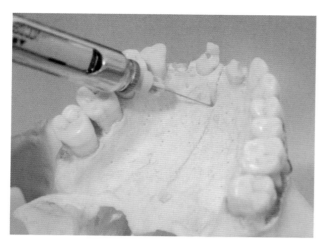

Figure 13-35. Target area for a nasopalatine nerve block.

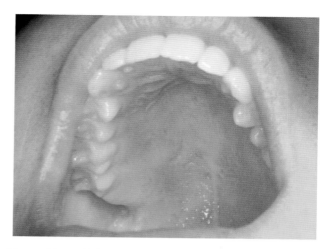

Figure 13-37. Palate when the patient is positioned properly.

7. Procedure
   a. Sit at the 9 or 10 o'clock position facing in the same direction as the patient (Fig. 13-36).
   b. Request the patient to do the following:
      (1) Open wide.
      (2) Extend the neck.
      (3) Turn the head to the left or right for improved visibility (Fig. 13-37).
   c. Prepare the tissue just lateral to the incisive papilla (Fig. 13-38).
      (1) Clean and dry with sterile gauze.
      (2) Apply topical antiseptic (optional).
      (3) Apply topical anesthetic for 2 minutes.
   d. After 2 minutes of topical anesthetic application, move the swab directly onto the incisive papilla (Figs. 13-38 and 13-39).
      (1) Apply pressure to the area of the papilla with the swab in your left hand (if right-handed).
      (2) Note ischemia at the injection site.

   e. Place the bevel against the ischemic soft tissues at the injection site. The needle must be well stabilized to prevent accidental penetration of tissues (see Fig. 13-39).
   f. With the bevel lying against the tissue:
      (1) Apply enough pressure to bow the needle slightly.
      (2) Deposit a small volume of anesthetic. The solution will be forced against the mucous membrane.
   g. Straighten the needle and permit the bevel to penetrate mucosa.
      (1) Continue to deposit small volumes of anesthetic throughout the procedure.
      2. Observe ischemia spreading into the adjacent tissues as solution is deposited.
   h. Continue to apply pressure with the cotton applicator stick while injecting the anesthetic.
   i. Slowly advance the needle toward the incisive foramen until bone is gently contacted (see Fig. 13-35).
      (1) The depth of penetration is approximately 5 mm.

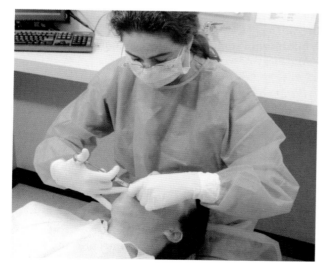

Figure 13-36. Position of the administrator for a nasopalatine nerve block.

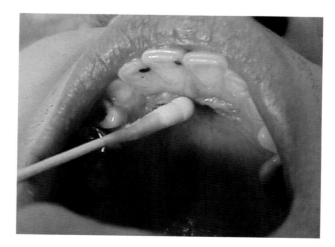

Figure 13-38. Topical anesthetic is applied lateral to the incisive papilla for 2 minutes, and then pressure is applied directly to the incisive papilla.

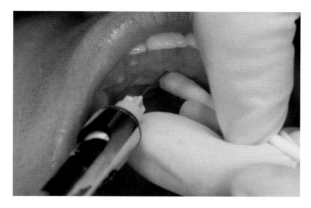

Figure 13-39. Pressure is maintained until the deposition of solution is completed. Needle penetration is just lateral to the incisive papilla.

    (2) Deposit small volumes of anesthetic while advancing the needle. As the tissue is entered, there is increased resistance to the deposition of solution, which is normal with the nasopalatine nerve block.

j. Withdraw the needle 1 mm (to prevent subperiosteal injection). The bevel now lies over the center of the incisive foramen.

k. Aspirate.

l. If negative, slowly deposit (15- to 30-second minimum) not more than one fourth of a cartridge (0.45 ml).

    (1) It is difficult in some patients to deposit 0.45 ml of anesthetic solution in this injection. Injection of anesthetic can cease when the area of ischemia noted at the injection site has increased from that produced by the application of pressure alone.

m. Slowly withdraw the syringe.

n. Make the needle safe.

o. Wait 2 to 3 minutes before commencing the dental procedure.

Signs and Symptoms

1. Subjective: numbness in the anterior portion of the palate
2. Objective: no pain during dental therapy

Safety Features

1. Contact with bone
2. Aspiration

Precautions

1. Against pain
   a. Do not insert directly into the incisive papilla (quite painful).
   b. Do not deposit solution too rapidly.
   c. Do not deposit too much solution.

2. Against infection
   a. If the needle is advanced more than 5 mm into the incisive canal and the floor of the nose is entered accidentally, infection may result. There is no reason for the needle to enter the incisive canal during a nasopalatine nerve block.

Failures of Anesthesia

1. Highly successful injection (>95% incidence of success)
2. Unilateral anesthesia
   a. If solution is deposited to one side of the incisive canal, unilateral anesthesia may develop.
   b. To correct: Reinsert the needle into the already anesthetized tissue and reinject solution into the unanesthetized area.
3. Inadequate palatal soft-tissue anesthesia in the area of the maxillary canine and first premolar
   a. If fibers from the greater palatine nerve overlap those of the nasopalatine nerve, anesthesia of the soft tissues palatal to the canine and first premolar could be inadequate.
   b. To correct: Local infiltration may be necessary as a supplement in the area inadequately anesthetized.

Complications

1. Few of significance
2. Hematoma possible but extremely rare because of the density and firm adherence of palatal soft tissues to bone
3. Necrosis of soft tissues possible when highly concentrated vasoconstricting solution (e.g., norepinephrine) is used for hemostasis over a prolonged period (not available in local anesthetics in the United States or Canada)
4. Because of the density of soft tissues, anesthetic solution may "squirt" back out the needle puncture site either during administration or after needle withdrawal. (This is of no clinical significance. However, do not let it surprise you into uttering a statement such as "whoops!" that might frighten the patient.)

Technique (Multiple Needle Penetrations)

1. A 27-gauge short needle is recommended.
2. Areas of insertion
   a. Labial frenum in the midline between the maxillary central incisors (Fig. 13-40, *B*)
   b. Interdental papilla between the maxillary central incisors (Fig. 13-40, *C*)
   c. If needed, palatal soft tissues lateral to the incisive papilla (Fig. 13-40, *D*)
3. Target area: incisive foramen, beneath the incisive papilla
4. Landmarks: central incisors and incisive papilla
5. Path of insertion
   a. First injection: infiltration into the labial frenum
   b. Second injection: needle held at a right angle to the interdental papilla

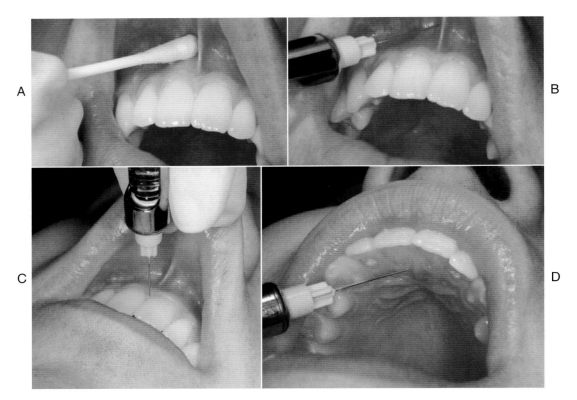

Figure 13-40. A, Topical anesthetic is applied to mucosa of the frenum. **B,** First injection, into the labial frenum. **C,** Second injection, into the interdental papilla between the central incisors. **D,** Third injection, when anesthesia of the nasopalatine area is inadequate after the first two injections.

c. Third injection: needle held at a 45-degree angle to the incisive papilla
6. Orientation of the bevel
   a. First injection: toward bone
   b. Second injection: not relevant
   c. Third injection: not relevant
7. Procedure
   a. First injection: infiltration of 0.3 ml into the labial frenum (see Fig. 13-40, *B*)
     (1) Prepare the tissue at the injection site.
       (a) Clean and dry with sterile gauze.
       (b) Apply topical antiseptic (optional).
       (c) Apply topical anesthetic for 1 minute (Fig. 13-40, *A*).
     (2) Retract the upper lip to stretch tissues and improve visibility. (Be careful not to overstretch the frenum.)
     (3) Gently insert the needle into the frenum and deposit 0.3 ml of anesthetic in approximately 15 seconds. (The tissue may balloon as solution is injected.)
     (4) Anesthesia of soft tissue develops immediately.
   b. Second injection: penetration through the labial aspect of the papilla between the maxillary central incisors toward the incisive papilla (see Fig. 13-40, *C*)
     (1) Retract the upper lip gently to increase visibility. (Do not overstretch the labial frenum.)

     (2) If a right-handed administrator, sit at 11 or 12 o'clock facing in the same direction as the patient. Tilt the patient's head toward the right to provide a proper angle for needle penetration.
     (3) Holding the needle at a right angle to the interdental papilla, insert it into the papilla just above the level of crestal bone.
       (a) Direct it toward the incisive papilla (on the palatal side of the interdental papilla).
       (b) Soft tissues on the labial surface have previously been anesthetized so there is no discomfort. However, as the needle penetrates toward the unanesthetized palatal side it becomes necessary to administer minute amounts of local anesthetic to prevent discomfort.
       (c) With the patient's head extended backward, you can see the ischemia produced by the local anesthetic and see the needle tip as it approaches the palatal aspect of the incisive papilla. Care must be taken to avoid needle puncture through the papilla into the oral cavity on the palatal side.
     (4) Aspirate when ischemia is noted in the incisive papilla or the needle tip becomes visible just beneath the tissue surface. If negative, administer no more than 0.3 ml of anesthetic solution in approximately 15 seconds. There is considerable

resistance to the deposition of solution but no patient discomfort.

(5) Stabilization of the syringe in this second injection is somewhat awkward, but critical. Use of a finger from the other hand to stabilize the needle is recommended (Fig. 13-41). However, the syringe barrel must be held such that it remains within the patient's line of sight, which is potentially disconcerting to some patients.

(6) Slowly withdraw the syringe.

(7) Make the needle safe.

(8) Anesthesia within the distribution of the right and left nasopalatine nerves usually develops in 2 to 3 minutes.

(9) If the area of clinically effective anesthesia proves to be less than adequate (as frequently happens), proceed to the third injection.

c. Third injection: use only when the second injection does not provide adequate palatal anesthesia

(1) Dry the tissue just lateral to the incisive papilla.

(2) Request the patient to open wide.

(3) Extend the patient's neck.

(4) Place the needle into soft tissue adjacent to the (diamond-shaped) incisive papilla, aiming toward the most distal portion of the papilla.

(5) Advance needle until contact is made with bone.

(6) Withdraw needle 1 mm to avoid subperiosteal injection.

(7) Aspirate.

(8) If negative, slowly deposit not more than 0.3 ml of anesthetic in approximately 15 seconds. *Note:* Use of topical and pressure anesthesia is unnecessary in the second and third injections because the tissues that the needle penetrates already have been anesthetized (by the first and second injections, respectively).

(9) Withdraw the syringe.

(10) Make the needle safe.

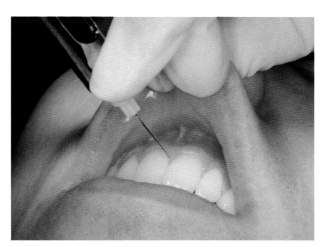

Figure 13-41. Use a finger of the opposite hand to stabilize the syringe during the second injection.

(11) Wait 2 to 3 minutes for the onset of anesthesia before beginning dental treatment.

Signs and Symptoms
1. Subjective: numbness of the upper lip (in the midline) and anterior portion of the palate
2. Objective: no pain during dental therapy

Safety Features
1. Aspiration
2. Contact with bone (third injection)

Advantage. Entirely or relatively atraumatic

Disadvantages
1. Requires multiple injections (two or three)
2. Difficult to stabilize the syringe during the second injection
3. Syringe barrel usually within the patient's line of sight during the second injection

Precautions
1. Against pain: If each injection is performed as recommended, the entire technique should be atraumatic.
2. Against infection: If a third injection is necessary, do not advance the needle into the incisive canal. With accidental penetration of the nasal floor, the risk of infection is increased.

Failures of Anesthesia
1. A highly successful (>95%) injection
2. Incomplete palatal anesthesia after the second injection
   a. To correct: A third injection may be necessary.
3. Inadequate anesthesia around the canine and first premolar because of overlapping fibers from the greater palatine nerve
   a. To correct: Local infiltration may be necessary as a supplement in the area.

Complications
1. Few of significance
2. Necrosis of soft tissues is possible when a highly concentrated vasoconstrictor solution, such as norepinephrine, is used for hemostasis over a prolonged period (not available in local anesthetics in the United States or Canada)
3. Interdental papilla between the maxillary incisors sometimes are tender for several days after injection.

Local Infiltration of the Palate

Other Common Names. None

Nerves Anesthetized. Terminal branches of the nasopalatine and greater palatine

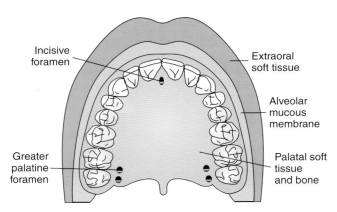

Figure 13-42. Area anesthetized by a palatal infiltration.

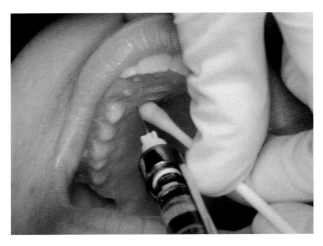

Figure 13-43. Area of insertion and target area for a palatal infiltration.

Areas Anesthetized Soft tissues in the immediate vicinity of injection (Fig. 13-42)

Indications
1. Primarily for achieving hemostasis during surgical procedures
2. Palatogingival pain control when limited areas of anesthesia are necessary for application of a rubber dam clamp, packing retraction cord in the gingival sulcus, or operative procedures on not more than two teeth

Contraindications
1. Inflammation or infection at the injection site
2. Pain control in soft-tissue areas involving more than two teeth

Advantages
1. Provides acceptable hemostasis when a vasoconstrictor is used
2. Provides a minimum area of numbness, thereby minimizing patient discomfort

Disadvantage. Potentially traumatic injection

Positive Aspiration. Negligible

Alternatives
1. For hemostasis: none
2. For pain control: nasopalatine or greater palatine nerve block, maxillary nerve block

Technique
1. A 27-gauge short needle is recommended, although the 25-gauge short also may be used.
2. Area of insertion: the attached gingiva 5 to 10 mm from the free gingival margin (Fig. 13-43)
3. Target area: gingival tissues 5 to 10 mm from the free gingival margin
4. Landmark: gingival tissue in the estimated center of the treatment area
5. Pathway of insertion: approaching the injection site at a 45-degree angle
6. Orientation of the bevel: toward palatal soft tissues
7. Procedure
   a. If a right-handed administrator, sit at the 10 o'clock position.
      (1) Face toward the patient for palatal infiltration on the right side.
      (2) Face in the same direction as the patient for palatal infiltration on the left side.
   b. Request the patient to do the following:
      (1) Open wide.
      (2) Extend the neck.
      (3) Turn the head to the left or right for improved visibility.
   c. Prepare the tissue at the site of injection.
      (1) Clean and dry with sterile gauze.
      (2) Apply topical antiseptic (optional).
      (3) Apply topical anesthetic for 2 minutes.
   d. After 2 minutes of topical anesthetic application, place the swab on the tissue immediately adjacent to the injection site.
      (1) With the swab in your left hand (if right-handed) apply pressure to the palatal soft tissues.
      (2) Observe the ischemia at the injection site.
   e. Place the bevel of the needle against the ischemic soft tissue at the injection site. The needle must be well stabilized to prevent accidental penetration of tissues.
   f. With the bevel lying against tissue:
      (1) Apply enough pressure to bow the needle slightly.
      (2) Deposit a small volume of local anesthetic. The solution is forced against the mucous membrane, forming a droplet.
   g. Straighten the needle and permit the bevel to penetrate mucosa.

(1) Continue to deposit small volumes of local anesthetic throughout this procedure.

(2) Ischemia of the tissues spreads as additional anesthetic is deposited. (When this injection is used for hemostasis, the vasoconstrictor in the local anesthetic produces intense ischemia of tissues.)

h. Continue to apply pressure with the cotton applicator stick throughout the injection.

i. Continue to advance the needle and deposit anesthetic until bone is gently contacted. Tissue thickness is only 3 to 5 mm in most patients.

j. If hemostasis is the goal in this technique, continue to administer solution until ischemia encompasses the surgical site. In usual practice, 0.2 to 0.3 ml of solution are adequate.

k. For hemostasis of larger surgical sites:

(1) Remove the needle from the first injection site.

(2) Place it in the new injection site at the periphery of the previously anesthetized tissue (Fig. 13-44).

(3) Penetrate the tissues and deposit anesthetic as in Step *j*. Topical anesthetic may be omitted for subsequent injections because the tissue penetrated is already anesthetized.

(4) Continue this overlapping procedure until adequate hemostasis develops over the entire surgical area.

l. Withdraw the syringe.

m. Make the needle safe.

n. Commence the dental procedure immediately.

Signs and Symptoms
1. Subjective: numbness, ischemia of the palatal soft tissues
2. Objective: no pain during dental therapy

Safety Feature. Anatomically safe area for injection

Precaution. Highly traumatic procedure if performed improperly

Failure of Hemostasis
1. There is a higher percentage of success if vasoconstrictor is included in the anesthetic solution; however, inflamed tissues may continue to hemorrhage despite the use of vasoconstrictor.

Complications
1. Few of significance.
2. Necrosis of soft tissues may be observed when a highly concentrated vasoconstricting solution is used for hemostasis over a prolonged period (e.g., norepinephrine) (not available in local anesthetics in the United States or Canada).

Anterior Middle Superior Alveolar Nerve Block

The anterior middle superior alveolar (AMSA) injection represents a newly described maxillary nerve block injection. It was first reported by Friedman and Hochman in 1997 during development of a CCLAD system.[5,9] This technique provides pulpal anesthesia on multiple maxillary teeth (incisors, canine, and premolars) from a single injection site. The injection site is on the hard palate about halfway along an imaginary line connecting the midpalatal suture to the free gingival margin. The location of the line is at the contact point between the first and second premolars (Fig. 13-45).

Because the local anesthetic is deposited on the palate, the muscles of facial expression and upper lip are not anesthetized. A minimal volume of local anesthetic is necessary to provide pulpal anesthesia from the central incisor to the second premolar on the side of the injection. This injection can be performed with little to no pain after injection techniques that have been outlined.[5] The use of a CCLAD system aids in the atraumatic administration of this injection.

The AMSA injection is most accurately described as a field block of the terminal branches (subneural dental plexus) of the ASA nerve that innervates the incisors to premolar teeth. In spite of the fact that studies suggest that the MSA nerve may be absent in 30% to 54% of individuals, a complete subneural

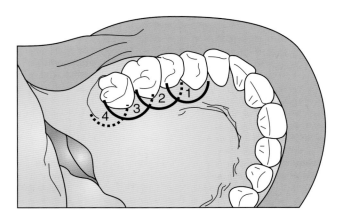

Figure 13-44. Overlapping of sequential palatal infiltrations and needle penetration sites.

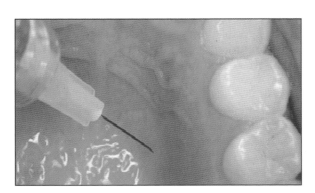

Figure 13-45. Location of injection site for anterior middle superior alveolar (AMSA) nerve block.

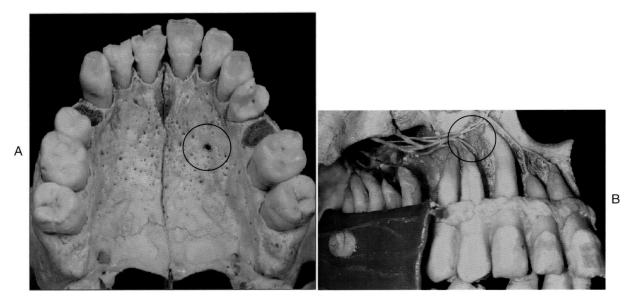

Figure 13-46. Anatomy of anterior middle superior alveolar (AMSA) nerve block. **A,** Palatal aspect—local anesthetic injected in area of circle. **B,** Buccal aspect—local anesthetic injected on palatal side in area of circle.

dental plexus must be present to provide innervation to the premolars and incisor teeth on all patients. It is the subneural dental plexus of the ASA nerve that is anesthetized in the AMSA injection. Two anatomical structures, the nasal aperture and maxillary sinus, cause the convergence of branches of the anterior and middle superior alveolar nerves and associated subneural dental plexus in the region of the apices of the premolars (Fig. 13-46). The injection site is at this region of convergence of these neural structures. Depositing a sufficient volume of local anesthetic allows it to diffuse through nutrient canals and porous cortical bone to envelope the concentrated subneural dental plexus at this location.

The AMSA injection may be particularly useful for aesthetic-restorative (cosmetic) dental procedures in which the dentist wishes to evaluate the smile line during treatment.[5] In addition, this injection has been found to be very useful for periodontal scaling and root planing of the maxillary region.[10] It provides profound soft-tissue anesthesia and anesthesia of the attached gingiva of the associated teeth. Perry and Loomer demonstrated a patient preference for the AMSA compared with supraperiosteal infiltration injections.[10] Subjects found the AMSA to be as effective as multiple maxillary infiltrations in the maxilla.

Several important procedures should be followed to perform this injection comfortably. These techniques are most easily accomplished when performed with a CCLAD system; however, this injection also has been successful using a standard aspirating dental syringe.

Other Common Name. Palatal approach anterior middle superior alveolar (AMSA).

Nerves Anesthetized
1. ASA nerve
2. MSA nerve, when present
3. Subneural dental nerve plexus of the anterior and middle superior alveolar nerves

Areas Anesthetized (Fig. 13-47)
1. Pulpal anesthesia of the maxillary incisors, canine, and premolars
2. Buccal attached gingiva of these same teeth
3. Attached palatal tissues from midline to free gingival margin on the associated teeth

Indications
1. Is easier performed with a CCLAD system
2. When dental procedures involving the maxillary anterior teeth or soft tissues are to be performed

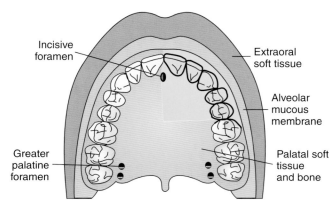

Figure 13-47. Anterior middle superior alveolar (AMSA) extent of anesthesia.

3. When anesthesia to multiple maxillary anterior teeth is desired from a single site injection
4. When scaling and root planing of the anterior teeth are to be performed
5. When anterior cosmetic procedures are to be performed and a smile-line assessment is important to a successful outcome
6. When a facial approach supraperiosteal injection has been ineffective because of dense cortical bone

Contraindications

1. Patients with unusually thin palatal tissues
2. Patients who cannot tolerate the 3- to 4-minute administration time
3. Procedures requiring more than 90 minutes

Advantages

1. Provides anesthesia of multiple maxillary teeth with a single injection
2. Comparatively simple technique
3. Comparatively safe; minimizes the volume of anesthetic and number of punctures required compared with traditional maxillary infiltrations of these teeth
4. Allows effective soft-tissue and pulpal anesthesia for periodontal scaling and root planing of the associated maxillary teeth
5. Allows for an accurate smile-line assessment to be performed after anesthesia has occurred, which may be helpful during cosmetic dentistry procedures
6. Eliminates the postoperative inconvenience of numbness to the upper lip and muscles of facial expression
7. Can be performed comfortably with a CCLAD system

Disadvantages

1. Requires a slow administration (0.5 ml/min) time
2. Can cause operator fatigue with a manual syringe because of extended injection time
3. May be uncomfortable for the patient if administered improperly
4. May need supplemental anesthesia for central and lateral incisor teeth
5. May cause excessive ischemia if administered too rapidly
6. Caution should be used when performing this injection with 4% local anesthetics (prilocaine HCl and articaine HCl). Reducing the recommended dosage by half is warranted.*
7. Use of local anesthetic containing epinephrine with a concentration of 1:50,000 is contraindicated.

Positive Aspirations. Less than 1%

---

*Self-limiting soft tissue ulceration and transient paresthesia from the administration, at a single palatal site, of 1.8 ml of 4% drug have been reported.

Alternatives

1. Multiple supraperiosteal or PDL injections for each tooth
2. ASA and MSA nerve blocks
3. Maxillary nerve block

Technique

1. Although a 27-gauge short needle is recommended, the authors of the AMSA papers recommend use of a 30-gauge extra-short needle.[5]
2. Area of insertion: on the hard palate about halfway along an imaginary line connecting the midpalatal suture to the free gingival margin; the location of the line is at the contact point between the first and second premolars.
3. Target area: palatal bone at injection site
4. Landmarks: the intersecting point midway along a line from the midpalatine suture to the free gingival margin intersecting the contact point between the first and second premolar
5. Orientation of the bevel: The bevel of the needle is placed against the epithelium. The needle is typically held at a 45-degree angle to the palate.
6. Procedure
   a. Sit at the 9 or 10 o'clock position facing same direction as the patient.
   b. Position the patient supine with slight hyperextension of head and neck to visualize nasopalatine papilla more easily.
   c. Use preparatory communication to inform the patient that the injection may take several minutes to administer and it may produce a sensation of firm pressure in the palate.
   d. Use comfortable arm and finger rests to avoid fatigue during the extended administration time.
   e. The use of a CCLAD system is suggested as it makes this injection easier to administer.
   f. Initial orientation of bevel is "face down" toward the epithelium holding the needle at approximately a 45-degree angle with a tangent to the palate.
   g. The final target is the bevel in contact with the palatal bone.
   h. A prepuncture technique can be utilized. Apply the bevel of the needle toward the palatal tissue. Place a sterile cotton applicator on top of the needle tip (Fig. 13-48). Apply light pressure on the cotton applicator to create a "seal" of the needle bevel against the outer surface. Initiate delivery of the local anesthetic to the surface of the epithelium. The objective is to force the solution through the outer epithelium into the surface tissue. The cotton applicator provides stabilization of the needle and prevents any excess local anesthetic solution from dripping into the patient's mouth. When using a CCLAD system, a slow rate of delivery (approximately 0.5 ml/min) is maintained during the entire injection. Maintain this position and pressure on the surface of the epithelium for 8 to 10 seconds.

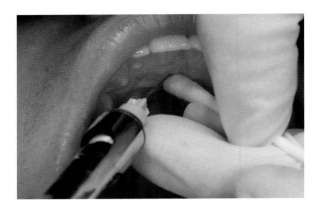

Figure 13-48. Prepuncture technique.

i. An "anesthetic pathway technique" can be utilized. Very slowly advance the needle tip into the tissue. Rotating the needle allows the needle to penetrate the tissue more efficiently.[11] Advance the needle 1 to 2 mm every 4 to 6 seconds while administering the anesthetic solution at the recommended slow rate. Attempt not to expand the tissue or advance the needle too rapidly if performing this with a manual syringe. Use of a CCLAD system makes this process easier to achieve.

j. After initial blanching is observed (approximately 30 seconds), pause for several seconds to allow for onset of superficial anesthesia.

k. Continue the slow insertion technique into the palatal tissue. Orientation of the handpiece should be from the contralateral premolars (Fig. 13-49). The needle is advanced until contact with bone occurs.

l. Ensure that the needle contact is maintained with bony surface of the palate. The bevel of the needle should face the surface of the bone.

m. Aspirate.

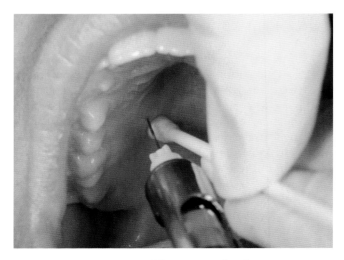

Figure 13-49. Anterior middle superior alveolar (AMSA) nerve block. Note syringe angulation from opposite side of mouth.

n. Anesthetic is delivered at a rate of approximately 0.5 ml during the injection for a final dosage of approximately 1.4 to 1.8 ml.

o. Advise the patient that he or she will experience a sensation of firm pressure.

Signs and Symptoms

1. Subjective: A sensation of firmness and numbness is immediately experienced on the palatal tissues.
2. Subjective: Numbness of the teeth and associated soft tissues extends from the central incisor to the second premolar on the side of the injection.
3. Objective: Blanching of the soft tissues (if a vasoconstrictor is used) of the palatal and facial attached gingiva is evident extending from the central incisor to the premolar region.
4. Objective: There is no pain during dental therapy.
5. Objective: No anesthesia of the face and upper lip occurs. *Note:* In some patients additional anesthetic may be necessary to supplement the incisor teeth. This can be performed from a palatal approach or as individual PDL injections.

Safety Features

1. Contact with the bone
2. Aspiration
3. Slow insertion (1 to 2 mm every 4 to 6 seconds)
4. Slow administration (0.5 ml/min)
5. Less anesthetic than necessary for a traditional facial approach

Precautions

1. Against pain
   a. Extremely slow insertion
   b. Slow administration during insertion with simultaneous administration of anesthetic solution
   c. Consider use of a CCLAD device.
2. Against tissue damage
   a. When using a 4% local anesthetic, reduce the volume of local anesthetic by one half (0.7 to 0.9 ml).
   b. Avoid excessive ischemia by not using local anesthetics containing epinephrine vasoconstricting solutions of with a concentration of 1:50,000.

Failure of Anesthesia

1. May need supplemental anesthesia for central and lateral incisors.
   a. Adequate volume of anesthetic may not reach dental branches.
   b. To correct, add more anesthetic or supplement in proximity to these teeth from the palatal approach.

Complications

1. Palatal ulcer at injection site developing 1 to 2 days postoperative
   a. Self-limiting
   b. Heals in 5 to 10 days
   c. Prevention includes slow administration to avoid excessive ischemia.

2. Unexpected contact with the nasopalatine nerve
3. Density of injection site causing squirt-back of anesthetic and bitter taste
   a. Aspirate while withdrawing syringe from tissue.
   b. Pause 3 to 4 seconds before withdrawing the needle to allow pressure to dissipate.
   c. Instruct assistant to suction any excess anesthetic that escapes during administration.

Palatal Approach-Anterior Superior Alveolar

The palatal approach-anterior superior alveolar (P-ASA) injection, as with the AMSA injection, was defined by Friedman and Hochman in conjunction with the clinical use and development of CCLAD system in the mid 1990s.[4,5,8] The P-ASA injection shares several common elements with the nasopalatine nerve block, but differs sufficiently to be considered a distinct identity. The P-ASA uses a similar tissue point of entry (lateral aspect of the incisive papilla) to the nasopalatine but differs in its final target; that is, needle position within the incisive canal. The volume of anesthetic recommended for the P-ASA is 1.4 to 1.8 ml, administered at a rate of 0.5 ml per minute.

The distribution of anesthesia differs between these injections as well. The nasopalatine nerve block provides anesthesia to the anterior palatal gingiva and mucoperiosteum and is recommended for surgical procedures on the anterior palate. It also may serve as a supplemental technique for achieving pulpal anesthesia to the incisor teeth. In contrast, the P-ASA is recommended as a primary method to achieving bilateral pulpal anesthesia of the anterior six maxillary teeth (incisors and canines). The P-ASA also provides profound soft-tissue anesthesia of the gingiva and mucoperiosteum in the region of the anterior palatal one third innervated by the nasopalatine nerve. In addition, soft-tissue anesthesia of the facial attached gingiva of the six anterior teeth are noted. Therefore the P-ASA is an attractive alternative for pain control before scaling and root planing, esthetic restorative procedures, and minor surgical procedures involving the premaxilla region. The P-ASA can be noted as the first dental injection to produce bilateral pulpal anesthesia from a single injection as its primary objective, making this a unique characteristic of this injection technique.

It is well documented in the dental literature that the subjective pain associated with injections into the nasopalatine region is typical associated with a significant degree of discomfort when performed with a manual syringe.[12-14] The introduction of CCLAD system has demonstrated that injections even into the dense highly innervated tissues of the palate can be performed predictably with little or no pain.[15] The P-ASA injection may be performed with a traditional manual syringe; however, a comfortable injection is more easily achieved with a CCLAD system.[16-19]

The P-ASA is useful when anesthesia to the maxillary anterior teeth is desired, without collateral anesthesia to the lip and muscles of facial expression. It has been shown to be desirable during scaling and root planing of the anterior teeth. It is also beneficial when anterior esthetic dentistry procedures are to be performed. The smile-line and the interrelationship between the lips, teeth, and soft tissues cannot be accurately assessed when a traditional (mucobuccal fold) approach to anesthesia is utilized because of paralysis of the upper lip. The palatal approach allows anesthesia to be limited to the subneural plexus for the maxillary anterior teeth and nasopalatine nerve. The minimum volume for this injection is 1.8 ml delivered at a slow rate of 0.5 ml per minute.

Other Common Name. Palatal approach ASA or palatal approach maxillary anterior field block

Nerves Anesthetized
1. Nasopalatine
2. Anterior branches of the ASA

Areas Anesthetized (Fig. 13-50)
1. Pulps of the maxillary central incisors, lateral incisors, and (to a lesser degree) the canines
2. Facial periodontal tissue associated with these same teeth
3. Palatal periodontal tissues associated with these same teeth

Indications
1. Procedure is easier with a CCLAD system.
2. Dental procedures involving the maxillary anterior teeth and soft tissues are to be performed.
3. Bilateral anesthesia of the maxillary anterior teeth is desired from a single site injection.
4. Scaling and root planing of the anterior teeth are to be performed.
5. When anterior cosmetic procedures are to be performed and a smile-line assessment is important to a successful outcome

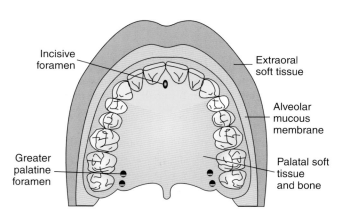

Figure 13-50. Palatal approach-anterior superior alveolar (P-ASA) extent of anesthesia.

6. When a facial approach supraperiosteal injection has been ineffective because of dense cortical bone

Contraindications
1. Patients with extremely long canine roots may not achieve profound anesthesia of these teeth from a palatal approach alone.
2. Patients who cannot tolerate the 3 to 4 minutes administration time
3. Procedures requiring more than 90 minutes

Advantages
1. Provides bilateral maxillary anesthesia from a single site injection
2. Comparatively simple technique to perform
3. Comparatively safe; minimizes the volume of anesthetic and number of punctures necessary compared with traditional maxillary infiltrations of these teeth
4. Allows for accurate smile-line assessment to be performed after anesthesia has occurred, which may be useful during cosmetic dentistry procedures
5. Eliminates the postoperative inconvenience of numbness to the upper lip and muscles of facial expression
6. Can be performed comfortably with a CCLAD system

Disadvantages
1. Requires slow administration (0.5 ml/min)
2. Operator fatigue with a manual syringe because of extended injection time
3. May be uncomfortable for the patient if administered improperly
4. May need supplemental anesthesia for canine teeth
5. May cause excessive ischemia if administered too rapidly
6. Caution should be used when performing this injection with 4% local anesthetics: prilocaine HCl and articaine HCl. Reducing the recommended dosage by half is warranted.*
7. Use of local anesthetic containing epinephrine with a concentration of 1:50,000 is contraindicated.

Positive Aspiration.
Less than 1% (assumed from data on nasopalatine block)

Alternatives
1. Supraperiosteal or PDL injections for each tooth
2. Right and left (bilateral) ASA nerve blocks
3. Right and left (bilateral) maxillary nerve block

Technique
1. A 27-gauge short needle is recommended. (Authors of the P-ASA papers suggest a 30-gauge extra-short needle.)[8]

---

*Self-limiting soft-tissue ulceration and transient paresthesia from the administration, at a single palatal site, of 1.8 ml of 4% drug have been reported.

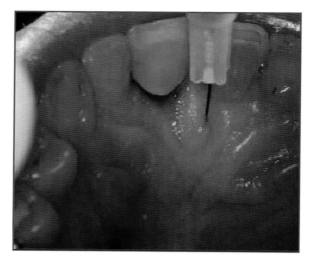

Figure 13-51. Palatal approach-anterior superior alveolar (P-ASA) area of needle insertion.

2. Area of insertion: just lateral to the incisive papilla in the papillary groove (Fig. 13-51)
3. Target area: nasopalatine foramen
4. Landmarks: nasopalatine papilla
5. Orientation of the bevel: The bevel of the needle is placed against the epithelium. The needle is typically held at a 45-degree angle to the palate.
6. Procedure
   a. Sit at the 9 or 10 o'clock position facing in the same direction as the patient.
   b. Position the patient supine with slight hyperextension of head and neck to visualize nasopalatine papilla more easily.
   c. Use preparatory communication to inform the patient that the injection may take several minutes to administer and may produce a sensation of firm pressure in the palate.
   d. Use comfortable arm and finger rests to prevent fatigue during the extended administration time.
   e. The use of a CCLAD system is recommended because it makes this injection easier to administer.
   f. Initial orientation of bevel is "face down" toward the epithelium, holding the needle at approximately a 45-degree angle with a tangent to the palate.
   g. A prepuncture technique can be utilized. Place the bevel of the needle against the palatal tissue. Place a sterile cotton applicator on top of the needle tip (see Fig. 13-48). Apply light pressure on the cotton applicator to create a "seal" of the needle bevel against the outer surface. Initiate delivery of the anesthetic solution to the surface of the epithelium. The objective is to force the solution through the outer epithelium into the tissue. Allow anesthetic solution to be delivered through the layer of the outer epithelium. The cotton applicator provides stabilization of the needle and prevents any excess dripping of anesthetic solution into the patient's

mouth. When using a CCLAD device, a slow rate of delivery (approximately 0.5 ml/min) is maintained during the entire injection. Maintain this position and pressure on the surface of the epithelium for 8 to 10 seconds.

h. An anesthetic pathway technique can be utilized. Very slowly advance the needle into the tissue. Rotating needle allows the needle to penetrate the tissue more efficiently. Advance the needle 1 to 2 mm every 4 to 6 seconds while administering the anesthetic solution at the recommended (slow) rate. Avoid expanding the tissue or advancing the needle too rapidly if performing the P-ASA with a manual syringe. It is at this step where use of a CCLAD system makes the process easier to achieve.

i. After initial blanching is observed (approximately 30 seconds), pause for several seconds to permit onset of superficial anesthesia.

j. Continue the slow insertion technique into the nasopalatine canal. Orientation of the needle should be parallel to the long axis of the central incisors. The needle is advanced to a depth of 6 to 10 mm (Fig. 13-52). *Note:* If resistance is encountered before final depth of penetration is reached, do not force the needle forward. Withdraw it slightly and reorient it to minimize the risk of penetration of the floor of the nose.

k. Ensure that the needle is in contact with the inner bony wall of the canal. (A well-defined nasopalatine canal may not be present in some patients.)

l. Aspirate within the canal space to avoid intravascular injection.

m. Anesthetic is delivered at a rate of approximately 0.5 ml during the injection for a final dosage of approximately 1.4 to 1.8 ml. Advise the patient that he or she will experience a sensation of firm pressure. *Note:* It has been reported that in a small percentage of cases needle insertion can stimulate the nasopalatine nerve (similar to contacting a nerve during an inferior alveolar block). This may be an unsettling surprise to the patient (and the operator) if it occurs. Reassure the patient with verbal support that this is not uncommon and is not a problem. If this should occur, reposition the needle and continue to administer the anesthetic before advancing further.

Signs and Symptoms

1. Subjective: A sensation of firmness and anesthesia is immediately experienced in the anterior palate.
2. Subjective: Numbness of the teeth and associated soft tissues extends from the right to the left canine.
3. Objective: Ischemia (blanching) of the soft tissues (if a vasoconstrictor is used) of the palatal and the facial attached gingiva is evident extending from the right to the left canine region.
4. Objective: There is no pain during dental therapy.
5. Objective: No anesthesia of the face and upper lip occurs. *Note:* In patients with long canine roots, additional local anesthetic may be needed. This can be performed from a palatal approach at a point that approximates the canine root tips.
   a. In rare instances, a facial approach (traditional) supraperiosteal injection may be necessary for the canine teeth.

Safety Features

1. Contact with the bone
2. Aspiration
3. Slow insertion (1 to 2 mm every 4 to 6 seconds)
4. Slow administration (0.5 ml/min)
5. Less anesthetic than necessary for a traditional facial approach

Precautions

1. Against pain:
   a. Extremely slow insertion
   b. Slow administration during insertion with simultaneous administration of anesthetic solution (anesthetic pathway)
   c. Consider using a CCLAD system.
2. Against tissue damage
   a. When using a 4% local anesthetic, reduce the volume of medications by one half (0.7 to 0.9 ml).
   b. Avoid excessive ischemia by not using drugs containing epinephrine in a concentration of 1:50,000.

Failure of Anesthesia

1. Highly successful injection for maxillary incisors
2. May need supplemental anesthesia for canines in patients with long roots
   a. Adequate volume of anesthetic may not reach dental branches.

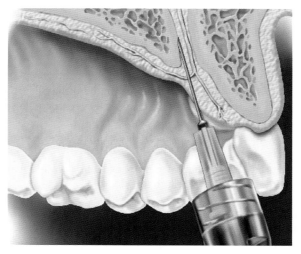

Figure 13-52. Palatal approach–anterior superior alveolar (P-ASA) orientation of syringe.

b. To correct, add more anesthetic or supplement in proximity to the canine teeth from the palatal approach.
3. Unilateral anesthesia
   a. Look for bilateral blanching.
   b. To correct, add more anesthetic.

Complications
1. Palatal ulcer at injection site developing 1 to 2 days postoperative
   a. Self-limiting
   b. Heals in 5 to 10 days
   c. Prevention includes slow administration to avoid excessive ischemia.
2. Unexpected nerve contact of the nasopalatine nerve
3. Density of injection site causing squirt-back of anesthetic and bitter taste
   a. Aspirate while withdrawing syringe from tissue.
   b. Pause 3 to 4 seconds before withdrawing the needle to allow pressure to dissipate.
   c. Instruct assistant to suction any excess local anesthetic that escapes during administration.

Maxillary Nerve Block

The maxillary (or second division) nerve block is an effective method of achieving profound anesthesia of a hemimaxilla. It is useful in procedures involving quadrant dentistry or in extensive surgical procedures. Two approaches are presented here. Both are effective, and the author does not maintain a preference for either one. The major difficulties in the greater palatine canal approach occur in locating the canal and negotiating it successfully. The major difficulty in the high tuberosity approach is the higher incidence of hematoma.

Other Common Names. Second division block, V_2 nerve block

Nerve Anesthetized. Maxillary division of the trigeminal nerve

Areas Anesthetized (Fig. 13-53).
1. Pulpal anesthesia of the maxillary teeth on the side of the block
2. Buccal periodontium and bone overlying these teeth
3. Soft tissues and bone of the hard palate and part of the soft palate, medially to the midline
4. Skin of the lower eyelid, side of the nose, cheek, and upper lip

Indications
1. Pain control before extensive oral surgical, periodontal, or restorative procedures requiring anesthesia of the entire maxillary division

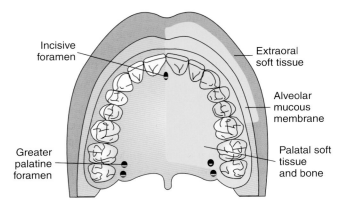

Figure 13-53. Areas anesthetized by a maxillary nerve block.

2. When tissue inflammation or infection precludes the use of other regional nerve blocks (e.g., PSA, ASA, AMSA, P-ASA) or supraperiosteal injection
3. Diagnostic or therapeutic procedures for neuralgias or tics of the second division of the trigeminal nerve

Contraindications
1. Inexperienced administrator
2. Pediatric patients
   a. More difficult because of smaller anatomical dimensions
   b. Need a cooperative patient
   c. Usually unnecessary in children because of the high success rate of other regional block techniques
3. Uncooperative patients
4. Inflammation or infection of tissues overlying the injection site
5. When hemorrhage is risky (e.g., a hemophiliac)
6. In the greater palatine canal approach: inability to gain access to the canal; bony obstructions may be present in 5% to 15% of canals

Advantages
1. Atraumatic injection via the high tuberosity approach
2. High success rate (>95%)
3. Minimizes the number of needle penetrations necessary for successful anesthesia of the hemimaxilla (minimum of four via PSA, infraorbital, greater palatine, and nasopalatine)
4. Minimizes total volume of local anesthetic solution injected to 1.8 versus 2.7 ml
5. Neither high tuberosity nor greater palatine canal approach usually is traumatic

Disadvantages
1. Risk of hematoma, primarily with the high tuberosity approach.
2. High-tuberosity approach is relatively arbitrary. Overinsertion is possible because of the absence of bony landmarks if proper technique is not followed.

3. Lack of hemostasis. If necessary, this necessitates infiltration with vasoconstrictor-containing local anesthetic at the surgical site.
4. Pain. The greater palatine canal approach is potentially (although not usually) traumatic.
5. Positive aspiration is less than 1% (greater palatine canal approach).

Alternatives. To achieve the same distribution of anesthesia present with a maxillary nerve block, all of the following must be administered:
1. PSA nerve block
2. ASA nerve block
3. Greater palatine nerve block
4. Nasopalatine nerve block

Technique (High-tuberosity Approach) (Fig. 13-54)
1. A 25-gauge long needle is recommended.
2. Area of insertion: height of the mucobuccal fold above the distal aspect of the maxillary second molar
3. Target area
   a. Maxillary nerve as it passes through the pterygopalatine fossa
   b. Superior and medial to the target area of the PSA nerve block
4. Landmarks
   a. Mucobuccal fold at the distal aspect of the maxillary second molar
   b. Maxillary tuberosity
   c. Zygomatic process of the maxilla
5. Orientation of the bevel: toward bone
6. Procedure
   a. Measure the length of a long needle from the tip to the hub (average 32 mm, but varies by manufacturer).
   b. Assume the correct position.
      (1) For a left high-tuberosity injection, a right-handed administrator should sit at the 10 o'clock position facing the patient (see Fig. 13-8, *A*).
      (2) For a right high-tuberosity injection, a right-handed administrator should sit at the 8 o'clock position facing the patient (see Fig. 13-8, *B*).
   c. Position the patient supine or semisupine for the right or left block.
   d. Prepare the tissue in the height of the mucobuccal fold at the distal of the maxillary second molar.
      1. Dry with sterile gauze.
      2. Apply topical antiseptic (optional).
      3. Apply topical anesthetic.
   e. Partially open the patient's mouth; pull the mandible toward the side of injection.
   f. Retract the cheek in the injection area with your index finger to increase visibility.
   g. Pull the tissues taut with this finger.
   h. Place the needle into the height of the mucobuccal fold over the maxillary second molar.
   i. Advance the needle slowly in an upward, inward, and backward direction as described for the PSA nerve block (p. 192).

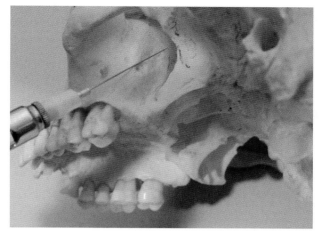

Figure 13-54. Maxillary nerve block, high-tuberosity approach.

   j. Advance the needle to a depth of 30 mm.
      (1) No resistance to needle penetration should be felt. If resistance is felt, the angle of the needle in toward the midline is too great.
      (2) At this depth (30 mm) the needle tip should lie in the pterygopalatine fossa in proximity to the maxillary division of the trigeminal nerve.
   k. Aspirate.
      (1) Rotate the syringe (needle bevel) one-fourth turn and reaspirate.
      (2) If negative:
         (a) Slowly (more than 60 seconds) deposit 1.8 ml.
         (b) Aspirate several times during injection.
   l. Withdraw the syringe.
   m. Make the needle safe.
   n. Wait 3 to 5 minutes before commencing the dental procedure.

Technique (Greater Palatine Canal Approach) (Fig. 13-55)
1. A 25-gauge long needle is recommended.
2. Area of insertion: palatal soft tissue directly over the greater palatine foramen
3. Target area: the maxillary nerve as it passes through the pterygopalatine fossa; the needle passes through the greater palatine canal to reach the pterygopalatine fossa
4. Landmark: greater palatine foramen, junction of the maxillary alveolar process and palatine bone
5. Orientation of the bevel: toward palatal soft tissues
6. Procedure
   a. Measure the length of a long needle from the tip to the hub (average 32 mm but varies by manufacturer).
   b. Assume the correct position.
      (1) For a right greater palatine canal maxillary block, sit facing toward the patient at the 7 or 8 o'clock position.
      (2) For a left greater palatine canal maxillary block, sit facing in the same direction as the patient at the 10 or 11 o'clock position.

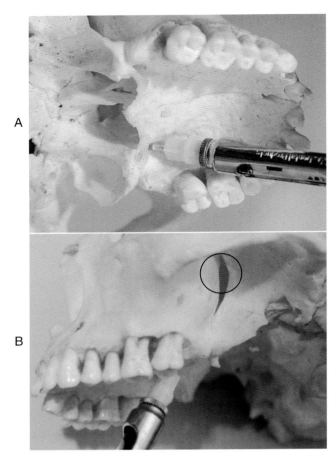

Figure 13-55. A, Maxillary nerve block, greater palatine canal approach. Notice the direction of the needle and syringe barrel into the canal. **B,** Second division nerve block (V₂), greater palatine canal approach. Note location of needle tip in pterygopalatine fossa *(circle).*

c. Request the patient, who is supine, to do the following:
   (1) Open wide.
   (2) Extend the neck.
   (3) Turn the head to the left or right (to improve visibility).
d. Locate the greater palatine foramen.
   (1) Place a cotton swab at the junction of the maxillary alveolar process and hard palate.
   (2) Start in the region of the second molar and palpate by pressing posteriorly into the tissues with the swab.
   (3) The swab "falls" into the depression created by the greater palatine foramen.
   (4) The foramen is most frequently located at the distal aspect of the maxillary second molar (see Table 13-2).
e. Prepare the tissues directly over the greater palatine foramen.
   (1) Clean and dry with sterile gauze.
   (2) Apply topical antiseptic (optional).

(3) Apply topical anesthetic for 2 minutes.
f. After 2 minutes of topical anesthetic application, move the swab posteriorly so it lies just behind the greater palatine foramen.
   (1) Apply pressure to the tissue with the cotton swab, held in the left hand (if right-handed).
   (2) Note ischemia at the injection site.
g. Direct the syringe into the mouth from the opposite side with the needle approaching the injection site at a right angle (Fig. 13-56).
h. Place the bevel against the ischemic soft tissue at the injection site. The needle must be well stabilized to prevent accidental penetration of the tissues.
i. With the bevel lying against the tissue:
   (1) Apply enough pressure to bow the needle slightly.
   (2) Deposit a small volume of local anesthetic. The solution is forced against the mucous membrane, forming a droplet.
j. Straighten the needle and permit the bevel to penetrate the mucosa.
   (1) Continue to deposit small volumes of anesthetic throughout the procedure.
   (2) Ischemia spreads into the adjacent tissues as the anesthetic is deposited.
k. Continue to apply pressure with the cotton applicator stick during this part of the procedure. The greater palatine nerve block is now complete.
l. Probe gently for the greater palatine foramen.
   (1) The patient feels no discomfort because of the previously deposited anesthetic solution.
   (2) The angle of the needle and syringe may be changed if needed.
   (3) The needle usually must be held at a 45-degree angle to facilitate entry into the greater palatine foramen (Table 13-3).
m. After locating the foramen, very slowly advance the needle into the greater palatine canal to a depth of 30 mm. Approximately 5% to 15% of

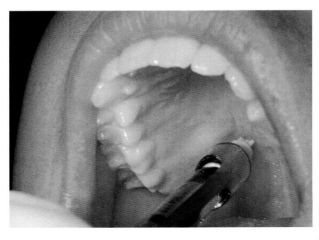

Figure 13-56. Maxillary nerve block, greater palatine canal approach.

greater palatine canals have bony obstructions that prevent passage of the needle.
(1) Never attempt to force the needle against resistance.
(2) If resistance is felt, withdraw the needle slightly and slowly attempt to advance it at a different angle.
(3) If the needle cannot be advanced further and the depth of penetration is almost adequate, continue with the next steps; however, if the depth is considerably deficient, withdraw the needle and discontinue the attempt.
n. Aspirate.
(1) Rotate the needle one-fourth turn and reaspirate.
(2) If negative, slowly deposit 1.8 ml of solution over a minimum of 1 minute.
o. Withdraw the syringe.
p. Make the needle safe.
q. Wait 3 to 5 minutes before commencing the dental procedure.

Signs and Symptoms
1. Subjective: pressure behind the upper jaw on the side being injected; this usually subsides rapidly, progressing to tingling and numbness of the lower eyelid, side of the nose, and upper lip
2. Subjective: sensation of numbness in the teeth and buccal and palatal soft tissues on the side of injection
3. Objective: no pain during dental therapy

Safety Feature. Careful adherence to technique

Precautions
1. Pain on insertion of the needle, primarily with the greater palatine canal approach; prevent by using atraumatic palatal injection protocol
2. Overinsertion of the needle; can occur in both approaches (although much less likely with the greater

palatine canal approach); prevent through careful adherence to protocol
3. Resistance to needle insertion in the greater palatine canal approach; never try to advance a needle against resistance

Failures of Anesthesia
1. Partial anesthesia; may result from underpenetration by needle. To correct: Reinsert the needle to proper depth and reinject.
2. Inability to negotiate the greater palatine canal. To correct:
   a. Withdraw the needle slightly and reangulate it.
   b. Reinsert carefully to the proper depth.
   c. If unable to bypass the obstruction easily, withdraw the needle and terminate the injection.
      (1) The high tuberosity approach may prove more successful in this situation.
   d. The greater palatine canal approach usually is successful if the needle has been advanced at least two thirds of its length into the canal.

Complications
1. Hematoma develops rapidly if the maxillary artery is punctured during maxillary nerve block via the high tuberosity approach. (Refer to "PSA Nerve Block, Complications," p. 192.)
2. Penetration of the orbit may occur during a greater palatine foramen approach if the needle goes in too far; more likely to occur in the smaller-than-average skull
3. Complications produced by injection of local anesthetic into the orbit include:*
   a. Volume displacement of the orbital structures, producing periorbital swelling and proptosis
   b. Regional block of the sixth cranial nerve (abducens), producing diplopia
   c. Classic retrobulbar block, producing mydriasis, corneal anesthesia, and ophthalmoplegia
   d. Possible optic nerve block with transient loss of vision
   e. Possible retrobulbar hemorrhage
   f. To prevent intraorbital injection: Strictly adhere to protocol and modify your technique for the smaller patient
3. Penetration of the nasal cavity
   a. If the needle deviates medially during insertion through the greater palatine canal, the paper-thin medial wall of the pterygopalatine fossa is penetrated and the needle enters the nasal cavity.
      (1) On aspiration, large amounts of air appear in the cartridge.
      (2) On injection, the patient complains that local anesthetic solution is running down the throat.

TABLE **13-3**
Angle of the Greater Palatine Foramen to the Hard Palate

Angle (°)	n = 199	Percent
20 to 22.5	2	1.005
25 to 27.5	4	2.01
30 to 32.5	18	9.045
35 to 37.5	28	14.07
40 to 42.5	25	12.56
45 to 47.5	34	17.08
50 to 52.5	34	17.08
55 to 57.5	29	14.57
60 to 62.5	17	8.54
65 to 67.5	7	3.51
70	1	0.50

From Malamed SF, Trieger N: Intraoral maxillary nerve block: an anatomical and clinical study, *Anesth Prog* 30:44-48, 1983.

*It has been reported that complications *a, b,* and *c* were most common after intraorbital injection; complications *d* and *e* were never encountered.[20,21]

TABLE **13-4**

Maxillary Teeth and Available Local Anesthetic Techniques

Teeth	Pulpal Anesthesia	Soft-Tissue	
		Buccal	Palatal
Incisors	Infraorbital (IO)	Infraorbital (IO)	Nasopalatine
	Infiltration	Infiltration	Infiltration
	AMSA	AMSA	AMSA
	P-ASA	P-ASA	P-ASA
	V_2	V_2	V_2
Canines	Infraorbital	Infraorbital	Nasopalatine
	Infiltration	Infiltration	Infiltration
	AMSA	AMSA	AMSA
	P-ASA	P-ASA	P-ASA
	V_2	V_2	V_2
Premolars	Infraorbital	Infraorbital	Greater palatine
	Infiltration	Infiltration	Infiltration
	MSA	MSA	AMSA
	AMSA	AMSA	V_2
	V_2	V_2	
Molars	PSA	PSA	Greater palatine
	Infiltration	Infiltration	Infiltration
	V_2	V_2	V_2

TABLE **13-5**

Recommended Volumes of Local Anesthetic for Maxillary Techniques

Technique	Volume (ml)
Supraperiosteal (infiltration)	0.6
Posterior superior alveolar (PSA)	0.9 to 1.8
Middle superior alveolar (MSA)	0.9 to 1.2
Anterior superior alveolar (ASA, infraorbital)	0.9 to 1.2
Anterior middle superior alveolar (AMSA)	1.4 to 1.8
Palatal approach-anterior superior alveolar (P-ASA)	1.4 to 1.8
Greater (anterior) palatine	0.45 to 0.6
Nasopalatine	0.45 (maximum)
Palatal infiltration	0.2 to 0.3
Maxillary (V_2) nerve block	1.8

(3) To prevent: Keep the patient's mouth wide open and take care during penetration that the advancing needle stays in the correct plane.

• • •

Table 13-4 summarizes the indications for maxillary local anesthesia. Table 13-5 includes volumes of solutions recommended for maxillary injections.

SUMMARY

Providing clinically adequate anesthesia in the maxilla is seldom a problem. The thin and porous bone of the maxilla permits the ready diffusion of local anesthetic to the apex of the tooth to be treated. For this reason many dentists rely solely on supraperiosteal (or "infiltration") anesthesia for most treatment in the maxilla.

It is only on rare occasion that difficulty arises with maxillary pain control. Most notable, of course, is the pulpally involved tooth; because of infection or inflammation, the use of supraperiosteal anesthesia is contraindicated or ineffective for this. In nonpulpally involved teeth the most often observed problems in obtaining adequate pulpal anesthesia via supraperiosteal injection develop in the central incisor (whose apex may lie beneath the denser bone and cartilage of the nose), the canine (whose root length may be considerable, with the local anesthetic deposited below the apex), and the maxillary molars (whose buccal root apices may be covered by denser bone of the zygomatic arch, a problem more often noted in patients 6 to 8 years of age, and whose palatal root may flare toward the palate, making the distance that local anesthetic must diffuse too great). In such situations the use of regional nerve block anesthesia is essential to clinical success in pain control. In reality, two safe and simple nerve blocks—the posterior superior alveolar and the anterior superior alveolar—enable dental care to be provided painlessly in virtually all patients.

Palatal anesthesia, although commonly thought of as being highly traumatic, can be provided in most cases with little or no discomfort to the patient.

REFERENCES

1. Adatia AK: Effects of cytotoxic chemotherapy on dental development, *J R Soc Med* 80:784-785, 1987 (letter).

2. Loetscher CA, Melton DC, Walton RE: Injection regimen for anesthesia of the maxillary first molar, *J Am Dent Assoc* 117:337-340, 1988.
3. Frazer M: Contributing factors and symptoms of stress in dental practice, *Br Dent J* 173(2):211, 1992.
4. Friedman MJ, Hochman MN: A 21(st) century computerized injection system for local pain control, *Compend Contin Educ Dent* 18(10):995-1000, 1002-1004, 1997.
5. Friedman MJ, Hochman MN: The AMSA injection: a new concept for local anesthesia of maxillary teeth using a computer-controlled injection system, *Quint Int* 29: 297-303, 1998.
6. Melzack R: *The puzzle of pain*, New York, 1973, Basic Books.
7.
8. Friedman MJ, Hochman MN: P-ASA block injection: a new palatal technique to anesthetize maxillary anterior teeth, *J Esthet Dent* 11(2):63-71, 1999.
9. Friedman MJ, Hochman MN: 21(st) century computerized injection for local pain control, *Compend Contin Educ Dent* 18:995-1003, 1997.
10. Perry DA, Loomer PM: Maximizing pain control. The AMSA injection can provide anesthesia with few injections and less pain, 49:28-33, 2003.
11. Hochman MN, Friedman MJ: In vitro study of needle deflection: a linear insertion technique versus a bidirectional rotation insertion technique, *Quint Int* 31(1):33-39, 2000.
12. Malamed SF: *Handbook of local anesthesia*, ed 4, St Louis, 1997, Mosby.
13. Jastak JT, Yagiela JA, Donaldson D: *Local anesthesia of the oral cavity*, Philadelphia, 1995, WB Saunders.
14. McArdle BF: Painless palatal anesthesia, *J Am Dent Assoc* 128:647, 1997.
15. Nicholson JW, Berry TG, Summitt JB, et al: Pain perception and utility: a comparison of the syringe and computerized local injection techniques, *Gen Dent* 49:167-172, 2001.
16. Hochman MN, Chiiarello D, Hochman C, et al: Computerized local anesthesia vs traditional syringe technique: Subjective pain response, *NYSDJ* 63(7):24-29, 1997.
17. Nicholson JW, Berry TG, Summitt JB, et al: Pain perception and utility: a comparison of the syringe and computerized local injection techniques, *Gen Dent* 49:167-172, 2001.
18. Perry DA, Loomer PM: Maximizing pain control. The AMSA injection can provide anesthesia with few injections and less pain, 49:28-33, 2003.
19. Fukayama H, Yoshikawa F, Kohase H, et al: Efficacy of AMSA anesthesia using a new injection system, the Wand, *Quint Int* 34:573-541, 2003.
20. Malamed SF, Trieger N: Intraoral maxillary nerve block: an anatomical and clinical study, *Anesth Prog* 30:44-48, 1983.
21. Poore TE, Carney FMT: Maxillary nerve block: a useful technique, *J Oral Surg* 31:749-755, 1973.

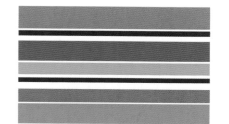

Techniques of Mandibular Anesthesia

Any practicing dentist or dental hygienist is well aware that a major clinical difference exists in the success rates for maxillary nerve blocks (e.g., posterior superior alveolar and anterior superior alveolar) and that for the inferior alveolar nerve block.

Achieving clinically acceptable anesthesia in the maxilla is rarely a problem, except in instances of anatomical anomalies or pathological conditions. Less dense bone covers the apices of maxillary teeth, and the relatively easy access to large nerve trunks provides the well-trained administrator with success rates of 95% or higher.

Not so in the adult mandible. Successful pulpal anesthesia of mandibular teeth is a bit more difficult to achieve on a consistently reliable basis. Success rates of 80% to 85% for the inferior alveolar nerve block, the most frequently administered mandibular injection, attest to this fact.[1] Reasons for these lower success rates include the greater density of the buccal alveolar plate (which precludes supraperiosteal injection [in the adult patient]), limited accessibility to the inferior alveolar nerve, and the wide variation in anatomy. Although an 80% rate of success does not seem particularly low, consider that one out of every five patients requires reinjection to achieve clinically adequate anesthesia.

Six nerve blocks are described in this chapter. Two of these—involving the mental and buccal nerves—provide regional anesthesia to soft tissues only and have exceedingly high success rates. In both instances the nerve anesthetized lies directly beneath the soft tissues, not encased in bone. The four remaining blocks—the inferior alveolar, incisive, Gow-Gates mandibular, and Vazirani-Akinosi (closed-mouth) mandibular—provide regional anesthesia to the pulps of some or all of the mandibular teeth in a quadrant. Three other injections that are of importance in mandibular anesthesia—the periodontal ligament, intraosseous, and intraseptal—are described

in Chapter 15. Although these techniques can be used successfully in either the maxilla or mandible, their greatest utility lies in the mandible, because in the mandible they can provide pulpal anesthesia of a single tooth without the lingual and facial soft-tissue anesthesia that occurs with other mandibular nerve block techniques.

The success rate of the *inferior alveolar* nerve block is lower than for most other nerve blocks. Because of anatomical considerations in the mandible (primarily the density of bone), the administrator must accurately deposit local anesthetic solution to within 1 mm of the target nerve. The inferior alveolar nerve block has a significantly lower success rate because of two factors—(1) anatomical variation in the height of the mandibular foramen on the lingual side of the ramus and (2) the greater depth of soft-tissue penetration necessary—that consistently lead to greater inaccuracy. Fortunately, the *incisive nerve block* provides pulpal anesthesia to the teeth anterior to the mental foramen (e.g., the incisors, canines, first premolars, and [in most instances] second premolars). The incisive nerve block is a valuable alternative to the inferior alveolar nerve block when treatment is limited to these teeth. To achieve anesthesia of the mandibular molars, however, the inferior alveolar nerve must be anesthetized, and this frequently entails (with all its attendant disadvantages) a lower incidence of successful anesthesia.

The third injection technique that provides pulpal anesthesia to mandibular teeth, the *Gow-Gates mandibular nerve block*, is a true mandibular block injection because it provides regional anesthesia to virtually all the sensory branches of V_3. In actual fact, the Gow-Gates may be thought of as a high inferior alveolar nerve block. When used, two beneficial effects are noted: (1) the problems associated with anatomical variations in the height of the mandibular foramen are obviated and (2) anesthesia of the other sensory branches of V_3 (e.g., the lingual, buccal, and mylohyoid nerves) is usually obtained along with that of the inferior alveolar nerve. With proper adherence to protocol (and experience using this technique), a success rate in excess of 95% can be achieved.

Another V_3 nerve block, the *closed-mouth mandibular nerve block*, is included in this discussion, primarily because it allows the doctor to achieve clinically adequate anesthesia in an extremely difficult situation—one in which a patient has limited mandibular opening as a result of infection, trauma, or postinjection trismus. It is also known as the Vazirani-Akinosi technique (after the two doctors who developed it). Some practitioners use it routinely for anesthesia in the mandibular arch. The closed-mouth technique is described mainly because with experience it can provide a success rate of better than 80% in situations (extreme trismus) in which the inferior alveolar and Gow-Gates nerve blocks have little or no likelihood of success.

In ideal circumstances the individual who is to administer the local anesthetic should be familiar with each of these techniques. The greater the number of techniques at one's disposal with which to attain mandibular anesthesia, the less likely it is that a patient will be dismissed from an office because of adequate pain control. More realistically, however, the administrator should become proficient with at least one of these procedures and have a working knowledge of the others to be able to use them with a good expectation of success should the appropriate situation arise.

INFERIOR ALVEOLAR NERVE BLOCK

The inferior alveolar nerve block (IANB), commonly (but inaccurately) referred to as the *mandibular nerve block*, is the most frequently used and possibly the most important injection technique in dentistry. Unfortunately, it also proves to be the most frustrating, with the highest percentage of clinical failures (approximately 15% to 20%) even when properly administered.[1]

It is an especially useful technique for quadrant dentistry. A supplemental block (buccal nerve) is needed only if soft-tissue anesthesia in the buccal posterior region is necessary. On rare occasion a supraperiosteal injection (infiltration) may be needed in the lower incisor region to correct partial anesthesia caused by the overlap of sensory fibers from the contralateral side. A periodontal ligament (PDL) injection might be necessary when isolated portions of mandibular teeth (usually the mesial root of a first mandibular molar) remain sensitive after an otherwise successful inferior alveolar nerve block.

The administration of bilateral IANBs should be rarely called for in dental treatments other than bilateral mandibular surgeries. They produce considerable discomfort, primarily from the lingual soft-tissue anesthesia, which usually persists for several hours after injection (the duration is dependent on the particular local

anesthetic used). The patient feels unable to swallow and, because of the lack of all sensation, is more likely to self-injure the anesthetized soft tissues, as well as being unable to enunciate well. Whenever possible, it is preferable to treat the entire right or left side of a patient's oral cavity (maxillary and mandibular) at one appointment rather than administer a bilateral IANB. Patients are much more capable of handling the posttreatment discomfort (e.g., feeling of anesthesia) associated with bilateral maxillary than with bilateral mandibular anesthesia.

One situation in which bilateral mandibular anesthesia frequently is used involves the patient who presents with six, eight, or ten lower anterior teeth (e.g., canine to canine; premolars to premolars) requiring restorative or soft-tissue procedures. Two excellent alternatives to *bilateral* IANBs are bilateral incisive nerve blocks (where lingual soft-tissue anesthesia is not necessary) and *unilateral* inferior alveolar blocks on the side that has the greater number of teeth requiring restoration or requires the greater degree of lingual intervention, combined with an *incisive* nerve block on the opposite side. It must be remembered that the incisive nerve block does *not* provide lingual soft-tissue anesthesia; thus lingual infiltration may be necessary.

In the following description of the inferior alveolar nerve block, the injection site is noted to be slightly higher than that usually depicted. The success rate of this technique, taught for many years at the University of Southern California School of Dentistry, approaches 85% to 90% and higher with experience.[2]

Other Common Name. Mandibular block

Nerves Anesthetized
1. Inferior alveolar, a branch of the posterior division of the mandibular
2. Incisive
3. Mental
4. Lingual (commonly)

Areas Anesthetized (Fig. 14-1)
1. Mandibular teeth to the midline
2. Body of the mandible, inferior portion of the ramus
3. Buccal mucoperiosteum, mucous membrane anterior to the mandibular first molar (mental nerve)
4. Anterior two thirds of the tongue and floor of the oral cavity (lingual nerve)
5. Lingual soft tissues and periosteum (lingual nerve)

Indications
1. Procedures on multiple mandibular teeth in one quadrant
2. When buccal soft-tissue anesthesia (anterior to the first molar) is necessary
3. When lingual soft-tissue anesthesia is necessary

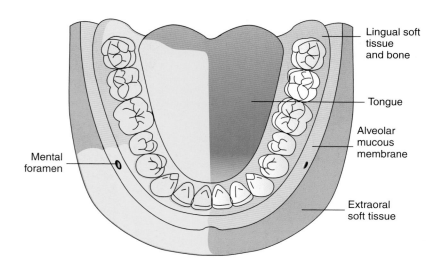

Mental foramen

Lingual soft tissue and bone

Tongue

Alveolar mucous membrane

Extraoral soft tissue

Figure 14-1. Area anesthetized by an inferior alveolar nerve block.

Contraindications
1. Infection or acute inflammation in the area of injection (rare)
2. Patients who might bite either the lip or the tongue; for instance, a very young child or a physically or mentally handicapped adult or child

Advantages. One injection provides a wide area of anesthesia (useful for quadrant dentistry)

Disadvantages
1. Wide area of anesthesia (not necessary for localized procedures)
2. Rate of inadequate anesthesia (15% to 20%)
3. Intraoral landmarks not consistently reliable
4. Positive aspiration (10% to 15%, highest of all intraoral injection techniques)
5. Lingual and lower lip anesthesia, discomfiting to many patients and possibly dangerous for certain individuals
6. Partial anesthesia possible where a bifid inferior alveolar nerve and bifid mandibular canals are present

Positive Aspiration. 10% to 15%

Alternatives
1. Mental nerve block, for buccal soft-tissue anesthesia anterior to the first molar
2. Incisive nerve block, for pulpal and buccal soft-tissue anesthesia of teeth anterior to the mental foramen
3. Supraperiosteal injection, for pulpal anesthesia of the central and lateral incisors, and sometimes the premolars (success rate extremely variable)
4. Gow-Gates mandibular nerve block
5. Vazirani-Akinosi mandibular nerve block
6. PDL injection for pulpal anesthesia of any mandibular tooth

7. Intraosseous (IO) injection for osseous and soft-tissue anesthesia of any mandibular region, but especially molars
8. Intraseptal injection for osseous and soft-tissue anesthesia of any mandibular region

Technique
1. A 25-gauge long needle is recommended for the adult patient.
2. Area of insertion: mucous membrane on the medial side of the mandibular ramus, at the intersection of two lines: one horizontal, representing the height of injection, and the other vertical, representing the anteroposterior plane of injection
3. Target area: inferior alveolar nerve as it passes downward toward the mandibular foramen but before it enters into the foramen
4. Landmarks (Figs. 14-2 and 14-3)
   a. Coronoid notch (greatest concavity on the anterior border of the ramus)
   b. Pterygomandibular raphe
   c. Occlusal plane of the mandibular posterior teeth
5. Orientation of the needle bevel: less critical than with other nerve blocks, because the needle approaches the inferior alveolar nerve at roughly a right angle
6. Procedure
   a. Assume the correct position.
      (1) For a right IANB, a right-handed administrator should sit at the 8 o'clock position *facing* the patient (Fig. 14-4, *A*).
      (2) For a left IANB, a right-handed administrator should sit at the 10 o'clock position facing in the *same direction* as the patient (Fig. 14-4, *B*).
   b. Position the patient supine (recommended) or semisupine. The mouth should be opened wide to permit greater visibility of and access to the injection site.

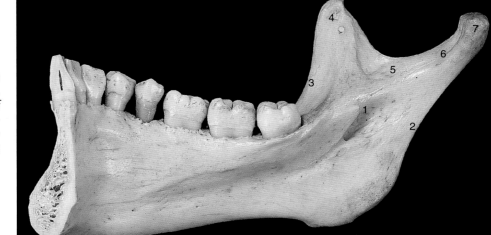

Figure 14-2. Osseous landmarks for inferior alveolar nerve block. *1,* Lingula; *2,* distal border of ramus; *3,* coronoid notch; *4,* coronoid process; *5,* sigmoid (mandibular) notch; *6,* neck of condyle; *7,* head of condyle.

c. Locate the needle penetration (injection) site.

There are three parameters that must be considered during the administration of the IANB: the *height* of the injection, the *anteroposterior* placement of the needle (which helps to locate a precise needle entry point), and the *depth* of penetration (which determines the location of the inferior alveolar nerve).

(1) HEIGHT OF INJECTION: Place the index finger or thumb of your left hand in the coronoid notch.

    (a) An imaginary line extends posteriorly from the finger tip in the coronoid notch to the deepest part of the pterygomandibular raphe (as it turns vertically upward toward the maxilla) determining the height of injection. This imaginary line should be parallel with the occlusal plane of the mandibular molar teeth. In most

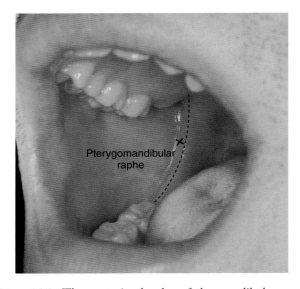

Figure 14-3. The posterior border of the mandibular ramus can be approximated intraorally by using the pterygomandibular raphe as it turns superiorly toward the maxilla.

patients this line lies 6 to 10 mm above the occlusal plane.

    (b) The finger on the coronoid notch is used to pull the tissues laterally, stretching them over the injection site, making them taut, enabling needle insertion to be less traumatic while also providing better visibility.

    (c) The needle insertion point lies three fourths of the anteroposterior distance from the coronoid notch back to the deepest part of the pterygomandibular raphe (Fig. 14-5). *Note:* The line should begin at the midpoint of the notch and terminate at the deepest (most posterior) portion of the pterygomandibular raphe as the raphe bends vertically upward toward the palate.

    (d) The posterior border of the mandibular ramus can be approximated intraorally by using the pterygomandibular raphe as it bends vertically upward toward the maxilla* (see Fig. 14-3).

    (e) An alternative method of approximating the length of the ramus is to place your thumb on the coronoid notch and your index finger extraorally on the posterior border of the ramus and estimate the distance between these points. However, many practitioners (including this author) have difficulty envisioning the width of the ramus in this manner.

    (f) Prepare tissue at the injection site:
    Dry with sterile gauze.
    Apply topical antiseptic (optional).
    Apply topical anesthetic for 1 to 2 minutes.
Place the barrel of the syringe in the corner of the mouth on the contralateral side (Figs. 14-5 and 14-6).

---

*The pterygomandibular raphe continues posteriorly in a horizontal plane from the retromolar pad before turning vertically toward the palate; *only the vertical portion of the pterygomandibular raphe is used as an indicator of the posterior border of the ramus.*

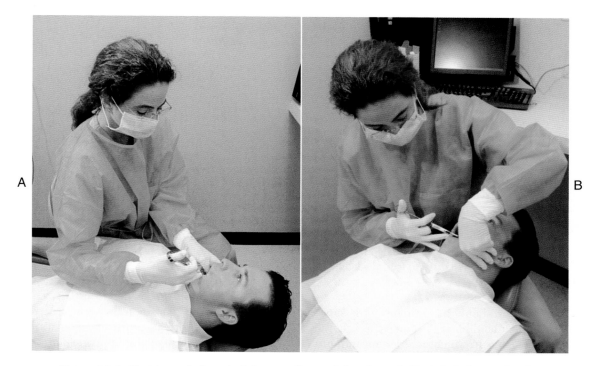

Figure 14-4. Position of the administrator for a right, **A,** and, **B,** left inferior alveolar nerve block.

(2) ANTEROPOSTERIOR SITE OF INJECTION: Needle penetration occurs at the intersection of two points.
  (a) Point 1 falls along the horizontal line from the coronoid notch to the deepest part of the pterygomandibular raphe as it ascends vertically toward the palate as just described.
  (b) Point 2 is on a vertical line through point 1 about three fourths of the distance from the anterior border of the ramus. This determines the anteroposterior site of the injection.

(3) PENETRATION DEPTH: In the third parameter of the IANB, *bone must be contacted.* Slowly advance the needle until you can feel it meet bony resistance.
  (a) For most patients it is not necessary to inject any local anesthetic solution as soft tissue is penetrated.
  (b) For anxious or sensitive patients it may be advisable to deposit small volumes as the needle is advanced.
  (c) The average depth of penetration to bony contact will be 20 to 25 mm, approximately two thirds to three fourths the length of a long dental needle (Fig. 14-7).

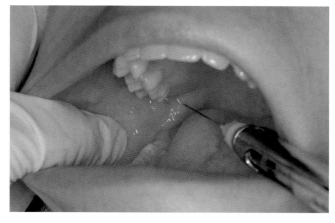

Figure 14-5. Notice the placement of the syringe barrel at the corner of the mouth, usually corresponding to the premolars. The needle tip gently touches the most distal end of the pterygomandibular raphe.

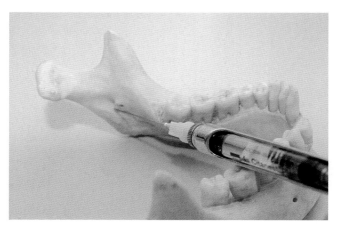

Figure 14-6. Placement of the needle and syringe for an inferior alveolar nerve block.

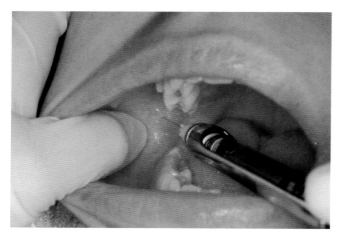

Figure 14-7. Inferior alveolar nerve block. The depth of penetration is 20 to 25 mm (two thirds to three fourths the length of a long needle).

(d) The needle tip should be located slightly superior to the mandibular foramen (where the inferior alveolar nerve enters [disappears] into bone). The foramen cannot be seen or palpated clinically.

(e) If *bone is contacted too soon* (less than half the length of a long dental needle), the needle tip is usually located too far *anteriorly* (laterally) on the ramus (Fig. 14-8). To correct:
  (i) Withdraw the needle slightly but do *not* remove it from the tissue.
  (ii) Bring the syringe barrel around toward the front of the mouth, over the canine or lateral incisor on the contralateral side.
  (iii) Redirect the needle until a more appropriate depth of insertion is obtained. The needle tip is now located *posteriorly* in the mandibular sulcus.

(f) If *bone is not contacted*, the needle tip is usually located too far *posterior* (medial) (Fig. 14-9). To correct:
  (i) Withdraw it slightly in tissue (leaving approximately one fourth its length in tissue) and reposition the syringe barrel more posteriorly (over the mandibular molars).
  (ii) Continue the insertion until contact with bone is made at an appropriate depth (20 to 25 mm).

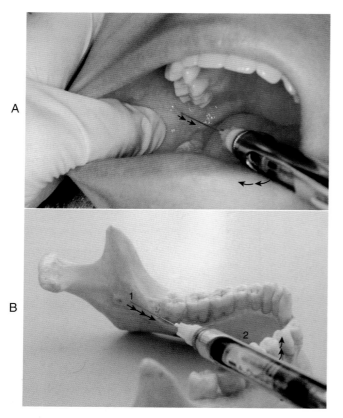

Figure 14-8. A, The needle is located too far anteriorly (laterally) on the ramus. **B,** To correct: Withdraw it slightly from the tissues *(1)* and bring the syringe barrel anteriorly toward the lateral incisor or canine *(2)*; reinsert to proper depth.

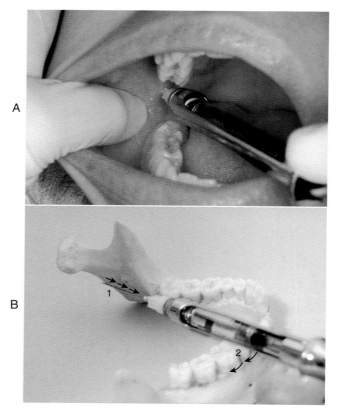

Figure 14-9. A, Overinsertion with no contact of bone. The needle is usually posterior (medial) to the ramus. **B,** To correct: Withdraw it slightly from the tissues *(1)* and reposition the syringe barrel over the premolars *(2)*; reinsert.

d. Insert the needle. When bone is contacted, withdraw approximately 1 mm to prevent subperiosteal injection.

e. Aspirate. If negative, slowly deposit 1.5 ml of anesthetic over a minimum of 60 seconds. (Because of the high incidence of positive aspiration and the natural tendency to deposit solution too rapidly, the sequence of slow injection, reaspiration, slow injection, reaspiration is strongly recommended.)

f. Slowly withdraw the syringe, and when approximately half its length remains within tissues, reaspirate. If negative, deposit a portion of the remaining solution (0.1 ml) to anesthetize the *lingual nerve*.

   (1) In most patients this deliberate injection for lingual nerve anesthesia *is not necessary*, because local anesthetic from the IANB anesthetizes the lingual nerve.

g. Withdraw the syringe slowly and make the needle safe.

h. After approximately 20 seconds, return the patient to the upright or semiupright position.

i. Wait 3 to 5 minutes before commencing the dental procedure.

Signs and Symptoms

1. Subjective: Tingling or numbness of the lower lip indicates anesthesia of the mental nerve, a terminal branch of the inferior alveolar nerve. It is a good indication that the inferior alveolar nerve is anesthetized, although *not* a reliable indicator of the depth of anesthesia.

2. Subjective: Tingling or numbness of the tongue indicates anesthesia of the lingual nerve, a branch of the posterior division of V_3. It usually accompanies IANB but may be present without anesthesia of the inferior alveolar nerve.

3. Objective: No pain is felt during dental therapy.

Safety Feature. The needle contacts bone preventing overinsertion, with its attendant complications.

Precautions

1. Do *not* deposit local anesthetic if bone is not contacted. The needle tip may be resting within the parotid gland near the facial nerve (cranial nerve VII), and a transient paralysis of the facial nerve is produced if solution is deposited.

2. Avoid pain by not contacting bone too forcefully.

Failures of Anesthesia. The most common causes of absent or incomplete IANB follow:

1. Deposition of anesthetic *too low* (below the mandibular foramen). To correct: Reinject at a higher site.

2. Deposition of anesthetic *too far anteriorly* (laterally) on the ramus. This is diagnosed by a lack of anesthesia except at the injection site and by the minimum depth of penetration before contact with bone (e.g., the needle

is usually less than halfway into tissue). To correct: Redirect the needle tip posteriorly.

3. Accessory innervation to the mandibular teeth

a. The primary symptom is isolated areas of incomplete pulpal anesthesia encountered on the mandibular molars (most commonly the mesial portion of the mandibular first molar) or premolars.

b. Although it has been postulated that several nerves provide the mandibular teeth with accessory sensory innervation (e.g., the cervical accessory and mylohyoid nerves), current thinking supports the mylohyoid nerve as the prime candidate.[3-5] The Gow-Gates mandibular nerve block, which routinely blocks the mylohyoid nerve, is *not* associated with problems of accessory innervation (unlike the IANB, which normally *does not* block the mylohyoid nerve).

c. To correct:

   (1) Technique #1

      (a) Use a 25-gauge long needle.

      (b) Retract the tongue toward the midline with a mirror handle or tongue depressor to provide access and visibility to the lingual border of the body of the mandible (Fig. 14-10).

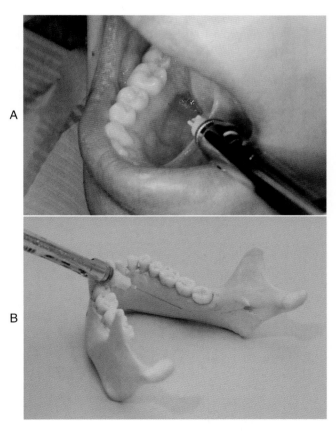

Figure 14-10. A, Retract the tongue to gain access to, and increase the visibility of, the lingual border of the mandible. **B,** Direct the needle tip below the apical region of the tooth immediately posterior to the tooth in question.

(c) Place the syringe in the corner of mouth on the opposite side and direct the needle tip to the apical region of the tooth immediately *posterior* to the tooth in question (e.g., the apex of the second molar if the first molar is the problem).

(d) Penetrate the soft tissues and advance the needle until bone (e.g., the lingual border of the body of the mandible) is contacted. Topical anesthesia is unnecessary if lingual anesthesia is already present. The depth of penetration to bone is 3 to 5 mm.

(e) Aspirate. If negative, slowly deposit approximately 0.6 ml (one third cartridge) of anesthetic (in about 20 seconds).

(f) Withdraw the syringe and make the needle safe.

(2) Technique #2. In any situation in which partial anesthesia of a tooth occurs, the PDL or IO injection may be administered; both techniques have a high expectation of success. (See Chapter 15 for discussion of PDL and IO techniques.)

d. Whenever a bifid inferior alveolar nerve is detected on the radiograph, incomplete anesthesia of the mandible may develop after IANB. In many such cases a second mandibular foramen, located more inferiorly, exists. To correct: Deposit a volume of solution *inferior* to the normal anatomical landmark.

4. Incomplete anesthesia of the central or lateral incisors
   a. This may comprise isolated areas of incomplete pulpal anesthesia.
   b. Often it is due to innervation from the mylohyoid nerve, though it may also arise from overlapping fibers of the contralateral inferior alveolar nerve.
   c. To correct:
      (1) Technique #1
         (a) Infiltrate supraperiosteally into the mucobuccal fold below the apex of the tooth in question (Fig. 14-11). This generally is

effective in the lateral incisor and (less often) central incisor region of the mandible because of the many small nutrient canals in cortical bone near the region of the incisive fossa.

(b) A 27-gauge short needle is recommended.

(c) Direct the needle tip toward the apical region of the tooth in question. Topical anesthesia is not necessary if mental nerve anesthesia is present.

(d) Aspirate.

(e) If negative, slowly deposit not more than 0.6 ml of local anesthetic solution in approximately 20 seconds.

(f) Wait 2 to 3 minutes before starting the dental procedure.

(2) As an alternate technique the PDL injection may be used. The PDL has great success in the mandibular anterior region.

Complications

1. Hematoma (rare)
   a. Swelling of tissues on the medial side of the mandibular ramus after the deposition of anesthetic
   b. Management: pressure and cold (e.g., ice) to the area for a minimum of 3 to 5 minutes

2. Trismus
   a. Muscle soreness or limited movement
      (1) A slight degree of soreness when opening the mandible is extremely common after IANB (when anesthesia has dissipated).
      (2) More severe soreness associated with limited mandibular opening is rare.
   b. Causes and management of limited mandibular opening after injection are discussed in Chapter 17.

3. Transient facial paralysis (facial nerve anesthesia)
   a. Produced by the deposition of local anesthetic into the body of the parotid gland. Signs and symptoms include an inability to close the lower eyelid and drooping of the upper lip on the affected side.

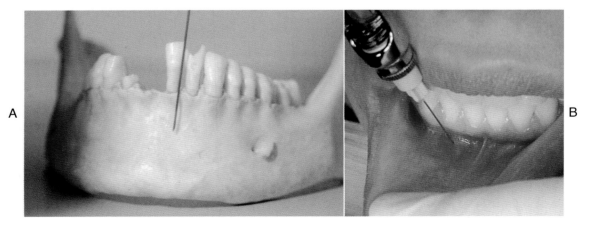

A   B

Figure 14-11. With supraperiosteal injection the needle tip is directed toward the apical region of the tooth in question. **A,** On a skull. **B,** In the mouth.

b. Management of transient facial nerve paralysis is discussed in Chapter 17.

BUCCAL NERVE BLOCK

The buccal nerve is a branch of the anterior division of V_3 and consequently is not anesthetized during IANB. Nor is anesthesia of this nerve necessary for most restorative dental procedures. The buccal nerve provides sensory innervation to the buccal soft tissues adjacent to the mandibular molars only. The sole indication for administration of a buccal nerve block therefore is when manipulation of these tissues is contemplated (e.g., with scaling or curettage, the use of a rubber dam clamp on soft tissues, the removal of subgingival caries, subgingival tooth preparation, placement of gingival retraction cord, and the placement of matrix bands).

It is common for the buccal nerve to be blocked routinely after IANB, even when buccal soft-tissue anesthesia in the molar region is not necessary. There is absolutely no indication for this injection in such a situation.

The buccal nerve block, commonly referred to as the *long buccal injection*, has a success rate approaching 100%. The reason for this is the buccal nerve is ready accessibility immediately beneath mucous membrane and not hidden within bone.

Other Common Names. Long buccal nerve block, buccinator nerve block

Nerve Anesthetized. Buccal (a branch of the anterior division of the mandibular)

Area Anesthetized. Soft tissues and periosteum buccal to the mandibular molar teeth (Fig. 14-12)

Indication. When buccal soft-tissue anesthesia is necessary for dental procedures in the mandibular molar region

Contraindication. Infection or acute inflammation in the area of injection

Advantages
1. High success rate
2. Technically easy

Disadvantages. Potential for pain if the needle contacts periosteum during injection

Positive Aspiration. 0.7%

Alternatives
1. Buccal infiltration
2. Gow-Gates mandibular nerve block
3. Vazirani-Akinosi mandibular nerve block
4. PDL injection
5. Intraosseous injection
6. Intraseptal injection

Technique
1. A 25-gauge long needle is recommended. This is most often used because the buccal nerve block is usually administered immediately after an IANB. A 27-gauge long needle also may be used. The long needle is recommended because of the posterior deposition site, not the depth of tissue insertion (which is minimal).
2. Area of insertion: mucous membrane distal and buccal to the most distal molar tooth in the arch
3. Target area: buccal nerve as it passes over the anterior border of the ramus
4. Landmarks: mandibular molars, mucobuccal fold
5. Orientation of the bevel: *toward* bone during the injection

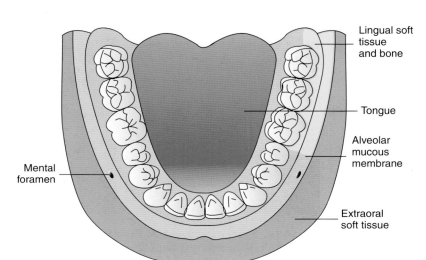

Lingual soft tissue and bone

Tongue

Alveolar mucous membrane

Mental foramen

Extraoral soft tissue

Figure 14-12. Area anesthetized by a buccal nerve block.

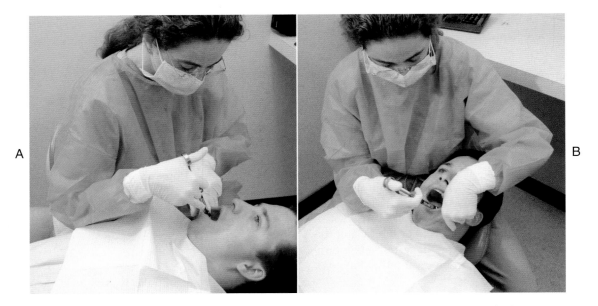

Figure 14-13. Position of the administrator for a right, **A,** and, **B,** left buccal nerve block.

6. Procedure
   a. Assume the correct position.
      (1) For a right buccal nerve block, a right-handed administrator should sit at the 8 o'clock position directly facing the patient (Fig. 14-13, *A*).
      (2) For a left buccal nerve block, a right-handed administrator should sit at 10 o'clock facing in the same direction as the patient (Fig. 14-13, *B*).
   b. Position the patient supine (recommended) or semisupine.
   c. Prepare the tissues for penetration distal and buccal to the most posterior molar.*
      (1) Dry with sterile gauze.
      (2) Apply topical antiseptic (optional).
      (3) Apply topical anesthetic for 1 to 2 minutes.
   d. With your left index finger (if right-handed), pull the buccal soft tissues in the area of injection laterally so that visibility will be improved. Taut tissues permit an atraumatic needle penetration.
   e. Direct the syringe toward the injection site with the bevel facing down toward bone and the syringe aligned parallel with the occlusal plane on the side of injection but buccal to the teeth (Fig. 14-14, *A*).
   f. Penetrate mucous membrane at the injection site, *distal* and *buccal* to the last molar (Fig. 14-14, *B*).
   g. Advance the needle slowly until mucoperiosteum is gently contacted.
      (1) To prevent pain when the needle contacts mucoperiosteum, deposit a few drops of local anesthetic just before contact.

---

*Because the buccal nerve block most often immediately follows an inferior alveolar nerve block, Steps (1), (2), and (3) of tissue preparation are usually completed before the inferior alveolar block.

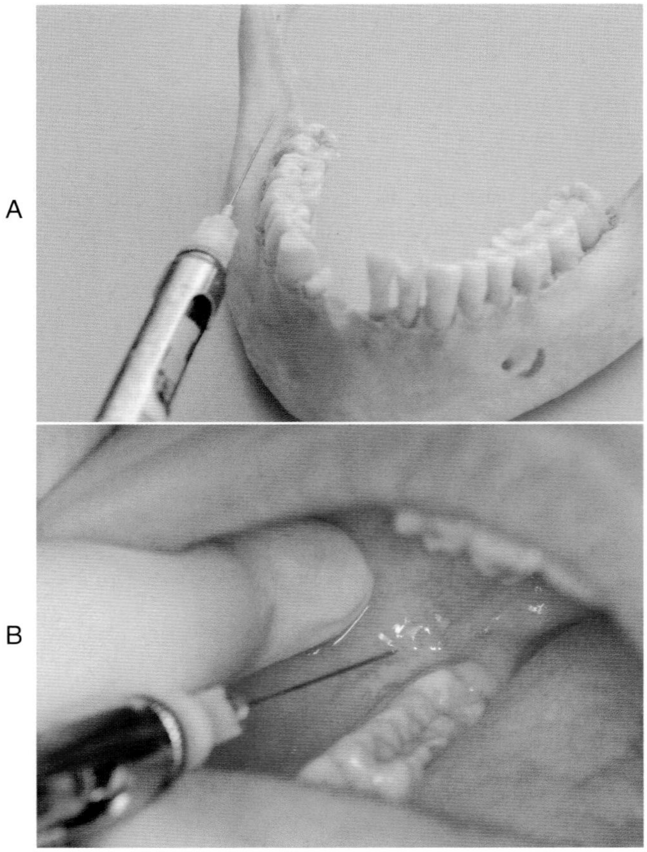

A

B

Figure 14-14. Syringe alignment. **A,** Parallel with the occlusal plane on the side of injection but buccal to it. **B,** Distal and buccal to the last molar.

(2) The depth of penetration is seldom more than 2 to 4 mm, and usually only 1 or 2 mm.
h. Aspirate.
i. If negative, slowly deposit 0.3 ml (approximately one eighth of a cartridge) over 10 seconds.
   (1) If tissue at the injection site balloons (becomes swollen during injection), stop depositing solution.
   (2) If solution runs out the injection site (back into the patient's mouth) during deposition
      (a) Stop the injection.
      (b) Advance the needle deeper into the tissue.*
      (c) Reaspirate.
      (d) Continue the injection.
j. Withdraw the syringe slowly and immediately make the needle safe.
k. Wait approximately 1 minute before commencing the planned dental procedure.

Signs and Symptoms
1. Because of the location and small size of the anesthetized area, the patient rarely experiences any subjective symptoms.
2. Objective: Instrumentation in the anesthetized area without pain indicates satisfactory pain control.

Safety Features
1. Needle contacting bone and preventing overinsertion
2. Minimum positive aspiration

Precautions
1. Pain on insertion from striking unanesthetized periosteum. This can be prevented by depositing a few drops of local anesthetic before contacting the periosteum.
2. Local anesthetic solution not being retained at the injection site. This generally means that needle penetration is not deep enough, the bevel of the needle is only partially in tissues, and solution is escaping during the injection.
   a. To correct:
      (1) Stop the injection.
      (2) Insert the needle to a greater depth.
      (3) Reaspirate.
      (4) Continue the injection.

Failures of Anesthesia. Rare with the buccal nerve block
1. Inadequate volume of anesthetic retained in the tissues

Complications
1. Few of any consequence
2. Hematoma (bluish discoloration and tissue swelling at the injection site). Blood may exit the needle puncture

point into the buccal vestibule. To treat: Apply pressure with gauze directly to the area of bleeding for a minimum of 3 to 5 minutes.

MANDIBULAR NERVE BLOCK: THE GOW-GATES TECHNIQUE

Successful anesthesia of the mandibular teeth and soft tissues is more difficult to achieve than anesthesia of maxillary structures. Failure rates of up to 20% are not uncommon with the traditional IANB technique previously described. Primary factors for this failure rate are the greater anatomical variation in the mandible and the need for deeper soft-tissue penetration. In 1973 George Albert Edwards Gow-Gates (1910–2001),[6] a general practitioner of dentistry in Australia, described a new approach to mandibular anesthesia. He had used this technique in his practice for approximately 30 years, with an astonishingly high success rate (approximately 99% *in his experienced hands*).

The Gow-Gates technique is a true mandibular nerve block because it provides sensory anesthesia to virtually the entire distribution of V_3. The inferior alveolar, lingual, mylohyoid, mental, incisive, auriculotemporal, and buccal nerves are all blocked in the Gow-Gates injection.

Significant advantages of the Gow-Gates technique over the IANB include its higher success rate, its lower incidence of positive aspiration (approximately 2% versus 10% to 15% with the IANB),[6,7] and the absence of problems with accessory sensory innervation to the mandibular teeth.

The only apparent disadvantage is a relatively minor one: an administrator experienced with the IANB may feel uncomfortable while learning the Gow-Gates mandibular nerve block (GGMNB). Indeed, the incidence of unsuccessful anesthesia with GGMNB may be as high as (if not higher than) that for the IANB until the administrator gains clinical experience with it. Thereafter, success rates of more than 95% are common. A new student of local anesthesia usually does not encounter as much difficulty as the more experienced administrator. This is the result of the strong bias of the experienced administrator to deposit the anesthetic drug "lower" (e.g., in the "usual" place). Two approaches are suggested for becoming accustomed with the GGMNB. The first is to begin to use the technique on all patients requiring mandibular anesthesia. Allow at least 1 to 2 weeks to gain clinical experience. The second approach is to continue using the conventional IANB but to use the GGMNB technique whenever clinically inadequate anesthesia occurs. Reanesthetize the patient using the GGMNB. Although experience is accumulated more slowly with this latter approach, its effectiveness is more dramatic because patients previously difficult to anesthetize now may be more easily managed.

---

*If an inadequate volume of solution remains in the cartridge, it may be necessary to remove the syringe from the patient's mouth and reload it with a new cartridge.

Other Common Names. Gow-Gates technique, third division nerve block, V_3 nerve block

Nerves Anesthetized
1. Inferior alveolar
2. Mental
3. Incisive
4. Lingual
5. Mylohyoid
6. Auriculotemporal
7. Buccal (in 75% of patients)

Areas Anesthetized (Fig. 14-15)
1. Mandibular teeth to the midline
2. Buccal mucoperiosteum and mucous membranes on the side of injection
3. Anterior two thirds of the tongue and floor of the oral cavity
4. Lingual soft tissues and periosteum
5. Body of the mandible, inferior portion of the ramus
6. Skin over the zygoma, posterior portion of the cheek, and temporal regions

Indications
1. Multiple procedures on mandibular teeth
2. When buccal soft-tissue anesthesia, from the third molar to the midline, is necessary
3. When lingual soft-tissue anesthesia is necessary
4. When a conventional inferior alveolar nerve block is unsuccessful

Contraindications
1. Infection or acute inflammation in the area of injection (rare)
2. Patients who might bite either their lip or their tongue, such as young children and physically or mentally handicapped adults

3. Patients who are unable to open their mouth wide (e.g., trismus)

Advantages
1. Requires only one injection; a buccal nerve block is usually unnecessary (accessory innervation has been blocked)
2. High success rate (>95%), with experience
3. Minimum aspiration rate
4. Few postinjection complications (e.g., trismus)
5. Provides successful anesthesia where a bifid inferior alveolar nerve and bifid mandibular canals are present

Disadvantages
1. Lingual and lower lip anesthesia is uncomfortable for many patients and possibly dangerous for certain individuals.
2. The time to onset of anesthesia is somewhat longer (5 min) than with an IANB (3 to 5 min), primarily because of the size of the nerve trunk being anesthetized and the distance of the nerve trunk from the deposition site (approximately 5 to 10 mm).
3. There is a learning curve with the Gow-Gates technique. Clinical experience is necessary to learn the technique and to fully take advantage of its greater success rate. This learning curve may prove to be frustrating for some persons.

Positive Aspiration. 2%

Alternatives
1. IANB and buccal nerve block
2. Vazirani-Akinosi closed-mouth mandibular block
3. Incisive nerve block: pulpal and buccal soft tissue anterior to the mental foramen
4. Mental nerve block: buccal soft tissue anterior to the first molar

Figure 14-15. Area anesthetized by a mandibular nerve block (Gow-Gates).

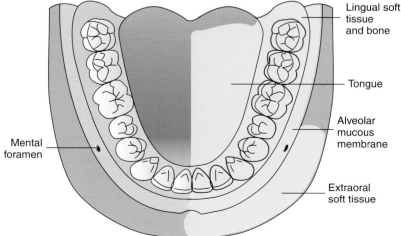
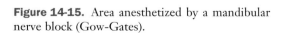

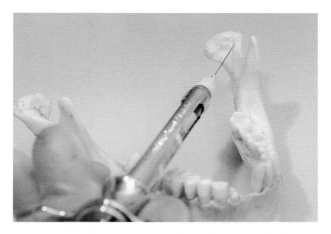

Figure 14-16. Target area for a Gow-Gates mandibular nerve block—neck of the condyle (corner of mouth, intertragic notch, tragus).

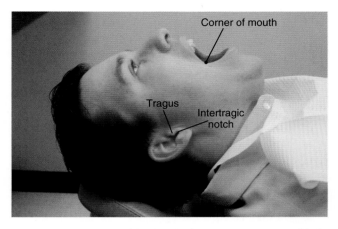

Figure 14-17. Extraoral landmarks for a Gow-Gates mandibular nerve block.

5. Buccal nerve block: buccal soft tissue from the third to the first molar region
6. Supraperiosteal injection: for pulpal anesthesia of the central and lateral incisors, and in some instances the canine
7. Intraosseous technique (see Chapter 15 for discussion)
8. PDL injection technique (see Chapter 15 for discussion)

Technique
1. 25-Gauge long needle recommended
2. Area of insertion: mucous membrane on the mesial of the mandibular ramus, on a line from the intertragic notch to the corner of the mouth, just distal to the maxillary second molar
3. Target area: lateral side of the condylar neck, just below the insertion of the lateral pterygoid muscle (Fig. 14-16)
4. Landmarks
   a. Extraoral
      (1) Lower border of the tragus (intertragic notch); the correct landmark is the center of the external auditory meatus, which is concealed by the tragus; therefore its lower border is adopted as a visual aid (Fig. 14-17)
      (2) Corner of the mouth
   b. Intraoral
      (1) Height of injection established by placement of the needle tip just below the mesiolingual (mesiopalatal) cusp of the maxillary second molar (Fig. 14-18, *A*)
      (2) Penetration of soft tissues just distal to the maxillary second molar at the height established in the preceding step (Fig. 14-18, *B*)
5. Orientation of the bevel: not critical
6. Procedure
   a. Assume the correct position.
      (1) For a right GGMNB, a right-handed administrator should sit in the 8 o'clock position *facing* the patient.

(2) For a left GGMNB, a right-handed administrator should sit in the 10 o'clock position facing the *same direction* as the patient.
   (3) These are the same positions used for a right and a left IANB (Fig. 14-4).
   b. Position the patient (Fig. 14-19).
      (1) Supine is recommended, although semisupine also may be used.
      (2) Request the patient to extend his or her neck and to open wide for the duration of the technique. The condyle then assumes a more frontal position and is closer to the mandibular nerve trunk.
   c. Locate the extraoral landmarks.
      (1) Intertragic notch
      (2) Corner of the mouth
   d. Place your left index finger or thumb on the coronoid notch; determination of the coronoid notch is *not* essential to the success of Gow-Gates, but in the author's experience palpation of this familiar intraoral landmark provides a sense of security besides enabling the tissues to be retracted, and it aids in determining the site of needle penetration.
   e. Visualize the intraoral landmarks.
      (1) Mesiolingual (mesiopalatal) cusp of the maxillary second molar
      (2) Needle penetration site is just distal to the maxillary second molar
   f. Prepare tissues at the site of penetration.
      (1) Dry tissue with sterile gauze.
      (2) Apply topical antiseptic (optional).
      (3) Apply topical anesthetic for minimum of 1 minute.
   g. Direct the syringe (held in your right hand) toward the site of injection from the corner of the mouth on the opposite side (as in IANB).
   h. Insert the needle gently into tissues at the injection site just distal to the maxillary second molar at the height of its mesiolingual (mesiopalatal) cusp.

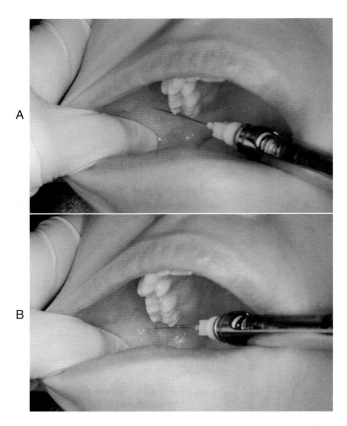

Figure 14-18. Intraoral landmarks for a Gow-Gates mandibular block. The tip of the needle is placed just below the mesiolingual cusp of the maxillary second molar, **A,** and is moved to a point just distal to the molar, **B,** maintaining the height established in the preceding step. This is the insertion point for the Gow-Gates mandibular nerve block.

i. Align the needle with the plane extending from the corner of the mouth to the intertragic notch on the side of injection. It should be parallel with the angle between the ear and the face (Fig. 14-20).
j. Direct the syringe toward the target area on the tragus.

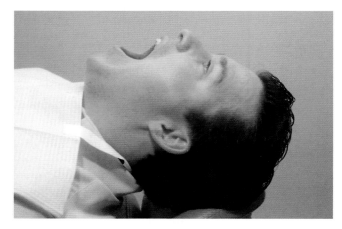

Figure 14-19. Position of the patient for a Gow-Gates mandibular nerve block.

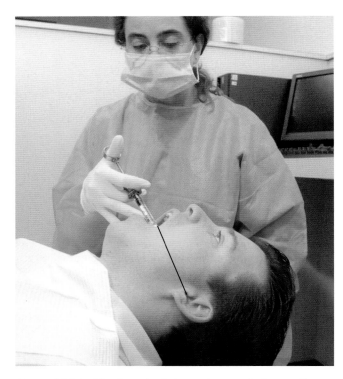

Figure 14-20. The barrel of the syringe and the needle are held parallel with a line connecting the corner of the mouth and the intertragic notch.

(1) The syringe barrel lies in the corner of the mouth over the premolars, but its position may vary from molars to incisors, depending on the divergence of the ramus as assessed by the angle of the ear to the side of the face (Fig. 14-21).
(2) The height of insertion above the mandibular occlusal plane is considerably greater (10 to 25 mm, depending on the patient's size) than that noted with the IANB.
(3) When a maxillary third molar is present in a normal occlusion, the site of needle penetration is just distal to that tooth.
k. Slowly advance the needle until bone is contacted.
  (1) Bone contacted is the neck of the condyle.
  (2) The average depth of soft-tissue penetration to bone is 25 mm, although some variation is observed. For a given patient the depth of soft-tissue penetration with the GGMNB approximates that with the IANB.
  (3) If bone is not contacted, withdraw the needle slightly and redirect. (Experience with the Gow-Gates technique has demonstrated that *medial* deflection of the needle is the most common cause of failure to contact bone.) Move the barrel of the syringe somewhat more distally, thereby angulating the needle tip anteriorly, and readvance the needle until bony contact is made.

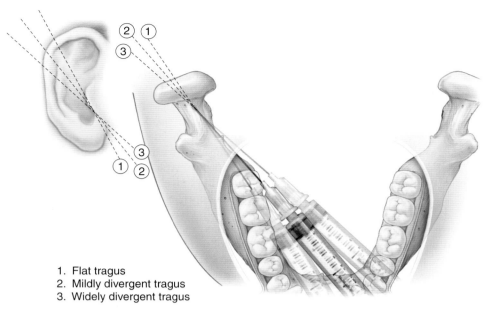

1. Flat tragus
2. Mildly divergent tragus
3. Widely divergent tragus

Figure 14-21. The location of the syringe barrel depends on the divergence of the tragus.

(a) A second cause of failure to contact bone is a partial closure of the patient's mouth (see step 6, b-2). Once the patient closes even slightly, two negatives occur: (1) the thickness of soft tissue increases and (2) the condyle moves in a distal direction. Both of these make it more difficult to locate the condylar neck with the needle.

(4) Do not deposit any local anesthetic if bone has not been contacted.

l.   Withdraw the needle 1 mm.

m. Aspirate.

n. If positive, withdraw the needle slightly, angle it superiorly, reinsert, reaspirate, and, if now negative, deposit the solution. Positive aspiration usually occurs in the internal maxillary artery, which is found *inferior* to the target area. The positive aspiration rate with the GGMNB technique is approximately 2%.[6,7]

o. If negative, slowly deposit 1.8 ml of solution over 60 to 90 seconds. Gow-Gates originally recommended that 3 ml of anesthetic be deposited.[6] However, 27 years of experience using the technique indicates that 1.8 ml usually is adequate to provide clinically acceptable anesthesia in virtually all cases. When partial anesthesia develops after administration of 1.8 ml, a second injection of approximately 1.2 ml is recommended.

p. Withdraw the syringe and make the needle safe.

q. Request that the patient keep the mouth open for 1 to 2 minutes after the injection to permit diffusion of the anesthetic solution.

(1) Use of a rubber bite block may assist the patient in keeping the mouth open.

r. After completion of the injection, return the patient to the upright or semiupright position.

s. Wait at least 3 to 5 minutes before commencing the dental procedure. The onset of anesthesia with the GGMNB may be somewhat slower, requiring 5 minutes or longer for the following reasons:

(1) Greater diameter of the nerve trunk at the site of injection

(2) Distance (5 to 10 mm) from the anesthetic deposition site to the nerve trunk

Signs and Symptoms

1. Subjective: Tingling or numbness of the lower lip indicates anesthesia of the mental nerve, a terminal branch of the inferior alveolar nerve. It is also a good indication that the inferior alveolar nerve may be anesthetized.

2. Subjective: Tingling or numbness of the tongue indicates anesthesia of the lingual nerve, a branch of the posterior division of the mandibular nerve. It is always present in a successful Gow-Gates mandibular block.

3. Objective: No pain is felt during dental therapy.

Safety Features

1. Needle contacting bone and preventing overinsertion

2. Very low positive aspiration rate; minimizes the risk of intravascular injection (the internal maxillary artery lies *inferior* to the injection site)

Precautions. Do not deposit local anesthetic if bone is not contacted; the needle tip usually is distal and medial to the desired site.

1. Withdraw slightly.

2. Redirect the needle laterally.

3. Reinsert the needle. Make gentle contact with bone.

4. Withdraw 1 mm and aspirate.

5. Inject if aspiration is negative.

Failures of Anesthesia. Rare with the Gow-Gates mandibular block once the administrator becomes familiar with the technique

1. Too little volume. The greater diameter of the mandibular nerve may require a larger volume of anesthetic solution. Deposit up to 1.2 ml in a second injection if the depth of anesthesia is inadequate after the initial 1.8 ml.
2. Anatomical difficulties. *Do not* deposit anesthetic unless bone is contacted.

Complications

1. Hematoma (<2% incidence of positive aspiration)
2. Trismus (extremely rare)
3. Temporary paralysis of cranial nerves III, IV, and VI. In a case of cranial nerve paralysis after a right Gow-Gates mandibular block, diplopia, right-sided blepharoptosis, and complete paralysis of the right eye persisted for 20 minutes after the injection. This has occurred after the accidental rapid intravenous administration of local anesthetic.[8] The recommendations of Dr. Gow-Gates include placing the needle on the lateral side of the anterior surface of the condyle, aspirating carefully, and depositing slowly.[6,7] If bone is not contacted, anesthetic solution should not be administered.

VAZIRANI-AKINOSI CLOSED-MOUTH MANDIBULAR BLOCK

The introduction of the Gow-Gates mandibular nerve block in 1973 spurred interest in alternative methods of achieving anesthesia in the lower jaw. In 1977 Dr. Joseph Akinosi reported on a closed-mouth approach to mandibular anesthesia.[9] Although this technique can be used whenever mandibular anesthesia is desired, its primary indication remains those situations in which limited mandibular opening precludes the use of other mandibular injection techniques. Such situations include the presence of spasm of the muscles of mastication (trismus) on one side of the mandible after numerous attempts at IANB, as might occur with a "hot" mandibular molar. In this instance, multiple injections have been necessary to provide anesthesia adequate to extirpate the pulpal tissues of the involved mandibular molar. When the anesthetic effect resolves hours later, the muscles into which the anesthetic solution was deposited become tender, producing some discomfort on opening the jaw. During a period of sleep, when the muscles are not in use, the muscles go into spasm (the same way one's leg muscles go into spasm after strenuous exercise, making it difficult to stand or walk the next morning), leaving the patient with significantly reduced occlusal opening in the morning. The management of trismus is reviewed in Chapter 17.

If it is necessary to continue dental care in the patient with significant trismus, the options for providing mandibular anesthesia are extremely limited. The inferior alveolar and Gow-Gates mandibular nerve blocks cannot be attempted when significant trismus is present. Extraoral mandibular nerve blocks can be attempted and, indeed, possess a significantly high success rate in experienced hands. Extraoral mandibular blocks can be administered either through the sigmoid notch or inferiorly from the chin (Fig. 14-22).[10,11] Because the mandibular division of the trigeminal nerve provides motor innervation to the muscles of mastication, a third division block (V_3) will relieve trismus that is produced secondary to muscle spasm (there are other causes of trismus). Although dentists are permitted to administer extraoral nerve blocks, few actually do so in clinical practice. The Vazirani-Akinosi technique is an intraoral approach to providing both anesthesia and motor blockade in cases of severe unilateral trismus.

In early editions of this textbook the technique described in the following was termed the *Akinosi closed-mouth mandibular block.* However, it appears that a very similar technique was initially described in 1960 by Vazirani.[12] The name *Vazirani-Akinosi closed-mouth mandibular block* was adopted for the fourth edition, giving recognition to both of the doctors who devised and publicized this closed-mouth approach to mandibular anesthesia.

In 1992 Wolfe described a modification of the original Vazirani-Akinosi technique.[13] The technique described was identical to the original technique except that the author recommended bending the needle at a 45-degree angle to enable it to remain in close proximity to the medial (lingual) side of the mandibular ramus as the needle is advanced through the tissues. Because the potential for needle breakage is increased when it is bent, bending any needle that is to be inserted into tissues to any significant depth is not recommended. The Vazirani-Akinosi closed-mouth mandibular block can be administered successfully without bending the needle.

Other Common Names. Akinosi technique, closed-mouth mandibular nerve block, tuberosity technique

Nerves Anesthetized

1. Inferior alveolar
2. Incisive
3. Mental
4. Lingual
5. Mylohyoid

Areas Anesthetized (Fig. 14-23)

1. Mandibular teeth to the midline
2. Body of the mandible and inferior portion of the ramus
3. Buccal mucoperiosteum and mucous membrane in front of the mental foramen
4. Anterior two thirds of the tongue and floor of the oral cavity (lingual nerve)
5. Lingual soft tissues and periosteum (lingual nerve)

Indications

1. Limited mandibular opening
2. Multiple procedures on mandibular teeth

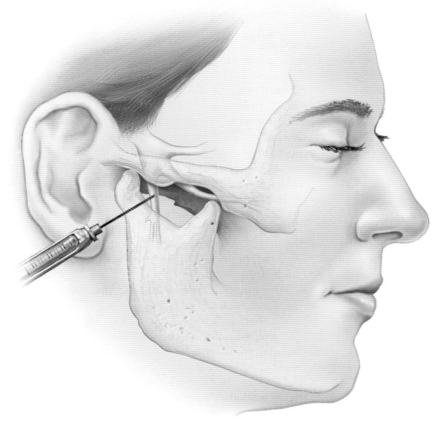

Figure 14-22. Extraoral mandibular block using lateral approach through the sigmoid notch. (Redrawn from Bennett CR: *Monheim's local anesthesia and pain control in dental practice,* ed 6, St. Louis, 1978, Mosby.)

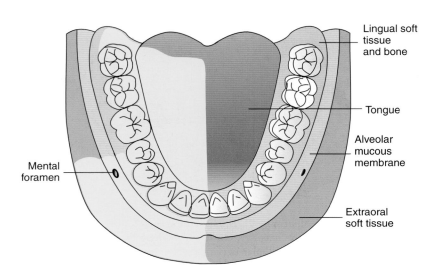

Lingual soft tissue and bone

Tongue

Alveolar mucous membrane

Mental foramen

Extraoral soft tissue

Figure 14-23. Area anesthetized by a Vazirani-Akinosi closed-mouth mandibular nerve block.

3. Inability to visualize landmarks for IANB (because of large tongue)

Contraindications
1. Infection or acute inflammation in the area of injection (rare)
2. Patients who might bite either their lip or their tongue, such as young children and physically or mentally handicapped adults
3. Inability to visualize or gain access to the lingual aspect of the ramus

Advantages
1. Relatively atraumatic
2. Patient need not be able to open the mouth
3. Fewer postoperative complications (e.g., trismus)
4. Lower aspiration rate (<10%) than with the inferior alveolar nerve block
5. Provides successful anesthesia where a bifid inferior alveolar nerve and bifid mandibular canals are present

Disadvantages
1. Difficult to visualize the path of the needle and the depth of insertion
2. No bony contact; depth of penetration somewhat arbitrary
3. Potentially traumatic if the needle is too close to periosteum

Alternatives. No intraoral nerve blocks are available. If a patient is unable to open his or her mouth because of trauma, infection, or postinjection trismus, there are no other suitable intraoral techniques available. The extraoral mandibular nerve block may be used when the doctor is well versed in the procedure.

Technique
1. A 25-gauge long needle is recommended (although a 27-gauge long may be preferred in patients whose ramus flares laterally more than usual).
2. Area of insertion: soft tissue overlying the medial (lingual) border of the mandibular ramus directly adjacent to the maxillary tuberosity at the height of the mucogingival junction adjacent to the maxillary third molar (Fig. 14-24)
3. Target area: soft tissue on the medial (lingual) border of the ramus in the region of the inferior alveolar, lingual, and mylohyoid nerves as they run inferiorly from the foramen ovale toward the mandibular foramen (the height of injection with the Vazirani-Akinosi being *below* that of the GGMNB but *above* that of the IANB)
4. Landmarks
   a. Mucogingival junction of the maxillary third (or second) molar
   b. Maxillary tuberosity
   c. Coronoid notch on the mandibular ramus
5. Orientation of the bevel (bevel orientation in the closed-mouth mandibular block is *very important*): The bevel must be oriented *away* from the bone of the mandibular ramus (e.g., bevel faces toward the midline)
6. Procedure
   a. Assume the correct position. For either a right or a left Vazirani-Akinosi, a right-handed administrator should sit at the 8 o'clock position *facing* the patient.

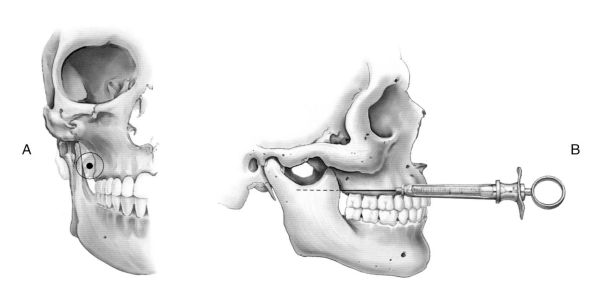

Figure 14-24. A, Area of needle insertion for a Vazirani-Akinosi block. **B,** Hold the syringe and needle at the height of the mucogingival junction above the maxillary third molar. (Redrawn from Gustanis JF, Peterson LJ: An alternative method of mandibular nerve block, *J Am Dent Assoc* 103:33-36, 1981.)

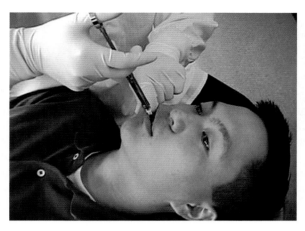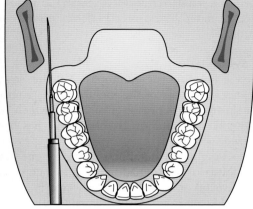

Figure 14-25. Vazirani-Akinosi closed-mouth mandibular nerve block. Barrel of syringe is held parallel to maxillary occlusal plane with needle at level of mucogingival junction of the second or third maxillary molar.

b. Position the patient supine (recommended) or semisupine.

c. Place your left index finger or thumb on the coronoid notch, reflecting the tissues on the medial aspect of the ramus laterally. Reflecting the soft tissues aids in visualization of the injection site and decreases trauma during needle insertion.

d. Visualize landmarks.
   (1) Mucogingival junction of the maxillary third or second molar
   (2) Maxillary tuberosity

e. Prepare the tissues at the site of penetration.
   (1) Dry with sterile gauze.
   (2) Apply topical antiseptic (optional).
   (3) Apply topical anesthetic for minimum of 1 minute.

f. Ask the patient to occlude gently with the cheeks and muscles of mastication relaxed.

g. Reflect the soft tissues on the medial border of the ramus laterally.

h. The barrel of the syringe is held parallel with the maxillary occlusal plane, the needle at the level of the mucogingival junction of the maxillary third (or second) molar (Fig. 14-24).

i. Direct the needle posteriorly and slightly laterally, so it advances at a tangent to the posterior maxillary alveolar process and parallel with the maxillary occlusal plane.

j. Orient the bevel *away* from the mandibular ramus; thus as the needle advances through tissues, needle deflection occurs *toward* the ramus and the needle remains in close proximity to the inferior alveolar nerve (Fig. 14-25).

k. Advance the needle 25 mm into tissue (for an average-sized adult). This distance is measured from the maxillary tuberosity. The tip of the needle should lie in the midportion of the pterygomandibular space, close to the branches of V_3 (Fig. 14-26).

l. Aspirate.

m. If negative, deposit 1.5 to 1.8 ml of anesthetic solution in approximately 60 seconds.

n. Withdraw the syringe slowly and immediately make the needle safe.

o. After the injection, return the patient to an upright or semiupright position.

p. Motor nerve paralysis develops as quickly as or more quickly than sensory anesthesia. The patient with trismus begins to notice increased ability to open the jaws shortly after the deposition of anesthetic.

q. Anesthesia of the lip and tongue is noted in 40 to 90 seconds; the dental procedure usually can start within 5 minutes.

r. When motor paralysis is present but sensory anesthesia is inadequate to permit the dental procedure to begin, readminister the Vazirani-Akinosi block or, because the patient can now open the jaws,

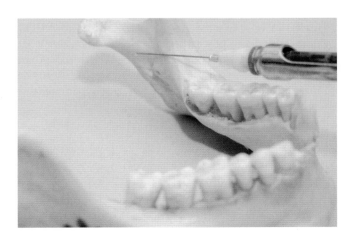

Figure 14-26. Advance the needle posteriorly into tissues on the medial side of the mandibular ramus.

perform the standard inferior alveolar, Gow-Gates, or incisive nerve block, or a PDL or intraosseous injection.

Signs and Symptoms
1. Subjective: Tingling or numbness of the lower lip indicates anesthesia of the mental nerve, a terminal branch of the inferior alveolar nerve, which is a good sign that the inferior alveolar nerve has been anesthetized.
2. Subjective: Tingling or numbness of the tongue indicates anesthesia of the lingual nerve, a branch of the posterior division of the mandibular nerve.
3. Objective: No pain is felt during dental treatment.

Safety Feature. Decreased risk of positive aspiration (compared with the IANB)

Precaution. Do not overinsert the needle (>25 mm). Decrease the depth of penetration in smaller patients; the depth of insertion will vary with the anteroposterior size of the patient's ramus.

Failures of Anesthesia
1. Almost always because of failure to appreciate the flaring nature of the ramus. If the needle is directed medially, it rests medial to the sphenomandibular ligament in the pterygomandibular space, and the injection fails. This is more common when a right-handed administrator uses the left-side Vazirani-Akinosi injection (or a left-handed administrator uses the right-side Vazirani-Akinosi injection). It may be prevented by directing the needle tip parallel with the lateral flare of the ramus and by using a 27-gauge needle in place of a 25-gauge.
2. Needle insertion point too low. To correct: Insert the needle at or slightly above the level of the mucogingival junction of the last maxillary molar. The needle also must remain parallel with the occlusal plane as it advances through the soft tissues.
3. Underinsertion or overinsertion of the needle. Because no bone is contacted in the Vazirani-Akinosi technique, the depth of soft-tissue penetration is somewhat arbitrary. Akinosi recommended a penetration depth of 25 mm in the *average-sized* adult, measuring from the maxillary tuberosity. In smaller or larger patients this depth of penetration should be altered.

Complications
1. Hematoma (<10%)
2. Trismus (rare)
3. Transient facial nerve (VII) paralysis
   a. This is caused by overinsertion and injection of the local anesthetic solution into the body of the parotid gland.
   b. It can be prevented by modifying the depth of needle penetration based on the length of the mandibular ramus. The 25-mm depth of penetration is the average for a normal-sized adult.

MENTAL NERVE BLOCK

The mental nerve is a terminal branch of the inferior alveolar nerve. Exiting the mental foramen at or near the apices of the mandibular premolars, it provides sensory innervation to the buccal soft tissues lying anterior to the foramen and the soft tissues of the lower lip and chin on the side of injection.

For most dental procedures there is very little indication for use of the mental nerve block. Indeed, of the techniques described in this section, the mental nerve block is the least frequently employed. It is used primarily for buccal soft-tissue procedures, such as suturing of lacerations or biopsies. Its success rate approaches 100% because of the ease of accessibility to the nerve.

Other Common Names. None

Nerve Anesthetized. Mental, a terminal branch of the inferior alveolar

Areas Anesthetized. Buccal mucous membranes anterior to the mental foramen (around the second premolar) to the midline and skin of the lower lip (Fig. 14-27) and chin

Indication. When buccal soft-tissue anesthesia is necessary for procedures in the mandible anterior to the mental foramen, such as the following:
1. Soft-tissue biopsies
2. Suturing of soft tissues

Contraindication. Infection or acute inflammation in the area of injection

Advantages
1. High success rate
2. Technically easy
3. Usually entirely atraumatic

Disadvantage. Hematoma

Positive Aspiration. 5.7%

Alternatives
1. Local infiltration
2. Inferior alveolar nerve block
3. Gow-Gates mandibular nerve block
4. Vazirani-Akinosi nerve block

Technique
1. A 25- or 27-gauge short needle is recommended.
2. Area of insertion: mucobuccal fold at or just anterior to the mental foramen

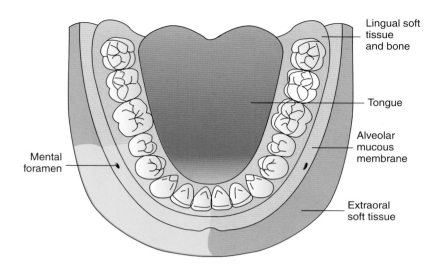

Figure 14-27. Area anesthesized by mental nerve block.

Labels on figure: Lingual soft tissue and bone; Tongue; Alveolar mucous membrane; Extraoral soft tissue; Mental foramen

3. Target area: mental nerve as it exits the mental foramen (usually located between the apices of the first and second premolars)
4. Landmarks: mandibular premolars and mucobuccal fold
5. Orientation of the bevel: *toward* bone during the injection
   a. Assume the correct position.
      (1) For a right or left mental nerve block. a right-handed administrator should sit comfortably in front of the patient so that the syringe may be placed into the mouth below the patient's line of sight (Fig. 14-28).
      (2) The recommended position for this injection has been changed in this edition. Many comments were received from doctors using this injection mentioning that the "old" position of

choice—sitting behind the patient—was psychologically traumatic for the patient. The syringe was always in the patient's line of sight (Fig. 14-29).
   b. Position the patient.
      (1) Supine is recommended, but semisupine is acceptable.
      (2) Have the patient partially close. This permits greater access to the injection site.
   c. Locate the mental foramen.
      (1) Place your index finger in the mucobuccal fold and press against the body of the mandible in the first molar area.
      (2) Move your finger slowly anteriorly until the bone beneath your finger feels irregular and somewhat concave (Fig. 14-30).

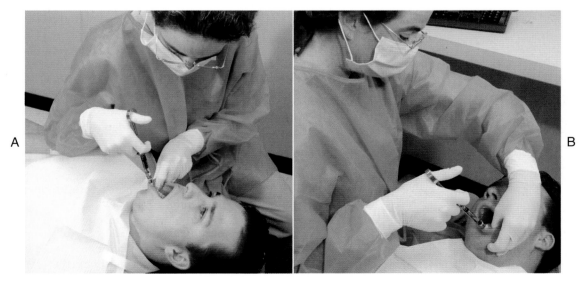

A   B

Figure 14-28. Position of the administrator for a right, **A,** and, **B,** left mental/incisive nerve block.

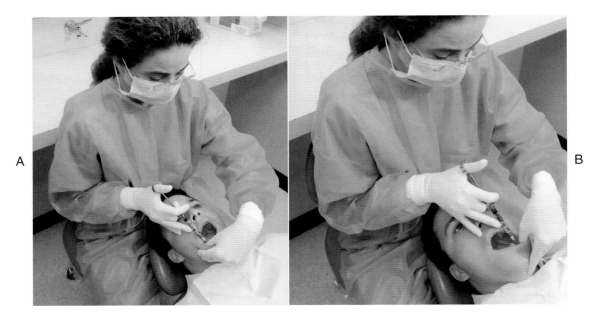

Figure 14-29. Sitting position behind patient keeps syringe in line of sight during, **A,** right and, **B,** left mental/incisive nerve block.

(a) The bone posterior and anterior to the mental foramen is smooth; however, the bone immediately around the foramen is rougher to the touch.

(b) The mental foramen usually is found around the apex of the second premolar. However, it may be found either anterior or posterior to this site.

(c) The patient may comment that finger pressure in this area produces soreness as the mental nerve is compressed against bone.

(3) If radiographs are available, the mental foramen may be located easily (Fig. 14-31).

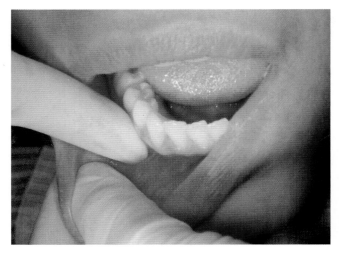

Figure 14-30. Locate the mental foramen by moving the fleshy pad of your finger anteriorly until the bone beneath becomes irregular and somewhat concave.

d. Prepare tissue at the site of penetration.
   (1) Dry with sterile gauze.
   (2) Apply topical antiseptic (optional).
   (3) Apply topical anesthetic for minimum of 1 minute.

e. With your left index finger pull the lower lip and buccal soft tissues laterally.
   (1) Visibility is improved.
   (2) Taut tissues permit an atraumatic penetration.

f. Orient the syringe with the bevel directed *toward* bone.

g. Penetrate the mucous membrane at the injection site, at the canine or first premolar, directing the syringe toward the mental foramen (Fig. 14-32).

h. Advance the needle slowly until the foramen is reached. The depth of penetration is 5 to 6 mm. For the mental nerve block to be successful there is no need to enter the mental foramen.

i. Aspirate.

j. If negative, slowly deposit 0.6 ml (approximately one third cartridge) over 20 seconds. If tissue at the injection site balloons (swells as the anesthetic is injected), stop the deposition and remove the syringe.

k. Withdraw the syringe and immediately make the needle safe.
   (1) Wait 2 to 3 minutes before commencing the procedure.

Signs and Symptoms
1. Subjective: Tingling or numbness of the lower lip
2. Objective: No pain during treatment

Safety Feature. The region is anatomically "safe."

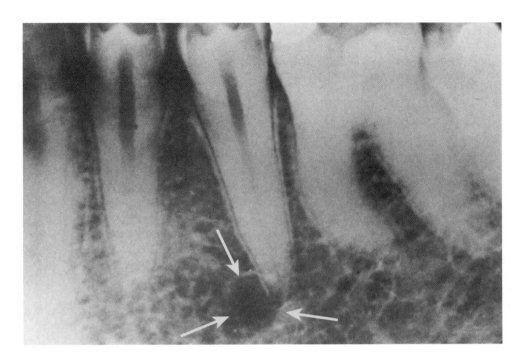

Figure 14-31. Radiographs can assist in locating the mental foramen *(arrows)*. (Courtesy of Dr. Robert Ziehm.)

Precautions. Striking the periosteum produces discomfort. To prevent: Avoid contact with the periosteum *or* deposit a small amount of solution before contacting the periosteum.

Failures of Anesthesia. Rare with the mental nerve block

Complications
1. Few of consequence
2. Hematoma (bluish discoloration and tissue swelling at the injection site). Blood may exit the needle puncture point into the buccal fold. To treat: Apply pressure with gauze directly to the area of bleeding for at least 2 minutes (see Fig. 17-2).

INCISIVE NERVE BLOCK

The incisive nerve is a terminal branch of the inferior alveolar nerve. Originating as a direct continuation of the inferior alveolar nerve at the mental foramen, the incisive nerve continues anteriorly in the incisive canal, providing sensory innervation to those teeth located anterior to the mental foramen. The nerve is always anesthetized when an inferior alveolar or mandibular nerve block is successful; therefore the incisive nerve block is not necessary when these blocks are administered.

The premolars, canine, and lateral and central incisors, including their buccal soft tissues and bone, are anesthetized when the incisive nerve block is administered.*

An important indication for the incisive nerve block is when the contemplated procedure involves both the right and left sides of the mandible. It is believed that bilateral inferior alveolar or mandibular nerve blocks are rarely needed (except in the case of bilateral surgical procedures in the mandible) because of the degree of discomfort and the inconvenience experienced by the patient both during and after the procedure. Where dental treatment involves bilateral procedures on mandibular premolars and anterior teeth, bilateral incisive nerve blocks can be administered. Pulpal, buccal soft-tissue, and bone anesthesia is readily obtained. Lingual

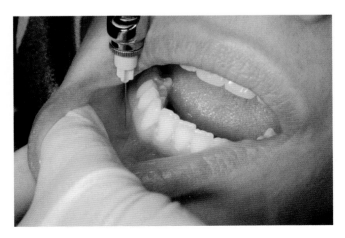

Figure 14-32. Mental nerve block—needle penetration site.

*The second premolar may not be anesthestized with this technique if the mental foramen lies beneath the first premolar.

soft tissues are *not* anesthetized with this block. If lingual soft tissues in very isolated areas require anesthesia, local infiltration can be accomplished readily by inserting a 27-gauge short needle through the interdental papilla on *both the mesial and distal aspect on the tooth being treated.* Because the buccal soft tissues are already anesthetized (incisive nerve block), the penetration is atraumatic. Local anesthetic solution should be deposited as the needle is advanced through the tissue toward the lingual (Fig. 14-33). This technique provides lingual soft-tissue anesthesia adequate for deep curettage, root planing, and subgingival preparations. Where there is a significant requirement for lingual soft-tissue anesthesia, an inferior alveolar or mandibular nerve block should be administered on that side, with the incisive nerve block administered on the contralateral side. In this manner the patient does not have to endure bilateral anesthesia of the tongue, which is a very disconcerting experience for many patients.

Another method of obtaining lingual anesthesia after the incisive nerve block is to administer a partial lingual nerve block (Fig. 14-34). Using a 25-gauge long needle, deposit 0.3 to 0.6 ml of local anesthetic under the lingual mucosa just distal to the last tooth to be treated. This provides lingual soft-tissue anesthesia adequate for any dental procedure in this area.

It is not necessary for the needle to enter into the mental foramen for an incisive nerve block to be successful. The first edition of this book and other textbooks of local anesthesia for dentistry recommended insertion of the needle into the foramen.[11,14,15] There are at least two disadvantages to the needle entering into the mental foramen: (1) the administration of an incisive nerve block becomes technically more difficult and (2) the risk of traumatizing the mental or incisive nerves and their associated blood vessels is increased. As described in the following, for the incisive nerve block to be successful the anesthetic should be deposited

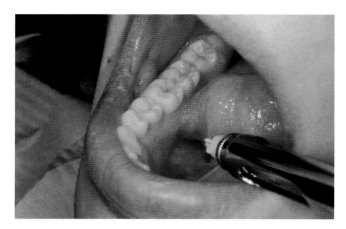

Figure 14-34. Retract the tongue to gain access to, and increase the visibility of, the lingual border of the mandible.

just outside the mental foramen and, under pressure, directed into the foramen. Indeed, the incisive nerve block may be considered the mandibular equivalent of the anterior superior alveolar nerve block, with the mental nerve block the equivalent of the infraorbital nerve block. Both of the disadvantages just mentioned are minimized by not entering into the mental foramen.

Other Common Name. Mental nerve block (inappropriate)

Nerves Anesthetized. Mental and incisive

Areas Anesthetized. (Fig. 14-35)
1. Buccal mucous membrane anterior to the mental foramen, usually from the second premolar to the midline
2. Lower lip and skin of the chin
3. Pulpal nerve fibers to the premolars, canine, and incisors

Indications
1. Dental procedures requiring pulpal anesthesia on mandibular teeth anterior to the mental foramen
2. When IANB is not indicated
   a. When six, eight, or ten anterior teeth (e.g., canine to canine or premolar to premolar) are treated, the incisive nerve block is recommended in place of bilateral IANBs.

Contraindication. Infection or acute inflammation in the area of injection

Advantages
1. Provides pulpal and hard tissue anesthesia *without* lingual anesthesia (which is uncomfortable and unnecessary for many patients); useful in place of bilateral IANBs
2. High success rate

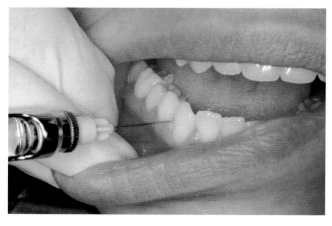

Figure 14-33. To obtain lingual anesthesia, after the incisive nerve block, insert needle interproximally from buccal and deposit anesthetic as the needle is advanced toward lingual.

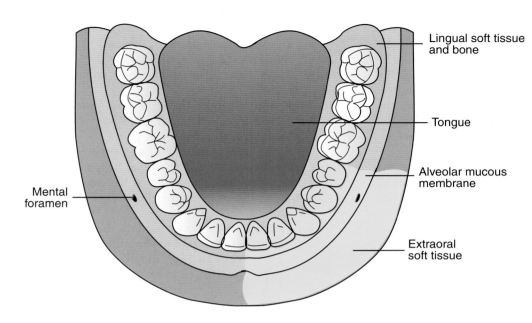

Figure 14-35. Area anesthetized by an incisive nerve block.

Disadvantages
1. Does not provide lingual anesthesia. The lingual tissues must be injected directly if anesthesia is desired.
2. Partial anesthesia may develop at the midline because of nerve fiber overlap with the opposite side (extremely rare). Local infiltration on the buccal of the mandibular central incisors may be necessary for complete pulpal anesthesia to be obtained.

Positive Aspiration. 5.7%

Alternatives
1. Local infiltration for buccal soft tissues and pulpal anesthesia of the central and lateral incisors
2. Inferior alveolar nerve block
3. Gow-Gates mandibular nerve block
4. Vazirani-Akinosi mandibular nerve block
5. Periodontal ligament injection

Technique
1. A 25-gauge short needle is recommended (although a 27-gauge short is more commonly used and is perfectly acceptable).
2. Area of insertion: mucobuccal fold at or just anterior to the mental foramen
3. Target area: mental foramen, through which the mental nerve exits and inside of which the incisive nerve is located
4. Landmarks: mandibular premolars and mucobuccal fold
5. Orientation of the bevel: *toward* bone during the injection
6. Procedure
   a. Assume the correct position.
      (1) For a right or left incisive nerve block and a right-handed administrator, sit comfortably in front of the patient so that the syringe may be placed into the mouth below the patient's line of sight (see Fig. 14-28).
      (2) The recommended position for this injection has been changed in this edition. Many comments were received from doctors using this injection mentioning that the "old" position of choice—sitting behind the patient—was psychologically traumatic for the patient. The syringe was always in the patient's line of sight (see Fig. 14-29).
   b. Position the patient.
      (1) Supine is recommended, but semisupine is acceptable.
      (2) Request that the patient partially close; this will permit greater access to the injection site.
   c. Locate the mental foramen.

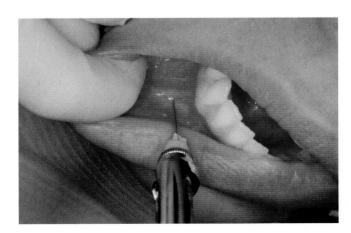

Figure 14-36. Retract the lip to improve access and permit atraumatic needle insertion.

(1) Place your thumb or index finger in the mucobuccal fold against the body of the mandible in the first molar area.

(2) Move it slowly anteriorly until you feel the bone become irregular and somewhat concave.

   (a) The bone posterior and anterior to the mental foramen feels smooth; however, the bone immediately around the foramen feels rougher to the touch.

   (b) The mental foramen is usually found at the apex of the second molar. However, it may be found either anterior or posterior to this site.

   (c) The patient may comment that finger pressure in this area produces soreness as the mental nerve is compressed against bone.

(3) If radiographs are available, the mental foramen may be located easily (see Fig. 14-31).

d. Prepare tissues at the site of penetration.

   (1) Dry with sterile gauze.

   (2) Apply topical antiseptic (optional).

   (3) Apply topical anesthetic for minimum of 1 minute.

e. With your left index finger pull the lower lip and buccal soft tissue laterally (Fig. 14-36).

   (1) Visibility is improved.

   (2) Taut tissues permit atraumatic penetration.

f. Orient the syringe with the bevel *toward* bone.

g. Penetrate mucous membrane at the canine or first premolar, directing the needle toward the mental foramen.

h. Advance the needle slowly until the mental foramen is reached. The depth of penetration is 5 to 6 mm. There is no need to enter the mental foramen for the incisive nerve block to be successful.

TABLE **14-1**
Mandibular Teeth and Available Local Anesthetic Techniques

Teeth	Pulpal	Soft-Tissue	
		Buccal	**Lingual**
Incisors	Incisive (Inc)	IANB	IANB
	Inferior alveolar (IANB)	GG	GG
	Gow-Gates (GG)	VA	VA
	Vazirani-Akinosi (VA)	Inc	PDL
	Periodontal ligament (PDL) injection	IS	IS
	Intraseptal (IS)	Mental	Inf
	Intraosseous (IO)	PDL	IO
	Infiltration (lateral incisor only)	Inf	
		IO	
Canines	Inferior alveolar	IANB	IANB
	Gow-Gates	GG	GG
	Vazirani-Akinosi	VA	VA
	Incisive	Inc	PDL
	Periodontal ligament injection	PDL	IS
	Intraseptal	IS	Inf
	Intraosseous	IO	IO
		Inf	
		Mental	
Premolars	Inferior alveolar	IANB	IANB
	Gow-Gates	GG	GG
	Vazirani-Akinosi	VA	VA
	Incisive	Inc	PDL
	Periodontal ligament injection	PDL	IS
	Intraseptal	IS	IO
	Intraosseous	IO	Inf
		Mental	
		Inf	
Molars	Inferior alveolar	IANB	IANB
	Gow-Gates	GG	GG
	Vazirani-Akinosi	VA	VA
	Periodontal ligament injection	PDL	PDL
	Intraseptal	IS	IS
	Intraosseous	IO	IO
		Inf	Inf

TABLE 14-2
Recommended Volumes of Local Anesthetic Solution for Mandibular Injection Techniques

Technique	Volume (ml)
Inferior alveolar	1.5
Buccal	0.3
Gow-Gates	1.8
Vazirani-Akinosi	1.5 to 1.8
Mental	0.6
Incisive	0.6 to 0.9

i. Aspirate.
j. If negative, slowly deposit 0.6 ml (approximately one third of a cartridge) over 20 seconds.
   (1) During the injection, maintain gentle finger pressure directly over the injection site to increase the volume of solution entering into the mental foramen. This may be accomplished with either intraoral or extraoral pressure.
   (2) Tissues at the injection site should balloon, but very slightly.
k. Withdraw the syringe and immediately make the needle safe.
l. Continue to apply pressure at the injection site for 2 minutes.
m. Wait 3 to 5 minutes before commencing the dental procedure.
   (1) Anesthesia of the mental nerve (lower lip, buccal soft tissues) is observed within seconds of the deposition.
   (2) Anesthesia of the incisive nerve requires additional time.

Signs and Symptoms
1. Subjective: Tingling or numbness of the lower lip
2. Objective: No pain during dental therapy

Safety Feature. Anatomically "safe" region

Precaution. Usually an atraumatic injection unless the needle contacts periosteum or solution is deposited too rapidly

Failures of Anesthesia
1. Inadequate volume of anesthetic solution in the mental foramen, with subsequent lack of pulpal anesthesia. To correct: Reinject into the proper region and apply pressure to the injection site.
2. Inadequate duration of pressure after injection. It is necessary to apply firm pressure over the injection site for a minimum of 2 minutes to force the local anesthetic into the mental foramen and provide anesthesia of the second premolar, which may be *distal* to the foramen. Failure to achieve anesthesia of the second premolar is

usually caused by inadequate application of pressure after the injection.

Complications
1. Few of any consequence
2. Hematoma (bluish discoloration and tissue swelling at injection site). Blood may exit the needle puncture site into the buccal fold. To treat: Apply pressure with gauze directly to the area for 2 minutes. This is rarely a problem, because proper incisive nerve block protocol includes the application of pressure at the injection site for 2 minutes.

• • •

Table 14-1 summarizes the various injection techniques applicable for mandibular teeth. Table 14-2 summarizes the recommended volumes for the various injection techniques.

REFERENCES

1. Kaufman E, Weinstein P, Milgrom P: Difficulties in achieving local anesthesia, *J Am Dent Assoc* 108:205-208, 1984.
2. Malamed SF: Unpublished clinical surveys at University of Southern California School of Dentistry, 1995.
3. Wilson S, Johns PI, Fuller PM: The inferior alveolar and mylohyoid nerves: an anatomic study and relationship to local anesthesia of the anterior mandibular teeth, *J Am Dent Assoc* 108:350-352, 1984.
4. Frommer J, Mele FA, Monroe CW: The possible role of the mylohyoid nerve in mandibular posterior tooth sensation, *J Am Dent Assoc* 85:113-117, 1972.
5. Roda RS, Blanton PL: The anatomy of local anesthesia, *Quint Intern* 25(1):27-38, 1994.
6. Gow-Gates GAE: Mandibular conduction anesthesia: a new technique using extraoral landmarks, *Oral Surg* 36:321-328, 1973.
7. Malamed SF: The Gow-Gates mandibular block: evaluation after 4275 cases, *Oral Surg* 51:463, 1981.
8. Fish LR, McIntire DN, Johnson L: Temporary paralysis of cranial nerves III, IV, and VI after a Gow-Gates injection, *J Am Dent Assoc* 119:127-130, 1989.
9. Akinosi JO: A new approach to the mandibular nerve block, *Br J Oral Surg* 15:83-87, 1977.
10. Murphy TM: Somatic blockade. In Cousins MJ, Bridenbaugh PO, editors: *Neural blockade in clinical anesthesia and management of pain*, Philadelphia, 1980, JB Lippincott.
11. Bennett CR: *Monheim's local anesthesia and pain control in dental practice*, ed 6, St Louis, 1978, Mosby.
12. Vazirani SJ: Closed mouth mandibular nerve block: a new technique, *Dent Dig* 66:10-13, 1960.
13. Wolfe SH: The Wolfe nerve block: a modified high mandibular nerve block, *Dent Today* 11:34-37, 1992.
14. Malamed SF: *Handbook of local anesthesia*, St Louis, 1980, Mosby.
15. Jastak JT, Yagiela JA, Donaldson D: *Local anesthesia of the oral cavity*, Philadelphia, 1995, WB Saunders.

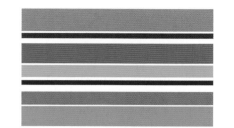

Supplemental Injection Techniques

CHAPTER
15

In this chapter a number of injections are described that are used in specialized clinical situations. Some may be used as the sole technique for pain control for certain types of dental treatment. For example, the periodontal ligament (PDL) injection, intraseptal, and intraosseous (IO) techniques provide effective pulpal anesthesia without the need for other injections. On the other hand, use of the intrapulpal injection is almost always reserved for situations in which other injection techniques have failed or are contraindicated for use. The PDL, intraseptal, and IO injections also are frequently used to supplement failed or only partially successful traditional injection techniques.

INTRAOSSEOUS ANESTHESIA

IO anesthesia involves the deposition of local anesthetic solution into the cancellous bone that supports the teeth. Although not new (IO anesthesia dates back to the early 1900s), a resurgence of interest in this technique in dentistry has taken place over the past 15 years.[1-5] Three techniques are discussed, two of which—the PDL injection and the intraseptal injection—are modifications of traditional IO anesthesia.

Periodontal Ligament Injection

Because of the thickness of the cortical plate of bone it is not possible to achieve profound pulpal anesthesia on a solitary tooth in the adult mandible with the techniques described in Chapter 14. On rare occasion, a supraperiosteal injection in the apical region of a mandibular lateral incisor provides pulpal anesthesia. However, a regional nerve block must be administered to obtain pulpal anesthesia in other regions of the mandible. An old technique has been repopularized. The PDL injection

(also known as the *intraligamentary injection* [ILI]), was originally described as the *peridental injection* in local anesthesia textbooks dating from 1912 to 1923.[6,7]

The peridental injection was not well received in those early years because it was claimed that the risk of producing blood-borne infection and septicemia was too great to warrant its use in patients. The technique never became popular but was used clinically by many doctors, although it was not referred to as the peridental technique. In clinical situations in which an inferior alveolar nerve block failed to provide adequate pulpal anesthesia to the first molar (usually its mesial root), the doctor inserted a needle along the long axis of the mesial root as far apically as possible and deposited a small volume of local anesthetic solution under pressure. This invariably provided effective pain control.

It was not until the early 1980s that the intraligamentary or PDL injection regained popularity. Credit for its increased interest must go to the manufacturers of syringe devices designed to make the injection easier to administer. These original devices, the Peripress and Ligmaject (Fig. 15-1), provide a mechanical advantage that allows the administrator to deposit the anesthetic more easily (and sometimes too easily). They appear similar to the Wilcox-Jewett Obtunder (Fig. 15-2), which was widely advertised to the dental profession in a 1905 catalog, *Dental Furniture, Instruments, and Materials*, perhaps reconfirming the adage that there is "nothing new under the sun."[8]

Why has the PDL (née peridental) injection enjoyed a renewal of popularity? Perhaps it is because the primary thrust of the advertising for the new syringes focused on being able to "avoid the mandibular block" injection with the PDL or intraligamentary technique; a concept to which the dental profession is receptive, given the fact that virtually all dentists have experienced periods when they have been unable to achieve adequate anesthesia with the inferior alveolar nerve block (a "mandibular slump").

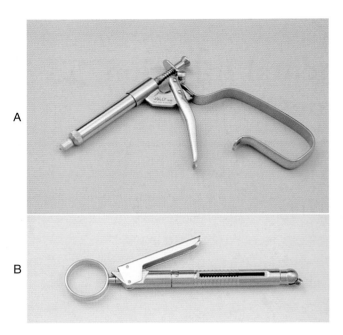

Figure 15-1. A, Original pressure syringe designed for a periodontal ligament or intraligamentary injection. **B,** Second-generation syringe for a periodontal ligament injection.

The PDL injection also may be used successfully in the maxillary arch; however, with the ready availability of other highly effective and atraumatic techniques, such as the supraperiosteal (infiltration) injection, and drugs such as articaine HCl to provide single-tooth pulpal anesthesia, there has been little compelling reason for use of the PDL in the upper jaw (although there is absolutely no other reason not to recommend it in this area). Possibly the greatest potential benefit of the PDL injection lies in the fact that it provides pulpal and soft-tissue anesthesia in a localized area (one tooth) of the mandible without producing extensive soft-tissue (e.g., tongue and lower lip) anesthesia as well. Virtually all dental patients prefer this technique to any of the "mandibular nerve blocks." In a clinical trial, Malamed reported that 74% of patients preferred the PDL injection primarily because of its lack

THE WILCOX-JEWETT OBTUNDER.

Lee S. Smith & Son, Pittsburg.

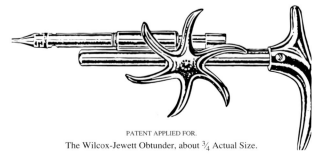

PATENT APPLIED FOR.
The Wilcox-Jewett Obtunder, about ¾ Actual Size.

Figure 15-2. Pressure syringe (1905) designed for a peridental injection.

of lingual and labial soft-tissue anesthesia.[9] It is interesting that those preferring the inferior alveolar nerve block did so for an important reason: with the inferior alveolar nerve block (IANB), once the lip and tongue became numb, patients were able to relax, knowing that the remainder of the dental treatment would not hurt. Without lingual and labial soft-tissue anesthesia in the PDL technique, they were unable to fully relax because they were not certain they had been adequately anesthetized.

Primary indications for the PDL injection include: (1) the need for anesthesia of but one or two mandibular teeth in a quadrant; (2) treatment of isolated teeth in both mandibular quadrants (to avoid bilateral inferior alveolar nerve block); (3) treatment of children (because residual soft-tissue anesthesia increases the risk of self-mutilation); (4) treatment in which nerve block anesthesia is contraindicated (e.g., in hemophiliacs); and (5) its use as a possible aid in the diagnosis (e.g., localization) of mandibular pain.

Contraindications to the PDL injection include infection or severe inflammation at the injection site, and primary teeth. Brannstrom and associates reported the development of enamel hypoplasia or hypomineralization or both in 15 permanent teeth after the administration of the periodontal ligament injection.[10] Fortunately there is little need for this technique in the primary dentition; other techniques, such as infiltration and nerve blocks, are effective and easy to administer.

Several concerns have been expressed about this technique, most of which were addressed in a status report on the PDL injection in the *Journal of the American Dental Association*.[11] Two concerns were: (1) the effect of the injection and deposition of the local anesthetic under pressure into the confined space of the PDL; and (2) the effect of the drug or vasoconstrictor on pulpal tissues. Walton and Garnick concluded that the PDL injection (administered with a conventional syringe) causes slight damage to tissues in the region of needle penetration only.[12] Apical areas appeared normal; the epithelial and connective tissue attachment to enamel and cementum was not disturbed by the needle puncture; slight resorption of nonvital bone occurred in the crestal regions, forming a wedge-shaped defect; soft-tissue damage was minimal; the disruption of tissue that did occur showed repair in 25 days, with absence of inflammation, and with the formation of new bone in the regions of resorption; the injection of the solution was not in itself damaging. Damage produced by needle penetration alone (no drug administered) appeared similar to that seen when a drug also had been deposited. The authors concluded that the PDL injection is safe to the periodontium.[12] In addition, there is no evidence to date that the inclusion of a vasoconstrictor in the local anesthetic solution has any detrimental effect on pulpal microcirculation after the PDL injection.

It appears that the mechanism whereby the local anesthetic solution reaches the periapical tissues with the

PDL injection is diffused apically and into the marrow spaces surrounding the teeth. The solution is not forced apically through the periodontal tissues, a procedure that might lead (as Nelson reported) to avulsion of a tooth (premolar) because of the increased hydrostatic pressure being exerted in a confined space.[13] Therefore the PDL injection appears to produce anesthesia in much the same way as the IO and intraseptal injections, by diffusion of anesthetic solution apically through marrow spaces in the intraseptal bone (Fig. 15-3).[14,15]

Postinjection complications are also of concern with the PDL injection. Reported complications have included mild to severe postoperative discomfort, swelling and discoloration of soft tissues at the injection site, and prolonged ischemia of the interdental papilla followed by sloughing and exposure of crestal bone.[16,17] Some of these complications result directly from poor operator technique, lack of familiarity with the pressure syringe, and injection of excessive volumes of local anesthetic into the PDL. The most frequently voiced postinjection complications are mild discomfort and sensitivity to biting and percussion for 2 or 3 days. The most common causes of postinjection discomfort are: (1) too rapid injection (producing edema and slight extrusion of the tooth, thus sensitivity on biting); and (2) injection of excessive volumes of local anesthetic into the site.

Before the PDL technique is described, it must be mentioned that although "special" PDL syringes can be used effectively and safely, usually there is no need for them. A conventional local anesthetic syringe is equally effective in providing PDL anesthesia. The use of a conventional syringe requires that the administrator apply significant force to deposit the local anesthetic into the periodontal tissues. Virtually all doctors and most hygienists are able to produce PDL anesthesia successfully without a special PDL syringe. Only when a doctor or hygienist is unable to achieve adequate PDL anesthesia with a conventional syringe is use of a PDL syringe recommended.

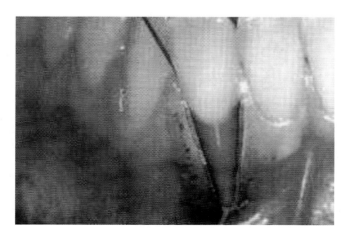

Figure 15-3. Periodontal ligament injection is intraosseous. Note dispersion of ink into surrounding bone.

Arguments against using the conventional syringe for PDL injections (and my rebuttals) include the following:

1. It is too difficult to administer the solution with a conventional syringe.
   Comment: Slow administration of the local anesthetic makes the PDL injection atraumatic. Improper use (fast injection) of the PDL syringe produces both immediate and postinjection pain.
2. The extreme pressure applied to the glass may shatter the cartridge. The PDL syringes provide a metal or plastic covering for the glass cartridge, thereby protecting the patient from shards of glass should the cartridge shatter during injection.
   Comment: Although I have read and heard of cartridges shattering during PDL injection, I have yet to experience this personally. However, there are several ways to minimize the risk: Because only small volumes of solution are injected (0.2 ml per root), a full, 1.8-ml cartridge is not necessary. Eliminate all but about 0.6 ml of solution before starting the PDL injection. This minimizes the area of glass being subjected to the increased pressures, decreasing the risk of breakage. In addition, glass cartridges have a thin Mylar plastic label that covers most or all of the glass. If a cartridge breaks, the glass will not shatter but will be contained by the plastic covering. A piece of transparent adhesive tape also might be placed over the exposed glass portions of the metal or plastic syringe.
3. Many manufacturers of PDL syringes recommend use of 30-gauge short or ultrashort needles in this technique.
   Comment: In my early experience with the PDL technique, I used the 30-gauge needle only to find that whenever pressure was applied to it (as in pushing it apically into the PDL) the 30-gauge needle bent easily. It was too fragile to withstand pressure without bending. PDL injection failure rates were excessive. A 30-gauge ultrashort needle was manufactured specifically for use with this injection technique (10-mm length). Although somewhat more effective than the 30-gauge short, there was no need to use a "special" needle for this injection. I have had great clinical success, with no increase in patient discomfort, using the more readily available 27-gauge short needle.

In summary, the PDL injection is an important component of the armamentarium of local anesthetic techniques for providing mandibular and, to a lesser degree, maxillary pain control.

Other Common Names. Peridental (original name) injection, intraligamentary injection (ILI)

Nerves Anesthetized. Terminal nerve endings at the site of injection and at the apex of the tooth

Areas Anesthetized. Bone, soft tissue, and apical and pulpal tissues in the area of injection (Fig. 15-4)

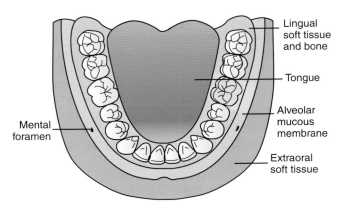

Figure 15-4. Area anesthetized by a periodontal ligament injection.

Indications
1. Pulpal anesthesia of one or two teeth in a quadrant
2. Treatment of isolated teeth in two mandibular quadrants (to avoid bilateral IANB)
3. Patients for whom residual soft-tissue anesthesia is undesirable
4. Situations in which regional block anesthesia is contraindicated
5. As a possible aid in diagnosis of pulpal discomfort
6. As an adjunctive technique after nerve block anesthesia if partial anesthesia is present

Contraindications
1. Infection or inflammation at the site of injection
2. Primary teeth, when the permanent tooth bud is present[10]
   a. Enamel hypoplasia has been reported to occur in a developing permanent tooth when a PDL injection was administered to the primary tooth above it.
   b. There appears to be little reason for use of the PDL technique in primary teeth because infiltration anesthesia and the incisive nerve block are effective in primary dentition.
3. Patient who requires a "numb" sensation for psychological comfort

Advantages
1. Prevents anesthesia of the lip, tongue, and other soft tissues, thus facilitating treatment in multiple quadrants during a single appointment
2. Minimum dose of local anesthetic necessary to achieve anesthesia (0.2 ml per root)
3. An alternative to partially successful regional nerve block anesthesia
4. Rapid onset of profound pulpal and soft-tissue anesthesia (30 seconds)
5. Less traumatic than conventional block injections
6. Well suited for procedures in children, extractions, and periodontal and endodontic single-tooth and multiple quadrant procedures

Disadvantages
1. Proper needle placement is difficult to achieve in some areas (e.g., distal of the second or third molar).
2. Leakage of local anesthetic solution into the patient's mouth produces an unpleasant taste.
3. Excessive pressure or overly rapid injection may break the glass cartridge.
4. A special syringe may be necessary.
5. Excessive pressure can produce focal tissue damage.
6. Postinjection discomfort may persist for several days.
7. The potential for extrusion of a tooth exists if excessive pressure or volumes are used.

Positive Aspiration. 0%

Alternative. Supraperiosteal injection (entire maxilla and the mandibular lateral incisor region)

Technique
1. A 27-gauge short needle is recommended.
2. Area of insertion: long axis of the tooth to be treated on its mesial or distal of the root (one-rooted tooth) or on the mesial and distal roots (of multirooted tooth) interproximally (Fig. 15-5)
3. Target area: depth of the gingival sulcus
4. Landmarks
   a. Root(s) of the tooth
   b. Periodontal tissues

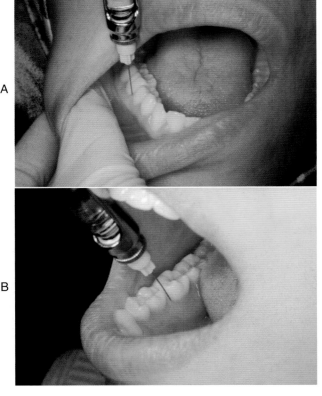

Figure 15-5. Area of insertion for a periodontal ligament injection. **A,** Buccal. **B,** Lingual.

5. Orientation of the bevel: Although not significant to success of the technique, it is recommended that the bevel of the needle face toward the root to permit easy advancement of the needle in an apical direction.
6. Procedure
   a. Assume the correct position. (This varies significantly with PDL injections on different teeth.) Sit comfortably, have adequate visibility of the injection site, and maintain control over the needle. It may be necessary to bend the needle to achieve proper angle, especially on the distal aspects of second and third molars.*
   b. Position the patient supine or semisupine, with the head turned to maximize access and visibility.
   c. Stabilize the syringe and direct it along the long axis of the root to be anesthetized.
      (1) The bevel faces the root of the tooth.
      (2) If interproximal contacts are tight, the syringe should be directed from either the lingual or buccal surface of the tooth but maintained as close to the long axis as possible.
      (3) Stabilize the syringe and your hand against the patient's teeth, lips, or face.
   d. With the bevel of the needle on the root, advance the needle apically until resistance is met.
   e. Deposit 0.2 ml of local anesthetic solution in a minimum of 20 seconds.
      (1) When using a conventional syringe, notice that the thickness of the rubber stopper in the local anesthetic cartridge is equal to 0.2 ml of solution. This may be used as a gauge for the volume of local anesthetic administration.
      (2) With the PDL syringe, each squeeze of the "trigger" provides a dose of 0.2 ml.
   f. There are two important indicators of success of the injection:
      (1) Significant resistance to the deposition of the local anesthetic solution
         (a) This is especially noticeable when the conventional syringe is used; resistance is similar to that felt with the nasopalatine injection.
         (b) The local anesthetic should not flow back into the patient's mouth. If this happens, repeat the injection at the same site but from a different angle. Two tenths of a milliliter of solution must be deposited and must remain within the tissues for the PDL to be effective.

      (2) Ischemia of the soft tissues adjacent to the injection site. (This is noted with all local anesthetic solutions but is more prominent with vasoconstrictor-containing local anesthetics.)
   g. If the tooth has only one root, remove the syringe from the tissue and cap the needle. Dental treatment usually may start within 30 seconds.
   h. If the tooth is multirooted, remove the needle and repeat the procedure on the other root(s).

Signs and Symptoms
1. Subjective and objective: There are no signs that absolutely assure adequate anesthesia; the anesthetized area is too circumscribed. When the following two signs are present, there is an excellent chance that profound anesthesia is present:
   a. Ischemia of soft tissues at the injection site
   b. Resistance to injection of solution

Safety Feature. Intravascular injection is extremely unlikely to occur.

Precautions
1. Keep the needle against the tooth to prevent overinsertion into soft tissues on the lingual aspect.
2. Do not inject too rapidly (minimum 20 seconds for 0.2 ml).
3. Do not inject too much solution (0.2 ml per root retained within tissues).
4. Do not inject directly into infected or highly inflamed tissues.

Failures of Anesthesia
1. Infected or inflamed tissues. The pH and vascularity changes at the apex and periodontal tissues minimize the effectiveness of the local anesthetic.
2. Solution not retained. In this case, remove the needle and reenter at a different site(s) until 0.2 ml of local anesthetic is deposited and retained in the tissues.
3. Each root must be anesthetized with 0.2 ml of solution.

Complications
1. Pain during insertion of the needle
   Cause #1: The needle tip is in soft tissues. *Correction:* Keep the needle against tooth structure.
   Cause #2: The tissues are inflamed. *Correction:* Avoid use of the PDL technique or apply a small amount of topical anesthetic for a minimum of 1 minute before injection.
2. Pain during injection of solution
   Cause: Too rapid injection of local anesthetic solution. *Correction:* Slow down the rate of injection to a minimum 20 seconds for a 0.2-ml solution regardless of the syringe being used.
3. Postinjection pain
   Cause: Too rapid injection, excessive volume of solution, too many tissue penetrations (the patient usually

---

*Although the author dislikes bending needles for most injections, it may become necessary for the success of the PDL and intrapulpal injections to bend the needle to gain access to certain areas of the oral cavity. Because the needle does not enter into tissues more than a few millimeters, bending it is not as risk-prone as when the needle enters more completely into tissues.

complains of soreness and premature contact when occluding). *Correction:* Manage symptomatically with warm saline rinses and mild analgesics, if necessary (usually resolves within 2 to 3 days).

Duration of Expected Anesthesia. The duration of pulpal anesthesia obtained with a successful PDL injection is extremely variable and not related to the drug administered. Administration of lidocaine with 1:100,000 epinephrine, for example, provides pulpal anesthesia ranging in duration from 5 to 55 minutes. The PDL injection may be repeated if necessary to permit the completion of the dental procedure. It appears that the volume of anesthetic solution used with the PDL is too small to provide the usually expected duration of anesthesia of the drug.

• • •

Intraseptal Injection

The intraseptal injection is similar in technique and design to the PDL injection. It is included for discussion because it is useful in providing osseous and soft-tissue anesthesia and hemostasis for periodontal curettage and surgical flap procedures. In addition, it may be effective when the condition of the periodontal tissues in the gingival sulci precludes use of the PDL injection (e.g., infection or acute inflammation). Saadoun and Malamed have shown that the path of diffusion of the anesthetic solution is through the medullary bone, as in the PDL injection.[19]

Other Common Names. None

Nerves Anesthetized. Terminal nerve endings at the site of injection and in the adjacent soft and hard tissues

Areas Anesthetized. Bone, soft tissue, root structure in the area of injection (Fig. 15-6)

Indication. When both pain control and hemostasis are desired for soft-tissue and osseous periodontal treatment

Contraindication. Infection or severe inflammation at the injection site

Advantages
1. Lack of lip and tongue anesthesia (appreciated by most patients)
2. Minimum volumes of local anesthetic necessary
3. Minimized bleeding during the surgical procedure
4. Atraumatic
5. Immediate (<30-second) onset of action
6. Few postoperative complications
7. Useful on periodontally involved teeth (avoids infected pockets)

Disadvantages
1. Multiple tissue punctures may be necessary
2. Bitter taste of the anesthetic drug (if leakage occurs)
3. Short duration of pulpal anesthesia; limited area of soft-tissue anesthesia (may necessitate reinjection)
4. Clinical experience necessary for success

Positive Aspiration. 0%

Alternatives
1. PDL injection in the absence of infection or severe periodontal involvement
2. IO anesthesia
3. Regional nerve block with local infiltration for hemostasis

Technique
1. A 27-gauge short needle is recommended.
2. Area of insertion: center of the interdental papilla adjacent to the tooth to be treated (Fig. 15-7)
3. Target area: same
4. Landmarks: papillary triangle, about 2 mm below the tip, equidistant from adjacent teeth
5. Orientation of the bevel: not significant, although Saadoun and Malamed recommend toward the apex[19]
6. Procedure
   a. Assume the correct position, which varies significantly from tooth to tooth. The administrator should be comfortable, have adequate visibility of

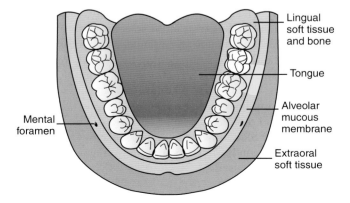

Figure 15-6. Area anesthesized by an intraseptal injection.

Labels: Lingual soft tissue and bone; Tongue; Alveolar mucous membrane; Extraoral soft tissue; Mental foramen

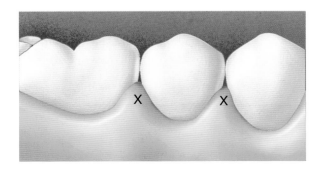

Figure 15-7. Area of insertion for an intraseptal injection.

CHAPTER 15 Supplemental Injection Techniques

the injection site, and maintain control over the needle.
b. Position the patient supine or semisupine with the head turned to maximize access and visibility.
c. Prepare tissue at the site of penetration.
(1) Dry with sterile gauze.
(2) Apply topical antiseptic (optional).
(3) Apply topical anesthetic for minimum of 1 minute.
d. Stabilize the syringe and orient the needle correctly (Fig. 15-8).
(1) Frontal plane: 45 degrees to the long axis of the tooth
(2) Sagittal plane: at right angle to the soft tissue
(3) Bevel facing the apex of the tooth
e. Slowly inject a few drops of local anesthetic as the needle enters soft tissue and advance the needle until contact with bone is made.
f. Applying pressure to the syringe, push the needle slightly deeper (1 to 2 mm) into the interdental septum.
g. Deposit 0.2 to 0.4 ml of local anesthetic in a minimum of 20 seconds.
(1) With a conventional syringe, the thickness of the rubber plunger is equivalent to 0.2 ml.
h. Two important items indicate success of the intraseptal injection:
(1) Significant resistance to the deposition of solution
(a) This is especially noticeable when a conventional syringe is used. Resistance is similar to that felt with the nasopalatine and PDL injections.
(b) Anesthetic solution should not come back into the patient's mouth. If this occurs, repeat the injection with the needle slightly deeper.
(2) Ischemia of soft tissues adjacent to the injection site (although noted with all local anesthetic

solutions, this is more prominent with local anesthetics containing a vasoconstrictor)
i. Repeat the injection as needed during the surgical procedure.

Signs and Symptoms
1. As with the PDL injection, there are *no objective symptoms* that ensure adequate anesthesia. The anesthetized area is too circumscribed.
2. Subjective: Ischemia of soft tissues is noted at the injection site.
3. Subjective: Resistance to the injection of solution is felt.
4. Objective: There is absence of pain during treatment.

Safety Feature. Intravascular injection is extremely unlikely to occur.

Precautions
1. Do not inject into infected tissue.
2. Do not inject rapidly (minimum 20 seconds).
3. Do not inject too much solution (0.2 to 0.4 ml per site).

Failures of Anesthesia
1. Infected or inflamed tissues. Changes in tissue pH minimize the effectiveness of the local anesthetic.
2. Solution not retained in tissue. To correct: Advance the needle further into the septal bone and readminister 0.2 to 0.4 ml.

Complication. Postinjection pain is unlikely to develop because the injection site is within the area of surgical treatment. Saadoun and Malamed demonstrated that postsurgical periodontal discomfort after the use of intraseptal anesthesia is no greater than that after a regional nerve block.[19]

Duration of Expected Anesthesia. The duration of osseous and soft-tissue anesthesia is variable after an intraseptal injection. Using an epinephrine concentration of 1:50,000, Saadoun and Malamed found pain control and hemostasis adequate for completion of the planned procedure without reinjection in most patients.[19] However, some patients require a second intraseptal injection.

• • •

Intraosseous Injection

Deposition of local anesthetic solution into the interproximal bone between two teeth has been practiced in dentistry since the start of the twentieth century.[20] Originally IO anesthesia necessitated the use of a half-round bur to provide entry into interseptal bone that had been surgically exposed. Once the hole had been made, a needle would be inserted into this hole and local anesthetic deposited.

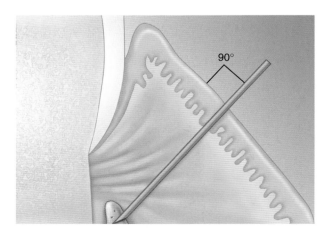
Figure 15-8. Orientation of the needle for an intraseptal injection.

261

The PDL and intraseptal injections already described are variations of IO anesthesia. In the PDL injection the local anesthetic enters interproximal bone through the periodontal tissues surrounding a tooth, whereas in intraseptal anesthesia the needle is gently embedded into the interproximal bone without the use of a bur.

In recent years the IO technique has been modified with the introduction of several devices* that simplify the procedure. The Stabident System was introduced, followed later by the X-Tip and most recently by the IntraFlow. The Stabident System consists of two parts: a perforator, a solid needle that perforates the cortical plate of bone with a conventional slow-speed contra-angle handpiece, and an 8-mm long, 27-gauge needle that is inserted into this predrilled hole for anesthetic administration (Fig. 15-9).

Experience with the IO technique has shown that the perforation of the interproximal bone is almost always entirely atraumatic. However, initially some persons had difficulty placing the needle of the local anesthetic syringe back into the previously drilled hole in the interproximal bone. Introduction of the X-Tip eliminated this problem. The X-Tip is composed of a drill and guide sleeve (Fig. 15-10). The drill leads the guide sleeve through the cortical plate of bone, after which it is separated and withdrawn. The guide sleeve remains in the bone and easily accepts a 27-gauge ultrashort needle, which is recommended for injection of the local anesthetic into the cancellous bone. The "Alternative Stabident System" introduced shortly thereafter eliminated the problem of locating the "hole" by inserting a conical-shaped "guide-sleeve" into the hole. The 27-gauge ultrashort needle could then be easily placed into the hole (Fig. 15-11).

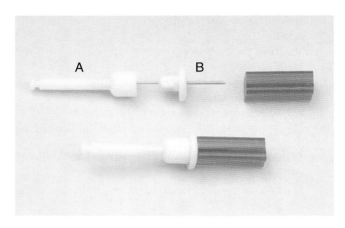

Figure 15-10. Intraosseous anesthesia—X-Tip. Components: **A,** drill; **B,** guide sleeve.

Recently introduced, the IntraFlow IO system combines the two steps previously described into one (Fig. 15-12).[3] The anesthetic cartridge is attached to a standard four-hole air hose on a treatment room delivery unit and is controlled by a foot rheostat. The IntraFlow is a specially modified slow-speed handpiece that consists of four main parts:

1. A needle or drill that makes the perforation through the bone and delivers the local anesthetic
2. A transfuser that acts as a conduit from the local anesthetic cartridge to the needle or drill
3. A latch tip or clutch that drives and governs the rotation of the needle or drill
4. A motor or infusion drive that powers the rotation of the needle or drill and, while holding the local

***Stabident Local Anesthesia System,** Fairfax Dental, Inc, 2601 S. Bayshore Drive, Suite 875, Miami, Florida 33133 USA, 1-800-233-2305. *www.stabident.com.*
X-Tip, (1) CE-Magic, 877-478-9748. (2) Dentsply, 1-800-877-0020. *www.dentsply.com.*
IntraFlow, IntraVantage, Inc, 2950 Xenium Lane, Suite 148, Plymouth, Minn 55441, 1-877-476-4299. *www.intravantageinc.com.*

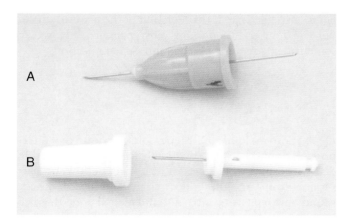

Figure 15-9. Intraosseus anesthesia—Stabident. Components: **A,** needle; **B,** perforator.

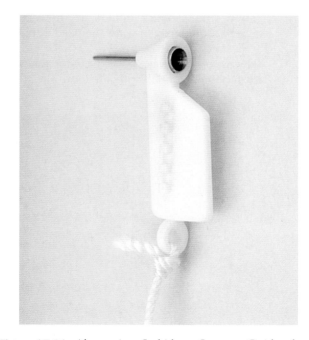

Figure 15-11. Alternative Stabident System. Guide sleeve remains in hole in bone, permitting easy access for needle.

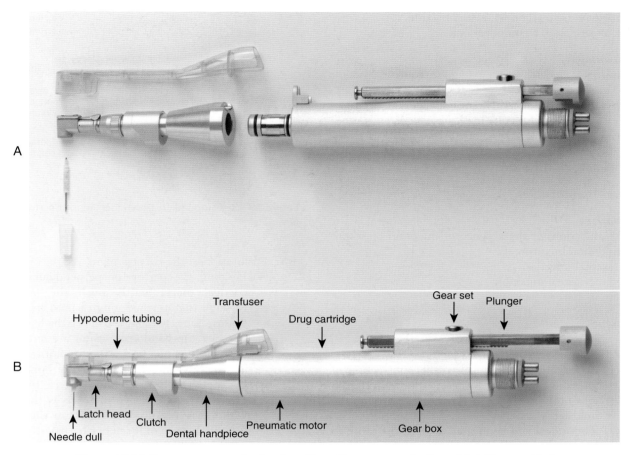

A

B

Gear set   Plunger

Transfuser

Hypodermic tubing   Drug cartridge

Latch head
Needle dull   Clutch   Pneumatic motor   Gear box
              Dental handpiece

Figure 15-12. Intraosseous anesthesia—IntraFlow. Components: **A,** dissembled; **B,** assembled.

anesthetic cartridge in place, powers the infusion plunger. A 24-gauge dual-beveled needle is used.

The IO injection technique can provide anesthesia of a single tooth or multiple teeth in a quadrant. To a significant degree the area of anesthesia is dependent on both the site of injection and the volume of local anesthetic deposited. It is recommended that 0.45 to 0.6 ml of anesthetic be administered when treatment is to be confined to not more than one or two teeth. Greater volumes (up to 1.8 ml) may be administered when treatment of multiple teeth in one quadrant is contemplated. The IO injection may be used when managing six or eight mandibular anterior teeth (e.g., first premolar to first premolar bilaterally). Bilateral IO injections are necessary, the perforation being made between the canine and first premolar on both sides. This provides pulpal anesthesia of eight teeth. It should be remembered, however, that the incisive nerve block provides pulpal anesthesia of these same teeth without the need for perforation of bone.

Because the IO injection site is relatively vascular, it is suggested that the volume of local anesthetic delivered be kept to the recommended minimum to avoid possible overdose.[21] In addition, because of the high incidence of palpitations noted when vasopressor-containing local

anesthetics are used, a "plain" local anesthetic is recommended in the IO injection. However, discussion with endodontists who use IO frequently indicates that the quality and depth of anesthesia are not as great when plain local anesthetics are used.

Other Common Names. None

Nerves Anesthetized. Terminal nerve endings at the site of injection and in the adjacent soft and hard tissues

Areas Anesthetized. Bone, soft tissue, and root structure in the area of injection

Indication. Pain control for dental treatment on single or multiple teeth in a quadrant

Contraindication. Infection or severe inflammation at the injection site

Advantages
1. Lack of lip and tongue anesthesia (appreciated by most patients)
2. Atraumatic

3. Immediate (<30 seconds) onset of action
4. Few postoperative complications

Disadvantages
1. Requires a special syringe (e.g., Stabident System, X-Tip, IntraFlow)
2. Bitter taste of the anesthetic drug (if leakage occurs)
3. Occasional (rare) difficulty in placing anesthetic needle into predrilled hole
4. High occurrence of palpitations when vasopressor-containing local anesthetic is used

Positive Aspiration. 0%

Alternatives
1. PDL injection, in the absence of infection or severe periodontal involvement
2. Intraseptal injection
3. Supraperiosteal injection
4. Regional nerve block

Technique*
1. Selection of site for injection
   a. Lateral perforation
      (1) At a point 2 mm apical to the intersection of lines drawn horizontally along the gingival margins of the teeth and a vertical line through the interdental papilla
      (2) The site should be located *distal* to the tooth to be treated, if possible, although the technique provides anesthesia in most cases when injected anterior to the tooth being treated.
      (3) Avoid injecting in the mental foramen area (increased risk of nerve damage).
   b. Vertical perforation (for edentulous areas)
      (1) Perforate at a point on the alveolar crest either mesial or distal to the treatment area (also called the *crestal anesthesia technique*).
2. Technique
   a. Remove the X-Tip from its sterile vial.
      (1) Hold the protective cover as you insert the X-Tip onto the slow speed handpiece (20,000 rpm).
   b. Prepare soft tissues at perforation site
      (1) Prepare tissue at the injection site with 2 × 2 inch sterile gauze.
      (2) Apply topical anesthetic to the injection site for minimum of 1 minute.
      (3) Place bevel of needle against gingiva, injecting a small volume of local anesthetic until blanching occurs.
      (4) Check soft-tissue anesthesia using a cotton pliers.
         (a) Cotton pliers leave a slight dimple. Mark the perforation site (Fig. 15-13).
      (5) Inject a few drops of local anesthetic into the dimple.

*From the instruction manual, CE-Magic, 1-877-478-9748. www.CE-Magic.com.

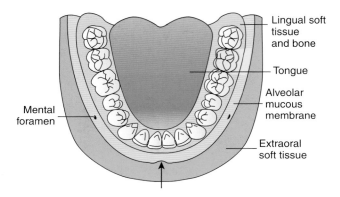

Figure 15-13. Cotton pliers leave indentation at perforation site *(arrow)*.

   c. Perforation of the cortical plate
      (1) Holding the perforator perpendicular to the cortical plate, gently push the perforator through the attached gingiva until its tip rests against bone (without activating the handpiece).
      (2) Activate the handpiece, using a gentle "pecking" motion on the perforator until a sudden loss of resistance is felt. Cortical bone will be perforated within 2 seconds (Fig 15-14).
      (3) Hold the guide sleeve in place as the drill is withdrawn (Fig. 15-15). Withdraw the perforator and dispose of it safely (sharps).
         (a) The guide sleeve remains in place until you are certain you have adequate anesthesia.
   d. Injection into cancellous bone
      (1) It is easy to insert the needle into the hole using an ultrashort needle (Fig. 15-16).
      (2) Press the tapered needle gently against the guide sleeve to minimize local anesthetic leakage.
         (a) Compress a cotton roll or 2 × 2 sterile gauze against the mucosa to absorb any excess local anesthetic.
      (3) Slowly and *gently* inject the local anesthetic solution

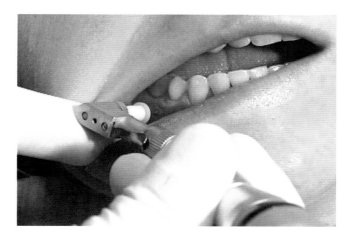

Figure 15-14. Drill hole using a gentle "pecking" motion.

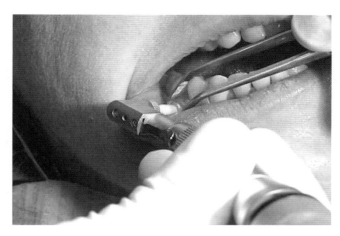

Figure 15-15. Hold the guide sleeve in place as the drill is withdrawn.

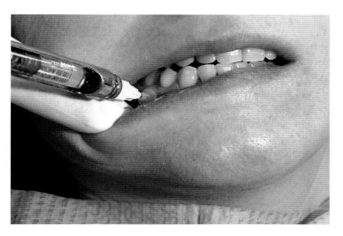

Figure 15-16. Insert needle into guide sleeve and inject local anesthetic solution.

   e. X-Tip doses: Recommended dosages for the X-Tip are the same for each local anesthetic solution as is recommended for other injections.
   f. Stabident doses (Table 15-1)
   g. Recommended technique for the IntraFlow IO syringe system is presented in Box 15-1.

Signs and Symptoms
1. As with the PDL injection, there are no objective signs that ensure adequate anesthesia. The anesthetized area is too circumscribed.
2. Subjective: ischemia of soft tissues at the injection site
3. Objective: absence of pain during treatment

Safety Feature. Intravascular injection is extremely unlikely, although the area injected into is vascular. Slow injection of the recommended volume of solution is important to keeping IO anesthesia safe.

Precautions
1. Do not inject into infected tissue.
2. Do not inject rapidly.
3. Do not inject too much solution. (See recommended dosages in Table 15-1.)
4. Do not use a vasopressor-containing local anesthetic unless necessary, and then only 1:200,000 or 1:100,000. Do not use 1:50,000 epinephrine.

Failures of Anesthesia
1. Infected or inflamed tissues. Changes in tissue pH minimize the effectiveness of the anesthetic.

TABLE 15-1
Stabident Dosages

	STABIDENT MANDIBULAR DOSAGES	
TO ANESTHETIZE	**INJECTION SITE**	**DOSE (number of 1.8 ml cartridges)**
One tooth	Immediately distal OR immediately mesial	1/4 1/3
Two adjacent teeth	Between the two teeth OR immediately distal to the more distal tooth	1/3 1/2
Three adjacent teeth	Immediately distal to the middle tooth	1/2
Six front teeth plus the first premolars (e.g., total of eight teeth)	Give two injections, one on each side, between the canine and the first premolar	1/2 on each side (total of one)
	STABIDENT MAXILLARY DOSAGES	
TO ANESTHETIZE	**INJECTION SITE**	**DOSE (number of 1.8 ml cartridges)**
One tooth	Immediately distal OR immediately mesial	1/4
Two adjacent teeth	Between the two teeth	1/4
Four adjacent teeth (e.g. 1, 2, 3 and 4)	Midway (e.g., two teeth distal and two teeth mesial to the injection site)	1/2
Up to eight teeth on one side	Midway (e.g., four teeth distal and four teeth mesial to the injection site)	1

(*From *www.stabident.com/manualall.htm.*)

BOX 15-1

Recommended Technique for the IntraFlow Intraosseous Syringe System

1. Select injection site, and then prepare tissue with topical anesthetic and soft-tissue anesthesia.
2. Depress foot pedal to perforate tissue and bone and begin injection.
3. Engage clutch when full depth of perforation is reached to stop rotation of the perforator (Fig. 15-12).
4. Continue injecting anesthetic.
5. Disengage clutch to start rotation and remove drill.
6. Wait 1 minute, then begin procedure.

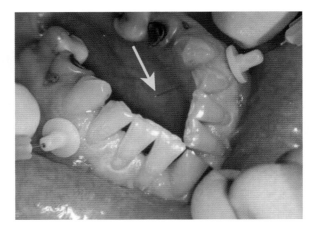

Figure 15-17. Accidental perforation of lingual plate *(arrow)*.

2. Inability to perforate cortical bone. If cortical bone is not perforated within 2 seconds, it is recommended that drilling be stopped and an alternative site be used.

Complications

1. Palpitation: This reaction frequently occurs when a vasopressor-containing local anesthetic is used. To minimize the risk, use a "plain" local anesthetic, if possible, or the most dilute epinephrine concentration available (e.g., 1:200,000).
2. Postinjection pain is unlikely after IO anesthesia. The use of mild analgesics (nonsteroidal antiinflammatory drugs) is recommended if discomfort occurs in the postinjection period.
3. Fistula formation at the site of perforation has been reported on several occasions. In most instances this can be prevented by employing a gentle "pecking" motion with the handpiece as the perforator goes through the cortical plate of bone. Application of a constant pressure against the bone presumably leads to the build-up of heat and possible fistula formation.
4. Separation of the perforator or cannula: Rare, but reported. The metal shaft of the bur or cannula separates and remains in bone. Usually easy to remove with a hemostat.
5. Perforation of lingual plate of bone (Fig. 15-17). Prevented by proper technique.

Duration of Expected Anesthesia. Pulpal anesthesia of between 15 and 30 minutes can be expected. If a vasopressor-containing solution is used, the duration approaches 30 minutes. If a plain solution is used, a 15-minute duration is usual. The depth of anesthesia is greater with a vasopressor-containing local anesthetic.

• • •

INTRAPULPAL INJECTION

Obtaining profound anesthesia in the pulpally involved tooth was a significant problem before the rediscovery of IO anesthesia. Specifically the problem occurred with mandibular molars because there were few alternative anesthetic techniques available with which the doctor could obtain profound anesthesia. Maxillary teeth usually are anesthetized with a supraperiosteal injection or nerve block such as the posterior superior alveolar (PSA), anterior superior alveolar (ASA), or (rarely) a maxillary (second division; V_2) nerve block. Mandibular teeth anterior to the molars are anesthetized with the incisive nerve block. Anesthesia of mandibular molars, however, usually is limited to nerve block anesthesia, which may prove to be ineffective in the presence of infection and inflammation. Methods of obtaining anesthesia for endodontics are described in Chapter 16.

Deposition of local anesthetic directly into the pulp chamber of a pulpally involved tooth provides effective anesthesia for pulpal extirpation and instrumentation where other techniques have failed. The intrapulpal injection may be used on any tooth when difficulty in providing profound pain control exists, but from a practical view it is necessary most commonly on mandibular molars.

The intrapulpal injection provides pain control both by the pharmacological action of the local anesthetic and applied pressure. This technique may be used once the pulp chamber is exposed, either surgically or pathologically.

Other Common Names. None

Nerves Anesthetized. Terminal nerve endings at the site of injection in the pulp chamber and canals of the involved tooth

Areas Anesthetized. Tissues within the injected tooth

Indication. When pain control is necessary for pulpal extirpation or other endodontic treatment in the absence of adequate anesthesia from other techniques

Contraindication. None. The intrapulpal injection may be the only local anesthetic technique available in some clinical situations.

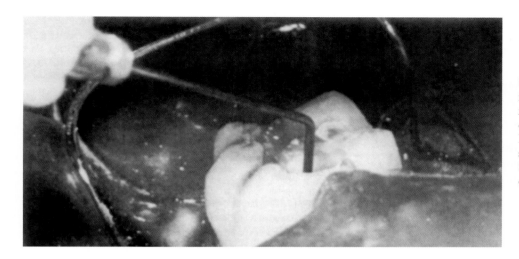

Figure 15-18. For the intrapulpal injection a 25-gauge 1- or 1⅝-inch needle is inserted into the pulp chamber or specific root canal. Bending the needle may be necessary to gain access. (From Cohen S, Burns RC: *Pathways of the pulp*, ed 8, St Louis, 2001, Mosby.)

Advantages
1. Lack of lip and tongue anesthesia (appreciated by most patients)
2. Minimum volumes of anesthetic solution necessary
3. Immediate onset of action
4. Very few postoperative complications

Disadvantages
1. Traumatic
   a. The intrapulpal injection is associated with a brief period of pain as anesthetic is deposited.
2. Bitter taste of the anesthetic drug (if leakage occurs)
3. May be difficult to enter certain root canals
   a. Bending of the needle may be necessary
4. Need a small opening into the pulp chamber for optimum effectiveness
   a. Large areas of decay make it more difficult to achieve profound anesthesia with the intrapulpal injection.

Positive Aspiration. 0%

Alternatives. IO. However, when IO fails, intrapulpal injection may be the only viable alternative to provide clinically adequate pain control.

Technique
1. Insert a 25- or 27-gauge short or long needle into the pulp chamber or the root canal as needed (Fig. 15-18).
2. Ideally, wedge the needle firmly into the pulp chamber or root canal.
   a. Occasionally the needle does not fit snugly into the canal. In this situation the anesthetic can be deposited in the chamber or canal. Anesthesia in this case is produced only by the pharmacological action of the local; there is no pressure anesthesia.
3. Deposit anesthetic solution under pressure.
   a. A small volume of anesthetic (0.2 to 0.3 ml) is necessary for successful intrapulpal anesthesia, if the anesthetic stays within the tooth. In many

situations the anesthetic simply flows back out of the tooth into the aspirator tip.
4. Resistance to the injection of the drug should be felt.
5. Bend the needle, if necessary, to gain access to the canal (Fig. 15-19).
   a. Although there is a greater risk of breakage with a bent needle, this is not a problem during intrapulpal anesthesia because the needle is inserted into the tooth itself, not into soft tissues. Retrieval is relatively simple if the needle breaks.
6. When the intrapulpal injection is performed properly, a brief period of sensitivity (ranging from mild to very painful) usually accompanies the injection. Pain relief usually occurs immediately thereafter, permitting instrumentation to proceed atraumatically.
7. Instrumentation may begin approximately 30 seconds after the injection.

Signs and Symptoms
1. As with the PDL, intraseptal, and IO injections, there are *no subjective symptoms* that ensure adequate anesthesia. The area is too circumscribed.

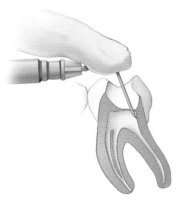

Figure 15-19. The needle may have to be bent to gain access to a canal. (Modified from Cohen S, Burns RC: *Pathways of the pulp*, ed 8, St Louis, 2001, Mosby.)

2. Objective: The endodontically involved tooth may be treated painlessly.

Safety Features
1. Intravascular injection is extremely unlikely to occur.
2. Small volumes of anesthetic are administered.

Precautions
1. Do not inject into infected tissue.
2. Do not inject rapidly (minimum 20 seconds).
3. Do not inject too much solution (0.2 to 0.3 ml).

Failures of Anesthesia
1. Infected or inflamed tissues. Changes in tissue pH minimize the effectiveness of the anesthetic. However, intrapulpal anesthesia invariably works to provide effective pain control.
2. Solution not retained in tissue. To correct: Try to advance the needle further into the pulp chamber or root canal and readminister 0.2 to 0.3 ml of anesthetic drug.

Complication. Discomfort during the injection of anesthetic. The patient may experience a brief period of intense discomfort as the injection of the anesthetic drug is started. Within a second (literally) the tissue is anesthetized and the discomfort ceases. The use of inhalation sedation (nitrous oxide or oxygen) can help to minimize or alter the feeling experienced.

Duration of Expected Anesthesia. The duration of anesthesia is variable after intrapulpal injection. The duration is adequate to permit atraumatic extirpation of the pulpal tissues in most instances.

REFERENCES

1. Masselink BH: The advent of painless dentistry, *Dent Cosmos* 52(8):868-872, 1910.
2. Magnes GD: Intraosseous anesthesia, *Anesth Prog* 15(9):264-267, 1968.
3. Klebber CH: Intraosseous anesthesia: implications, instrumentation and techniques, *J Amer Dent Assoc* 134(4):487-491, 2003.
4. Brown R: Intraosseous anesthesia: a review, *J Calif Dent Assoc* 27(10):785-792, 1999.
5. Weathers A Jr: Taking the mystery out of endodontics, Part 6. Painless anesthesia for the "hot" tooth, *Dent Today* 18(12):90-93, 1999.
6. Bethel LP, editor: *Dental summary*, vol 32, Toledo, Ohio, 1912, Ranson & Randolph, p 167.
7. Fischer G: *Local anesthesia in dentistry*, ed 3, Philadelphia, 1923, Lea & Febiger, p 197.
8. *Illustrated catalogue of dental furniture, instruments, and materials*, ed 4, Pittsburgh, 1905, Lee S Smith & Son.
9. Malamed SF: The periodontal ligament (PDL) injection: an alternative to inferior alveolar nerve block, *Oral Surg* 53:117-121, 1982.
10. Brannstrom M, Lindskog S, Nordenvall KJ: Enamel hypoplasia in permanent teeth induced by periodontal ligament anesthesia of primary teeth, *J Am Dent Assoc* 109(5):735-736, 1984.
11. Council on Dental Materials, Instruments, and Equipment: Status report: the periodontal ligament injection, *J Am Dent Assoc* 106:222-224, 1983.
12. Walton RE, Garnick JJ: The periodontal ligament injection: histologic effects on the periodontium in monkeys, *J Endodod* 8:22-26, 1982.
13. Nelson PW: Injection system, *J Am Dent Assoc* 103:692, 1981 (letter).
14. Shepherd PA, Eleazer PD, Clark SJ, et al: Measurement of intraosseous pressures generated by the Wand, high-pressure periodontal ligament syringe, and the Stabident system, *J Endodont* 27(6):381-384, 2001.
15. Meechan JG: Supplementary routes to local anaesthesia, *Intern Endodont J* 35(11):885-896, 2002.
16. Wong JK: Adjuncts to local anesthesia: separating fact from fiction, *Can Dent Assoc* 67(7):391-397, 2001.
17. Quinn CL: Injection techniques to anesthetize the difficult tooth, *J Calif Dent Assoc* 26(9):665-667, 1998.
18. Brannstrom N, Nordenvall KJ, Hedstrom KG: Periodontal tissue changes after intraligamentary anesthesia, *ADSC J Dent Child* 49:417, 1982.
19. Saadoun A, Malamed SF: Intraseptal anesthesia in periodontal surgery, *J Am Dent Assoc* 111:249-256, 1985.
20. Fischer G: *Local anesthesia in dentistry*, ed 3, Philadelphia, 1923, Lea & Febiger, pp 244-248.
21. Leonard M: The efficacy of an intraosseous injection system of delivering local anesthetic, *J Am Dent Assoc* 126(1):81-86, 1995.

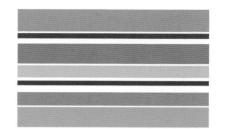

Local Anesthetic Considerations in Dental Specialties

CHAPTER
16

The techniques of local anesthesia described previously in this section are valuable to doctors in virtually all areas of dental practice. However, there are specific needs and problems associated with pain control in particular areas of dentistry. This chapter discusses the dental specialties listed below and their peculiar needs in the area of pain control:

Endodontics
Pediatric dentistry
Periodontics
Oral and maxillofacial surgery
Fixed prosthodontics
Long-duration anesthesia
Dental hygiene

ENDODONTICS

Effects of Inflammation on Local Anesthesia

Inflammation and infection lower tissue pH, altering the ability of a local anesthetic to provide clinically adequate pain control. As a review, most local anesthetics are weak bases (pKa, 7.5 to 9.5). Local anesthetics are injected in their acid–salt form (through combination with hydrochloric acid), improving both their water solubility and stability. When a local anesthetic is injected into tissue, it is rapidly neutralized by tissue fluid buffers, and a part of the cationic form (RNH+) is converted to the nonionized base (RN), according to the Henderson-Hasselbalch equation (see Chapter 1). The nonionized base is able to diffuse into the nerve. Pulpal and periapical inflammation or infection can cause tissue pH in the affected region to be lowered (e.g., pus has a pH of 5.5 to 5.6). Increased acidity does several things.[1] It limits the

formation of nonionized base (RN), favoring formation of the cationic form (RNH+). The RN that does penetrate the nerve once again encounters a normal tissue pH 7.3 inside the nerve and reequilibrates to both the RN and RNH+ forms. This RNH+ is available to block sodium channels, but with fewer cations available inside the nerve sheath, there is a greater likelihood of incomplete anesthesia developing. The overall effect of ion entrapment is to delay the onset of anesthesia and possibly interfere with nerve blockade.[2] It changes the products of inflammation so they inhibit anesthesia by directly affecting the nerve. Brown demonstrated that inflammatory exudates enhance nerve conduction by lowering the response threshold of the nerve,[1] which may inhibit local anesthesia. It causes blood vessels in the region of inflammation to become unusually dilated, allowing for a more rapid uptake of anesthetic from the site of injection. Thus there is an increased possibility that local anesthetic blood levels may be elevated (from those seen in normal tissue).[2]

There are two primary methods of obtaining adequate nerve block anesthesia in the presence of tissue inflammation. First, administer the local anesthetic away from the area of inflammation. It is undesirable to inject anesthetic solutions into areas of infection because of the possibility of spreading the infection to uninvolved regions.[3,4] The administration of local anesthetic solution into a site distant from the involved tooth is more likely to provide adequate pain control because of the presence of more normal tissue conditions. *Regional nerve block anesthesia is a major factor in pain control for pulpally involved teeth.* Second, deposit a larger volume of anesthetic into the region. This provides a greater number of uncharged base molecules able to diffuse through the nerve sheath, with the increased likelihood of a satisfactory anesthetic block.[5,6]

Methods of Achieving Anesthesia

The following techniques are recommended for providing pain control in pulpally involved teeth: local infiltration (supraperiosteal injection), regional nerve block, intrapulpal injection, periodontal ligament injection, intraseptal injection, and intraosseous injection. The order in which these techniques are discussed is the typical sequence in which they are normally used to achieve pain control.

Local Infiltration (Supraperiosteal Injection). Local infiltration is commonly used to provide pulpal anesthesia in maxillary teeth. It is usually effective in endodontic procedures when severe inflammation or infection is not present. Local infiltration should *not* be attempted in a region where infection is obviously (clinically or radiographically) present because of the possible spread of infection to other regions and a greatly decreased rate of success. When infection is present, other techniques of pain control should be relied on. Infiltration anesthesia is often effective at subsequent endodontic visits, if adequate débridement and shaping of the canals have been accomplished previously.

Regional Nerve Block. Regional nerve block anesthesia is recommended where infiltration anesthesia may be ineffective or contraindicated. These techniques are discussed in detail in Chapters 13 and 14. Regional nerve block is likely to be effective because the anesthetic solution is deposited at a distance from the inflammation, where tissue pH and other factors are more normal.

Periodontal Ligament Injection. The periodontal ligament (PDL) injection may be an effective method of providing anesthesia in pulpally involved teeth if infection and severe inflammation are not present. This technique is discussed in Chapter 15. By way of review, a 27-gauge short needle is firmly placed between the interproximal bone and the tooth to be anesthetized. The bevel of the needle should face the tooth (although bevel orientation is not critical to success). It is appropriate to bend the needle if necessary to gain access. A small volume (0.2 ml) of local anesthetic is deposited under pressure. It may be necessary to repeat the PDL injection on all four sides of the tooth.

Intraosseous Injection. The intraosseous (IO) injection has experienced a resurgence of enthusiasm in recent years.[7-15] It can produce anesthesia deep enough to permit access into the pulp chamber, at which time intrapulpal anesthesia can be administered (if necessary). The technique for the IO injection is described in Chapter 15 and is reviewed here (Figs. 16-1 and 16-2):
1. Apply topical anesthetic at the site of the injection to anesthetize the soft tissue.

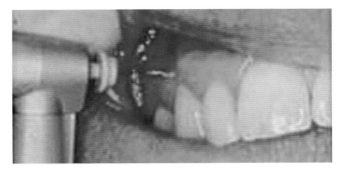

Figure 16-1. Stabident intraosseous injection technique.

2. Holding the perforator perpendicular to the cortical plate, gently push it through the attached gingiva until its tip rests against bone.
3. Activate the handpiece in short spurts, applying light pressure on the perforator until a sudden loss of resistance is felt.
4. Withdraw the perforator and dispose of it safely.
5. Insert the local anesthetic needle into the hole and deposit the volume of local anesthetic appropriate for the procedure (see charts in Chapter 15).

Cardiovascular absorption of the local anesthetic after IO injection is more rapid than after the other techniques described.[16,17] Transient elevations in heart rate were noted in 67% (28/42) of healthy patients receiving 2% lidocaine with 1:100,000 epinephrine via IO injection. No significant increase was noted when 3% mepivacaine was injected IO in the same patients.[17] The heart rate returned to within 5 beats of normal within 4 minutes in 79% of the patients.

The use of epinephrine-containing local anesthetics in the IO technique is not contraindicated in healthy, non–cardiovascular risk patients. However, where significant cardiovascular risk or other contraindications to the administration of epinephrine exist, a "plain" local anesthetic is a good alternative for IO anesthesia.

Intraseptal Injection. This is a variation of the IO and PDL injections and may be used as an alternative to these techniques. It is more successful in younger patients

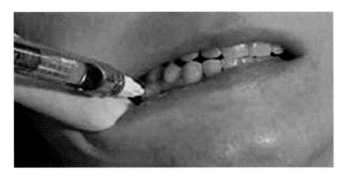

Figure 16-2. X-Tip intraosseous injection technique.

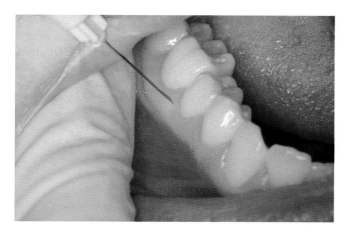

Figure 16-3. For the intraseptal injection a 27-gauge, short needle is inserted into the intraseptal bone distal to the tooth to be anesthetized.

because of the decreased density of bone. Intraseptal anesthesia is described in Chapter 15 and proceeds as follows:[18]

1. Anesthetize the soft tissues at the injection site via local infiltration.
2. Insert a 27-gauge short needle into the intraseptal bone distal to the tooth to be anesthetized (Fig. 16-3).
3. Advance the needle firmly into the cortical plate of bone.
4. Inject about 0.2 ml of anesthetic. Considerable resistance must be encountered as the anesthetic is being deposited. If the administration is easy, the needle tip is most likely in soft tissue, not bone.

Intrapulpal Injection. The intrapulpal injection provides pain control both by the pharmacological action of the local anesthetic and by applied pressure. This technique may be used once the pulp chamber is exposed, either surgically or pathologically. The technique is described in Chapter 15.

When intrapulpal injections are administered properly, a brief period of sensitivity, ranging from mild to severe, may accompany the injection. Clinical pain relief follows almost immediately, permitting instrumentation to proceed atraumatically.

Occasionally the anesthetic needle does not fit snugly into the canal, preventing the increased pressure normally found in the intrapulpal injection. In this situation the anesthetic can be deposited in the chamber or canal. Anesthesia is produced only by the pharmacological action of the local; there is no pressure anesthesia. Instrumentation may begin approximately 30 seconds after the injection.

With the growing popularity of IO anesthesia, the need for intrapulpal injections to provide profound pain control in cases of irreversible pulpitis has decreased.

• • •

Today there are few, if any, occasions when all the discussed techniques fail to provide clinically acceptable pain control, and intrapulpal anesthesia cannot be attempted until the pulp is exposed. The following sequence of treatment then may be of value:

1. Use slow-speed high-torque instrumentation (which is usually less traumatic than the high-speed low-torque option).
2. Use conscious sedation (which helps to moderate the patient's response to painful stimuli). Nitrous oxide–oxygen inhalation sedation is a readily available, safe, and highly effective method of elevating a patient's pain reaction threshold.
3. If, after Steps 1 and 2, the pulp chamber is opened, administer direct intrapulpal anesthesia. Usually this is effective despite the brief period of pain associated with its administration.
4. If a high level of pain persists and it is still not possible to enter the pulp chamber, then the following sequence should be considered:
   a. Place a cotton pellet saturated with local anesthetic loosely on the pulpal floor of the tooth.
   b. Wait 30 seconds, after which press the pellet more firmly into the dentinal tubules or the area of pulpal exposure. This area initially may be sensitive but should become insensitive within 2 to 3 minutes.
   c. Remove the pellet and continue use of the slow-speed drill until pulpal access is gained, at which time direct injection into the pulp can be performed.

In most endodontic procedures there may be difficulty in providing adequate anesthesia only at the first appointment. Once the pulp tissue has been extirpated, the need for pulpal anesthesia disappears. Soft-tissue anesthesia may be necessary at ensuing appointments for comfortable placement of the rubber dam clamp, but if adequate tooth structure remains, even that may not be necessary. Some patients respond unfavorably to instrumentation of their root canals, even when the canals have been thoroughly débrided. If this occurs, infiltration (in the maxilla) or intrapulpal anesthesia, or topical anesthetic, may be used. Apply a small amount of topical anesthetic ointment onto the file or reamer before inserting it into the canal. This helps to desensitize the periapical tissues during instrumentation of canals. Patients also may react to filling the canals. Local anesthesia should be considered before this stage of treatment is started.

PEDIATRIC DENTISTRY

Pain control is one of the most important aspects of behavioral management in children undergoing dental treatment. Unpleasant childhood experiences have made many adults acutely phobic with regard to dental treatment. Today, however, many local anesthetic drugs are available to make pain management relatively easy. Special concerns in pediatric dentistry relevant to local anesthetic include anesthetic overdose, complications related to the prolonged duration of soft-tissue anesthesia, and technique variations related to the smaller skulls and differing anatomy of younger patients.

Local Anesthetic Overdose

Overdose from a drug develops when its blood level in a target organ (e.g., brain) becomes excessive (see Chapter 18). Undesirable (toxic) effects may be caused by intravascular injection or the administration of large volumes of the drug. Local anesthetic toxicity develops when the blood level of the drug in the brain or heart becomes too high. Therefore local anesthetic toxicity relates to the volume of drug reaching the cerebrovascular and cardiovascular systems and to the volume of blood in the patient. Once a drug has reached toxic levels, it exerts unwanted and possibly deleterious systemic actions. Local anesthetic toxicity produces central nervous system (CNS) and cardiovascular system (CVS) depression, with reactions ranging from mild tremor to tonic–clonic convulsions (CNS), from a slight decrease in blood pressure and cardiac output to cardiac arrest (CVS).

A disproportionately high number of deaths and serious morbidity caused by local anesthetic overdose have occurred in children, leading to the assumption that local anesthetics are more toxic in children than adults.[19,20] This is untrue; it is the safety margin of local anesthetics in small children that is low. Given an equal dose of local anesthetic, a healthy patient with a greater blood volume has a lower blood level of anesthetic than a patient with a lesser blood volume. Blood volume, to a large degree, relates to body weight: the greater the body weight, the greater the blood volume (except where the patient is markedly obese).

Maximum recommended doses (MRDs) of all drugs administered by injection should be calculated by body weight and should not be exceeded, unless it is absolutely essential to do so.[20] For example, two cartridges of 3% mepivacaine (54 mg per cartridge) exceed the MRD for a 15-kg (33-lb) child of 66 mg. Unfortunately, the lack of awareness of maximum doses has led to fatalities in children.[21-25] The ease with which a child may be overdosed with local anesthetics is compounded by the practice of multiple quadrant dentistry and the concomitant use of sedative drugs (especially opioids).[19] When treating a child, the dentist should maintain strict adherence to maximum doses (Table 16-1) and anesthetize only that quadrant currently being treated.

Cheatham and associates surveyed 117 dentists who regularly treated children about their local anesthetic usage.[26] They found that the lighter the weight of the patient, the more likely the doctor was to administer an overly large dose of the local anesthetic, based on milligrams per kilogram of body weight. For example, a 13-kg patient should receive no more than 91 mg of lidocaine (based on a high MRD of 7.0 mg/kg). The range of doses administered by dentists treating children was 0.9 to 19.3 mg/kg. As the patient's weight increased, the number of milligrams per pound or kilogram reached lower and safer levels, the maximum mg/kg range falling to 12.6 mg/kg in the 20-kg patient and to 7.2 mg/kg in the 35-kg patient. The mean dose of local anesthetic also fell when the patient's weight increased, from 5.4 mg/kg in the 13-kg patient to 4.8 mg/kg in the 20-kg patient to 3.8 mg/kg in the 35-kg patient (Table 16-2).

The administration of large volumes of local anesthetic is not necessary when seeking pain control in younger patients. Because of differences in anatomy (see "Techniques of Local Anesthesia in Pediatric Dentistry"), smaller volumes of local anesthetics provide the depth and duration of pain control usually necessary to successfully complete the planned dental treatment in younger patients.

Because all injectable local anesthetics possess vasodilating properties, leading to more rapid vascular uptake and a shorter duration of adequate anesthesia, it is strongly

TABLE 16-1
Maximum Recommended Doses (MRDs) of Local Anesthetics

Drug	Formulation	Manufacturer's MRD	mg/lb (mg/kg)	Author's MRD	mg/lb (mg/kg)
Articaine	4% with epinephrine	500	3.2 (7.0)	500	3.2 (7.0)
Lidocaine	Plain	300	2.0 (4.4)	300	2.0 (4.4)
Lidocaine	Epinephrine 1:100,000	500	3.3 (7.0)	300	2.0 (4.4)
Lidocaine	Epinephrine 1:50,000	500	3.3 (7.0)	300	2.0 (4.4)
Mepivacaine	Plain	400	2.6 (5.7)	300	2.0 (4.4)
Mepivacaine	With levonordefrin	400	2.6 (5.7)	300	2.0 (4.4)
Prilocaine	Plain	600	4.0 (8.8)	400	2.7 (6.0)
Prilocaine	With epinephrine	600	4.0 (8.8)	400	2.7 (6.0)
Bupivacaine	With epinephrine	90	1.3 (0.6)	90	1.3 (0.6)

TABLE 16-2
Local Anesthetic Administration by Dentists Who Treat Children (*n* = 117)

Age	Patient Weight (kg)	Mean Dose (mg/kg)	Mean (mg/kg)	Range (mg)	Range (mg/kg)	Recommended (MRD) mg/kg
2	13	69.9	5.4	12 to 252	0.9 to **19.3**	Lidocaine 4.4 to 7.0; Mepivacaine 4.4 to 6.0
5	20	96.5	4.8	18 to 252	0.9 to **12.6**	
10	35	135	3.8	36 to 252	1.0 to 7.2	

(Modified from Cheatham BD, Primosch RE, Courts FJ: A survey of local anesthetic usage in pediatric patients by Florida dentists, *J Dent Child* 59: 401-407, 1992.)

recommended that a vasopressor be included in the local anesthetic solution unless there is a compelling reason for it to be excluded.[27] Many treatment appointments in pediatric dentistry do not exceed 30 minutes in duration; therefore the use of a local anesthetic containing a vasopressor is considered to be unnecessary and unwarranted. It is thought that the increased duration of soft-tissue anesthesia, especially after inferior alveolar nerve block, increases the risk of the patient suffering self-inflicted injury to the soft tissues. A non–vasopressor-containing local anesthetic is frequently used (most often mepivacaine 3%). Providing 20 to 40 minutes of pulpal anesthesia, mepivacaine 3% is considered the appropriate drug for this group of patients; it is, provided that treatment is limited to one quadrant per visit. However, when multiple quadrants are to be treated (and anesthetized) in one visit on a smaller patient, the administration of a "plain" drug into multiple injection sites increases the potential risk of overdose. The use of a local anesthetic containing a vasopressor is strongly recommended whenever multiple quadrants are anesthetized in the smaller pediatric patient. Sixty-nine percent of doctors treating children administered lidocaine with epinephrine as their primary anesthetic (Table 16-3).[26]

Factors increasing the risk of local anesthetic overdosage in younger patients are presented in Box 16-1.[28]

TABLE 16-3
Local Anesthetic Choice by Dentists Who Treat Children (*n* = 117)

Anesthetic Formulation	Percent Employing
2% lidocaine + 1:100,000 epinephrine	69
3% mepivacaine	11
2% lidocaine	8
2% mepivacaine + 1:20,000 levonordefrin	8
Other anesthetics	4

(Adapted from Cheatham BD, Primosch RE, Courts FJ: A survey of local anesthetic usage in pediatric patients by Florida dentists, *J Dent Child* 59:401-407, 1992.)

Complications of Local Anesthesia

Accidental biting or chewing of the lip, tongue, or cheek is a complication of residual soft-tissue anesthesia (Fig. 16-4). Soft-tissue anesthesia always lasts longer than pulpal anesthesia and may be present for 4 to 5 hours or more after local anesthetic administration. Fortunately, most patients do not encounter problems related to

BOX 16-1

Factors Adding to Increased Risk of Local Anesthetic Overdose in Younger Patients

1. Treatment plan: all four quadrants treated using local anesthetic in one visit
2. Local anesthetic administered is a plain (no vasopressor) solution
3. Full cartridges (1.8 ml) administered with each injection
4. Local anesthetic administered to all four quadrants at one time
5. Exceeding the maximum dosage based on patient's body weight

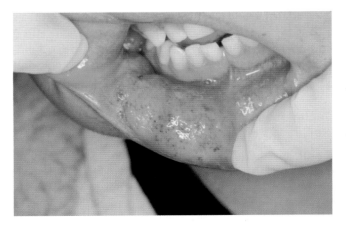

Figure 16-4. Lip trauma caused by biting while the area was anesthetized.

TABLE 16-4
Relative Durations of Pulpal and Soft Tissue Anesthesia

Drug	Approximate Pulpal Anesthesia (min)	Approximate Soft-tissue Anesthesia (hr)
Mepivacaine plain	20 to 40	3 to 4
Prilocaine plain	(infiltration) 10	1½ to 2
Lidocaine plain	5 to 10	1 to 1½

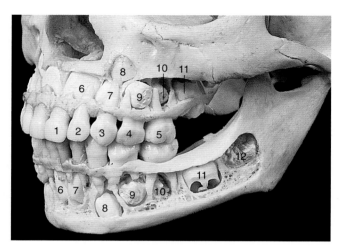

Figure 16-5. Upper and lower jaws in a 4-year-old child with erupted primary teeth and unerupted permanent teeth. *1,* First (central) incisor of primary dentition; *2,* second (lateral) incisor of primary dentition; *3,* canine of primary dentition; *4,* first molar of primary dentition; *5,* second molar of primary dentition; *6,* first (central) incisor of permanent dentition; *7,* second (lateral) incisor of permanent dentition; *8,* canine of permanent dentition; *9,* first premolar of permanent dentition; *10,* second premolar of permanent dentition; *11,* first molar of permanent dentition; *12,* second molar of permanent dentition. (From Abrahams PH, Marks SC Jr, Hutchings RT: *McMinn's color atlas of human anatomy,* ed 5, St Louis, 2003, Mosby.)

prolonged soft-tissue anesthesia, but the majority of those who do are young or mentally or physically disabled. Problems related to soft-tissue anesthesia most often involve the lower lip. Much less frequently the tongue is injured, and rarely the upper lip is involved.

Several preventive measures can be implemented:

1. Select a local anesthetic with a duration of action that is appropriate for the length of the planned procedure. There are drugs that provide pulpal anesthesia of adequate duration (20 to 40 minutes) for restorative procedures, with a relatively shorter duration of soft-tissue anesthesia (1 to 3 hours instead of 4 or 5) (Table 16-4). It should be kept in mind, however, that there is no research to demonstrate a relationship between reduced soft-tissue trauma and the use of plain local anesthetics. The clinician also must consider the advisability of using a local anesthetic with vasopressor in view of the decreased margin of safety of local anesthetics in smaller children.

2. Advise both the patient and accompanying adult about the possibility of injury if the patient bites, sucks, or chews on the lips, tongue, or cheeks or ingests hot substances while anesthesia persists.

3. Some doctors reinforce the verbal warning to the patient and adult by placing a cotton roll in the mucobuccal fold (held in position by dental floss through the teeth) if soft-tissue anesthesia is still present at the time of the patient's discharge. Warning stickers are also available to help prevent soft-tissue trauma.

The management of soft-tissue trauma involves reassuring the patient, allowing time for the anesthetic effects to diminish, and coating the involved area with a lubricant (petroleum jelly) to help prevent drying, cracking, and pain.

Techniques of Local Anesthesia in Pediatric Dentistry

Local anesthetic techniques in children do not differ greatly from those used in adults. Skulls of children do have some anatomical differences from those of adults, however. For instance, maxillary and mandibular bone in children is generally less dense, which works to the dentist's advantage (Fig. 16-5). Decreased density permits a more rapid and complete diffusion of the anesthetic solution. Children are also smaller; thus the standard injection techniques usually can be completed with a decreased depth of needle penetration.

Maxillary Anesthesia. All primary teeth and permanent molars can be anesthetized by supraperiosteal infiltration in the mucobuccal fold. The *posterior superior alveolar nerve block* often is not necessary because of the effectiveness of infiltration in children. However, in some individuals the morphology of the bone surrounding the apex of the permanent first molar does not permit effective infiltration of local anesthetic. This is because the zygomatic process lies closer to the alveolar bone in children. A posterior superior alveolar (PSA) nerve block may be warranted in this clinical situation. A short dental needle should be used and the depth of needle penetration modified to meet the smaller dimensions of the pediatric patient to minimize the risk of hematoma. As an alternative to the PSA, Rood[29] has suggested using buccal infiltrations on both the mesial and distal of the maxillary first molar to avoid a prominent zygomatic process. The *anterior superior alveolar nerve block* also can be used in children, as long as it is realized that the depth of penetration is probably just slightly greater than with a supraperiosteal injection (because of the lower height of the maxillae in children). Generally, there are few indications for either the posterior superior alveolar or anterior superior alveolar nerve block in children because of the lack of need for multiple restorations in one quadrant.

Occasionally a maxillary tooth remains sensitive after a supraperiosteal injection because of accessory innervation from the palatal nerves[30] or widely flared palatal roots. Palatal anesthesia can be obtained in children through the nasopalatine and greater (anterior) palatine nerve blocks. The technique for a *nasopalatine nerve block* proceeds exactly as described in Chapter 13. That for a *greater palatine nerve block* is as follows: The administrator visualizes a line from the gingival border of the most posterior molar that has erupted to the midline. The needle is inserted from the opposite side of the mouth, distal to the last molar, bisecting this line. If the child has only primary dentition, the needle is inserted approximately 10 mm posterior to the distal surface of the second primary molar, bisecting the line drawn toward the midline.

An intrapapillary injection also can be used to achieve palatal anesthesia in young children. Once buccal anesthesia is effective, the needle (27-gauge short) is inserted horizontally into the buccal papilla just above the interdental septum. Local anesthetic is injected as the needle is advanced toward the palatal side. This should cause ischemia of the soft tissue.[31]

Mandibular Anesthesia. *Supraperiosteal infiltration* usually is effective in providing pain control of mandibular primary teeth. Sharaf reported in 80 children (ages 3 to 9 years) that buccal infiltration in the mandible was as effective as inferior alveolar nerve block (IANB) anesthesia in all situations except when pulpotomy was performed on the primary second molar.[32] This is because of the decreased density of bone in the mandible in younger children. The rate of success of mandibular infiltration anesthesia decreases somewhat for primary mandibular molars as the child increases in age. The technique of supraperiosteal infiltration in the mandible is the same as in the maxilla. The tip of the needle is directed toward the apex of the tooth, in the mucobuccal fold, and approximately one fourth to one third (0.45 to 0.6 ml) cartridge is slowly deposited.

The IANB has a greater success rate in children than adults because of the location of the mandibular foramen. The mandibular foramen in children lies distal and more inferior to the occlusal plane. Benham[32] demonstrated that the mandibular foramen lies at the height of the occlusal plane in children and rises an average 7.4 mm above the occlusal plane in adults. He also found that there is no age-related difference as to the anteroposterior position of the foramen on the ramus.

The technique for an IANB is essentially identical for adults and children. Differences include placing the syringe barrel over the primary molars on the opposite side of the mouth and using an average penetration depth of 15 mm (although this varies with the size of the mandible and age of the patient). Bone should be contacted before any solution is deposited. In general, the more inferior location of the mandibular foramen in children provides a greater opportunity for successful anesthesia. "Low"

injections are more likely to be successful. In clinical situations the success rate for well-behaved children usually exceeds 90% to 95%.

Because of the decreased thickness of soft tissue overlying the inferior alveolar nerve (about 15 mm) a 25- or 27-gauge short needle may be recommended in the IANB in younger patients. A long needle should be used once the patient is of sufficient size that a short needle does not reach the injection site without entering tissue almost to its hub.

The *buccal nerve* may be anesthetized if anesthesia of the buccal tissues in the permanent molar region is necessary. The needle tip is placed distal and buccal to the most posterior tooth in the arch. Deposit approximately 0.3 ml of solution.

The *Vazirani-Akinosi* and *Gow-Gates mandibular nerve blocks* also can be used in children. Akinosi[33] advocates the use of short needles with this technique. He also states that the technique appears less reliable in children, which he relates to the difficulty of judging the depth of penetration necessary in a growing child. The Gow-Gates mandibular block can be used successfully in children.[34] However, these injections are rarely necessary in pediatric dentistry because of the relative ease with which one can achieve inferior alveolar and incisive nerve block anesthesia.

The *incisive nerve block* provides pulpal anesthesia of the five primary mandibular teeth in a quadrant. Deposition of anesthetic solution outside the mental foramen and the application of finger pressure for 2 minutes provide a very high degree of success. The mental foramen is usually located between the two primary mandibular molars.

The *PDL injection* has been well accepted in pediatric dentistry. It provides the doctor with the means to achieve anesthesia of proper depth and duration on one tooth, without unwanted residual soft-tissue anesthesia. The PDL is also useful when a child has discrete carious lesions in multiple quadrants. See Chapter 15 for a complete discussion of technique for the PDL injection. It is recommended that the described technique be scrupulously adhered to both to avoid physiological (pain) and psychological (fear) trauma to the patient. The PDL injection is not recommended for use on primary teeth because of the possibility of the development of enamel hypoplasia in the developing permanent tooth.[35]

PERIODONTICS

The special requirements for local anesthesia in periodontal procedures center on the use of vasopressors to provide hemostasis and the use of long-duration local anesthetics for postoperative pain control. Long-duration anesthesia is discussed as a separate subject later in this chapter.

Soft-tissue manipulation and surgical procedures are associated with hemorrhage, especially when the tissues involved are not healthy. Administration of local anesthetics without vasopressors proves to be counterproductive because the vasodilating property of the local anesthetic increases bleeding in the region of the injection.[36] Vasopressors are added to counteract this unwanted action.

The pharmacology of vasopressors is more completely discussed in Chapter 3. As a review, vasopressors produce arterial smooth muscle contraction by direct stimulation of α receptors located in the wall of the blood vessel. Consequently it follows that local anesthetics with vasopressors used for hemostasis must be injected directly into the region where the bleeding is to occur.

Pain control for periodontal procedures should be achieved through nerve block techniques, such as the posterior superior alveolar, inferior alveolar, and infraorbital nerve blocks. Saadoun[18] has shown that the *intraseptal technique* is very effective for periodontal flap surgical procedures. It decreases the total volume of administered anesthetic and volume of blood lost during the procedure. Local anesthetic solutions used for nerve blocks should include a vasopressor in a concentration not greater than 1:100,000 epinephrine or 1:20,000 levonordefrin. An epinephrine concentration of 1:50,000 is not recommended for pain control because depth, duration, and success rates are no greater than those seen with anesthetics containing 1:100,000 epinephrine.

Epinephrine is the drug of choice for local hemostasis. Norepinephrine can produce marked tissue ischemia, which can lead to necrosis and sloughing and is not recommended for use in hemostasis.[37,38] Epinephrine is most commonly used for hemostasis in a concentration of 1:50,000 (0.2 mg/ml). Generally, small volumes are deposited (not exceeding 0.1 ml) when it is used for hemostasis. Epinephrine also provides excellent hemostasis in a concentration of 1:100,000, although surgical bleeding is inversely proportional to the concentration of vasopressor administered. When plain local anesthetic is infiltrated (e.g., 3% mepivacaine) during periodontal surgery, blood loss is two to three times that noted when 2% lidocaine with 1:100,000 epinephrine is administered.[39] Buckley and associates demonstrated that the use of a 1:50,000 epinephrine concentration produced a 50% decrease in bleeding during periodontal surgery from that seen with a 1:100,000 concentration (with 2% lidocaine).[40] However, epinephrine is not a drug without systemic effects and some undesirable local effects. Studies have shown that even the small volumes of epinephrine used in dentistry can significantly increase the concentrations of plasma catecholamine and alter cardiac function.[41] Therefore it is prudent to administer the smallest volume of the least concentrated form of epinephrine that provides clinically effective hemostasis.

As tissue levels of epinephrine decrease after its injection for hemostasis, a rebound vasodilation develops. Sveen demonstrated that postsurgical bleeding (at 6 hours) occurred in 13 of 16 (81.25%) patients receiving 2% lidocaine with epinephrine for surgical removal of a third molar, whereas 0 of 16 patients who underwent surgery with 3% mepivacaine bled at 6 hours postsurgery.[39] Bleeding interfered with postoperative healing in 9 of 16 (56.25%) patients receiving lidocaine with epinephrine, compared with 25% of patients receiving no epinephrine. There is also evidence that the use of epinephrine in local anesthetics during surgery may produce an increase in postoperative pain.[42]

Many doctors use a 30-gauge short needle to deposit anesthetics for hemostasis. Their rationale is that the thinner needle produces a smaller defect (puncture) in the tissue. If a small puncture is important, then the 30-gauge needle should be used, but only for this purpose. The 30-gauge short needle should not be used if there is the possibility of positive aspiration of blood or if any depth of soft tissue must be penetrated. The aspiration of blood through a 30-gauge needle is difficult (although possible). A 27-gauge needle can be used for local infiltration to achieve hemostasis when vascularity is a problem, or in any other area of the oral cavity without any increase in patient discomfort.

ORAL AND MAXILLOFACIAL SURGERY

Pain control during surgical procedures is achieved through the administration of local anesthetics, either alone or in combination with inhalation sedation, intravenous sedation, or general anesthesia. As is the case with periodontal surgery, the long-duration local anesthetics play an important role in postoperative pain control and are discussed separately.

Local anesthetic techniques used in oral surgery do not differ from those employed in nonsurgical procedures. Therefore it should be expected that instances of either partial or incomplete anesthesia will develop. Oral surgeons frequently treat patients who have received intravenous sedation or general anesthesia before the start of the surgery. These techniques act to modify the patient's reaction to pain, tending to decrease the number of reported instances of inadequate local anesthesia.

Local anesthesia is administered almost routinely to patients for third molar extractions under general anesthesia. The reasons for this are as follows:

1. Pain control during the surgery permits a lessened exposure to general anesthetic agents, allowing for a faster postanesthetic recovery period and minimizing drug-related complications.
2. Hemostasis is possible if a vasopressor is included.
3. Residual local anesthesia in the postoperative period minimizes the requirement for oral opioid analgesics.

The volume of drug and the rate at which it is administered are important in all areas of dental practice, but probably most important during the extraction of teeth from multiple quadrants. When four third molars are extracted, effective pain control must be obtained in all four quadrants. This requires multiple injections of local anesthetics, which usually occur within a relatively short period of time. Four cartridges or more of local anesthetic are frequently used.* The rate at which these local anesthetics are administered must be closely monitored to lessen the occurrence of complications. Complications arising from the rapid administration of local anesthetic include any of the following:

1. Pain during the injection
2. Greater possibility of a serious overdose reaction, if the local anesthetic is administered intravascularly (speed of injection significantly affects the clinical manifestations of toxicity)
3. Postanesthetic pain caused by tissue trauma during the injection

These complications and their prevention, recognition, and management are discussed in greater depth in Chapters 17 and 18.

It should be noted that the inferoposterior border of the mandible is not innervated by the trigeminal nerve in some persons. Any of the mandibular nerve blocks described in Chapter 14 provide only partial anesthesia in this situation. The PDL injection usually corrects the lack of pain control in this circumstance.

FIXED PROSTHODONTICS

When preparing a tooth for full coverage (crown or bridge), it is necessary to place a provisional restoration over the prepared tooth. Although achieving pain control might not be difficult at the initial visit, there may be subsequent visits during which it is difficult to adequately anesthetize the prepared tooth. The reason for this is probably the provisional restoration. Overly high restorations produce traumatic occlusion, which can lead to considerable sensitivity after about a day. Poorly adapted gingival margins develop microleakage, which also causes sensitivity. The procedure itself also can cause tooth sensitivity, through desiccation of tooth structure, possible pulpal involvement, and periodontal irritation. The longer these sources of irritation are present, the greater the trauma to the tooth is likely to be and the more difficult it is to achieve adequate anesthesia. Usually a regional nerve block is effective. Supraperiosteal injections generally do not provide adequate pain control in these situations

(depth may be adequate, but duration is considerably shorter than that usually expected from the drug).

LONG-DURATION LOCAL ANESTHESIA

Prolonged Dental or Surgical Procedures

Several specialty areas of dental practice have a need for longer than usual pulpal or soft-tissue anesthesia. They are fixed prosthodontics, oral surgery, and periodontics. During longer procedures (2 or more hours) an adequate duration of pulpal anesthesia may be difficult to achieve with the more commonly used anesthetics: articaine, lidocaine, mepivacaine, and prilocaine. Bupivacaine (Marcaine) is a long-acting local anesthetic that can then be used. It is discussed more completely in Chapter 4.

Bupivacaine, a homologue of mepivacaine, has a long duration of clinical effectiveness when used for regional nerve block. Its duration of action when administered by supraperiosteal injection, although still long, is somewhat shorter (shorter even than that of lidocaine with epinephrine).[43] Its postoperative analgesic period lasts an average of 8 hours in the mandible and 5 hours in the maxilla.

Bupivacaine is available with a vasopressor (1:200,000 epinephrine). It is interesting to note that the addition of vasopressor to bupivacaine does not prolong its duration of action.[44]

Postprocedural Pain Control

Often, after extensive surgical procedures, the patient experiences considerable pain when the local anesthetic effect dissipates. It was, and still is in many cases, common practice to treat postoperative pain through the use of opioid analgesics. However, opioids have a high incidence of undesirable side effects such as nausea, vomiting, constipation, respiratory depression, and postural hypotension, especially in ambulatory patients.[45]

Long-acting local anesthetics administered to surgical patients offer a means of providing successful postoperative pain control with a minimal risk of developing adverse reactions. An advantage of using long-duration local anesthetics is their longer postoperative analgesia, which leads to a reduced need for the administration of postoperative opioid analgesic drugs.[46] Dentists often use an intermediate-acting local anesthetic, such as articaine, lidocaine, mepivacaine, or prilocaine with a vasopressor, during the surgical period and administer the long-acting local anesthetic just before the termination of the surgery. Danielsson and associates compared bupivacaine, etidocaine, and lidocaine with regard to their effect on postoperative pain, and found that both bupivacaine and etidocaine were more effective in controlling postoperative pain when compared with lidocaine.[43] They also reported that bupivacaine was more effective than etidocaine in

---

*Typical local anesthetic injections for extraction of four third molars include the following:
1. Right and left inferior alveolar nerve blocks, 1.8 ml each (3.6 ml)
2. Right and left posterior superior alveolar nerve blocks or supraperiosteal infiltration over each third molar, 1.3 to 1.8 ml each (2.6 to 3.6 ml)
3. Right and left palatal infiltration over the maxillary third molars, 0.45 ml each, or right and left greater palatine nerve block, 0.45 ml each (0.09 ml)
Total volume of local anesthetic: 8.1 ml or 162 mg or a 2% solution, 243 mg of a 3%, or 324 mg of a 4%.

providing postoperative analgesia and that patients receiving bupivacaine used significantly fewer analgesics.

It is pertinent to note that there appears to be a difference between etidocaine and bupivacaine with respect to their ability to provide adequate hemostasis, even though they contain the same concentration of vasopressor (1:200,000). Danielsson and associates noted that bupivacaine and lidocaine provided adequate hemostasis in 90% and etidocaine in only 75% of the procedures.[44] It is possible that a higher concentration of local anesthetic may necessitate a higher concentration of vasopressor to provide comparable hemostasis. Also keep in mind the different vasodilating properties of the solutions.[47]

Protocol for Perioperative and Postoperative Pain Control in Surgical Patients. Postoperative pain associated with most uncomplicated dental surgical procedures is mild and well managed by oral administration of nonsteroidal antiinflammatory drugs (NSAIDs) such as aspirin and ibuprofen. The preoperative administration of NSAIDs appears to delay the onset of postoperative pain and to lessen its severity.[46,48] When a patient is unable to

---

BOX 16-2

Pain Control Regimen for Surgical Procedures

Preoperative: Administer one or two oral doses of nonsteroidal antiinflammatory drug (NSAID), minimally 1 hour before the scheduled surgical procedure.

Perioperative: Administer local anesthetic of adequate duration for procedure (articaine, lidocaine, mepivacaine, prilocaine with or without vasopressor).

If surgery is planned at approximately 30-minute duration: *immediately* follow initial local anesthetic injection with long-acting local anesthetic (bupivacaine).

If surgery is planned at one hour or longer duration: at the *conclusion* of the surgical procedure reinject the patient with long-acting local anesthetic (bupivacaine).

Postoperative: Have patient continue to take oral NSAID on a timed basis (e.g., bid, tid, qid) for the number of days considered necessary by the surgeon.

Contact patient via telephone the evening of the surgery to determine level of comfort. *If considerable pain is present,* add opioid to NSAID: codeine, oxycodone, and propoxyphene.

(From Malamed SF: Local anesthetics: dentistry's most important drugs, *J Am Dent Assoc* 125:1571-1576, 1994.)

TABLE 16-5
Nonsteroidal Antiinflammatory Drugs

Generic	Proprietary	Availability	Dosage Regimen
Celecoxib	Celebrex	100-, 200-mg tablets	200 mg PO bid
Diclofenac	Cataflam, Voltaren	50-mg tablets, 50- and 75-mg delayed-release tablets, 100-mg extended-release tablets	50 mg PO tid
Etodolac	Lodine	200- and 400-mg capsules; 400- and 500-mg tablets; 400-, 500-, 600-mg extended-release tablets	200–400 mg PO q6–8h
Fenoprofen	Nalfon Pulvules	200-, 300-mg capsules; 600-mg tablets	200 mg PO q4–6h
Flurbiprofen	Ansaid	50- and 100-mg tablets	50–100 mg PO bid-tid
Ibuprofen	Various	100-, 200-mg tablets (OTC); 400-, 600-, 800-mg tablets (Rx); 200-mg capsules (OTC); 100 mg/5 ml suspension; 40 mg/ml oral drops (pediatric)	400 mg PO q4–6h
Indomethacin	Indocin	25- and 50-mg capsules; 75-mg sustained-release capsules	25–50 mg PO tid prn
Ketoprofen	Orudis	12.5-mg tablets (OTC); 25-, 50-, 75-mg capsules; 100-, 150-, and 200-mg extended-release capsule	25–50 mg PO q6–8h
Ketorolac	Toradol	10-mg tablets	10 mg PO q4–6h
Meclofenamate	Various	50- and 100-mg capsules	50–100 mg PO q4–6h
Mefenamic acid	Ponstel	250-mg capsule	50 mg PO q4–6h prn
Nabumetone	Relafen	500- and 750-mg tablets	1 g PO bid for 7–14 d
Naproxen	Aleve, Anaprox, Naprosyn	200-mg tablets (OTC); 250- and 500-mg tablets (Rx); 375- and 500-mg delayed-release tablets; 375- and 500-mg controlled-release tablets	250–500 mg PO bid
Oxaprozin	Daypro	600-mg tablets	1200 mg PO qd
Piroxicam	Feldene	10- and 20-mg capsules	20 mg PO qd
Rofecoxib	Vioxx	12.5- and 25-mg tablets 12.5 mg/5ml and 25 mg/5 ml suspension	50 mg PO qd
Sulindac	Clinoril	150- and 200-mg tablets	200 mg PO bid for 7–14 d

(Data from *Drug Facts and Comparisons 2004,* ed 8, St Louis, 2003, Facts and Comparisons.)
OTC, Over the counter.

tolerate aspirin or other NSAIDs, acetaminophen can provide acceptable analgesia.

Other dental surgical procedures, such as removal of bony impactions and osseous periodontal or endodontic surgery, are more traumatic and typically are associated with more intense and prolonged postoperative pain. The onset of such pain can be delayed by the presurgical administration of an NSAID followed by the administration of a long-acting local anesthetic (bupivacaine) at the completion of the surgery.[48]

When postoperative pain does emerge, it may require the addition of an opioid to the nonsteroidal regimen. Codeine, at a dosage level of 30 to 60 mg every 4 to 6 hours, is frequently prescribed and often very effective. Alternative opioids include propoxyphene or oxycodone administered in doses that are equianalgesic to 30 to 60 mg of codeine.[48]

Box 16-2 outlines a recommended protocol for the management of intraoperative and postoperative pain associated with dental surgical procedures.[49] Common NSAIDs and their recommended doses are listed in Table 16-5.

DENTAL HYGIENE

In 1997 when the fourth edition of this textbook was published, registered dental hygienists in 20 states in the United States and several provinces in Canada were permitted to administer local anesthesia to dental patients. This number increased to 32 in 2003 (Table 16-6).[50] The inclusion of this expanded function in the Dental Practice Act in these areas has proved of great benefit to the hygienist, doctor, and dental patient.[51,52]

Not all patients need local anesthesia for scaling, root planing, and subgingival curettage, but many do. The periodontal tissues being treated are normally sensitive to stimuli and are even more so when inflammation is present. Such is frequently the case when a patient is treated by the dental hygienist.

The hygienist who is permitted to administer local anesthetics to dental patients requires the same technique armamentarium as the doctor. Regional block anesthesia, especially in the maxilla (posterior superior or anterior superior alveolar nerve block), is an integral part of the hygienist's anesthetic armamentarium since hygienists usually treat whole quadrants in one appointment. The hygiene patient requires the same depth of anesthesia as that obtained by the doctor doing restorative dentistry or surgery. Root planing without discomfort requires pulpal anesthesia, along with soft-tissue and osseous anesthesia.[53]

Before dental hygienists were permitted to administer local anesthetics, pain control necessitated that the doctor administer local anesthesia or inhalation sedation (nitrous oxide and oxygen) for the hygienist's patients, or the hygienist applied topical anesthetic to the buccal and linguopalatal soft tissue in all four quadrants. Although these alternatives are workable, they do not compare with permitting a well-trained dental hygienist to administer local anesthetics to patients. More than 70% of respondents to a survey on dental hygiene patients' need for pain control reported that their patients needed anesthesia but did not receive it.[53]

Feedback from dentists whose hygienists administer local anesthesia has been uniformly positive, with negative comments extremely rare.[51,52] Dental patients themselves are aware of the difference in local anesthesia administered by the dental hygienist and that administered by the dentist. They frequently comment on the lack of discomfort when the hygienist injects the local anesthetic. Be it a slower rate of administration, more attention to the details of atraumatic injection technique, or greater empathy, it works.

TABLE **16-6**

States Permitting Administration of Local Anesthetics by Dental Hygienists

State and Year Implemented	Supervision Required	Block and/or Infiltration
AK 1981	Direct	Both
AZ 1976	Direct	Both
AR 1995	Direct	Both
CA 1976	Direct	Both
CO 1977	Direct	Both
HI 1987	Direct	Both
ID 1975	Direct	Both
IA 1998	Direct	Both
IL 2000	Direct	Both
KS 1993	Direct	Both
KY 2002	Direct	Both
LA 1998	Direct	Both
ME 1997	Direct	Both
MN 1995	Direct	Both
MO 1973	Direct	Both
MI 2002	Direct	Both
MT 1985	Direct	Both
ND 2003	Direct	Both
NE 1995	Direct	Both
NH 2002	Direct	Both
NV 1972	Direct	Both
NM 1972	Direct	Both
NY 2001	Direct	Infiltration
OK 1980	Direct	Both
OR 1975	General	Both
SC 1995	Direct	Infiltration
SD 1992	Direct	Both
UT 1983	Direct	Both
VT 1993	Direct	Both
WA 1971	Direct	Both
WI 1998	Direct	Both
WY 1991	Direct	Both

(Data from American Dental Hygienists Association, Chicago, 2003.)

REFERENCES

1. Brown RD: The failure of local anaesthesia in acute inflammation, *Br Dent J* 151:47-51, 1981.
2. Vandermeulen E: Pain perception, mechanisms of action of local anesthetics and possible causes of failure, *Rev Belge Medecine Dent* 55:19-40, 2000.
3. Kitay D, Ferraro N, Sonis ST: Lateral pharyngeal space abscess as a consequence of regional anesthesia, *J Am Dent Assoc* 122:56-59, 1991.
4. Connor JP, Edelson JG: Needle tract infection: a case report, *Oral Surg* 65:401-403, 1988.
5. Jeske AH: Local anesthetics: special considerations in endodontics, *Tex Dent J* 120:231-237, 2003.
6. Meechan JG: Supplementary routes to local anesthesia, *Intern Endodont J* 35:885-896, 2002.
7. Coggins R, Reader A, Nist R, et al: Anesthetic efficacy of the intraosseous injection in maxillary and mandibular teeth, *Oral Surg, Oral Med, Oral Path, Oral Radiol, Endodont* 81:634-641, 1996.
8. Reisman D, Reader A, Nist R, et al: Anesthetic efficacy of the supplemental intraosseous injection of 3% mepivacaine in irreversible pulpitis, *Oral Surg, Oral Med, Oral Path, Oral Radio, Endodont* 84:676-682, 1997.
9. Leonard M: The efficacy of an intraosseous injection system of delivering local anesthetic, *J Am Dent Assoc* 126: 11-86, 1995.
10. Coury KA: Achieving profound anesthesia using the intraosseous technique, *Tex Dent J* 114:34-39, 1997.
11. Nusstein J, Reader A, Nist R, et al: Anesthetic efficacy of the supplemental intraosseous injection of 2% lidocaine with 1:100,000 epinephrine in irreversible pulpitis, *J Endodont* 24:478-491, 1998.
12. Quinn CL: Injection techniques to anesthetize the difficult tooth, *J Calif Dent Assoc* 26:665-667, 1998.
13. Parente SA, Anderson RW, Herman WW, et al: Anesthetic efficacy of the supplemental intraosseous injection for teeth with irreversible pulpitis, *J Endodont* 24:826-828, 1998.
14. Brown R: Intraosseous anesthesia: a review, *J Calif Dent Assoc* 27:785-792, 1999.
15. Weathers A Jr: Taking the mystery out of endodontics, Part 6. Painless anesthesia for the "hot" tooth, *Dent Today* 18:90-93, 1999.
16. Stabile P, Reader A, Gallatin E, et al: Anesthetic efficacy and heart rate effects of the intraosseous injection of 1.5% etidocaine (1:200,000 epinephrine) after an inferior alveolar nerve block, *Oral Surg, Oral Med, Oral Path, Oral Radio, Endodont* 89:407-411, 2000.
17. Replogle K, Reader A, Nist R, et al: Cardiovascular effects of intraosseous injections of 2% lidocaine with 1:100,000 epinephrine and 3% mepivacaine, *J Am Dent Assoc* 130: 549-657, 1999.
18. Saadoun AP, Malamed SF: Intraseptal anesthesia in periodontal surgery, *J Am Dent Assoc* 111:249, 1985.
19. Goodsen JM, Moore PA: Life-threatening reactions after pedodontic sedation: an assessment of narcotic, local anesthetic, and antiemetic drug interaction, *J Am Dent Assoc* 107:239-245, 1983.
20. Moore PA: Preventing local anesthesia toxicity, *J Am Dent Assoc* 123:60-64, 1992.
21. Berquist HC: The danger of mepivacaine 3% toxicity in children, *Can Dent Assoc J* 3:13, 1975.
22. Malamed SF: Morbidity, mortality and local anesthesia, *Primary Dent Care* 6:11-15, 1999.
23. Meechan J: How to avoid local anaesthetic toxicity, *Br Dent J* 184:334-335, 1998.
24. Meechan JG, Rood JP: Adverse effects of dental local anaesthesia, *Dent Update* 24:315-318, 1997.
25. Davis MJ, Vogel LD: Local anesthetic safety in pediatric patients, *NY State Dent J* 62:22-35, 1996.
26. Cheatham BD, Primosch RE, Courts FJ: A survey of local anesthetic usage in pediatric patients by Florida dentists, *J Dent Child* 59:401-407, 1992.
27. Yagiela JA: Regional anesthesia for dental procedures, *Int Anesthesiol Clin* 27:28-82, 1989.
28. Malamed SF: Allergic and toxic reactions to local anesthetics, *Dent Today* 22(4):114-121, April 2003.
29. Rood JP: Notes on local analgesia for the child patient, *Dent Update* 8:377-381, 1981.
30. Kaufman L, Sowray JH, Rood JP: *General anaesthesia, local analgesia, and sedation in dentistry,* Oxford, UK, 1982, Blackwell Scientific.
31. O'Sullivan VR, Holland T, O'Mullane DM, et al: A review of current local anaesthetic techniques in dentistry for children, *J Irish Dent Assoc* 32:17-27, 1986.
32. Benham NR: The cephalometric position of the mandibular foramen with age, *J Dent Child* 43:233-237, 1976.
33. Akinosi JO: A new approach to the mandibular nerve block, *Br J Oral Surg* 15:83-87, 1977.
34. Yamada A, Jastak JT: Clinical evaluation of the Gow-Gates block in children, *Anesth Prog* 28:106-109, 1981.
35. Brannstrom M, Lindskog S, Nordenvall KJ: Enamel hypoplasia in permanent teeth induced by periodontal ligament anesthesia of primary teeth, *J Am Dent Assoc* 109: 535-736, 1984.
36. Davenport RE, Porcelli RJ, Iacono VJ, et al: Effects of anesthetics containing epinephrine on catecholamine levels during periodontal surgery. *J Periodontol* 61:553-558, 1990.
37. van der Bijl P, Victor AM: Adverse reactions associated with norepinephrine in dental local anesthesia, *Anesth Prog* 39: 37-89, 1992.
38. Jakob W: Local anaesthesia and vasoconstrictive additional components, *Newslett Int Fed Dent Anesthesiol Soc* 2:1, 1989.
39. Sveen K: Effect of the addition of a vasoconstrictor to local anesthetic solution on operative and postoperative bleeding, analgesia and wound healing, *Int J Oral Surg* 8:301-306, 1979.
40. Buckley JA, Ciancio SG, McMullen JA: Efficacy of epinephrine concentration in local anesthesia during periodontal surgery, *J Periodontol* 55:653-657, 1984.
41. Jastak JT, Yagiela JA: Vasoconstrictors and local anesthesia; a review and rationale for use, *J Am Dent Assoc* 107: 623-630, 1983.
42. Skoglund LA, Jorkjend L: Postoperative pain experience after gingivectomies using different combinations of local anaesthetic agents and periodontal dressings, *J Clin Periodontol* 18:204-209, 1991.
43. Danielsson K, Evers H, Nordenram A: Long-acting local anesthetics in oral surgery: an experimental evaluation of bupivacaine and etidocaine for oral infiltration anesthesia, *Anesth Prog* 32:65-68, 1985.
44. Danielsson K, Evers H, Holmlund A, et al: Long-acting local anaesthetics in oral surgery, *Int J Oral Maxillofac Surg* 15:119-126, 1986.

45. Hardman JG, Limbird LE, editors: *Goodman & Gilman's the pharmacological basis of therapeutics*, ed 10, New York, 2001, McGraw-Hill.

46. Jackson DL, Moore PA, Hargreaves KM: Pre-operative nonsteroidal antiinflammatory medication for the prevention of postoperative dental pain, *J Am Dent Assoc* 119:641-647, 1989.

47. Linden ET, Abrams H, Matheny J, et al: A comparison of postoperative pain experience following periodontal surgery using two local anesthetic agents, *J Periodontol* 57:637-642, 1986.

48. Acute Pain Management Guideline Panel: *Acute pain management: operative or medical procedures and trauma. Clinical practice guideline*, AHCPR Pub No 92-0032, Rockville, Md, 1992, Agency for Health Care Policy and Research, Public Health Service, US Department of Health and Human Services.

49. Malamed SF: Local anesthetics: dentistry's most important drugs, *J Am Dent Assoc* 125:1571-1576, 1994.

50. American Dental Hygienists Association, *www.adha.org*, Chicago, 2003.

51. Sisty-LePeau N, Boyer EM, Lutjen D: Dental hygiene licensure specifications on pain control procedures, *J Dent Hyg* 64:179-185, 1990.

52. DeAngelis S, Goral V: Utilization of local anesthesia by Arkansas dental hygienists, and dentists' delegation/satisfaction relative to this function, *J Dent Hyg* 74:196-204, 2000.

53. Sisty-LePeau N, Nielson-Thompson N, Lutjen D: Use, need and desire for pain control procedures by Iowa hygienists, *J Dent Hyg* 66(3):137-146, 1992.

IN THIS PART

PART FOUR

Complications, Legal Considerations, Future Trends, and Questions

In spite of careful patient evaluation, proper tissue preparation, and meticulous technique of administration, local and systemic complications associated with dental anesthesia occasionally develop. These problems are addressed in Chapters 17 and 18. Emphasis is placed on prevention, recognition, and management of the complications.

New to this edition is a discussion, by Dr. Daniel Orr II, of legal considerations associated with the administration of local anesthetics (Chapter 19).

Chapter 20, Future Trends in Pain Control, first appeared in the third edition and is updated here. There has been considerable interest demonstrated in recent years in improving local anesthesia as "the" technique of pain control. Examples include the computer-controlled local anesthetic delivery systems described in Chapter 5. In addition, alternative techniques for providing clinically pain-free dental and medical care are continually sought. In the 1980s electronic dental anesthesia (EDA) was shown to be a viable alternative to injectable local anesthetics in certain types of dental care. Although EDA is not employed by many United States dentists, it remains a part of the pain control armamentarium. A relatively new consideration, presently undergoing clinical trials, is the ability to "reverse" local anesthesia at the completion of a procedure. Most dental treatment does not possess considerable postoperative discomfort, and numerous patients complain about the prolonged soft-tissue anesthesia associated with local anesthetic injections. Research is being conducted into methods of "unanesthetizing" patients at the conclusion of treatment.

Chapter 21 presents a series of questions related to local anesthesia and pain control in dentistry. These frequently asked questions (FAQs) come from doctors who have had peculiar situations arise in connection with local anesthetic administration. The more common questions are presented here as a matter of interest and in the hope that the answers to specific questions or problems might be included.

Local Complications

CHAPTER 17

A number of potential complications are associated with the administration of local anesthetics:

- Needle breakage
- Persistent anesthesia or paresthesia
- Facial nerve paralysis
- Trismus
- Soft-tissue injury
- Hematoma
- Pain on injection
- Burning on injection
- Infection
- Edema
- Sloughing of tissues
- Postanesthetic intraoral lesions

For purposes of convenience these complications may be separated into those that occur *locally* in the region of the injection and those that are *systemic*. Systemic complications associated with the administration of local anesthesia are discussed in Chapter 18, and include overdosage (toxic reaction), allergy, and psychogenic reactions; localized complications are described in this chapter.

It must be emphasized that with any complication associated with the administration of a local anesthetic, a written note should be entered onto the patient's dental chart. For complications that become chronic, a note should appear whenever the patient is reevaluated.

NEEDLE BREAKAGE

Breakage and retention of needles within tissues has become an extremely rare occurrence because of the introduction of disposable needles. However, reports of needle breakage still appear, despite the fact that virtually all such instances are preventable (Fig. 17-1).[1–9]

It is estimated (conservatively) that dentists in the United States administer in excess of 300 million local anesthetic cartridges annually. Given that in many instances multiple injections are administered with one cartridge, the number of actual needle penetrations of intraoral mucous membranes occurring in dental patients in the United States is exceedingly high, probably in excess of 500 million a year.

In the 30 years (1973–2003) that this author has been involved in the teaching of local anesthesia, he has been involved with 34 instances in which litigation has resulted from a broken dental needle retained in the patient's mouth. In 33 of these cases the inferior alveolar nerve block was the injection being administered at the time of needle breakage. The remaining incident occurred during a posterior superior alveolar nerve block. The gauge and length of needle used by the dentist in all but one case was a 30-gauge short. A 27-gauge short needle was used in the other instance.

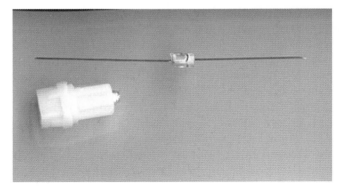

Figure 17-1. Metal disposable needle, disassembled.

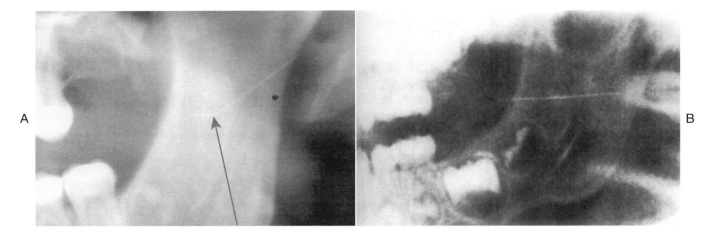

A   B

Figure 17-2. A, Radiograph of a broken dental needle (note bend in needle: *arrow*). **B,** Radiograph of a broken dental needle in the pterygomandibular space. (**B,** From Marks RB, Carlton DM, McDonald S: Management of a broken needle in the pterygomandibular space: report of a case, *J Am Dent Assoc* 109:263-264, 1984. Reprinted by permission.)

Separate data, received from a major local anesthetic needle manufacturer,[10] reports 27 instances of broken dental needles over a 5-year period. These reports are in addition to those referred to previously. The injection being administered at the time of needle breakage was not documented. However, the needle employed was a 30-gauge short in all reported instances.

Disposable dental needles as used in most countries, including the United States and Canada, are extremely well manufactured (see Chapter 6). The needle itself is composed of one continuous strand of metal that starts at the needle tip and continues into the hub to exit on the opposite side as the portion of the needle that penetrates the cartridge (see Fig. 17-1). Needles do not "separate" (as in two pieces of metal separating at the hub), as was claimed by doctors in some of these cases. The occurrence of truly "defective" dental needles is so low as to be a nonentity.[11,12]

In many of the cases of retained broken dental needles there is strong clinical and scientific evidence that the needle had been bent (by the doctor) before its insertion into the patient's mouth (Figs. 17-2, *A* and 17-3).

In each and every case of retained broken dental needles there was one factor universally present: The needle had been inserted into the soft tissues its entire length. Inferior alveolar nerve block (IANB) in the typical adult patient requires soft-tissue penetration to a depth of 20 to 25 mm. Because the tip-to-hub length of a short dental needle is approximately 20 mm (some 30-gauge needles are even shorter; see Table 6-4), it is evident that these needles had to be inserted to their hub to reach the inferior alveolar nerve. Needles, when they break, *always* break at the hub (the most rigid portion of the needle). If the needle is inserted into soft tissue to the hub when it breaks, the elasticity of the soft tissues produces a rebound and the needle is buried. The syringe is removed from the mouth with the needle no longer present (Fig. 17-4).

If a long dental needle had been used for the injection in question, and the needle had still broken (at the hub) there would remain, still visible in the patient's mouth, approximately 7 to 12 mm of needle that could then easily be removed from the mouth with a forceps.

If a 25- or 27-gauge needle had been employed instead of a 30-gauge needle, the likelihood of the needle breaking at all would have been negligible.

Causes

The primary cause of needle breakage is *weakening of the dental needle by bending it* before its insertion into the

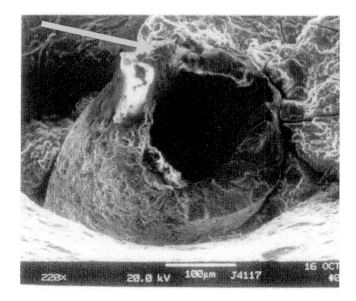

Figure 17-3. Scanning electron microscopy of broken dental needle. Arrow at 11 o'clock position indicates area where needle was bent superiorly before injection, per court testimony of forensic metallurgist.

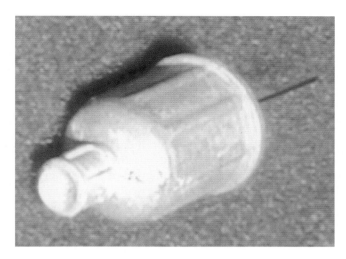

Figure 17-4. Hub of broken needle from Figure 17-2, *B*.

patient's mouth. Another potential cause is *sudden unexpected movement* by the patient as the needle penetrates muscle or contacts periosteum.[6] If the patient's movement is opposite that of the needle, the force of contact may prove adequate to break the needle (especially if previously bent and if the needle is "finer" [e.g., 30 gauge]). This is more likely to occur in the pediatric dental patient.

1. Smaller needles (e.g., 30 gauge) are far more likely to break than larger needles (e.g., 25 gauge).
2. Needles that have previously been *bent* (in an attempt to direct them more accurately into the tissue) are weakened and more likely to break than unbent needles.
3. Needles may prove to be defective in manufacture (an exceedingly rare, and unlikely, cause of needle breakage).

Problem

Needle breakage per se is not a significant problem. If a broken needle can be retrieved without surgical intervention, no emergency exists. A Magill intubation forceps or hemostat can be used to grasp the visible proximal end of the needle fragment and remove it from the soft tissue.

Needles that break off within tissues and cannot readily be retrieved do not migrate more than a few millimeters. They become encased in scar tissue within a few weeks. Localized or systemic infection produced by such needles is extremely rare. Electing to leave a needle fragment in the tissue instead of attempting its removal usually leads to fewer problems than the extensive, involved, and often traumatic surgical procedure necessary for its removal. More recently, however, removal of the broken needle has been considered to be warranted, primarily because of the patient's (and doctor's) fear of needle migration, but also because of legal considerations.[4,6] In

addition, removal of the needle allays the psychological worries of both the patient and practitioner.

Prevention

Use larger-gauge needles for techniques requiring penetration of significant depths of soft tissue; 25-gauge needles are appropriate for an inferior alveolar, mandibular, posterior superior alveolar (PSA), anterior superior alveolar (ASA), and maxillary nerve block.

Use long needles for injections requiring penetration of significant (>18 mm) depths of soft tissues.

Do not insert a needle into tissues to its hub, unless it is absolutely essential for the success of the technique; the point at which the needle shaft meets the hub is the least flexible, weakest part of the needle and the site at which needle breakage occurs. Select a needle of adequate length for the contemplated procedure.

Do not redirect a needle once it is inserted into tissues. Excessive lateral force on the needle is a factor in breakage. Withdraw the needle *almost* completely before redirecting it.

Management

Shira has presented a description of the management of broken needles.[13] A summary of his prudent suggestions follows:

1. When a needle breaks:
   a. Remain calm; do not panic.
   b. Instruct the patient not to move. Do not remove your hand from the patient's mouth; keep the patient's mouth open. If available, place a bite block in the patient's mouth.
   c. If the fragment is visible, try to remove it with a small hemostat or a Magill intubation forceps. (See Chapter 8.)
2. If the needle is lost (not visible) and cannot be readily retrieved:
   a. Do *not* proceed with an incision or probing.
   b. Calmly inform the patient; attempt to allay fears and apprehension.
   c. Note the incident on the patient's chart. Keep the remaining needle fragment. Inform your insurance carrier immediately.
   d. Refer the patient to an oral and maxillofacial surgeon for *consultation*, not for removal of the needle.
3. When a needle breaks, consideration should be given to its immediate removal, *under the following conditions:*
   a. The needle is superficial *and* easily located through radiological and clinical examination; removal by a competent dental surgeon is possible.
   b. Despite its superficial location, attempted retrieval is unsuccessful within a reasonable length of time; it is then prudent to abandon the attempt and allow the needle fragment to remain.

c. The needle is located in deeper tissues or is hard to locate; it should be permitted to remain *without* an attempt at removal.

In many instances, attempted removal of the broken needle is performed in the operating room under general anesthesia.

There is considerable precedent to justify the retention of a broken needle if removal appears difficult.

Unfortunately, the likelihood of litigation ensuing after a broken needle incident is high.

PERSISTENT ANESTHESIA OR PARESTHESIA

On occasion a patient reports feeling numb ("frozen") many hours or days after a local anesthetic injection. Normal distribution of patient response to drugs allows for the rare individual (e.g., hyperreactor) who may experience prolonged soft-tissue anesthesia after local anesthetic administration persisting for many hours longer than that which is expected. This is not a problem.

When anesthesia persists for days, weeks, or months there is an increased potential for the development of problems. Paresthesia or persistent anesthesia is a disturbing yet sometimes unpreventable complication of local anesthetic administration. Paresthesia is also one of the most frequent causes of dental malpractice litigation.

A patient's clinical response to this can be many and varied, including sensations of numbness, swelling, tingling, and itching. There may be associated oral dysfunction, including tongue biting, drooling, loss of taste, and speech impediment.[14–17]

Paresthesia is defined as *persistent anesthesia* (anesthesia well beyond the expected duration), or *altered sensation* well beyond the expected duration of anesthesia. In addition, the definition of paresthesia should also include *hyperesthesia* and *dysesthesia*, in which the patient experience both pain and numbness.[18]

Causes

Trauma to any nerve may lead to paresthesia. Paresthesia is a not uncommon complication of oral surgical procedures and mandibular dental implants.[15,19–21] In an audit of 741 third mandibular molar extractions, Bataineh found postoperative lingual nerve anesthesia in 2.6%; inferior alveolar nerve paresthesia was 3.9%, developing in 9.8% of patients under age 20 years. There was also a significant correlation between incidence of paresthesia and the experience of the operator.[21]

Injection of a local anesthetic solution contaminated by alcohol or sterilizing solution near a nerve produces irritation, resulting in edema and increased pressure in the region of the nerve, leading to paresthesia. These contaminants, especially alcohol, are neurolytic and can produce long-term trauma to the nerve (paresthesia lasting for months to years).

Trauma to the nerve sheath can be produced by the needle during injection. The patient reports the sensation of an "electric shock" throughout the distribution of the involved nerve. Although it is exceedingly difficult (and a highly unlikely possibility) to actually sever a nerve trunk or even its fibers with the small needles used in dentistry, trauma to a nerve produced by contact with the needle is all that may be needed to produce paresthesia.[15,16] Insertion of a needle into a foramen, as in the second division (maxillary) nerve block via the greater palatine foramen, also increases the likelihood of nerve injury.

Hemorrhage into or around the neural sheath is another cause. Bleeding increases pressure on the nerve, leading to paresthesia.[14–16,18]

The local anesthetic solution itself may contribute to the development of paresthesia after local anesthetic injection. Haas and Lennon published a retrospective study of paresthesia after the injection of local anesthetic in dentistry in Canada over a 20-year period (1973–1993).[14] Only cases where no surgery was performed were considered. One hundred forty-three cases of paresthesia unrelated to surgery were reported in this period. All reported cases involved either the inferior alveolar or lingual nerve or both, with anesthesia of the tongue reported most often, followed by anesthesia of the lip. Pain (hyperesthesia) was reported by 22% of the patients. Paresthesia was reported most often after the administration of a 4% local anesthetic, either prilocaine HCl and articaine HCl. The observed frequencies of paresthesia after the administration of articaine HCl and prilocaine HCl were significantly greater than the expected frequencies for these drugs, based on the distribution of local anesthetic use in Ontario in 1993 (Table 17-1).[22] According to Haas the incidence of permanent paresthesia resulting from

TABLE **17-1**
Local Anesthetic Use by Ontario Dentists

Local Anesthetic	Vasoconstrictor	% Using Formulation
2% Lidocaine HCl	Epinephrine 1:100,000	23.4
4% Articaine HCl	Epinephrine 1:200,000	19.9
4% Articaine HCl	Epinephrine 1:100,000	17.9
4% Prilocaine HCl	Epinephrine 1:200,000	16.4
2% Mepivacaine HCl	Levonordefrin 1:20,000	6.4
3% Mepivacaine HCl	—	6.3
0.5% Bupivacaine HCl	Epinephrine 1:200,000	2.1

(Data from Haas DA, Lennon D: Local anesthetic use by dentists in Ontario. *J Canad Dent Assoc* 61(4):297-304, 1995.)

all local anesthetics is approximately 1:785,000; for 0.5%, 2%, and 3% local anesthetics it is approximately 1:1,200,000, and for 4% local anesthetics it is approximately 1:500,000.[23]

It is apparent that all local anesthetics are, to varying degrees, neurotoxic.[24] The concentration of the local anesthetic may have some bearing on the observed incidence of paresthesia. Prilocaine HCl is a good example: It is used as a 4% solution in many countries, whereas in others it is employed as a 3% concentration. Reports of paresthesia associated with the administration of prilocaine HCl most often derive from areas where it is used as the 4% solution.

Until more data can be gathered as to the incidence of paresthesia to local anesthetic drugs it appears that some caution must be advised when considering the use of 4% local anesthetics for nerve blocks in the mandible. As with all procedures considered for use by a "doctor," as well as drugs considered for administration by a "doctor," the benefit to be gained from use of the drug or therapeutic procedure must be weighed against the risks involved in their use. Only when the benefit to be gained clearly outweighs the risk should the drug or procedure be used.

Problem

Persistent anesthesia, rarely total, in most cases partial, can lead to self-inflicted injury. Biting or thermal or chemical insult can occur without a patient's awareness, until the process has progressed to a serious degree. When the lingual nerve is involved, the sense of taste (via the chorda tympani nerve) also may be impaired.

In some instances a loss of sensation (paresthesia) is not the clinical manifestation of nerve injury. *Hyperesthesia* (an increased sensitivity to noxious stimuli) and *dysesthesia* (a painful sensation occurring to usually nonnoxious stimuli) also may be noted. Haas and Lennon reported that pain was present in 22% of the 143 cases of paresthesia they reviewed.[14]

Prevention

Strict adherence to injection protocol and proper care and handling of dental cartridges help minimize the risk of paresthesia. Nevertheless, cases of paresthesia still occur despite care taken during injection.

Management

Most paresthesias resolve within approximately 8 weeks without treatment.[25] Only if damage to the nerve is severe will the paresthesia be permanent, and then only rarely. In most situations paresthesia is minimal, with the patient retaining most sensory function to the affected area. Therefore the risk of self-inflicted tissue injury is minimal. Haas and Lennon, in a 21-year retrospective study of Canadian dentists, reported that most paresthesias

involved the tongue, with the lower lip the next most common site of involvement.[14]

McCarthy has recommended the following sequence in managing the patient with a persistent sensory deficit after local anesthesia:[26]

1. Be reassuring. The patient usually telephones the office the day after the dental procedure complaining of still being a little numb.
   a. Speak with the patient personally! Do not relegate the duty to an auxiliary. Remember that if patients cannot get through to speak to their doctor, they can always get the doctor's attention through litigation!
   b. Explain that paresthesia is not uncommon after local anesthetic administration. Sisk and associates have reported that paresthesia may develop in up to 22% of patients in very selected circumstances.[27]
   c. Arrange an appointment to examine the patient.
   d. Record the incident on the dental chart.
2. Examine the patient.
   a. Determine the degree and extent of paresthesia.
   b. Explain to the patient that paresthesia normally persists for at least 2 months before resolution begins and that it may last up to a year or longer.
   c. "Tincture of time" is the recommended medicine.
   d. Record all findings on the patient's chart.
3. Reschedule the patient for examination every 2 months for as long as the sensory deficit persists.
4. If sensory deficit is still evident 1 year after the incident, consultation with an oral surgeon or neurologist is recommended. Consultation should be considered earlier if the patient or doctor considers it prudent.
5. Dental treatment may continue, but avoid readministering local anesthetic into the region of the previously traumatized nerve. Use alternate local anesthetic techniques if possible.

FACIAL NERVE PARALYSIS

The seventh cranial nerve carries motor impulses to the muscles of facial expression, of the scalp and external ear, and of other structures. Paralysis of some of its terminal branches occurs whenever an infraorbital nerve block is administered or when maxillary canines are infiltrated. Muscle droop is also observed when, occasionally, the motor fibers are anesthetized by inadvertent deposition of local anesthetic into their vicinity. This may occur when anesthetic is introduced into the deep lobe of the parotid gland, through which terminal portions of the facial nerve extend (Fig. 17-5).

The facial nerve branches and the muscles they innervate are listed below:
1. Temporal branches
   a. Frontalis
   b. Orbicularis oculi
   c. Corrugator supercilii

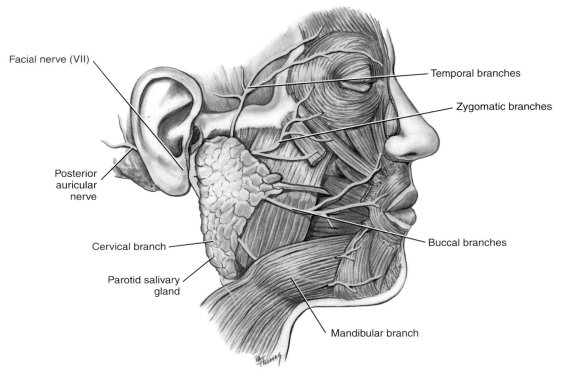

Figure 17-5. Facial nerve distribution.

2. Zygomatic branches
   a. Orbicularis oculi
3. Buccal branches: supplying the region inferior to the eye and around the mouth
   a. Procerus
   b. Zygomaticus
   c. Levator labii superioris
   d. Buccinator
   e. Orbicularis oris
4. Mandibular branch: supplying muscles of the lower lip and chin
   a. Depressor anguli oris
   b. Depressor labii inferioris
   c. Mentalis

Cause

Transient facial nerve paralysis is commonly caused by the introduction of local anesthetic into the capsule of the parotid gland, which is located at the posterior border of the mandibular ramus, clothed by the medial pterygoid and masseter muscles.[27–31] Directing the needle posteriorly or inadvertently deflecting it in a posterior direction during an IANB, or overinsertion during a Vazirani-Akinosi nerve block, may place the tip of the needle within the body of the parotid gland. If local anesthetic is deposited, transient paralysis can result. Duration of the paralysis is equal to that of the soft-tissue anesthesia usually noted for that drug.

Problem

Loss of motor function to the muscles of facial expression produced by local anesthetic deposition is normally *transitory*. It lasts no more than several hours depending on the local anesthetic formulation used, volume injected, and proximity to the facial nerve. There is usually minimal or no sensory loss.

During this time the patient has unilateral paralysis and be unable to use these muscles (Fig. 17-6). The primary problem associated with transient facial nerve paralysis is cosmetic: The person's face appears lopsided. There is no treatment other than waiting until the action of the drug resolves.

A secondary problem is that the patient is unable to voluntarily close one eye. The protective lid reflex of the eye is abolished. Winking and blinking become impossible. The cornea, however, does retain its innervation; thus, if it is irritated, the corneal reflex is intact and tears lubricate the eye.

Prevention

Transient facial nerve paralysis is almost always preventable by adhering to protocol with the inferior alveolar and Vazirani-Akinosi nerve blocks (as described in Chapter 14), although in some situations branches of the facial nerve may lie close to the site of local anesthetic deposition in the IANB and Vazirani-Akinosi nerve blocks.

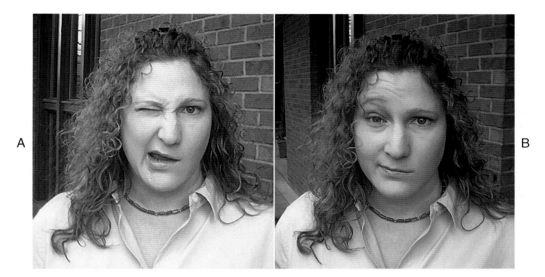

Figure 17-6. Facial nerve paralysis. Note, **A,** inability to close eyelid and, **B,** drooping of lip on affected side (patient's left).

A needle tip in contact with bone (medial aspect of the ramus) before depositing local anesthetic solution virtually precludes the possibility that anesthetic will be deposited into the parotid gland during an IANB. If the needle deflects posteriorly during this block and bone is not contacted, the needle should be withdrawn *almost entirely* from the soft tissues, the barrel of the syringe brought posteriorly (therefore, the needle tip being directed more anteriorly), and the needle readvanced until it contacts bone.

Because there is no contact with bone during the Vazirani-Akinosi nerve block, overinsertion of the needle, either absolute (>25 mm) or relative (25 mm in a smaller patient), should be avoided, if possible.

Management

Within seconds to minutes after the deposition of local anesthetic into the parotid gland, the patient senses a weakening of the muscles on the affected side of the face. Sensory anesthesia is *not* present in this situation. Management includes the following:

1. Reassure the patient. Explain that the situation is transient, will last for a few hours, and will resolve without residual effect. Mention that it is produced by the normal reaction to local anesthetic drugs on the facial nerve, which is a motor nerve to the muscles of facial expression.
2. Contact lenses should be removed until muscular movement returns.
3. An eye patch should be applied to the affected eye until muscle tone returns. If resistance is offered by the patient, advise the patient to manually close the lower eyelid periodically to keep the cornea lubricated.
4. Record the incident on the patient's chart.
5. Although there is no contraindication to reanesthetizing the patient to achieve mandibular anesthesia, it

may be prudent to forego further dental care at this appointment.

TRISMUS

Trismus, from the Greek *trismos,* is defined as a prolonged, tetanic spasm of the jaw muscles by which the normal opening of the mouth is restricted (locked jaw). The designation was originally used only in tetanus, but as an inability to open the mouth may be seen in a variety of conditions, the term is currently used in restricted jaw movement regardless of etiology.[32] Although postinjection pain is the most common local complication of local anesthesia, trismus can become one of the more chronic and complicated problems to manage.[33–35]

Causes

Trauma to muscles or blood vessels in the infratemporal fossa is the most common etiological factor in trismus associated with dental injections of local anesthetics.

Local anesthetic solutions into which alcohol or cold sterilizing solutions have diffused produce irritation of tissues (e.g., muscle), leading potentially to trismus.

Local anesthetics have been demonstrated to have slight mycotoxic properties on skeletal muscles. The injection of local anesthetic solution either intramuscularly or supramuscularly leads to a rapidly progressive necrosis of the exposed muscle fibers.[36–38]

Hemorrhage is another cause of trismus. Large volumes of extravascular blood can produce tissue irritation, leading to muscle dysfunction as the blood is slowly resorbed.

A low-grade infection after injection can also cause trismus.[39]

Every needle insertion produces some insult to the tissue through which it passes. It stands to reason, then, that multiple needle penetrations correlate with a greater incidence of postinjection trismus. In addition, Stacy and Hajjar found that of 100 needles used for the administration of the IANB, 60% were barbed on removal from the tissues. The barb occurred when the needle came into contact with the medial aspect of the mandibular ramus. Withdrawal of the needle from tissue increased the likelihood of involvement of the lingual or inferior alveolar nerve and the development of trismus.[40]

Excessive volumes of local anesthetic solution deposited into a restricted area produce distention of tissues, which may lead to postinjection trismus. This is more common after multiple missed IANBs.

Problem

Although the limitation of movement associated with postinjection trismus is usually minor, it is possible for much more severe limitation to develop. The average interincisal opening in cases of trismus is 13.7 mm (range 5 to 23 mm).[37] Stone and Kaban reported four cases of severe trismus after multiple inferior alveolar (IA) or PSA nerve blocks, three of which required surgical intervention.[41] Before surgery the patients had limited mandibular openings of approximately 2 mm, despite usual treatment regimens.

In the acute phase of trismus, pain produced by hemorrhage leads to muscle spasm and limitation of movement.[42,43] The second, or chronic, phase usually develops if treatment is not begun. Chronic hypomobility is secondary to organization of the hematoma, with subsequent fibrosis and scar contracture.[44] Infection also may produce hypomobility through increased pain, increased tissue reaction (irritation), and scarring.[39]

Prevention

1. Use a sharp, sterile, disposable needle.
2. Properly care for and handle dental local anesthetic cartridges.
3. Use aseptic technique. Contaminated needles should be changed immediately.
4. Practice atraumatic insertion and injection technique.
5. Avoid repeat injections and multiple insertions into the same area through knowledge of anatomy and proper technique. Use regional nerve blocks instead of local infiltration (supraperiosteal injection) wherever possible and rational.
6. Use minimum effective volumes of local anesthetic. Refer to specific protocols for recommendations.
   Trismus is not always preventable.

Management

In most instances of trismus the patient reports pain and some difficulty opening his or her mouth on the day after dental treatment in which a posterior superior alveolar or inferior alveolar nerve block was administered. Hinton and associates reported that the onset of trismus occurred 1 to 6 days posttreatment (average 2.9 days).[37] The degree of discomfort and dysfunction varies but is usually mild.

With mild pain and dysfunction the patient reports minimum difficulty opening his or her mouth. Arrange an appointment for examination. In the interim, prescribe heat therapy, warm saline rinses, analgesics and, if necessary, muscle relaxants to manage the initial phase of muscle spasm.[45,46] *Heat therapy* consists of applying hot, moist towels to the affected area for approximately 20 minutes every hour. For a *warm saline rinse*, a teaspoon of salt is added to a 12-ounce glass of warm water and held in the mouth on the involved side (and spit out) to help relieve the discomfort of trismus. Aspirin (325 mg) is usually adequate as an *analgesic* in managing pain associated with trismus. Its antiinflammatory properties also are beneficial. On rare occasion, codeine may be necessary (30 to 60 mg q6h) if the discomfort is more intense. Diazepam (approximately 10 mg bid) or other benzodiazepine is used for *muscle relaxation* if deemed necessary.

The patient should be advised to initiate physiotherapy consisting of opening and closing the mouth, as well as lateral excursions of the mandible for 5 minutes every 3 to 4 hours. Chewing gum (sugarless, of course!) is yet another means of providing lateral movement of the temporomandibular joint.

Record the incident, findings, and treatment on the patient's dental chart. Avoid further dental treatment in the involved region until symptoms resolve and the patient is more comfortable.

If continued dental care in the area is urgent, as with an infected painful tooth, it may prove difficult to achieve effective pain control when trismus is present. The Vazirani-Akinosi mandibular nerve block usually provides relief of the motor dysfunction, permitting the patient to open his or her mouth and allow the administration of the appropriate injection for clinical pain control, if needed.

In virtually all cases of trismus related to intraoral injections that are managed as described, patients report improvement within 48 to 72 hours. Therapy should be continued until the patient is free of symptoms. If pain and dysfunction continue unabated beyond 48 hours, consider the possibility of infection. Antibiotics should be added to the treatment regimen described and continued 7 full days. Complete recovery from injection-related trismus takes about 6 weeks, with a range of 4 to 20 weeks.[37]

For severe pain or dysfunction if no improvement is noted within 2 or 3 days without antibiotics or within 5 to 7 days with antibiotics, or if the ability to open the mouth has become limited, the patient should be referred to an oral and maxillofacial surgeon for evaluation. Other therapies, including the use of ultrasound or appliances, are available for use in these situations.[47,48]

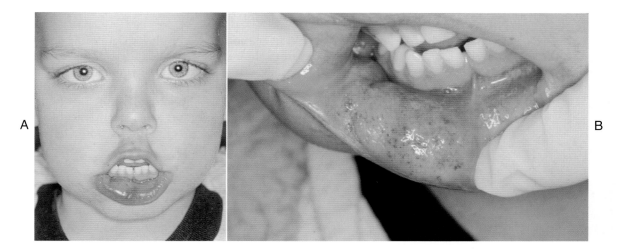

Figure 17-7. A and **B,** Traumatized lip caused by inadvertent biting while it was still anesthetized.

Temporomandibular joint involvement is rare in the first 4 to 6 weeks after injection. Surgical intervention to correct chronic dysfunction may be indicated in some instances.[37,41]

SOFT-TISSUE INJURY

Self-inflicted trauma to the lips and tongue is frequently caused by the patient inadvertently biting or chewing these tissues while still anesthetized (Fig. 17-7).

Cause

Trauma occurs most frequently in younger children and in mentally or physically disabled children or adults; however, it can and does occur in patients of all ages. The primary cause is the fact that soft-tissue anesthesia lasts significantly longer than does pulpal anesthesia. Dental patients receiving local anesthetic during their treatment usually are dismissed from the dental office with residual soft-tissue numbness. (See the discussion in Chapter 20 on the possibility of "unanesthetizing" the patient at the conclusion of treatment.)

Problem

Trauma to anesthetized tissues can lead to swelling and significant pain when the anesthetic effects resolve. A young child or handicapped individual may have difficulty coping with the situation, and this may lead to behavioral problems. The possibility that infection will develop is remote in most instances.

Prevention

A local anesthetic of appropriate duration should be selected if dental appointments are brief. (Refer to the discussion of lip chewing and duration of anesthesia for specific drugs, p. 275.)

A cotton roll can be placed between the lips and teeth if they are still anesthetized at the time of discharge. Secure the roll with dental floss wrapped around the teeth (this also prevents inadvertent aspiration of the roll) (Fig. 17-8).

Warn the patient and guardian against eating, drinking hot fluids, and biting on the lips or tongue to test for anesthesia.

A self-adherent warning sticker may be used on children. It states, "Watch me, my lips and cheeks are numb." The sticker is placed on the patient's forehead (Fig. 17-9).

Management

Management of the patient with self-inflicted soft-tissue injury secondary to lip or tongue biting or chewing is symptomatic:
1. Analgesics for pain, as necessary
2. Antibiotics, as necessary, in the unlikely situation that infection results
3. Lukewarm saline rinses to aid in decreasing any swelling that may be present

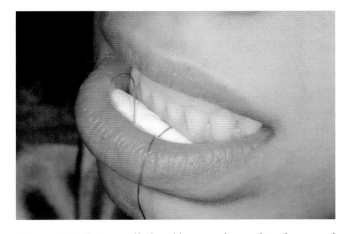

Figure 17-8. Cotton roll placed between lips and teeth, secured with dental floss, minimizes risk of accidental mechanical trauma, to anesthetized tissues.

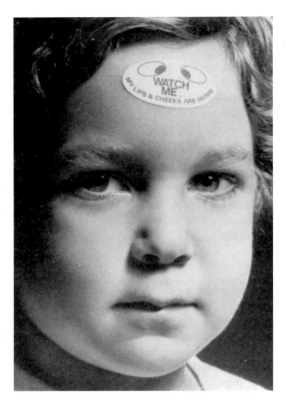

Figure 17-9. Self-adherent warning sticker to help prevent accidental trauma to anesthetized tissues in children.

4. Petroleum jelly or other lubricant to cover a lip lesion and minimize irritation

HEMATOMA

The effusion of blood into extravascular spaces can result from inadvertently nicking a blood vessel (artery or vein) during the injection of a local anesthetic. A hematoma developing subsequent to the nicking of an artery usually increases rapidly in size until treatment is instituted, because of the significantly greater blood pressure within the artery. Nicking a vein may or may not result in the formation of a hematoma. Tissue density surrounding the injured vessel is a determining factor.

Cause

Because of the density of tissue in the hard palate and its firm adherence to bone, hematoma rarely develops after a palatal injection. A rather large hematoma may result from either arterial or venous puncture after posterior superior alveolar or inferior alveolar nerve block. The tissues surrounding these vessels more readily accommodate significant volumes of blood. The blood effuses from vessels until extravascular exceeds intravascular pressure or clotting occurs. Hematomas after the inferior alveolar nerve block are usually only visible intraorally, whereas PSA hematomas are visible extraorally.

Problem

A hematoma rarely produces significant problems, aside from the resulting "bruise," which may or may not be visible extraorally. Possible complications of hematoma include trismus and pain. The swelling and discoloration of the region usually subside within 7 to 14 days.

A hematoma constitutes an inconvenience to the patient and an embarrassment to the person administering the drug (Fig. 17-10).

Prevention

1. Knowledge of the normal anatomy involved in the proposed injection is important. Certain techniques have a greater risk of visible hematoma. The PSA nerve block is the most common, followed by the IANB (a distant second) and the mental/incisive nerve block (a close third when the foramen is entered, a distant third if the technique described in Chapter 14 is adhered to).
2. Modify the injection technique as dictated by the patient's anatomy. For example, the depth of penetration for a PSA nerve block may be decreased in a patient with smaller facial characteristics.[49,50]
3. Use a short needle for the PSA nerve block to decrease the risk of hematoma.
4. Minimize the number of needle penetrations into tissue.
5. Never use a needle as a probe in tissues.
   Hematoma is not always preventable.

Management

Immediate. When swelling becomes evident during or immediately after a local anesthetic injection, direct pressure should be applied to the site of bleeding. For most injections the blood vessel lies between the skin and

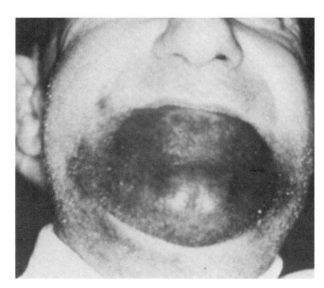

Figure 17-10. Hematoma that developed after bilateral mental nerve blocks.

bone, on which pressure should be applied for not less than 2 minutes. This effectively stops the bleeding.

Inferior alveolar nerve block. Pressure is applied to the medial aspect of the mandibular ramus. Clinical manifestations of the hematoma are intraoral: possible tissue discoloration and probable tissue swelling on the medial (lingual) aspect of the mandibular ramus.

Anterior superior alveolar (infraorbital) nerve block. Pressure is applied to the skin directly over the infraorbital foramen. Clinical manifestation is discoloration of the skin below the lower eyelid. Hematoma is unlikely to arise with ASA nerve block because the technique described requires application of pressure to the injection site throughout drug administration and for a period of 2 to 3 minutes after.

Incisive (mental) nerve block. Pressure is placed directly over the mental foramen, on the skin or mucous membrane. Clinical manifestations are discoloration of skin over the mental foramen or swelling in the mucobuccal fold in the region of the mental foramen (see Fig. 17-10). As with the ASA nerve block, pressure applied during the administration of the drug effectively minimizes the risk of hematoma formation during incisive (not mental) nerve block.

Buccal nerve block or any palatal injection. Place pressure at the site of bleeding. In these injections the clinical manifestations of hematoma are usually visible only within the mouth.

Posterior superior alveolar nerve block. The posterior superior alveolar (PSA) nerve block usually produces the largest and most esthetically unappealing hematoma. The infratemporal fossa, into which bleeding occurs, can accommodate a large volume of blood. The hematoma usually is not recognized until a colorless swelling appears on the side of the face (usually a few minutes after the injection is completed). It progresses over a period of days inferiorly and anteriorly toward the lower anterior region of the cheek. It is difficult to apply pressure to the site of bleeding in this situation because of the location of the involved blood vessels. It is also relatively difficult to apply pressure directly to the posterior superior alveolar artery (the primary source of bleeding), the facial artery, and the pterygoid plexus of veins. They are located posterior, superior, and medial to the maxillary tuberosity. Bleeding normally ceases when external pressure on the vessels exceeds the internal pressure or when clotting occurs. Digital pressure can be applied to the soft tissues in the mucobuccal fold as far distally as can be tolerated by the patient (without eliciting a gag reflex). Apply pressure in a medial and superior direction. If available, ice should be applied (extraorally) to increase pressure on the site and help constrict the vessel.

Subsequent. The patient may be discharged once bleeding stops. Note the hematoma on the patient's dental chart.

Advise the patient about possible soreness and limitation of movement (trismus). If either of these develops, begin treatment as described for trismus. There will likely be discoloration as a result of extravascular blood elements, which is gradually resorbed over 7 to 14 days.

If soreness develops, advise the patient to take an analgesic such as aspirin. *Do not apply heat* to the area for at least 4 to 6 hours after the incident. Heat produces vasodilation, which may further increase the size of the hematoma. Heat may be applied to the region beginning the next day. It serves as an analgesic, and its vasodilating properties may increase the rate at which blood elements are resorbed, although its benefits are debatable. The patient should apply warm moist towels to the affected area for 20 minutes every hour.

Ice *may* be applied to the region immediately on recognition of a developing hematoma. It acts as both an analgesic and a vasoconstrictor, and it may aid in minimizing the size of the hematoma.

Time (tincture of time) is the most important element in managing a hematoma. With or without treatment, a hematoma will be present for 7 to 14 days. Avoid additional dental therapy in the region until symptoms and signs resolve.

PAIN ON INJECTION

Pain on injection of a local anesthetic can best be prevented through careful adherence to the basic protocol of atraumatic injection. (See Chapter 11.)

Causes

1. Careless injection technique and callous attitude ("Palatal injections always hurt" or "This will hurt a little") all too often become self-fulfilling prophesies.
2. A needle can become dull from multiple injections.
3. Rapid deposition of the local anesthetic solution may cause tissue damage.
4. Needles with barbs (from impaling bone) may produce pain as they are withdrawn from tissue.[40]

Problem

Pain on injection increases patient anxiety and may lead to sudden unexpected movement, increasing the risk of needle breakage.

Prevention

1. Adhere to proper techniques of injection, both anatomical and psychological.
2. Use sharp needles.

3. Use topical anesthetic properly before injection.
4. Use sterile local anesthetic solutions.
5. Inject local anesthetics slowly.
6. Be certain that the temperature of the solution is correct. A solution that is too hot or too cold may be more uncomfortable than one at room temperature.

Management

No management is necessary. However, steps should be taken to prevent the recurrence of pain associated with the injection of local anesthetics.

BURNING ON INJECTION

Causes

A burning sensation occurring during injection of a local anesthetic is not uncommon. There are several potential causes.

The primary cause of a mild burning sensation is the pH of the solution being deposited into the soft tissues. The pH of local anesthetic solutions as prepared for injection is approximately 5, whereas that of solutions containing a vasopressor is even more acidic (around 3). Wahl and associates compared the pain on injection of prilocaine plain to lidocaine with epinephrine (1:100,000) and found no statistical difference in patient perception;[51] however, when bupivacaine with epinephrine (1:200,000) was compared to prilocaine plain, significantly more pain was reported by patients receiving bupivacaine.[52]

Rapid injection of local anesthetic, especially in the denser more adherent tissues of the palate, produces a burning sensation.

Contamination of the local anesthetic cartridges can result when they are stored in alcohol or other sterilizing solutions, leading to diffusion of these solutions into the cartridge.

Solutions warmed to normal body temperature usually are considered "too hot" by the patient.

Problem

Although usually transient, the sensation of burning on injection of a local anesthetic indicates that tissue irritation is occurring. If this is caused by the pH of the solution, it rapidly disappears as the anesthetic action develops. There is usually no residual sensitivity noted when the anesthetic action terminates.

When a burning sensation occurs as a result of rapid injection, contaminated solution, or overly warm solution, there is a greater likelihood that tissue may be damaged, with subsequent development of other complications such as postanesthetic trismus, edema, or possible paresthesia.

Prevention

It is difficult, if not impossible, to eliminate the mild burning sensation that some patients experience during injection of a local anesthetic solution. However, the duration of this sensation is but a few seconds, its intensity is low, and many patients are not even aware of it.

Slowing the injection should help. The *ideal* rate is 1 ml/min. Do not exceed the *recommended* rate of 1.8 ml in 1 minute.

The cartridge of anesthetic should be stored at room temperature either in the container in which it was shipped or in a suitable container *without* alcohol or other sterilizing agents. (See Chapter 7 for proper care and handling of dental cartridges.)

In ophthalmology and dermatology, surgeons commonly "alkalinize" the local anesthetics before their injection to make the injection more comfortable for the patient.[53,54] Cross published the results of a trial of alkalinization of local anesthetics in dentistry.[55]

Commercial manufacture of local anesthetic cartridges containing bicarbonate is unlikely because the stability of the local anesthetic solution (and therefore its marketable shelf life) decreases with increasing pH of the solution.

Management

Because most instances of burning on injection are transient and do not lead to prolonged tissue involvement, formal treatment is not usually indicated. In those few situations in which postinjection discomfort, edema, or paresthesia becomes evident, management of the specific problem is indicated.

INFECTION

Infection after the local anesthetic administration in dentistry has become an extremely rare occurrence since the introduction of sterile disposable needles and glass cartridges.

Causes

The major cause of postinjection infection is contamination of the needle before administration of the anesthetic. Contamination of a needle always occurs when the needle touches mucous membrane in the oral cavity. This cannot be prevented, nor is it a significant problem because the normal flora of the oral cavity does not lead to tissue infection.

Improper technique in the handling of the local anesthetic equipment and improper tissue preparation for injection are other possible causes of infection.

Injecting Local Anesthetic Solution into an Area of Infection. As discussed, local anesthetics are less effective when injected into infected tissues. However, if deposited under pressure, as in the periodontal ligament injection, the force of their administration might transport bacteria into adjacent, healthy tissues, spreading infection.

Problem

Contamination of needles or solutions may cause a low-grade infection when the needle or solution is placed in deeper tissue. This may lead to trismus if it is not recognized and proper treatment is not initiated.[39]

Prevention

1. Use sterile disposable needles.
2. Properly care for and handle needles. Take precautions to avoid contamination of the needle through contact with nonsterile surfaces; avoid multiple injections with the same needle, if possible.
3. Properly care for and handle dental cartridges of local anesthetic.
   a. Use a cartridge only once (one patient).
   b. Store cartridges aseptically in their original container, covered at all times.
   c. Cleanse the diaphragm with a sterile disposable alcohol wipe immediately before use.
4. Properly prepare the tissues before penetration. Dry them and apply topical antiseptic (optional).

Management

Low-grade infection, which is rare, is seldom recognized immediately. The patient usually reports postinjection pain and dysfunction 1 or more days after dental care. There are rarely any overt signs and symptoms of infection. Immediate treatment consists of those procedures used to manage trismus: heat and analgesic if needed, muscle relaxant if needed, and physiotherapy. Trismus produced by factors other than infection normally responds with resolution or improvement within several days. If signs and symptoms of trismus do not begin to respond to conservative therapy within 3 days, the possibility of a low-grade infection should be entertained and the patient started on a 7- to 10-day course of antibiotics. Prescribe 29 (or 41, if 10 days) tablets of penicillin V (250-mg tablets). The patient takes 500 mg immediately and then 250 mg four times a day until all tablets have been taken. Erythromycin may be substituted if the patient is allergic to penicillin.

Record the progress and management of the patient on the dental chart.

EDEMA

Swelling of tissues is not a syndrome but a clinical sign of the presence of some disorder.

Causes

1. Trauma during injection
2. Infection
3. Allergy: Angioedema is a common response to ester-type topical anesthetics in an allergic patient; localized tissue swelling occurs as a result of vasodilation secondary to histamine release).
4. Hemorrhage (effusion of blood into soft tissues produces swelling)
5. Injection of irritating solutions (alcohol or cold sterilizing solution-containing cartridges)
6. Hereditary angioedema is a condition characterized by the sudden onset of brawny nonpitting edema affecting the face, extremities, and mucosal surfaces of the intestine and respiratory tract, often without obvious precipitating factors. Manipulation within the oral cavity, including local anesthetic administration, may precipitate an attack. Lips, eyelids, and the tongue are often involved.[56] Karlis and associates noted that 15% to 33% of untreated angioedema patients died from acute airway obstruction as a result of laryngeal edema.[57]

Problem

Edema related to local anesthetic administration is seldom intense enough to produce significant problems such as airway obstruction. Most instances of local anesthetic-related edema result in pain and dysfunction of the region and embarrassment for the patient.

Angioneurotic edema produced by topical anesthetic in an allergic individual can compromise the airway. Edema of the tongue, pharynx, or larynx may develop and represents a potentially life-threatening situation that requires vigorous management.[58]

Prevention

1. Properly care for and handle the local anesthetic armamentarium.
2. Use atraumatic injection technique.
3. Complete an adequate medical evaluation of the patient before drug administration.

Management

The management of edema is predicated on reduction of the swelling as quickly as possible and on the cause of the edema. When produced by traumatic injection or introduction of irritating solutions, edema is usually of minimal degree and resolves in several days without formal therapy. In this and all situations in which edema is present, it may be necessary to prescribe analgesics for pain.

After hemorrhage, edema resolves more slowly (over 7 to 14 days) as extravasated blood elements are resorbed into the vascular system. If signs of hemorrhage are evident (e.g., bluish discoloration progressing to green and other colors), management follows that discussed for hematoma.

Edema produced by infection does not resolve spontaneously but may, in fact, become progressively more intense if untreated. If signs and symptoms of infection (pain, mandibular dysfunction, edema, warmth) do not appear to resolve within 3 days, antibiotic therapy should be instituted as outlined.

Allergy-induced edema is potentially life threatening. Its degree and location are highly significant. If swelling develops in buccal soft tissues and there is absolutely no airway involvement, treatment consists of intramuscular and oral histamine-blocker administration and consultation with an allergist to determine the precise cause of the edema.

If edema occurs in any area where it compromises breathing, treatment consists of the following:
1. P (position): If unconscious, the patient is placed supine.
2. A-B-C (airway, breathing, circulation): Basic life support is administered, as needed.
3. D (definitive treatment): Emergency medical service (e.g., 911) is summoned.
4. Epinephrine is administered: 0.3 mg (adult), 0.15 mg (child), intramuscularly (IM) or intravenously (IV), every 10 to 15 minutes until respiratory distress resolves.
5. Histamine-blocker is administered IM or IV.
6. Corticosteroid is administered IM or IV.
7. Preparation is made for cricothyrotomy if total airway obstruction appears to be developing. This is extremely rare, but is the reason for summoning emergency medical services early.
8. The patient's condition is thoroughly evaluated before the next appointment to determine the cause of the reaction.

SLOUGHING OF TISSUES

Prolonged irritation or ischemia of gingival soft tissues may lead to a number of unpleasant complications, including epithelial desquamation and sterile abscess.

Causes

Epithelial Desquamation
1. Application of a topical anesthetic to the gingival tissues for a prolonged period
2. Heightened sensitivity of the tissues to a local anesthetic
3. Reaction in an area where a topical has been applied

Sterile Abscess
1. Secondary to prolonged ischemia resulting from the use of a local anesthetic with vasoconstrictor (usually norepinephrine)
2. Usually develops on the hard palate

Problem

Pain, at times severe, may be a consequence of epithelial desquamation or a sterile abscess. There is a remote possibility that infection may develop in these areas.

Prevention

Use topical anesthetics as recommended. Allow the solution to contact the mucous membranes for 1 to 2 minutes to maximize its effectiveness and minimize toxicity.

When using vasoconstrictors for hemostasis, do not use overly concentrated solutions. Norepinephrine (Levophed) 1:30,000 is the agent most likely to produce ischemia of sufficient duration to cause tissue damage and a sterile abscess (Fig. 17-11). Epinephrine (1:50,000) also may produce this problem, if reinjection of the solution occurs whenever ischemia resolves, over a long period of time. The palatal tissues are virtually the only place in the oral cavity where this phenomenon occurs.

Management

Usually no formal management is necessary for either epithelial desquamation or sterile abscess. Be certain to reassure the patient of this fact.

Management may be symptomatic. For pain, analgesics such as aspirin or codeine and a topically applied ointment (Orabase) to minimize irritation to the area are recommended.

Epithelial desquamation resolves within a few days; the course of a sterile abscess may run 7 to 10 days.

Record data on the patient's chart.

POSTANESTHETIC INTRAORAL LESIONS

Patients occasionally report that approximately 2 days after an intraoral injection of local anesthetic, ulcerations developed in their mouth, primarily around the site(s) of

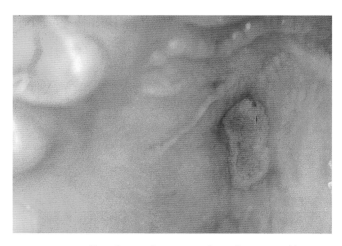

Figure 17-11. Sloughing of tissue on the palate caused by prolonged ischemia secondary to the use of local anesthetic with high concentration (1:50,000) of epinephrine.

the injection(s). The primary initial symptom is pain, usually of a relatively intense nature.

Cause

Recurrent aphthous stomatitis or herpes simplex can occur intraorally after a local anesthetic injection or after any trauma to the intraoral tissues.

Recurrent aphthous stomatitis (recurrent aphthous ulceration) is the most common oral mucosal disease known to human beings.[59] Recurrent aphthous stomatitis is more frequently observed than herpes simplex, typically developing on gingival tissues that are *not* attached to underlying bone (e.g., movable tissue), such as the buccal vestibule (Fig. 17-12). In spite of much continuing research, the causes remain poorly understood, the ulcers are not preventable, and treatment is symptomatic.

Herpes simplex also can develop intraorally, although more commonly it is observed extraorally. It is viral and becomes manifest as small bumps on tissues that are attached to underlying bone (e.g., fixed) such as the soft tissue of the hard palate (Fig. 17-13).

Trauma to tissues by a needle, local anesthetic solution, cotton swab, or any other instrument (e.g., rubber dam clamp or hand piece) may activate the latent form of the disease process that was present in the tissues before injection.

Problem

The patient complains of acute sensitivity in the ulcerated area. Many consider that the tissue has become infected as a result of the local anesthetic injection they received; however, the risk of a secondary infection developing in this situation is minimal.

Prevention

Unfortunately, there is no means of preventing these intraoral lesions from developing in susceptible patients. Extraoral herpes simplex, on occasion, may be prevented

or its clinical manifestations minimized if treated in its prodromal phase. The prodrome consists of a mild burning or itching sensation at the site where the virus is present (e.g., lip). Antiviral agents, such as *acyclovir*, applied qid to the affected area effectively minimize the acute phase of this process.

Management

Primary management is symptomatic. Pain is the major initial symptom, developing approximately 2 days after injection. Reassure the patient that the situation is *not* caused by a bacterial infection secondary to the local anesthetic injection but in fact is an exacerbation of a process that was present, in latent form, in the tissues before injection. Indeed, most of these patients have experienced this response before and are resigned to it happening again.

No management is necessary if the pain is not severe. However, if it causes the patient to complain, treatment can be instituted, usually with varying degrees of success. The objective is to keep the ulcerated areas covered or anesthetized.

Topical anesthetic solutions (e.g., viscous lidocaine) may be applied as needed to the painful areas. A mixture of equal amounts of diphenhydramine (Benadryl) and

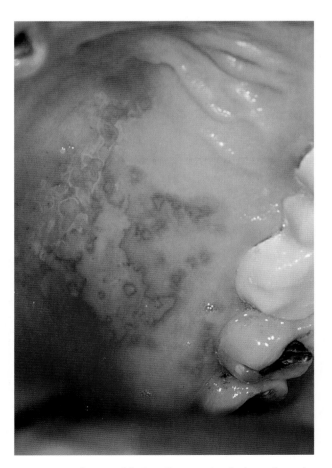

Figure 17-13. Intraoral lesion (herpes simplex) on the palate. (From Eisen D, Lynch D: The mouth: diagnosis and treatment, St Louis, 1998, Mosby.)

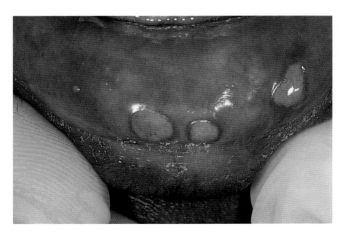

Figure 17-12. Aphthous stomatitis. (From Eisen D, Lynch D: The mouth: diagnosis and treatment, St Louis, 1998, Mosby.)

milk of magnesia rinsed in the mouth effectively coat the ulcerations and provide relief from pain. Orabase, a protective paste, *without* Kenalog can provide a degree of pain relief. Kenalog, a corticosteroid, is not recommended because its antiinflammatory actions increase the risk of viral or bacterial involvement. A tannic acid preparation (Zilactin) can be applied topically to the lesions either extraorally or intraorally (dry the tissues first). Studies from the University of Alabama have demonstrated that most patients achieve substantial pain relief with a duration of up to 6 hours.[60,61]

The ulcerations usually last 7 to 10 days with or without treatment.

Maintain records on the patient's chart.

REFERENCES

1. Orr DL II: The broken needle: report of a case, *J Am Dent Assoc* 107(4):603-604, 1983.
2. Burgess JO: The broken dental needle: a hazard, *Spec Care Dentist* 8(2):71-73, 1988.
3. Fox LJ, Belfiglio EK: Report of a broken needle, *Gen Dent* 34:102-106, 1986.
4. Marks RB, Carlton DM, McDonald S: Management of a broken needle in the pterygomandibular space: report of a case, *Am Dent Assoc* 109:263-264, 1984.
5. Pietruszka JF, Hoffman D, McGivern BE Jr: A broken needle and its surgical removal: a case report, *NY State Dent J* 52:28-31, 1986.
6. Bedrock RD, Skigen A, Dolwick F: Retrieval of a broken needle in the pterygomandibular space. Case report, *J Am Dent Assoc* 130:685-687, 1999.
7. Dhanrayani PJ, Jonaidel O: A forgotten entity: 'broken needle while inferior dental block.' *Dent Update* 27(2):101, 2000.
8. Murray M: A forgotten entity: 'broken needle while administering inferior dental block.' *Dent Update* 27(6):306, 2000 (letter).
9. Zeltser R, Cohen C, Casap N: The implications of a broken needle in the pterygomandibular space: clinical guidelines for prevention and retrieval, *Pediatr Dent* 24(2):153-156, 2002.
10. Dentsply-MPL Technologies, Franklin Park, Ill, personal communication, 2003.
11. Schein H: New York, personal communication, 2003.
12. Septodont Inc, New Castle, Del., personal communication, 2003.
13. Shira RB: Surgical emergencies. In McCarthy FM, editor: *Emergencies in dental practice*, ed 3, Philadelphia, 1979, WB Saunders.
14. Haas DA, Lennon D: A 21 year retrospective study of reports of paresthesia following local anesthetic administration, *J Can Dent Assoc* 61(4):319-320, 323-326, 329-330, 1995.
15. Pogrel MA, Thamby S: Permanent nerve involvement resulting from inferior alveolar nerve blocks, *J Am Dent Assoc* 131:901-907, 2000.
16. Pogrel MA, Thamby S: The etiology of altered sensation in the inferior alveolar, lingual, and mental nerves as a result of dental treatment, *J Calif Dent Assoc* 27:531-538, 1999.
17. Dower JS Jr: A review of paresthesia in association with administration of local anesthesia, *Dent Today* 22:64-69, 2003.
18. Haas DA: Localized complications from local anesthesia, *J Calif Dent Assoc* 26:677-682, 1998.
19. Malden NJ, Maidment YG: Lingual nerve injury subsequent to wisdom teeth removal: a 5-year retrospective audit from a High Street dental practice, *Br Dent J* 193(4):203-205, 2002.
20. Heller AA, Shankland WE II: Alternative to the inferior alveolar nerve block anesthesia when placing mandibular dental implants posterior to the mental foramen, *J Oral Implantol* 27(3):127-133, 2001.
21. Bataineh AB: Sensory nerve impairment following mandibular third molar surgery, *J Oral Maxillofac Surg* 59(9):1012-1017, 2001.
22. Haas DA, Lennon D: Local anesthetic use by dentists in Ontario, *J Can Dent Assoc* 61(4):297-304, 1995.
23. Haas DA: Personal communication, June, 2003.
24. Kasaba T, Onizuka S, Takasaki M: Procaine and mepivacaine have less toxicity in vitro than other clinically used local anesthetics, *Anesth Analg* 97(1):85-90, 2003.
25. Nickel AA Jr: A retrospective study of paresthesia of the dental alveolar nerves, *Anesth Prog* 37(1):42-45, 1990.
26. McCarthy FM: Personal communication, 1979.
27. Sisk AL, Hammer WB, Shelton DW, et al: Complications following removal of impacted third molars, *J Oral Maxillofac Surg* 44:855-859, 1986.
28. Cooley RL, Coon DE: Transient Bell's palsy following mandibular block: a case report, *Quint Int* 9:9, 1978.
29. Crean SJ, Powis A: Neurological complications of local anaesthetics in dentistry, *Dent Update* 26(8):344-349, 1999.
30. Malamed SF: The possible secondary effects in cases of local anesthesia, *Rev Belge Medec Dent* 55(1):19-28, 2000.
31. Haas DA: Localized complications from local anesthesia, *J Calif Dent Assoc* 26(9):677-682, 1998.
32. Tveter-as K, Kristensen S: The aetiology and pathogenesis of trismus, *Clin Otolaryngol* 11(5):383-387, 1986.
33. Dhanrajani PJ, Jonaidel O: Trismus: etiology, differential diagnosis and treatment, *Dent Update* 29(2):88-92, 94, 2002.
34. Leonard M: Trismus: what is it, what causes it, and how to treat it, *Dent Today* 18(6):74-77, 1999.
35. Marien M Jr: Trismus: causes, differential diagnosis, and treatment, *Gen Dent* 45(4):350-355, 1997.
36. Benoit PW, Yagiela JA, Fort NF: Pharmacologic correlation between local anesthetic-induced myotoxicity and disturbances of intracellular calcium distribution, *Toxic Appl Pharmacol* 52:187-198, 1980.
37. Hinton RJ, Dechow PC, Carlson DS: Recovery of jaw muscle function following injection of a myotonic agent (lidocaine-epinephrine), *Oral Surg Oral Med Oral Pathol* 59:247-251, 1986.
38. Jastak JT, Yagiela JA, Donaldson D: Complications and side effects. In Jastak JT, Yagiela JA, Donaldson D, editors: *Local anesthesia of the oral cavity*, Philadelphia, 1995, WB Saunders.
39. Kitay D, Ferraro N, Sonis ST: Lateral pharyngeal space abcess as a consequence of regional anesthesia, *J Am Dent Assoc* 122(7):56-59, 1991.
40. Stacy GC, Hajjar G: Barbed needle and inexplicable paresthesias and trismus after dental regional anesthesia, *Oral Surg Oral Med Oral Pathol* 77(6):585-588, 1994.

41. Stone J, Kaban LB: Trismus after injection of local anesthetic, *Oral Surg* 48:29-32, 1979.
42. Eanes WC: A review of the considerations in the diagnosis of limited mandibular opening, *Cranio* 9(2):137-144, 1991.
43. Luyk NH, Steinberg B: Aetiology and diagnosis of clinically evident jaw trismus, *Aust Dent J* 35(6):523-529, 1990.
44. Brooke RI: Postinjection trismus due to formation of fibrous band, *Oral Surg Oral Med Oral Pathol* 47:424-426, 1979.
45. Himel VT, Mohamed S, Luebke RG: Case report: relief of limited jaw opening due to muscle spasm, *LDA J* 47:6-7, 1988.
46. Kouyoumdjian JH, Chalian VA, Nimmo A: Limited mandibular movement: causes and treatment, *J Prosthet Dent* 59(3):330-333, 1988.
47. Carter EF: Therapeutic ultrasound for the relief of restricted mandibular movement, *Dent Update* 13(10):503, 504, 506, 508-509, 1986.
48. Lund TW, Cohen JI: Trismus appliances and indications for use, *Quint Int* 24(4):275-279, 1993.
49. Harn SD, Durham TM, Callahan BP, et al: The triangle of safety: a modified posterior superior alveolar injection technique based on the anatomy of the PSA artery, *Gen Dent* 50(6):554-557, 2002.
50. Harn SD, Durham TM, Callahan BP, et al: The posterior superior alveolar injection technique: a report on technique variations and complications, *Gen Dent* 50(6):544-550, 2002.
51. Wahl MJ, Overton D, Howell J, et al: Pain on injection of prilocaine plain vs. lidocaine with epinephrine. A prospective double-blind study, *J Am Dent Assoc* 132(10):1398-1401, 2001.
52. Wahl MJ, Schmitt MM, Overton DA, et al: Injection pain of bupivacaine with epinephrine vs. prilocaine plain, *J Am Dent Assoc* 133(12):1652-1656, 2002.
53. Hinshaw KD, Fiscella R, Sugar J: Preparation of pH-adjusted local anesthetics, *Ophthal Surg* 26(3):194-199, 1995.
54. Stewart JH, Chinn SE, Cole GW, et al: Neutralized lidocaine with epinephrine for local anesthesia, *J Dermatol Surg Oncol* 16(9):842-845, 1990.
55. Cross VW: Pain reduction in local anesthetic administration through pH buffering, *J Indiana Dent Assoc* 70(2): 24-25, 1991.
56. Nzeako U, Frigas E, Tremaine W: Hereditary angioedema: a broad review for clinicians, *Arch Intern Med* 161(20): 2417-2429, 2001.
57. Karlis V, Glickman RS, Stern R, et al: Hereditary angioedema: case report and review of management, *Oral Surg Oral Med Oral Path Oral Radiol Endodont* 83(4):462-464, 1997.
58. Hayes SM: Allergic reaction to local anesthetic: report of a case, *Gen Dent* 28(1):30-31, 1980.
59. Ship JA: Recurrent aphthous stomatitis. An update, *Oral Surg Oral Med Oral Path Oral Radiol Endodont* 82(2):118, 1996.
60. Raborn GW, McGaw WT, Grace M, et al: Herpes labialis treatment with acyclovir 5% modified aqueous cream: a double-blind randomized trial, *Oral Surg Oral Med Oral Pathol* 67(6):676-679, 1989.
61. Raborn GW, McGaw WT, Grace M, et al: Treatment of herpes labialis with acyclovir. Review of three clinical trials, *Am J Med* 85(2A):39-42, 1988.

Systemic Complications

CHAPTER 18

The therapeutic use of drugs is commonplace in dentistry, and the administration of local anesthetics is considered essential whenever potentially painful procedures are contemplated. It is estimated (conservatively) that dental professionals in the United States administer in excess of 6 million dental cartridges per week, or more than 300 million per year.

Local anesthetics are extremely safe drugs when used as recommended. However, whenever any drug, including local anesthetics, is used, the potential for development of unwanted responses exists. In this chapter systemic adverse reactions to drugs in general, and local anesthetics in particular, are reviewed.

Several general principles of toxicology (the study of the harmful effects of chemicals or drugs on biological systems) are presented to further an understanding of the material in this chapter.

Harmful effects of drugs range from those that are inconsequential to the patient and entirely reversible once the drug is withdrawn, to those that are uncomfortable but not seriously harmful, to those that can seriously incapacitate or prove fatal to the patient.

Whenever any drug is administered, two types of actions may be observed: (1) desirable actions, which are clinically sought and usually beneficial; and (2) undesirable actions, which are additional and not sought.

◆ **Principle 1: No drug ever exerts a single action.** All drugs exert many actions, desirable and undesirable. In ideal circumstances the right drug in the right dose is administered via the right route to the right patient at the right time for the right reason and does not produce any undesirable effects.[1] This ideal clinical situation is rarely, if ever, attained, because no drug is so specific that it produces only the desired actions in all patients.

◆ **Principle 2: No clinically useful drug is entirely devoid of toxicity.** The aim of rational drug treatment is to maximize the therapeutic and minimize the toxic effects of any given drug. No drug is completely safe or completely harmful. All drugs are capable of producing harm if handled improperly; conversely, any drug may be handled safely if proper precautions are observed.

◆ **Principle 3: The potential toxicity of a drug rests in the hands of the user.** A second factor in the safe use of drugs (after the drug itself) is the person to whom the drug is being administered. Individuals react differently to the same stimulus. Therefore patients vary in their reactions to a drug. Before administering any drug, the doctor must ask the patient specific questions about his or her medical and drug history. Physical evaluation and the ensuing dialogue history related to local anesthetic administration is presented in Chapters 4 and 10.

CLASSIFICATION OF ADVERSE DRUG REACTIONS

Classifying adverse drug reactions, in the past, has been the object of much confusion; reactions were labeled as side effects, adverse experience, drug-induced disease, diseases of medical progress, secondary effects, and intolerance. The term *adverse drug reaction* (ADR) is preferred at this time.

Box 18-1 outlines the three major methods by which drugs produce adverse reactions.

Overdose reactions, allergy, and idiosyncrasy are important topics in relation to local anesthetics and pain control in dentistry. A brief overview of each is presented, followed by an in-depth look at overdose and allergy.

Causes of Adverse Drug Reactions

TOXICITY CAUSED BY *DIRECT EXTENSION OF THE USUAL PHARMACOLOGICAL EFFECTS* OF THE DRUG:
1. Side effects
2. Overdose reactions
3. Local toxic effects

TOXICITY CAUSED BY *ALTERATION IN THE RECIPIENT* OF THE DRUG:
1. A disease process (hepatic dysfunction, congestive heart failure, renal dysfunction)
2. Emotional disturbances
3. Genetic aberrations (atypical plasma cholinesterase, malignant hyperthermia)
4. Idiosyncrasy

TOXICITY CAUSED BY *ALLERGIC RESPONSES* TO THE DRUG

Overdose reactions are those clinical signs and symptoms that manifest as a result of an absolute or relative overadministration of a drug (which leads to elevated blood levels). Signs and symptoms of overdose are related to a direct extension of the normal pharmacological actions of the drug in the various tissues and organs of the body. Local anesthetics are drugs that act to depress excitable membranes (e.g., the central nervous system [CNS] and myocardium). When administered properly and in therapeutic dosages, they cause little or no clinical evidence of CNS or CVS (cardiovascular system) depression. However, signs and symptoms of selective CNS and CVS depression develop with increased levels in the cerebral circulation or myocardium. *Toxic reaction* is a synonym for overdose. Toxins are poisons. All drugs are poisons when administered to excess; thus the term *toxic reaction.*

Allergy is a hypersensitive state acquired through exposure to a particular allergen (a substance capable of inducing altered bodily reactivity), reexposure to which brings about a heightened capacity to react. Clinical manifestations of allergy vary and include the following:
• Fever
• Angioedema
• Urticaria
• Dermatitis
• Depression of blood-forming organs
• Photosensitivity
• Anaphylaxis

In contrast to the overdose reaction, in which clinical manifestations are related directly to the pharmacological properties of the causative agent, the clinically observed reaction in allergy is always produced by an exaggerated response of the patient's immune system. Allergic responses to a local anesthetic, antibiotic, latex, shellfish, bee sting, peanuts, or strawberries are produced by the same mechanism and may present clinically similar signs and symptoms. All allergies require the same basic management. Overdose reactions to these substances appear clinically dissimilar, necessitating entirely different modes of emergency management.

Another point of contrast between overdose and allergic responses relates to the amount of drug necessary to produce or provoke the reaction. For an overdose reaction to develop, a large enough amount of the drug must have been administered so that excessive blood levels occur in the target organ(s) or tissues. *Overdose reactions are dose related.* In addition, the degree of intensity (severity) of the clinical signs and symptoms relates directly to the blood level of the administered drug. The greater the dose administered, the higher the blood level, and the more severe the reaction. By contrast, *allergic reactions are not dose related.* A large dose of a drug (e.g., "overdose") administered to a nonallergic patient does not provoke an allergic response, whereas a minuscule amount (e.g., 0.1 ml) of a drug to which the patient is allergic can provoke life-threatening anaphylaxis.

Idiosyncrasy, the third category of true adverse drug reactions, is a term used to describe a qualitatively abnormal, unexpected response to a drug, differing from its pharmacological actions and thus resembling hypersensitivity. However, the idiosyncratic reaction does not involve a proven, or even suspected, allergic mechanism. A second definition considers an idiosyncratic reaction to be any adverse response that is neither an overdose nor an allergic reaction. An example is stimulation or excitation that develops in some patients after administration of a CNS-depressant drug (e.g., a histamine-blocker). Unfortunately, it is virtually impossible to predict which persons will have such reactions or the nature of the resulting idiosyncrasy.

It is thought that virtually all instances of idiosyncratic reaction have an underlying genetic mechanism. These aberrations remain undetected until the individual receives

TABLE **18-1**
Comparison of Allergy and Overdose

	Allergy	Overdose
CLINICAL RESPONSE		
Dose	Non–dose related	Dose related
S&S	Similar, regardless of allergen	Relate to pharmacology of drug administered
Management	Similar (epinephrine, histamine blockers)	Different: specific for drug administered

S&S, Signs and symptoms.

a specific drug, which then produces its bizarre (non-pharmacological) clinical expression.

Specific management of idiosyncratic reactions is difficult to discuss because of the unpredictable nature of the response. Treatment is necessarily symptomatic: positioning, airway, breathing, circulation, and definitive care.

Table 18-1 compares allergy and overdose.

OVERDOSE

A drug overdose reaction has been defined as those clinical signs and symptoms that result from an overly high blood level of a drug in various target organs and tissues. Overdose reactions are the most common of all true adverse drug reactions, accounting for up to 99% in some estimates.[2]

For an overdose reaction to occur the drug must first gain access to the circulatory system in quantities sufficient to produce adverse effects on various tissues of the body. Normally there is both a constant absorption of the drug from its site of administration into the circulatory system and a steady removal of the drug from the blood as it undergoes redistribution (e.g., to skeletal muscle and fat) and biotransformation in other parts of the body (e.g., liver). Overly high drug levels in the blood and target organs rarely develop (Fig. 18-1) in this situation.

However, there are a number of ways in which this "steady state" can be altered, leading to either a rapid or more gradual elevation of the drug's blood level. In either case a drug overdose reaction is caused by a level of a drug in the blood sufficiently high to produce adverse effects in various organs and tissues of the body in which the drug exerts a clinical action (these are termed the *target organs* of the drug). The reaction continues only as long as the blood level of the drug in the target organs remains above the threshold for overdose.

Predisposing Factors

Overdose to local anesthetics is related to the blood level of the local anesthetic occurring in certain tissues after the drug is administered. Many factors influence the rate at which this level is elevated and the length of time it remains elevated. The presence of one or more of these factors predisposes the patient to the development of

overdose. The first group of factors relates to the patient; the second group to the drug and the area into which the drug is administered (Box 18-2).

Patient Factors

Age. Although ADRs, including overdose, can occur in persons of any age, individuals at either end of the age spectrum experience a higher incidence of such reaction.[3–8] The functions of absorption, metabolism, and excretion may be imperfectly developed in young persons and may be diminished in old persons, thereby increasing the half-life of the drug, elevating circulating blood levels, and increasing the risk of overdose.[9]

Weight. The greater the (lean) body weight of a patient (within certain limits), the larger the dose of a drug that can be tolerated before overdose reactions occur. Most drugs are distributed evenly throughout the body. Larger individuals have a greater blood volume and consequently a lower level of the drug per milliliter of blood. Maximum recommended doses (MRDs) of local anesthetics normally are calculated on the basis of milligram of drug per kilogram or pound of body weight. One of the major factors involved in producing local anesthetic overdose in the past was a lack of consideration of this

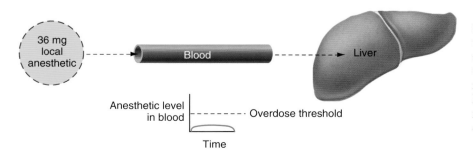

Figure 18-1. Under normal conditions there is both a constant absorption of local anesthetic from the site of deposition into the cardiovascular system and a constant removal of the drug from the blood by the liver. Local anesthetic levels in the blood remain low and below the threshold for overdose.

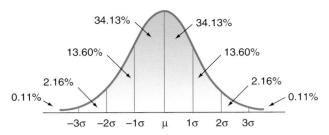

Figure 18-2. Normal distribution curve (bell curve). (From Freilich JD, Bennett CR: Conscious-sedation in a patient on combined tranylcypromine and lithium therapy: a case report, *Anesth Prog* 30:86-88, 1983.)

extremely important factor. Determination of maximum doses according to milligram per pound or kilogram of body weight is based on the responses of the "normal-responding" patient, which are calculated from the responses of thousands of patients. Individual patient response to drug administration, however, may demonstrate significant variation. The normal distribution curve (Fig. 18-2) illustrates this fact. The usual cerebral blood level of lidocaine necessary to induce seizure activity is approximately 7.5 µg/ml. However, patients on the hyporesponding side of this curve may not convulse until a significantly higher brain–blood level is reached, whereas others (hyperresponders) may convulse at a brain–blood level considerably below 7.5 µg/ml.

Other medications. Administration of concomitant medications may influence local anesthetic drug levels. Patients taking *meperidine* (Demerol), *phenytoin* (Dilantin), *quinidine* (an antidysrhythmic), and *desipramine* (a tricyclic antidepressant) have increased local anesthetic blood levels and thus may experience toxic actions of the local anesthetic at lower administered doses because of protein binding competition. The H_2 histamine blocker *cimetidine* slows the biotransformation of lidocaine by competing for hepatic oxidative enzymes with the local anesthetic, leading to somewhat elevated lidocaine blood levels.[10-12]

Sex. Studies in animals have shown that sex is a factor in drug distribution, response, and metabolism; although it is not of major significance in humans. In humans, the only instance of sexual difference affecting a drug response is pregnancy. During pregnancy, renal function may be disturbed, leading to impaired excretion of certain drugs, their accumulation in the blood, and increased risk of overdose. However, local anesthetic seizure thresholds for the fetus, newborn, and mother are significantly different.[11-15] In the adult woman the seizure threshold is reported to be 5.8 mg/kg, in the newborn 18.4, and in the fetus 41.9 mg/kg. This is thought to be a result of the efficient placental clearance of lidocaine into the mother's plasma.

Presence of disease. Disease may affect the ability of the body to transform a drug into an inactive product.

Hepatic and *renal dysfunction* impair the body's ability to break down and excrete the local anesthetic, leading to an increased anesthetic blood level, whereas *congestive heart failure* decreases liver perfusion (the volume of blood flowing through the liver during a specific period), thereby increasing the half-lives of amide local anesthetics and increasing the risk of overdose.[16,17]

Genetics. Genetic deficiencies may alter a patient's response to certain drugs. A genetic deficiency in the enzyme serum pseudocholinesterase (serum cholinesterase, plasma pseudocholinesterase, plasma cholinesterase) is an important example. This enzyme, produced in the liver, circulates in the blood and is responsible for the biotransformation of the ester local anesthetics. A deficiency in this enzyme either quantitatively or qualitatively can prolong the half-life of an ester local anesthetic and increase its blood level. Approximately 1 in 2820 persons, or 6% to 7% of patients in most surgical populations possess atypical serum pseudocholinesterase.[18]

Mental attitude and environment. A patient's psychological attitude influences the ultimate effect of a drug. Although of greater importance with regard to antianxiety or analgesic drugs, it is also important with regard to local anesthetics. Psychological attitude affects the patient's response to various stimuli. The apprehensive patient who overreacts to stimulation (experiencing pain when gentle pressure is applied) is more likely to receive a larger dose of local anesthetic. It also has been demonstrated that the local anesthetic seizure threshold is lower in patients who are fearful and apprehensive than in nonfearful patients.[19] Both of these factors—larger dose requirement and the lower seizure threshold—increase the likelihood of local anesthetic overdose. The concomitant judicious use of psychosedation techniques can minimize this risk.

Drug Factors

Vasoactivity. All local anesthetics currently used in dentistry have vasodilating properties. Injection into soft tissues increases perfusion in the area, leading to an increased rate of drug absorption from the site of injection into the cardiovascular system. This causes two undesirable effects: a shorter duration of clinical anesthesia and an increased blood level of the local anesthetic.

Concentration. The greater the concentration (percent solution injected) of the local anesthetic administered, the greater the number of milligrams per milliliter of solution and the greater the circulating blood volume of the drug in the patient. For example, 1.8 ml of a 4% solution is 72 mg of the drug, but 1.8 ml of a 2% solution represents only 36 mg. If the drug is clinically effective as a 2% concentration, higher concentrations should not be used. *The lowest concentration of a given drug that is clinically effective should be selected for use.* For the commonly used local anesthetics in dentistry these ideal concentrations have been determined and are represented in the commercially available forms of these drugs.

Dose. The larger the volume of a local anesthetic administered, the greater the number of milligrams injected and the higher the resulting circulating blood level. *The smallest dose of a given drug that is clinically effective should be administered.* For each of the injection techniques discussed in this book, a recommended dose has been presented. Whenever possible, this dose should not be exceeded. Although "dental" doses of local anesthetics are relatively small compared with those used in many nondental nerve blocks, significantly high blood levels of the local anesthetic can be achieved in dental situations because of the greater vascularity of the intraoral injection site or inadvertent intravascular injection.

Route of administration. Local anesthetics used to control pain produce their clinical effect in the area of injection. The drug should not enter into the cardiovascular system and reach a minimum therapeutic blood level, as most other drugs do. Local anesthetics administered for antidysrhythmic purposes must reach a therapeutic blood level to be effective. Indeed, one factor involved in terminating pain control by a local anesthetic is diffusion of the drug out of the nerve tissue, and its absorption into the CVS and removal from the area of injection.

A factor in local anesthetic overdose in dentistry is inadvertent *intravascular injection.* Extremely high drug levels can be reached in a short time, leading to serious overdose reactions.

Absorption of local anesthetics through oral mucous membranes is also potentially dangerous because of the rate at which some topically applied anesthetics enter the circulatory system. Lidocaine and tetracaine are absorbed well after topical application to mucous membranes, Benzocaine, on the other hand, is poorly absorbed.

Rate of injection. The rate at which a drug is injected is a very important factor in the causation or prevention of overdose reactions. (According to the author, rate of injection is *the* single most important factor.) Whereas intravascular injection may or may not produce signs and symptoms of overdose (indeed, lidocaine is frequently administered intravenously in doses of 1.0 to 1.5 mg/kg to treat ventricular ectopy), the rate at which the drug is injected is a major factor in determining whether drug administration will prove clinically safe or hazardous. Malagodi and associates demonstrated that the incidence of seizures with etidocaine went up when the rate of intravenous (IV) infusion was increased.[20]

Rapid intravenous (IV) administration (15 seconds) of 36 mg of lidocaine produces greatly elevated levels and virtually ensures an overdose reaction. Slow (60-second) IV administration produces significantly lower levels in the blood, with a lesser risk that a severe overdose reaction will develop.

Vascularity of the injection site. The greater the vascularity of the injection site, the more rapid the absorption of the drug from that area into the circulation. Unfortunately (in this regard) for dentistry, the oral cavity is one of the most highly vascular areas of the entire body. However, there are some areas within the oral cavity that are less well perfused (e.g., the site for the Gow-Gates nerve block), and these are usually more highly recommended than other, more well-perfused, sites (e.g., those for the inferior alveolar or posterior superior alveolar nerve blocks).

Presence of vasoconstrictors. The addition of vasoconstrictor to a local anesthetic produces a decrease in the perfusion of an area and a decreased rate of systemic absorption of the drug. This, in turn, decreases the clinical toxicity of the local anesthetic (see Table 3-1).

Causes

Elevated blood levels of local anesthetics may result from one or more of the following:
1. Biotransformation of the drug is unusually slow.
2. The unbiotransformed drug is too slowly eliminated from the body through the kidneys.
3. Too large a total dose is administered.
4. Absorption from the injection site is unusually rapid.
5. Inadvertent intravascular administration occurs.

Biotransformation and Elimination. *Ester* local anesthetics, as a group, undergo more rapid biotransformation in the liver and blood than the amides. Plasma pseudocholinesterase is primarily responsible for their hydrolysis to paraaminobenzoic acid.

Atypical pseudocholinesterase occurs in approximately 1 out of every 2820 individuals, or 6% to 7% of patients in a surgical population.[18] Patients with a familial history of this disorder may be unable to biotransform ester agents at the usual rate, and subsequently higher levels of ester anesthetics may develop in their blood.

Atypical pseudocholinesterase represents a *relative contraindication* to the administration of ester local anesthetics. Amide local anesthetics may be used without increased risk of overdose in patients with pseudocholinesterase deficiency.

Amide local anesthetics are biotransformed in the liver by hepatic microsomal enzymes. A history of liver disease, however, does not absolutely contraindicate their use. In an ambulatory patient with a history of liver disease (ASA II or III), amide local anesthetics may be used judiciously *(relative contraindication)* (Fig. 18-3).

Minimum effective volumes of anesthetic should be used. Average, even low-average, doses may be capable of producing an overdose if liver function is compromised

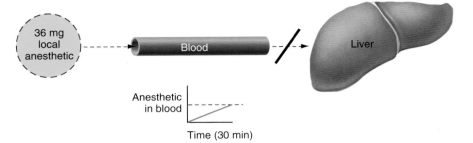

Figure 18-3. In patients with significant liver dysfunction, removal of a local anesthetic agent from the blood may be slower than its absorption into the blood, leading to a slow but steady rise in the blood anesthetic level.

to a great enough degree (ASA IV, V); however, this situation is unlikely to occur in an ambulatory patient.[17]

Renal dysfunction also can delay elimination of the active local anesthetic from the blood. A percentage of all anesthetics is eliminated unchanged through the kidneys: 2% procaine, 10% lidocaine, and 1% to 15% mepivacaine and prilocaine. Renal dysfunction may lead to a gradual increase in the level of active local anesthetic in the blood.[16]

Excessive Total Dose. Given in excess, *all* drugs are capable of producing signs and symptoms of overdose (Fig. 18-4). Precise milligram dosages or the blood levels at which clinical effects are noted are impossible to predict. Biological variability has a great influence on the manner in which persons respond to drugs.

The MRD of parenterally administered (injected) drugs is commonly calculated after consideration of a number of factors, including:

1. **Patient's age.** Individuals at either end of the age spectrum may be unable to tolerate normal doses, which should be decreased accordingly.
2. **Patient's physical status.** For medically compromised individuals (ASA III, IV, and V) the calculated MRD should be decreased.
3. **Patient's weight.** The larger the person (within limits), the greater is the distribution of the drug. With a normal dose the blood level of the drug is lower in the larger patient, and a larger milligram dose can be administered safely. Although this rule is generally valid, there are always exceptions; care must be exercised whenever any drug is administered.

Maximum recommended doses of local anesthetics should be determined after consideration of the patient's age, physical

status, and body weight. Table 18-2 provides maximum recommended doses based on body weight for lidocaine, mepivacaine, prilocaine, and articaine.

It is highly unlikely that the maximum figures indicated in Table 18-2 will be reached in the typical dental practice. There is rarely an occasion to administer more than three or four cartridges during a dental appointment. Regional block anesthesia is capable of obtunding the full mouth in an adult with six cartridges, and with two cartridges in the primary dentition. Yet despite this ability to achieve widespread anesthesia with minimum volumes of anesthetic, the administration of excessive volumes is the most frequently seen cause of local anesthetic overdose.[21,22]

Rapid Absorption into the Circulation. Vasoconstricting drugs are considered an integral component of all local anesthetics whenever depth and duration of anesthesia are important. There are few indications in dentistry for the use of local anesthetics without a vasoconstrictor. Vasoconstrictors increase the duration of anesthesia and reduce systemic toxicity of most local anesthetics by delaying their absorption into the CVS. Vasoconstrictors should be included in local anesthetic solutions unless specifically contraindicated by the medical status of the patient or the duration of the planned treatment.[23] The American Dental Association and the American Heart Association summarized this as follows: "Vasoconstrictor agents should be used in local anesthetic solutions during dental practice only when it is clear that the procedure will be shortened or the analgesia rendered more profound. When a vasoconstrictor is indicated, extreme care should be taken to avoid intravascular injection. The minimum possible amount of vasoconstrictor should be used."[24] Rapid absorption of local anesthetics also may occur after

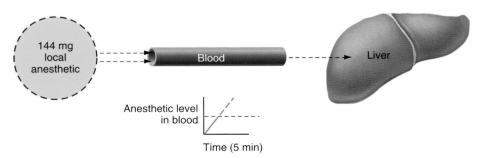

Figure 18-4. Even in a patient with normal liver function, a large dose of local anesthetic may be absorbed into the cardiovascular system more rapidly than the liver can remove it. This produces a relatively rapid elevation of the blood anesthetic level.

TABLE 18-2
Maximum Recommended Doses of Local Anesthetics

Drug	Formulation	MRD	mg/lb	(mg/kg)	Author's MRD	mg/kg[17,18]
Articaine	With epinephrine	500*	3.2	(7.0)	3.2	7.0
Lidocaine	Plain	300†	2.0	(4.4)†	300	4.4
	With epinephrine	500†	3.3	(7.0)†	300	4.4
Mepivacaine	Plain	400†	2.6	(5.7)†	300	4.4
	With levonordefrin	400†	2.6	(5.7)†	300	4.4
Prilocaine	Plain	600†	4.0	(8.8)†	400	6.0
	With epinephrine	600†	4.0	(8.8)†	400	6.0

*Manufacturer's recommendation. Prescribing information, New Castle, Del., 2000.
†Manufacturer's recommendation. Prescribing information: dental, Westborough, Mass, 1990, Astra Pharmaceutical Products.

their application to oral mucous membranes. Absorption of some topically applied local anesthetics into the circulation is rapid, exceeded in rate only by direct intravascular injection.[25] Local anesthetics designed for topical application are used in a greater concentration than formulations suitable for parenteral administration.

From the perspective of overdose, amide topical anesthetics, when applied to wide areas of mucous membrane, increase the risk of serious reactions. Benzocaine, an ester anesthetic, which is poorly, if at all, absorbed into the cardiovascular system, is less likely to produce an overdose reaction than amides, although cases of methemoglobinemia from excessive benzocaine administration have been reported.[26–28] The risk of allergy (more likely with esters than amides) must be addressed before using any drug.

Serious overdose reactions have been reported after topical application of amide local anesthetics.[29–32]

The area of application of a topical anesthetic should be limited. There are few indications for applying a topical to more than a full quadrant (buccal and lingual/palatal) at one time. Application of an amide topical to a wide area requires a large quantity of the agent and increases the likelihood of overdose.

The use of metered dosage forms of topical anesthetics is recommended whenever and wherever possible. Disposable nozzles now are available for metered sprays that make maintenance of sterility simpler (Fig. 18-5). Ointments or gels, if used in small amounts (as on the tip of a cotton applicator stick), may be applied with minimal risk of overdose.

Intravascular Injection. An intravascular injection may occur with any type of intraoral nerve block but is more likely with the following:[33]

Nerve block	Positive aspiration rate (%)
Inferior alveolar	11.7
Mental or incisive	5.7
Posterior superior alveolar	3.1
Anterior superior alveolar	0.7
(Long) buccal	0.5

Both IV and intraarterial (IA) injections are capable of producing overdose (Fig. 18-6). A rapidly administered IA injection can cause retrograde blood flow in the artery as the anesthetic drug is deposited (Fig. 18-7).[34] Intravascular injections within the usual practice of dentistry should not occur. With care and knowledge of the anatomy of the area to be anesthetized and proper technique of aspiration before injecting the anesthetic solution, overdose as a result of inadvertent intravascular injection is minimized.

Prevention. To prevent intravascular injection, *use an aspirating syringe.* In an unpublished survey the author conducted, 23% of dentists questioned stated that they routinely use nonaspirating syringes to administer local anesthetics. There is no justification for the use of nonaspirating syringes for any intraoral injection technique, because it is impossible to determine the precise location of the needle tip without aspirating.

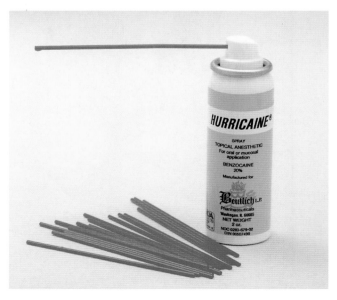

Figure 18-5. Metered spray with disposable nozzle.

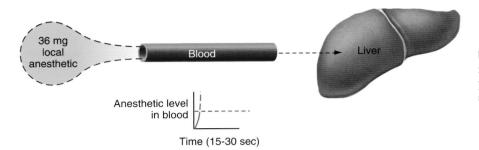

Figure 18-6. Direct intravascular administration of one cartridge of local anesthetic produces marked elevation of the blood anesthetic level in a very short time.

Use a needle no smaller than 25 gauge when the risk of aspiration is high. Although aspiration of blood is possible through smaller-gauge needles, there is an increase in resistance to the return of blood into the lumen of smaller-gauge needles, leading to an increased likelihood of an unreliable aspiration test. Therefore injection techniques with a greater likelihood of positive aspiration dictate the use of a 25-gauge needle.

Aspirate in at least two planes before injection. Figure 18-8 illustrates how an aspiration test may be negative even though the needle tip lies within the lumen of a blood vessel. Multiple aspiration tests before injecting solution, with the needle bevel in different planes, overcome this

potential problem. After aspiration, rotate the syringe about 45 degrees to reorient the needle bevel relative to the wall of the blood vessel and reaspirate.

Slowly inject the anesthetic. Rapid intravascular injection of 1.8 ml of a 2% local anesthetic solution produces a level in the blood greatly in excess of that necessary for overdose. *Rapid injection* is defined (by the author) as the administration of the entire volume of a dental cartridge in 30 seconds or less. The same volume of anesthetic deposited intravascularly slowly (minimum 60 seconds) produces blood levels below the minimum for serious overdose (seizure). In the event that the level does exceed this minimum, the onset of the reaction will be slower,

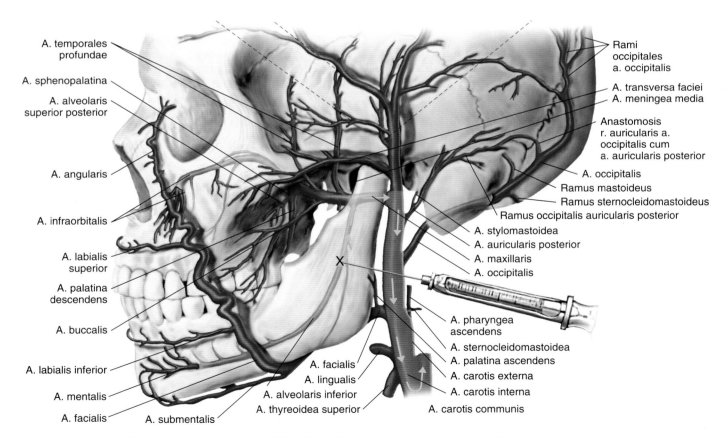

Figure 18-7. Reverse carotid blood flow. Rapid intraarterial deposition of local anesthetic into the inferior alveolar artery *(X)* produces an overdose reaction. Blood flow in the arteries is reversed because of the high pressure produced by the rate of injection. *Arrows* indicate the path of the solution into the cerebral circulation.

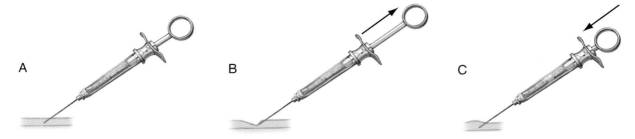

Figure 18-8. Intravascular injection of local anesthetic. **A,** Needle is inserted in the lumen of the blood vessel. **B,** Aspiration test is performed. Negative pressure pulls the vessel wall against the bevel of the needle; therefore no blood enters the syringe (negative aspiration). **C,** Drug is injected. Positive pressure on the plunger of the syringe forces local anesthetic solution out through the needle. Wall of the vessel is forced away from the bevel, and anesthetic solution is deposited directly into the lumen of the blood vessel.

with signs and symptoms less severe than those observed after a more rapid injection. Slow injection is the most important factor in preventing adverse drug reactions, even more so than aspiration. The ideal rate of local anesthetic administration is 1 ml/min. *Under no circumstances should the rate of drug deposition be less than 60 seconds for a 1.8-ml cartridge.* However, because the recommended volumes of local anesthetic for most intraoral injection techniques are considerably less than 1.8 ml, most injections can be administered safely in less than 1 minute.

* * *

The truth about local anesthetic overdosage in dentistry:[35] The *administration of too large a local anesthetic dose* in relation to the age and weight of the patient is the most common cause of serious local anesthetic overdose reactions in dentistry. Although some serious cases of local anesthetic overdose have occurred in adult patients,[5] the overwhelming majority of problems commonly develop in the child who is young (2 to 6 years), lightweight (15 to 40 kg), well behaved, requires multiple procedures in four quadrants, and is managed in the office of an inexperienced general dentist.[3]

Review of many of the cases that resulted in serious morbidity or death reveals a number of shared factors, none of which by themselves might pose a serious problem, but when added together act to produce clinical signs and symptoms of local anesthetic overdose. These factors are presented in Box 18-3.

1. *Treatment plan:* In interviews with trained pediatric dentists, it has been the author's experience that when presented with the patient described in the preceding (young, light-weight, well-behaved), the pediatric dentist will not treat all four quadrants at one visit using local anesthetic alone. Limiting treatment to one or two quadrants per visit represents a more rational approach to this patient's needs, and increases safety.

The dentist who is confronted with a (well-meaning) parent or grandparent who complains of the difficulties of getting to the dental office and the inconvenience of having to miss a half day of work, and wanting

to have their child's dental care accomplished in one visit (not two or more), might feel pressured into agreeing to this request, thus increasing the risk for local anesthetic overdose.

2. *Choice of local anesthetic:* In most instances where serious local anesthetic overdose has occurred in children, the local anesthetic administered has been a "plain" drug, either mepivacaine HCl 3% or prilocaine HCl 4%. Both of these are excellent local anesthetics when used properly. The rationale behind the clinician's selection of a short-acting drug for children includes: (1) most pediatric appointments are of short duration, and (2) "plain" local anesthetics have a shorter duration of posttreatment soft-tissue anesthesia, minimizing the likelihood of inadvertent soft-tissue injury as the child bites or chews his or her numb lip or tongue.

As a rule, the pediatric dentist administers a "plain" local anesthetic only when treatment is limited to one quadrant. When treatment extends to two quadrants or more in one visit, a vasopressor-containing local anesthetic is selected. Prolonged posttreatment soft-tissue anesthesia does lead to the increased possibility of soft-tissue damage; however, this risk is far outweighed by benefits accrued through delayed absorption of both the local anesthetic and vasopressor into

---

BOX 18-3

Factors Adding to Increased Risk of Local Anesthetic Overdose in Younger Patients

1. Treatment plan where all four quadrants are treated with local anesthetic in one visit
2. Local anesthetic administered is a plain (no vasopressor) solution
3. Full cartridges (1.8 ml) administered with each injection
4. Local anesthetic administered to all four quadrants at one time
5. Exceeding the maximum dosage based on patient's body weight

TABLE 18-3
Local Anesthetic of Choice for 117 Dentists Who Treat Children

Local Anesthetic Formulation	Percent Preferentially Employing Drug
2% lidocaine + epinephrine	69
3% mepivacaine	11
2% lidocaine	8
2% mepivacaine + levonordefrin	8
Other	4

(From Cheatham BD, Primosch RE, Courts FJ: A survey of local anesthetic usage in pediatric patients by Florida dentists, *J Dent Child* 59:401-407, 1992.)

the CVS (the risk of overdose is diminished). There are many ways of preventing postoperative soft-tissue injury, such as securing a cotton roll in the buccal fold and advising the parent to watch the child. (See Chapters 16 and 17.)

Table 18-3 presents primary local anesthetic of choice for 117 dentists who treat children.[36]

3. *Volume of local anesthetic administered:* Pain control for the entire primary dentition can be achieved with approximately two cartridges of local anesthetic. In the child patient there is rarely a compelling reason to administer a full 1.8-ml cartridge of local anesthetic in any one injection. Yet full cartridges tend to be routinely administered when children receive local anesthetic administered by nonpediatric dentists. In many of the instances where death resulted, a total of five, six, or seven cartridges were administered.[3]

In cases where local anesthetic *must* be administered to all four quadrants of a younger child, this can be achieved with no more than two cartridges, as follows: either one-fourth cartridge each for the right- and left-incisive nerve blocks (anesthetizing all mandibular teeth) or one-half cartridge each for right- and left-inferior alveolar nerve blocks; and one-quarter cartridge each for the right- and left-anterior superior alveolar nerve blocks. In lieu of the anterior superior alveolar nerve block, maxillary infiltrations may be administered with one-sixth cartridge per injection (Table 18-4).

TABLE 18-4
Recommended Volumes of Local Anesthetic for Intraoral Injections

Technique	Adult Volume (ml)	Pediatric Volume (ml)
Infiltration (supraperiosteal)	0.6	0.3
Inferior alveolar	1.5	0.9
Gow-Gates mandibular	1.8	0.9
Mental or incisive	0.6	0.45
Posterior superior alveolar	0.9	0.45
Anterior superior alveolar (infraorbital)	0.9	0.45
Greater (anterior) palatine	0.45	0.2
Nasopalatine	0.2	0.2
Maxillary (second division)	1.8	0.9

4. *Local anesthetic administered to all four quadrants at one time:* The administration, over 1 or 2 minutes, of four or more cartridges of a local anesthetic without a vasopressor to all four quadrants makes little therapeutic sense, while increasing the likelihood of an overdose. Administration of local anesthetic to one quadrant, treating that area, anesthetizing the next quadrant, and so on, makes considerably more sense both from a therapeutic and safety perspective. For equal amounts of local anesthetic, administration over a longer time frame (e.g., 1 to 2 hours) results in a lower blood level of the local anesthetic compared with the entire dose being administered at one time.

5. *Exceeding the maximum dosage based on patient's body weight:* An important factor, especially when managing younger, lighter-weight patients, is maximum dosage. Determine the weight of the patient (in pounds [lb] or kilograms [kg]) before the start of treatment. It is preferable to weigh the child on a scale, because parents frequently can offer only a rough estimate of their child's weight (usually underestimating). One must always remember that these figures are not absolutes. Exceeding the MRD of a drug does not guarantee that an overdose is going to happen (see Table 18-5 and discussion). On the other hand, administering dosages

TABLE 18-5
Maximum Recommended Dosages of Local Anesthetics

Drug	Clinical Percent mg / ml		mg/Cartridge (1.8 ml)	Recommended* mg/kg	mg/lb	Absolute Maximum* (mg)
Articaine	4	40	72	7.0	3.2	500
Lidocaine	2	20	36	4.4	2.0	300
Mepivacaine	2	20	36	4.4	2.0	300
Mepivacaine	3	30	54	4.4	2.0	300
Prilocaine	4	40	72	6.0	2.7	400
Bupivacaine	0.5	5	9	1.3	0.6	90

*Maximum recommended doses of local anesthetics are for local anesthetic solutions either containing vasoconstrictors or without vasoconstrictors.

TABLE 18-6
Local Anesthetic Administration for Removal of Third Molars

Procedure (Number of Third Molars Extracted at Visit)	N = (Number of Patients in Category)	Number of Cartridges (Range)	Number of Cartridges (Average)
1	5	4–10	6.2
2	13	4–23	12.18
3	8	10–20	15.33
4	39	6–26	19.24

(From Malamed SF: Unpublished data, 2002.)

below the maximum calculated by body weight is no guarantee that adverse reactions will not be seen. The likelihood of ADRs developing is dose-related. Smaller dosages minimize this risk; larger doses increase it.

Maximum recommended dosages of commonly administered local anesthetics are summarized in Table 18-5.

The intrinsic safety of local anesthetics is illustrated in Table 18-6, which presents the volume of local anesthetic administered on 65 occasions by a general dentist who removed third molars from college-aged individuals.

None of these patients experienced an adverse response to the local anesthetic, although many received dosages many times the MRD.[37] This is one indication that local anesthetics are extremely safe drugs when administered to healthy, adult patients. Unfortunately, when administered in overly large doses to younger, lightweight patients, overdose is a significant risk.

Virtually all local anesthetic overdose reactions are preventable if the clinician adheres to the very basic, simple recommendations presented in the preceding. In the unlikely situation where an overdose reaction develops, adherence to the basic steps of emergency management will lead to a successful outcome in virtually all cases.

Clinical Manifestations

Clinical signs and symptoms of local anesthetic overdose appear whenever the anesthetic blood level in an organ becomes overly high for that individual (Box 18-4). The rate of onset of signs and symptoms and, to an extent, their severity correspond to this level. Table 18-7 compares the various forms of local anesthetic overdose.

Note: It is also possible that the excitatory phase of the overdose reaction may be extremely brief or may not occur at all, in which case the first clinical manifestation of overdose may be drowsiness progressing to unconsciousness and respiratory arrest. This appears to be more common with lidocaine than other local anesthetics.[38]

The clinical manifestations of local anesthetic overdose continue until anesthetic blood levels in the affected organs (brain, heart) fall below the minimum value (through redistribution) or until clinical signs and symptoms are terminated through the use of appropriate drug therapy.

Pathophysiology

The blood or plasma level of a drug is the amount absorbed into the circulatory system and transported in plasma throughout the body. Levels are measured in micrograms per milliliter (μg/ml). Recall that 1000 μg equals 1 mg. Figure 18-9 illustrates clinical manifestations observed with increasing blood levels of lidocaine in the CNS and heart. Blood levels are estimated because significant individual variation can occur.

Local anesthetics exert a depressant effect on all excitable membranes. In the clinical practice of anesthesia

BOX 18-4

Overdose Levels

MINIMAL TO MODERATE OVERDOSE LEVELS

Signs	Symptoms (progressive with increasing blood levels)
Talkativeness	Lightheadedness and dizziness
Apprehension	Restlessness
Excitability	Nervousness
Slurred speech	Numbness
Generalized stutter, leading to muscular twitching and tremor in the face and distal extremities	Sensation of twitching before actual twitching is observed (see "Generalized stutter" under "Signs")
Euphoria	Metallic taste
Dysarthria	Visual disturbances (inability to focus)
Nystagmus	Auditory disturbances (tinnitus)
Sweating	Drowsiness and disorientation
Vomiting	Loss of consciousness

Failure to follow commands or be reasoned with
Disorientation
Loss of response to painful stimuli
Elevated blood pressure
Elevated heart rate
Elevated respiratory rate

MODERATE TO HIGH OVERDOSE LEVELS
Signs
Tonic–clonic seizure activity followed by:
   Generalized central nervous system depression
   Depressed blood pressure, heart rate, and respiratory rate

TABLE **18-7**
Comparison of Forms of Local Anesthetic Overdose

	Rapid Intravascular	Too Large a Total Dose	Rapid Absorption	Slow Bio-transformation	Slow Elimination
Likelihood of occurrence	Common	Most common	Likely with "high normal" doses if no vasoconstrictors are used	Uncommon	Least common
Onset of signs and symptoms	Most rapid (seconds); intraarterial faster than intravenous	3 to 5 min	3 to 5 min	10 to 30 min	10 min to several hr
Intensity of signs and symptoms **Duration of signs and symptoms**	Usually most intense 2 to 3 min	Gradual onset with increased intensity; may prove quite severe Usually 5 to 30 min; depends on dose and ability to metabolize or excrete		Gradual onset with slow increase in intensity of symptoms Potentially longest duration because of inability to metabolize or excrete agents	
Primary prevention	Aspirate, slow injection	Administer minimal doses	Use vasoconstrictor; limit topical anesthetic use or use nonabsorbed type (base)	Adequate pretreatment physical evaluation of patient	
Drug groups	Amides and esters	Amides; esters only rarely	Amides; esters only rarely	Amides and esters	Amides and esters

a local anesthetic is applied to a specific region of the body, where it produces its primary effect: a reversible depression of peripheral nerve conduction; other effects are related to its absorption into the circulation and its subsequent actions on excitable membranes, including smooth muscle, the myocardium, and the CNS.

After the intraoral administration of 40 to 160 mg of a local anesthetic (lidocaine) the blood level rises to a maximum of approximately 1 µg/ml. (The usual range is between 0.5 and 2 µg/ml, but remember that response to drugs varies according to the individual.) Adverse reactions to the anesthetic are extremely uncommon in most individuals at these normal blood levels.

Central Nervous System Actions. The CNS is extremely sensitive to the actions of local anesthetics. As the cerebral blood level of local anesthetic increases, clinical signs and symptoms are noted.

Local anesthetics cross the blood–brain barrier, producing CNS depression. At nonoverdose levels of lidocaine (<5 µg/ml) there are no clinical signs of adverse CNS effects. Indeed, therapeutic advantage may be taken of lidocaine at blood levels between 0.5 and 4 µg/ml, because then lidocaine possesses anticonvulsant properties.[39-41] Mechanism of this action is a depression of hyperexcitable neurons found in the amygdala of seizing patients.

Signs of CNS toxicity appear at a cerebral blood level greater than 4.5 µg/ml. There is generalized cortical sensitivity: agitation, talkativeness, and irritability.

Tonic–clonic seizures generally occur at levels greater than 7.5 µg/ml. With further increases in the local anesthetic blood level, seizure activity terminates and a state of generalized CNS depression develops. Respiratory depression and arrest are manifestations of this. Chapter 2 describes the method through which a CNS-depressant drug, such as a local anesthetic, produces clinical signs and symptoms of CNS stimulation.

Cardiovascular System Actions. The CVS is much less sensitive to the actions of local anesthetics. Adverse CVS responses do not usually develop until long after adverse CNS actions have appeared.

Local anesthetics, primarily lidocaine, have been used in the management of cardiac dysrhythmias, especially ventricular extrasystoles and ventricular tachycardias. The minimum effective level of lidocaine for this action is 1.8 µg/ml, and the maximum is 5 µg/ml, the level at which undesirable actions become more likely.[42]

Increased levels (5 to 10 µg/ml) lead to minor alterations on the electrocardiogram, myocardial depression, decreased cardiac output, and peripheral vasodilation. Above 10 µg/ml there is an intensification of these effects: primarily massive peripheral vasodilation, marked reduction in myocardial contractility, severe bradycardia, and possible cardiac arrest.[43,44]

Management

Management of a local anesthetic overdose is based on the severity of the reaction. In most cases the reaction is mild

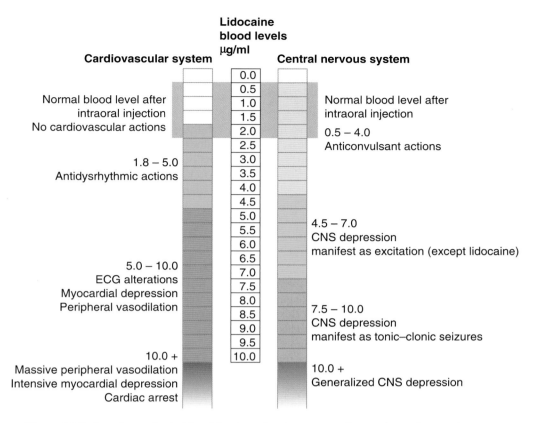

Figure 18-9. Local anesthetic blood levels and actions on cardiovascular and central nervous systems.

and transitory, requiring little or no specific treatment. In other instances, however, it may be more severe and longer lasting, in which case prompt therapy is necessary.

Most local anesthetic overdose reactions are self-limiting, because the blood level in the target organs (e.g., brain and heart) continues to decrease as the reaction progresses and redistribution and biotransformation take place (*if* the heart is still beating effectively). Only rarely are drugs other than oxygen necessary to terminate a local anesthetic overdose. When any of the signs and symptoms of overdose develop, do *not* simply label the patient "allergic" to local anesthetics, for this will further complicate future treatment (see p. 279).

Mild Overdose Reaction. Signs and symptoms of a mild overdose are retention of consciousness, talkativeness, and agitation, along with increased heart rate, blood pressure, and respiratory rate usually developing between 5 and 10 minutes after completion of the anesthetic injection(s).

Slow onset (≥5 minutes after administration). Possible causes of reactions with a slow onset are unusually rapid absorption, and too large a total dose. Management follows the usual P→A→B→C→D algorithm used in management of all medical emergencies. Box 18-5 summarizes basic emergency management.

BOX 18-5

Basic Emergency Management

P . . . POSITION
Unconscious . . . supine with feel elevated slightly
Conscious . . . based upon patient comfort

A . . . AIRWAY
Unconscious . . . assess and maintain airway
Conscious . . . assess airway

B . . . BREATHING
Unconscious . . . assess and ventilate if necessary
Conscious . . . assess breathing

C . . . CIRCULATION
Unconscious . . . assess and provide external cardiac compression if necessary
Conscious . . . assess circulation

D . . . DEFINITIVE CARE
Diagnosis:
Management: Emergency drugs and/or assistance (emergency medical services, dial 911).

Use the following protocol to deal with a slow onset of symptoms.

P→A→B→C. Position the conscious patient comfortably. A, B, and C are assessed as adequate (patient is conscious and talking).

D (definitive care):

1. Reassure the patient that everything is all right.
2. Administer oxygen via nasal cannula or nasal hood. This is indicated as a means of preventing acidosis, a situation in which the seizure level of local anesthetic is decreased. The greater the arterial carbon dioxide tension, the lower the local anesthetic blood level necessary to induce or perpetuate tonic–clonic activity.[45]
3. Monitor and record vital signs. Postexcitation depression is usually mild, with little or no therapy necessary.
4. (optional) If trained and if equipment is available, establish an IV infusion. Use of anticonvulsants (e.g., diazepam or midazolam) is usually not indicated at this time, although diazepam may be administered *slowly intravenously* and titrated at a rate of 5 mg/minute (midazolam at 1 mg/min) if CNS stimulation appears to be intensifying toward a more severe reaction.
5. Permit the patient to recover for as long as necessary. Dental care may or may not be continued after an evaluation of the patient's physical and emotional status. The patient may leave the dental office unescorted only if you are convinced that full recovery has occurred. Vital signs should be recorded and compared with baseline values, and the patient evaluated thoroughly before discharge. If an anticonvulsant drug was administered or doubt exists as to the level of recovery, do not permit the patient to leave the office; seek emergency medical assistance (e.g., dial 911).

Slower onset (≥15 minutes after administration). Possible causes of reactions of a slower onset are abnormal biotransformation and renal dysfunction. Follow this protocol for dealing with the slower onset of signs and symptoms in a conscious patient.

P→A→B→C. Position the conscious patient comfortably. A, B, and C are assessed as adequate (patient is conscious and talking).

D (definitive care):

1. Reassure the patient.
2. Administer oxygen.
3. Monitor vital signs.
4. Administer an anticonvulsant. Overdose reactions caused by abnormal biotransformation or renal dysfunction usually progress somewhat in intensity and last longer (because the drug cannot be eliminated rapidly). If venipuncture can be performed and if equipment is available, titrate 5 mg of diazepam/minute (or midazolam 1 mg/min) until the clinical signs and symptoms of overdose subside.

5. Summon medical assistance. When venipuncture is not practical or if an anticonvulsant drug has been administered, seek emergency medical assistance as soon as possible. Postexcitement depression usually is moderate after a mild excitement phase. Administration of diazepam, midazolam, or any other anticonvulsant will intensify this depression slightly. Monitoring of the patient's status and adherence to the steps of basic life support are normally more than adequate for this situation.
6. After termination of the reaction, be sure that the patient is examined by a physician or hospital staff member to determine possible causes. The examination should include blood tests and hepatic and renal function tests.
7. Do not let the patient leave the dental office alone. Arrangements should be made for an adult companion if hospitalization is not deemed necessary.
8. Determine the cause of the reaction before proceeding with therapy requiring additional local anesthetics.

Severe Overdose Reaction

Rapid onset (within 1 minute). Signs and symptoms are unconsciousness with or without convulsions. The probable cause is intravascular injection.

P→A→B→C. Place the unconscious patient in the supine position. A, B, and C are assessed and maintained, as necessary. Remove the syringe from the mouth (if still present) and place the patient supine with the feet elevated slightly. Subsequent management is based on the presence or absence of convulsions.

D (definitive care): In the presence of tonic–clonic convulsions:

1. Protect the patient's arms, legs, and head. Loosen tight clothing, such as ties, collars, and belts, and remove the pillow (or "doughnut") from the headrest.
2. Immediately summon emergency medical assistance.
3. Continue basic life support. Maintenance of an adequate airway and adequate ventilation are of the utmost importance during management of local anesthetic-induced tonic–clonic seizures. Increased oxygen utilization and hypermetabolism, with increased production of CO_2 and lactic acid, occur during the seizure and lead to acidosis; this, in turn, lowers the seizure threshold (the blood level at which local anesthetic-induced seizures begin), prolonging the reaction.[46] Cerebral blood flow during such a seizure is also increased, elevating still further local anesthetic blood levels within the CNS.
4. Administer an anticonvulsant. The blood level of the local anesthetic declines as the drug undergoes redistribution and, if acidosis is not present, seizures cease within 1 to 3 minutes. Anticonvulsant therapy is usually *not* indicated. If a seizure is protracted (4 to 5 minutes with no indication of terminating), consider administering an anticonvulsant. IV diazepam,

titrated at a rate of 5 mg/minute or midazolam (1 mg/min) until seizures cease is the preferred treatment.[47,48] If venipuncture is not feasible, 5 mg of midazolam may be given IM.[49,50] Intranasal (IN) midazolam may be administered at a dose of 0.25 mg/kg (up to 10 mg).[51] Seizures usually stop within 1 to 2 minutes after IN midazolam. Maintain basic life support and obtain the assistance of emergency medical personnel.

Postseizure (postictal) phase. CNS depression is usually present at an intensity equal that of the excitation phase (Fig. 18-10). The patient may be drowsy or unconscious; breathing may be shallow or absent; the airway may be partially or totally obstructed; blood pressure and heart rate may be depressed or absent. A more intense postseizure state is likely where anticonvulsants have been administered to terminate the seizure.

P→A→B→C. Implementation of the steps of basic life support is crucial: airway, breathing, and circulation must be provided as needed. In all postictal situations, maintenance of an adequate airway is necessary; in some other cases assisted or controlled ventilation may be indicated; for a small percentage of the most severe reactions, artificial circulation must be added to the first two steps of basic life support.

D (definitive care):
1. Additional management such as use of a vasopressor (phenylephrine or methoxamine) IM is indicated if hypotension persists for extended periods (30 minutes). Preferred initial management for hypotension in this situation is positioning of the patient and the administration of IV fluids.
2. Allow the patient to rest until recovery is sufficient to permit discharge. This means a return of vital signs to estimated baseline levels. Do not permit the patient to leave unescorted. In all situations in which local anesthetic induced seizures develop and

emergency medical services are necessary, evaluation of the patient in an emergency department of a hospital usually is necessary.

Slow onset (5 to 15 minutes). Possible causes of severe reactions of slow onset are too large a total dose, rapid absorption, abnormal biotransformation, and renal dysfunction. *Note:* Overdose reactions that develop very slowly (15 to 30 min) are unlikely to progress to severe clinical manifestations if the patient is continually observed and management is started promptly.

Terminate dental treatment as soon as the signs of toxicity first appear.

P→A→B→C. Provide basic life support (BLS) as necessary. As in the preceding protocol, the prevention of acidosis and hypoxia through airway management and adequate pulmonary ventilation is of primary importance to a successful outcome.

D (definitive care):
1. Administer an anticonvulsant. If symptoms are mild at the onset but progress in severity, and if an IV line can be established, definitive treatment with IV anticonvulsants and continued oxygen administration is indicated. IM or IN midazolam may be considered when the IV route is not available.
2. Summon emergency medical assistance immediately if seizures develop.
3. Postseizure management includes BLS and the IM or IV administration of a vasopressor for hypotension, as needed. The administration of IV fluids is recommended for management of hypotension.
4. Permit the patient to recover for as long as necessary before discharge to hospital. Completely evaluate the patient's condition before readministering a local anesthetic. The patient should be examined by a physician before discharge.

• • •

Overdose reactions are the most common "true" adverse drug reactions associated with the administration of the amide local anesthetics. Most overdose reactions are preventable through adequate pretreatment evaluation of the patient and rational use of these drugs. In the few instances in which clinical manifestations of overly high local anesthetic blood levels become evident, a successful outcome usually is noted if the condition is promptly recognized and the patient treated effectively. Primary among the steps of management are maintenance of a patent airway and adequate oxygenation. Data indicate that if local anesthetic-induced seizures are brief and well managed, no permanent neurological or behavioral sequelae remain postictally.[52] In other words, ischemic CNS damage is *not* inevitable with well-managed, brief, local anesthetic-induced seizures.

Epinephrine Overdose

Precipitating Factors and Prevention. With the withdrawal of levonordefrin from the dental market in 2003,

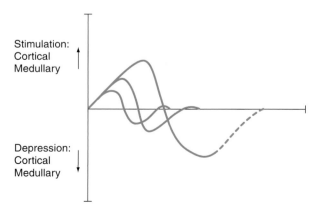

Figure 18-10. Effects of local anesthetics on the central nervous system. Notice that the intensity of depression is equal to the intensity of the preceding stimulation. (From Bennett CR: *Monheim's local anesthesia and pain control in dental practice,* ed 7, St Louis, 1984, Mosby.)

TABLE 18-8
Dilutions of Vasoconstrictors used in Dentistry

Dilution	Drug Available	mg/ml	mg per Cartridge (1.8 ml)	Maximum no. of Cartridges Used for Healthy Patient and Cardiac-Impaired Patient
1:1000	Epinephrine (emergency kit)	1.0	Not applicable	Not available in local anesthetic cartridge
1:10,000	Epinephrine (emergency kit)	0.1	Not applicable	Not available in local anesthetic cartridge
1:20,000	Levonordefrin	0.5	0.09	10 (H), 2 (C)
1:30,000	Levarterenol	0.034	0.06	5 (H), 2 (C)
1:50,000	Epinephrine	0.02	0.036	5 (H), 1 (C)
1:100,000	Epinephrine	0.01	0.018	10 (H), 2 (C)
1:200,000	Epinephrine	0.005	0.009	20 (H), 4 (C)

H, Healthy patient; *C,* cardiac-impaired patient.

epinephrine is the sole vasoconstrictor found in local anesthetics in the United States. Table 18-8 outlines the milligram per milliliter concentrations of vasoconstrictors currently used in dentistry.

The optimum concentration of epinephrine for prolongation of pain control (with lidocaine) appears to be 1:250,000.[53] Use of a 1:50,000 epinephrine concentration for pain control cannot be recommended. Epinephrine 1:50,000 or 1:100,000 is useful via local infiltration in the control of bleeding when applied directly to the surgical area. Epinephrine or local anesthetic overdose reactions occurring under these conditions are rare.

Epinephrine overdose is more common after its use in gingival retraction cord before impressions are taken for a crown and bridge procedure. Currently available cords contain approximately 225.5 μg of racemic epinephrine per inch of cord.[54] Epinephrine is readily absorbed through gingival epithelium that has been disturbed (abraded) by the dental procedure. About 64% to 94% of applied epinephrine is absorbed into the CVS.[54] There is extreme variability in absorption according to the degree and duration of vascular exposure (bleeding). With regard to vasoconstrictors used for gingival retraction purposes, the American Dental Association states in *Accepted Dental Therapeutics:* "Since effective agents which are devoid of systemic effects are available, it is not advisable to use epinephrine for gingival retraction, and its use is contraindicated in individuals with a history of cardiovascular disease."[55]

Clinical Manifestations. Clinical signs and symptoms of epinephrine or other vasopressor overdose are listed in Box 18-6.

Management. Most instances of epinephrine overdose are of such short duration that little or no formal management is necessary. On occasion, however, the reaction may be prolonged and some management is desirable.

Terminate the procedure. If possible, remove the source of epinephrine. Stopping the injection of local anesthetic does not remove epinephrine that has been deposited; however, endogenous epinephrine and norepinephrine release from the adrenal medulla and nerve endings is lessened once the anxiety-inducing stimulus is eliminated. Epinephrine-impregnated gingival retraction cord, if present, should be removed.

Basic management follows the usual **P→A→B→C→D** algorithm used in management of all medical emergencies.

P→A→B→C. Position the conscious patient comfortably. The supine position is not recommended, however, because it accentuates the CVS effects. A semisitting or erect position minimizes any further elevation in cerebral blood pressure. A, B, and C are assessed as adequate (patient is conscious and talking).

D (definitive care):
1. Reassure the patient that the signs and symptoms will subside momentarily. Anxiety and restlessness

BOX 18-6

Signs and Symptoms of Epinephrine or Other Vasopressor Overdose

Signs	Symptoms
Sharp elevation in blood pressure, primarily systolic	Fear, anxiety
Elevated heart rate	Tenseness
Possible cardiac dysrhythmias (premature ventricular contractions, ventricular tachycardia, ventricular fibrillation)	Restlessness
	Throbbing headache
	Tremor
	Perspiration
	Weakness
	Dizziness
	Pallor
	Respiratory difficulty
	Palpitations

are common clinical manifestations of epinephrine overdose.

2. Monitor vital signs and administer oxygen. The blood pressure and heart rate should be checked every 5 minutes during the episode. Striking elevations in both parameters are noted but gradually return toward baseline. Oxygen may be administered if necessary. The patient may complain of difficulty breathing. An apprehensive patient may hyperventilate (increased rate and depth of breathing). Oxygen is not indicated in the management of hyperventilation, because it can exacerbate symptoms and possibly lead to carpopedal tetany.

3. Recovery. Permit the patient to remain in the dental chair as long as necessary to recover. The degree of postexcitation fatigue and depression noted vary but are usually prolonged. Do not discharge the patient if any doubt remains about ability for self-care.

ALLERGY

Allergy is a hypersensitive state, acquired through exposure to a particular allergen, reexposure to which produces a heightened capacity to react. Allergic reactions cover a broad spectrum of clinical manifestations ranging from mild and delayed responses occurring as long as 48 hours after exposure to the allergen, to immediate and life-threatening reactions developing within seconds of exposure (Table 18-9).

Predisposing Factors

The incidence of allergy in the population is not low: about 15% of patients with allergy have conditions severe enough to require medical management, and some 33% of all chronic disease in children is allergic in nature.[56]

Allergy to local anesthetics does occur, but its incidence has decreased dramatically since the introduction of amide anesthetics in the 1940s. Brown and associates stated, "The advent of the amino-amide local anesthetics which are not derivatives of para-aminobenzoic acid markedly changed the incidence of allergic type reactions to local anesthetic drugs. Toxic reactions of an allergic type to the amino amides are extremely rare, although several cases have been reported in the literature in recent years which suggest that this class of agents can on rare occasions produce an allergic type of phenomenon."[57]

Allergic responses to local anesthetics include dermatitis (common in dental office personnel), bronchospasm (asthmatic attack), and systemic anaphylaxis. The most frequently encountered are localized dermatological

TABLE 18-9
Classification of Allergic Diseases (After Gell and Coombs)

Type	Mechanism	Principal Antibody or Cell	Time of Reactions	Clinical Examples
I	Anaphylactic (immediate, homocytotropic, antigen-induced, antibody-mediated)	IgE	Seconds to minutes	Anaphylaxis (drugs, insect venom, antisera) Atopic bronchial asthma Allergic rhinitis Urticaria Angioedema Hay fever
II	Cytotoxic (antimembrane)	IgG IgM (activate complement)	—	Transfusion reactions Goodpasture's syndrome Autoimmune hemolysis Hemolytic anemia Certain drug reactions Membranous glomerulonephrosis
III	Immune complex (serum sickness–like)	IgG (form complexes with complement)	6 to 8 hr	Serum sickness Lupus nephritis Occupational allergic alveolitis Acute viral hepatitis
IV	Cell-mediated (delayed) or tuberculin-type response	—	48 hr	Allergic contact dermatitis Infectious granulomas (tuberculosis, mycoses) Tissue graft rejection Chronic hepatitis

(Adapted from Krupp MA, Chatton MJ: *Current medical diagnosis and treatment*, Los Altos, Calif, 1994, Lange Medical.)

reactions. Life-threatening allergic responses related to local anesthetics are indeed rare.[58]

Hypersensitivity to the ester-type local anesthetics is much more frequent: procaine, propoxycaine, benzocaine, tetracaine, and related compounds such as procaine penicillin G and procainamide.

Amide-type local anesthetics are essentially free of this risk. However, reports from the literature and from medical history questionnaires indicate that *alleged* allergy to amide drugs appears to be increasing, despite the fact that subsequent evaluation of these reports usually finds them describing cases of overdose, idiosyncrasy, or psychogenic reactions.[59,60] Allergy to one amide local anesthetic does not preclude the use of other amides because cross-allergenicity does not occur.[61] With ester-type local anesthetic allergy, however, cross-allergenicity does occur; thus all ester-type local anesthetics are contraindicated with a documented history of ester allergy.[61]

Allergic reactions have been documented for the various contents of the dental cartridge. Table 18-10 lists the functions of these components. Of special interest with regard to allergy is the bacteriostatic agent *methylparaben*. The parabens (methyl, ethyl, and propyl) are included, as bacteriostatic agents, in all multiuse drugs, cosmetics, and some foods. Their increasing use has led to more frequent sensitization to them. In evaluating local anesthetic allergy, Aldrete and Johnson demonstrated positive reactions to methylparaben but negative reactions to the amide anesthetic without the bacteriostatic agent.[2] Table 18-11 presents Aldrete and Johnson's dermal reaction findings in patients exposed to various ester and amide local anesthetic solutions. The authors reported no signs of systemic anaphylaxis occurring in any of the subjects.

Sodium Bisulfite Allergy. Allergy to *sodium bisulfite* or *metabisulfite* is being reported today with increasing frequency.[62–65] Bisulfites are antioxidants, commonly sprayed

TABLE 18-10
Contents of Local Anesthetic Cartridge

Ingredient	Function
Local anesthetic agent	Conduction blockade
Vasoconstrictor	Decrease absorption of local anesthetic into blood, thus increasing duration of anesthesia and decreasing toxicity of anesthetic
Sodium metabisulfite	Antioxidant for vasoconstrictor
Methylparaben*	Preservative to increase shelf life; bacteriostatic
Sodium chloride	Isotonicity of solution
Sterile water	Diluent

*Methylparaben has been excluded from all local anesthetic cartridges manufactured in the United States since January 1984, although it is still found in multidose vials of medication.

TABLE 18-11
Frequency of Dermal Reactions in Patients Exposed to Various Local Anesthetic Agents

Agent	Nonallergic Patients (*n* = 60)	Allergic Patients (*n* = 11)
NaCl	0	0
Procaine	20	8
Chloroprocaine	11	8
Tetracaine	25	8
Lidocaine	0	0
Mepivacaine	0	0
Prilocaine	0	0
Methylparaben	8	NA

(From Aldrete JA, Johnson DA: Evaluation of intracutaneous testing for investigation of allergy to local anesthetic agents, *Anesth Analg* 49:173-183, 1970.)
NA, Not available.

onto fruits and vegetables to keep them appearing "fresh" for long periods of time. For example, apple slices sprayed with bisulfite do not turn brown (become oxidized). Persons allergic to bisulfites (most often steroid-dependent asthmatics) may develop a severe response (bronchospasm).[64,66] The U.S. Food and Drug Administration has enacted regulations that limit the use of bisulfites on foods. A history of allergy to bisulfites should alert the dentist to the possibility of this same type of response if sodium bisulfite or metabisulfite is included in the local anesthetic solution. Sodium bisulfite or metabisulfite is found in all dental local anesthetic cartridges that contain a vasoconstrictor, but is not found in "plain" local anesthetic solutions.

In the presence of a documented sulfite allergy it is suggested that a local anesthetic solution without a vasopressor ("plain local anesthetic") be used (e.g., mepivacaine HCl 3%; prilocaine HCl 4%) if possible. There is no cross-allergenicity between sulfites and the "sulfa-" type antibiotics (sulfonamides).

Epinephrine Allergy. Allergy to epinephrine cannot occur in a living person. Questioning of the "epinephrine-allergic" patient (see Dialogue History, p. 323) immediately reveals signs and symptoms related to increased blood levels of circulating catecholamines (tachycardia, palpitation, sweating, nervousness), likely the result of fear of receiving injections (release of endogenous catecholamines [epinephrine and norepinephrine]). Management of fears and anxieties about receipt of the injection is in order in most of these situations.

Latex Allergy. The thick plunger (also known as the *stopper*) on one end of the local anesthetic cartridge, and the thin diaphragm on the other end of the cartridge (see Fig. 7-1) through which the needle penetrates may contain latex. Because latex allergy is of growing concern among all healthcare professionals, the risk of provoking an allergic reaction in a latex-sensitive patient must be considered. A recent review of the literature on latex allergy and local anesthetic cartridges by Shojaei and Haas demonstrates that latex allergen can be released into the local anesthetic solution as the needle penetrates the diaphragm, but there were no reports or case studies in which an allergic response to the latex component of the cartridge containing a dental local anesthetic was documented.[65]

Topical Anesthetic Allergy. Topical anesthetics possess a potential to induce allergy. Most of the commonly used topical anesthetics in dentistry are esters, such as benzocaine and tetracaine. The incidence of allergy to this classification of local anesthetics far exceeds that of the amide local anesthetics. However, because benzocaine (an ester topical anesthetic) is not absorbed systemically, allergic responses that might develop in response to its application normally are limited to the site of application.[67] When other topical formulations, ester or amide, that are absorbed systemically are applied to mucous membranes, allergic responses may be either localized or systemic. Many also contain preservatives such as methylparaben, ethylparaben, or propylparaben.

Prevention

Medical History Questionnaire. The medical history questionnaire contains several questions related to allergy:

QUESTION: Are you allergic to (e.g., have itching, rash, swelling of hands, feet, or eyes) or made sick by penicillin, aspirin, codeine, or any other medications?

QUESTION: Have you ever had asthma, hay fever, sinus trouble, or allergies or hives?

These questions seek to determine if the patient has experienced any adverse drug reactions. ADR's are not uncommon; those most frequently reported are labeled as *allergy*. If the patient mentions any reaction to local anesthetics, the following protocol should be observed before use of the questionable drug is considered. If the patient relates a history of alleged local anesthetic allergy, it is imperative that the dentist consider the following factors:
1. Assume that the patient is truly allergic to the drug in question and then take whatever steps are necessary to determine whether the alleged "allergy" is indeed an allergy.
2. Any drug or closely related drug to which a patient claims to be allergic *must not* be used until the alleged allergy can be absolutely disproved.
3. For almost all drugs commonly implicated in allergic reactions, equally effective alternate drugs exist (e.g., antibiotics and analgesics).

4. The only drug group in which alternatives are not equally effective is the local anesthetics.

• • •

Two major components are useful for determining the veracity of a claim of allergy: (1) *dialogue history*, whereby additional information is sought directly from the patient, and (2) *consultation* for a more complete evaluation if doubt still persists.

Dialogue History. The following questions are included in the dialogue history between the dentist and a patient with an alleged allergy to local anesthetics. The first two questions are the most critical, for they immediately establish in the evaluator's mind a feeling that allergy either does or does not exist.[68]

QUESTION: Describe exactly what happened.

QUESTION: What treatment was given?

After these two questions the evaluator may consider others that will help elucidate the actual reaction.

QUESTION: What position were you in during the injection of the local anesthetic?

QUESTION: What was the time sequence of events?

QUESTION: Were the services of emergency personnel necessary?

QUESTION: What drug was used?

QUESTION: What volume of the drug was administered?

QUESTION: Did the local anesthetic solution contain a vasoconstrictor?

QUESTION: Were you taking any other drugs or medications at the time of the incident?

QUESTION: Can you provide the name, address, and telephone number of the doctor (dentist or physician) who was treating you when the incident occurred?

Answers to these questions provide enough information to permit a doctor to make an informed determination as to whether or not a true allergic reaction to a drug occurred. This is the initial step in managing alleged local anesthetic allergy. The dialogue history follows.

QUESTION: Describe exactly what happened.

This is probably the most important question, because it allows the patient to describe the actual sequence of events. The "allergy," in most instances, is explained by the answer to this question. The symptoms described by the patient should be recorded and evaluated to help in formulating a tentative diagnosis of the adverse reaction. Did the patient lose consciousness? Did convulsions occur? Was there skin involvement or respiratory distress? The manifestations of allergic reactions are discussed in the following. Knowing them can aid the evaluator in rapidly determining the nature of the reaction that occurred.

Allergic reactions involve one or more of the following: skin (itching, hives, rash, edema), gastrointestinal system (cramping, diarrhea, nausea, vomiting), exocrine glands (runny nose, watery eyes), respiratory system (wheezing, laryngeal edema), and cardiovascular system (angioedema, vasodilation, hypotension). Most patients describe their local anesthetic "allergy" as one in which they experienced palpitations, severe headache, sweating, and mild shaking (tremor). Such reactions are almost always of psychogenic origin or are related to the administration of overly large doses of vasoconstrictor (e.g., epinephrine). They are not allergic in nature. Hyperventilation, an anxiety-induced reaction in which patients lose control over their breathing (exhaling and inhaling rapidly and deeply), is accompanied by dizziness, lightheadedness, and peripheral paresthesias (fingers, toes, and lips). Complaints of itching, hives, rash, or edema lead to the conclusion that an allergic reaction actually may have occurred.

QUESTION: What treatment was given?

When the patient is able to describe his or her management, the evaluator usually can determine its cause. *Were drugs injected? If so, what drugs? Epinephrine, histamine blockers, corticosteroids, or anticonvulsants? Was aromatic ammonia used? Oxygen?* Knowledge of the specific management of these situations can lead to an accurate diagnosis.

Drugs used in the management of allergic reactions include three categories: *vasopressors* (epinephrine [Adrenalin]), *histamine blockers* (diphenhydramine [Benadryl] or chlorpheniramine [Chlor-Trimeton]), and *corticosteroids* (hydrocortisone sodium succinate [Solu-Cortef]).

Mention of the use of one or more of these drugs increases the likelihood that an allergic response did occur. *Anticonvulsants*, such as diazepam (Valium), midazolam (Versed), and pentobarbital (Nembutal), are administered intravenously to terminate seizures induced by overdose of local anesthetic. *Aromatic ammonia* is frequently used in the treatment of syncopal episodes. *Oxygen* may be administered in any or all of these reactions, but is not specific for allergy.

QUESTION: What position were you in when the reaction took place?

Injection of a local anesthetic into an upright patient is most likely to produce a psychogenic reaction (vasodepressor syncope). This does not exclude the possibility that another type of reaction may occur, but with the patient supine during the injection, vasodepressor syncope is a less likely etiology, even though the transient loss of consciousness may (on very rare occasion) develop in these circumstances.[69] In some of the evaluations of allergy to local anesthetics that the author carried out, the patient had been given an intracapsular injection of corticosteroid in the knee. Seated upright on a table in the physician's treatment room, the patient was able to watch the entire procedure, and it was profoundly disturbing. In an effort to make such injections more tolerable, lidocaine or another local anesthetic is added to the steroid mixture. In spite of this, however, the intracapsular injection of corticosteroid and lidocaine is extremely uncomfortable. Many patients experience their "allergic reaction" at this time. Therefore the supine position is recommended as being physiologically best tolerated for the administration of all local anesthetic injections.

QUESTION: What was the time sequence of events?

When, in relation to the administration of the local anesthetic, did the reaction occur? Most adverse drug reactions associated with local anesthetic administration occur during or immediately (within seconds) after the injection. Syncope, hyperventilation, overdose, and (sometimes) anaphylaxis are most likely to develop immediately during the injection or within minutes thereafter, although they all may occur later, during dental therapy. Also, seek to determine the amount of time that elapsed during the entire episode. *How long was it before the patient was discharged from the office? Did dental treatment continue after the episode?* The fact that dental treatment continued after this episode indicates that the response was probably minor and of a nonallergic nature.

QUESTION: Were the services of a physician, emergency medical services, or hospital necessary?

A positive response to this usually indicates the occurrence of a more serious reaction. Most psychogenic reactions are ruled out by a positive answer, although an overdose or allergic reaction indeed may have occurred.

QUESTION: What local anesthetic was administered?

A patient who is truly allergic to a drug should be told the exact (generic) name of the substance. Many persons with documented allergic histories wear a medical-alert tag or bracelet (Fig. 18-11) that lists specific items to which they are sensitive. However, some patients respond to this question with: "I'm allergic to local anesthetics" or "I'm allergic to Novocain" or "I'm allergic to all 'caine' drugs." Of 59 patients reporting allergy to local anesthetics, 54 could name one or more local anesthetics they believed were responsible. Five referred to only caine drugs.[70] Novocain (procaine) and other esters rarely are used today as injectable local anesthetics in dentistry (though the esters maintain some popularity in medicine),

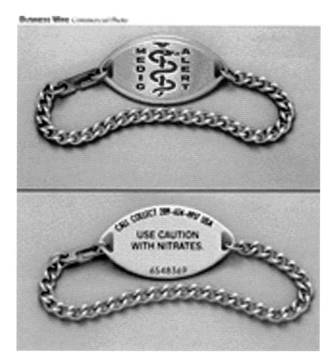

Figure 18-11. Medic-alert bracelet provides vital medical information about patient.

the amides having virtually replaced the esters in clinical practice. Yet patients throughout the world frequently call the local anesthetics they receive "shots of Novocain." Two reasons exist for this. First, many older patients at one time received Novocain as a dental local anesthetic, and its name has become synonymous with intraoral dental injections. Second, despite the fact that most dentists do not inject procaine or procaine-propoxycaine, many still describe local anesthetics as Novocain when talking with their patients. Thus the usual response of a patient to this question remains, "I'm allergic to Novocain." This response, received from a patient who has been managed properly in the past after an adverse reaction, indicates that the patient was sensitive to ester local anesthetics but not necessarily to amide local anesthetics. However, the answers usually are too general and vague for any conclusions to be drawn.

QUESTION: What amount of drug was administered?

This question seeks to determine whether there was a definite dose–response relationship, as might occur with an overdose reaction. The problem is that patients rarely know these details and can provide little or no assistance. The doctor who was involved in the prior episode(s) may be of greater assistance.

QUESTION: Did the anesthetic solution contain a vasoconstrictor or preservative?

The presence of vasoconstrictor might lead to the thought of an overdose reaction (relative or absolute) to

this component of the solution. A preservative, such as methylparaben or sodium bisulfite, in the solution might lead to the belief that an allergic reaction did occur to the preservative, not to the local anesthetic. Unfortunately, however, most patients are unable to furnish this information. Today, methylparaben is found only in multiple-dose vials of local anesthetics (and most other drugs). Bisulfites are found in all dental local anesthetic cartridges containing a vasopressor.

QUESTION: Were you taking any other drugs or medications at the time of the reaction?

This question seeks to determine the possibility of a drug–drug interaction or a side effect of other drugs as being responsible for the reported adverse response. Reidenburg and Lowenthal, reporting in 1968 on adverse *nondrug* reactions, demonstrated that "adverse" effects and side effects, which are so often blamed on medications, occur with considerable regularity in persons who have received no drugs or medications for weeks.[71] In other words, many so-called *adverse drug reactions* may be nothing more than a coincidental event: the person's becoming overly tired, irritable, nauseated, or dizzy for reasons unrelated to drugs. Unfortunately, however, it seems that whenever such symptoms develop in a patient taking a medication the drug is immediately thought to be responsible, with the label "allergy" often applied.

QUESTION: Can you provide the name and address of the doctor (dentist, physician, or hospital) who was treating you at the time of the incident?

If possible, it is usually valuable to speak to the person who managed the previous episode. In most instances this person is able to locate patient records and describe in detail what transpired. If it is not possible to locate or contact the doctor, the patient's primary care physician should be consulted. Direct discussion with the patient and doctor can provide a wealth of information that the knowledgeable dentist can use to determine more precisely the nature of the previous reaction.

Questions for the Patient with an Alleged Allergy to Local Anesthetic
1. **Describe your reaction:**
   Itching, hives, rash, feeling faint, dizzy, lightheaded, perspiration, shaking, palpitation
2. **How was your reaction treated?**
   Epinephrine, histamine blocker, corticosteroid, oxygen, spirits of ammonia ("smelling salts"), no treatment necessary
3. **What position were you in at the time of the reaction?**
   Supine, upright, partially reclined
4. **What is the name, address, and telephone number of the doctor in whose office this reaction occurred?**

Consultation and Allergy Testing. Consultation should be considered if any doubt remains as to the cause of the reaction after the dialogue history. Referral to a doctor who will test for allergy to local anesthetics is recommended.

Although no form of allergy testing is 100% reliable, skin testing is the primary mode of assessing a patient for local anesthetic allergy. Intracutaneous injections are among the most reliable means available, being 100 times more sensitive than cutaneous testing, and involve depositing 0.1 ml of test solution into the patient's forearm.[2,70,72–75] In all such instances, the local anesthetic solutions should contain neither vasoconstrictor nor preservative. Methylparaben, if evaluated, should be tested separately.[76]

The protocol for intracutaneous testing for local anesthetic allergy used at the University of Southern California School of Dentistry for the past 25 years involves the administration of 0.1 ml of each of the following: 0.9% sodium chloride, 1% or 2% lidocaine, 3% mepivacaine, and 4% prilocaine, without methylparaben, bisulfites, or vasopressors. After successful completion of this phase of testing, 0.9 ml of one of the previously noted local anesthetic solutions that produced no reaction is injected intraorally via supraperiosteal infiltration atraumatically (but without topical anesthesia) above a maxillary right or left premolar or anterior tooth. This is termed an *intraoral challenge test*, and it frequently provokes the "allergic" reaction: fainting, sweating, and palpitations.

After more than 210 local anesthetic allergy testing procedures, the author has encountered four allergic responses to the paraben preservative (before 1984 the protocol included testing for parabens) and none to the amide local anesthetic itself. Numerous psychogenic responses have been observed during either the intracutaneous or intraoral testing phases (syncope, hyperventilation, palpitations).

Such testing may be carried out by any person who is knowledgeable in the procedure and is also fully prepared to manage whatever adverse reactions may develop. It must be remembered that skin testing is not without risk. Severe immediate allergic reactions may be precipitated by as little as 0.1 ml of drug in a sensitized patient. Emergency drugs, equipment, and trained personnel always must be available whenever allergy testing is performed.

Intracutaneous allergy testing should be carried out only after an intensive dialogue history in which the evaluator has become convinced that the prior reaction to the local anesthetic was not allergy. The testing procedure is used to confirm this fact to the patient. The intraoral challenge test was added to the protocol when several patients with negative responses to intracutaneous testing stated, "But the dentist will give me a larger amount in the mouth." It was intended to provide the patient with the psychological support needed to receive intraoral local anesthetic injections safely.

Informed consent is obtained before allergy testing. The consent includes, among other possible complications, acute allergy (anaphylaxis), cardiac arrest, and death.

A continuous intravenous infusion is started before all allergy testing procedures, and emergency drugs and equipment are readily available throughout the testing.

Dental Management in the Presence of Alleged Local Anesthetic Allergy

When doubt persists concerning a history of allergy to local anesthetics, do not administer these drugs to the patient. *Assume that allergy exists. Do not use local anesthetics, including topical anesthetics, unless and until allergy has been absolutely disproved.*

Elective Dental Care. Dental treatment requiring local anesthesia (topical or injectable) should be postponed until a thorough evaluation of the patient's "allergy" is completed. Dental care not requiring local anesthesia may be completed during this time.

Emergency Dental Care. Pain or oral infection presents a more difficult situation in the "I am allergic to Novocain" patient. Commonly this patient is new to the office, requiring tooth extraction, pulpal extirpation, or incision and drainage (I&D) of an abscess, with a normal medical history except for their alleged "allergy to Novocain." If, after dialogue history, the "allergy" appears to have been a psychogenic reaction but some doubt remains, consider one of several courses of action.

Emergency protocol no. 1. The most practical approach to this patient is *no treatment of an invasive nature*. Arrange an appointment for immediate consultation and allergy testing. Do *not* carry out any dental care requiring the use of either injectable or topical local anesthetics. For incision and drainage of an abscess, inhalation sedation with nitrous oxide and oxygen might be an acceptable alternative.

Acute pain may be managed with oral analgesics; infection with oral antibiotics. These only constitute temporary measures. After complete evaluation of the "allergy," definitive dental care may proceed.

Emergency protocol no. 2. Use *general anesthesia* in place of local anesthesia for management of a dental emergency. When properly used, general anesthesia is a highly effective and relatively safe alternative. Its lack of availability is a major problem in most dental practices.

When general anesthesia is used, be careful to avoid local anesthetics in these procedures:
1. Topical application (via spray) to the pharynx and tracheal mucosa immediately before intubation
2. Infiltration of the skin with local anesthetic before venipuncture to decrease discomfort

General anesthesia, within either the dental office or a hospital operating room, is a viable alternative to local anesthetic administration in managing the "allergic" patient, provided adequate facilities and well-trained personnel are available.

Emergency protocol no. 3. *Histamine blockers as local anesthetics* should be considered if general anesthesia is not available and if it is deemed necessary to intervene physically in the dental emergency. Most injectable histamine blockers have local anesthetic properties. Diphenhydramine hydrochloride in a 1% solution with 1:100,000 epinephrine provides pulpal anesthesia for up to 30 minutes.[77] Although the quality of soft- and hard-tissue anesthesia obtained with diphenhydramine and lidocaine are equivalent, an undesirable side effect frequently noted during injection of diphenhydramine is a burning or stinging sensation, which limits the use of this agent for most patients to emergency procedures only.[78] Nitrous oxide and oxygen used along with diphenhydramine minimize patient discomfort while increasing their pain reaction threshold. Another (possibly positive) side effect of diphenhydramine and many histamine blockers is CNS depression (sedation, drowsiness), which may prove somewhat beneficial during treatment but mandates that an adult guardian be available to take the patient home after treatment.

Emergency protocol no. 4. *Electronic dental anesthesia* (EDA) or other nondrug techniques of pain control, such as hypnosis, may provide effective pain control in some situations in which local anesthetics are contraindicated. The adjunctive use of nitrous oxide–oxygen inhalation sedation increases the effectiveness of EDA and might permit the successful completion of painful procedures without the need for local anesthetic administration.[79,80]

Management of the Patient with Confirmed Allergy. Management of the dental patient with a confirmed allergy to local anesthetics varies according to the nature of the allergy. If the allergy is limited to ester anesthetics, an amide anesthetic may be used (provided it does not contain a paraben preservative, which is closely related to the esters). No dental cartridge manufactured in the United States since January 1984 contains methylparaben.

If, in the extremely unlikely case, a documented allergy to an amide local anesthetic exists, other amide local anesthetics may be employed because cross-allergenicity between amide locals does not occur.[61]

If allergy does truly exist to an ester local anesthetic (a much more likely situation), dental treatment may be safely completed via one of the following:
1. Administration of an amide local anesthetic
2. Use of histamine blockers as local anesthetics
3. General anesthesia
4. Alternative techniques of pain control
   a. Electronic dental anesthesia
   b. Hypnosis

On occasion it is reported that a patient is "allergic to all 'caine' drugs." Such a report should provoke close scrutiny by the dentist, and the method by which this conclusion was reached should be reexamined.

All too often patients are mislabeled "allergic to local anesthetics." Such patients ultimately must have dental treatment carried out in a hospital setting, usually under general anesthesia, when a proper evaluation might have saved the patient time and money and decreased the risk of dental care.[58]

Clinical Manifestations

Table 18-9 lists the various forms of allergic reactions. It is also possible to classify allergic reactions by the time elapsing between contact with the antigen and the onset of clinical manifestations of allergy. *Immediate reactions* develop within seconds to hours of exposure. (They include Types I, II, and III in Table 18-9.) With *delayed reactions*, clinical manifestations develop hours to days after antigenic exposure (Type IV).

Immediate reactions, particularly Type I, anaphylaxis, are significant. Organs and tissues involved in immediate allergic reactions include the skin, cardiovascular system, respiratory system, and gastrointestinal system. Generalized (systemic) anaphylaxis involves all these systems. Type I reactions also may involve only one system, in which case they are termed *localized allergy*. Examples of localized anaphylaxis and their "targets" are bronchospasm (respiratory system) and urticaria (skin).

Time of Onset of Symptoms

The time elapsing between a patient's exposure to the antigen and the development of clinical signs and symptoms is important. In general, the more rapidly signs and symptoms develop following antigenic exposure, the more intense the reaction is likely to be. Conversely, the more time between exposure and onset, the less intense the reaction. Cases have been reported of systemic anaphylaxis arising many hours after exposure.[81]

The rate of progression of signs and symptoms once they appear is also significant. Situations in which signs and symptoms rapidly increase in intensity are likely to be more life threatening than those progressing slowly or not at all once they appear.

Signs and Symptoms

Dermatological Reactions. The most common allergic drug reaction associated with local anesthetic administration is urticaria and angioedema.

Urticaria is associated with *wheals*, which are smooth, elevated patches of skin. Intense itching (pruritus) frequently is present.

Angioedema is localized swelling in response to an allergen. Skin color and temperature usually are normal (unless urticaria or erythema is present). Pain and itching are uncommon.

Angioedema most frequently involves the face, hands, feet, and genitalia, but it can also involve the lips, tongue, pharynx, and larynx. It is more common after the application of topical anesthetics to oral mucous membranes.

Within 30 to 60 minutes the tissue in contact with the allergen appears swollen.

Allergic skin reactions, if the sole manifestation of an allergic response, are normally not life threatening; however, those occurring rapidly after drug administration may be the first indication of a more generalized reaction to follow.

Respiratory Reactions. Clinical signs and symptoms of allergy may be solely related to the respiratory tract, *or* respiratory tract involvement may occur along with other systemic responses.

Bronchospasm is the classic respiratory allergic response. Following are its signs and symptoms:

- Respiratory distress
- Dyspnea
- Wheezing
- Flushing
- Cyanosis
- Perspiration
- Tachycardia
- Increased anxiety
- Use of accessory muscles of respiration

Laryngeal edema, an extension of angioneurotic edema to the larynx, is a swelling of the soft tissues surrounding the vocal apparatus with subsequent obstruction of the airway. Little or no exchange of air from the lungs is possible. Laryngeal edema represents the effects of allergy on the upper airway, whereas bronchospasm represents the effects on the lower airway (smaller bronchioles). Laryngeal edema is a life-threatening emergency.

Generalized Anaphylaxis. The most dramatic and acutely life-threatening allergic reaction is generalized anaphylaxis. Clinical death can occur within a few minutes. Generalized anaphylaxis can develop after the administration of an antigen by any route but is more common after parenteral administration (injection). Time of response is variable, but the reaction typically develops rapidly, reaching maximum intensity within 5 to 30 minutes. It is unlikely that this reaction will ever be noted after the administration of amide local anesthetics.

Signs and symptoms of generalized anaphylaxis, listed according to their typical progression, follow:

- Skin reactions
- Smooth muscle spasm of the gastrointestinal and genitourinary tracts and respiratory smooth muscle (bronchospasm)
- Respiratory distress
- Cardiovascular collapse

In fatal anaphylaxis, respiratory and cardiovascular disturbances predominate and are evident early in the reaction. The typical reaction progression is shown in Box 18-7.

In rapidly developing reactions *all signs and symptoms may occur within a very short time with considerable overlap.* In particularly severe reactions respiratory and cardiovascular signs and symptoms may be the only ones present.

BOX 18-7

Typical Reaction Progression of Generalized Anaphylaxis

1. Early phase: *skin reactions*
   a. Patient complains of feeling sick
   b. Intense itching (pruritus)
   c. Flushing (erythema)
   d. Giant hives (urticaria) over the face and upper chest
   e. Nausea and possibly vomiting
   f. Conjunctivitis
   g. Vasomotor rhinitis (inflammation of mucous membranes in the nose, marked by increased mucous secretion)
   h. Pilomotor erection (feeling of hair standing on end)
2. Associated with skin responses are various *gastrointestinal* or *genitourinary* disturbances related to smooth muscle spasm
   a. Severe abdominal cramps
   b. Nausea and vomiting
   c. Diarrhea
   d. Fecal and urinary incontinence
3. *Respiratory symptoms* usually develop next
   a. Substernal tightness or pain in chest
   b. Cough may develop
   c. Wheezing (bronchospasm)
   d. Dyspnea
   e. If the condition is severe, cyanosis of the mucous membranes and nail beds
   f. Possible laryngeal edema
4. The *cardiovascular system* is next to be involved
   a. Pallor
   b. Lightheadedness
   c. Palpitations
   d. Tachycardia
   e. Hypotension
   f. Cardiac dysrhythmias
   g. Unconsciousness
   h. Cardiac arrest

The reaction or any part of it can last from minutes to a day or more.[82]

With prompt and appropriate treatment the entire reaction may be terminated rapidly. However, hypotension and laryngeal edema may persist for hours to days despite intensive therapy. Death, which may occur at any time during the reaction, usually is secondary to upper airway obstruction produced by laryngeal edema.[83]

Management

Skin Reactions. Management is predicated on the rate at which the reaction appears after antigenic challenge.

Delayed skin reactions. Signs and symptoms developing 60 minutes or more after exposure usually do not progress and are not considered life threatening. Examples are a localized mild skin and mucous membrane reaction after application of topical anesthetic. In most instances the patient already may have left the dental office, calling back later describing these signs and symptoms; or the patient may still be in the dental office at the conclusion of his or her treatment.

Basic management follows the usual **P→A→B→C →D** algorithm used in management of all medical emergencies.

P→A→B→C. Position the conscious patient comfortably. A, B, and C are assessed as adequate (patient is conscious and talking).

D (definitive care):
1. Oral histamine blocker: 50 mg diphenhydramine or 10 mg chlorpheniramine; a prescription for diphenhydramine, 50 mg capsules, one q6 h for 3 to 4 days should be given to the patient.
2. The patient should remain in the office under observation for 1 hour before discharge to ensure that the reaction does not progress.
3. Obtain medical consultation, if necessary, to determine the cause of the reaction. A complete list of all drugs and chemicals administered to or taken by the patient should be compiled for use by the allergy consultant.
4. If drowsiness occurs after oral histamine blocker administration, the patient should not be permitted to leave the dental office unescorted.

Immediate skin reactions. Signs and symptoms of allergy developing within 60 minutes require more vigorous management. Examples are conjunctivitis, rhinitis, urticaria, pruritus, and erythema.

P→A→B→C. Position the conscious patient comfortably. A, B, and C are assessed as adequate (patient is conscious and talking).

D (definitive care):
1. Administer epinephrine. 0.3 mg (0.15 mg for a child) epinephrine IM or subcutaneously (SC).
2. Administer IM histamine blocker: 50 mg diphenhydramine (25 mg for a child) or 10 mg chlorpheniramine (5 mg for a child).
3. Obtain medical consultation with a physician, allergist, or hospital emergency room personnel *before discharge* from the dental office if epinephrine has been administered. It may be necessary to transfer the patient to the physician or hospital for observation before discharge. This should be done via emergency medical services (911).
4. Observe the patient a minimum of 60 minutes for evidence of recurrence. Discharge in the custody of an adult if any parenteral drugs have been given.
5. Prescribe an oral histamine blocker for 3 days.
6. Fully evaluate the patient's reaction before further dental care.

Respiratory Reactions

Bronchospasm. P→A→B→C. Position the conscious patient comfortably. Most persons experiencing respiratory distress prefer to be seated upright to varying degrees. A, B, and C are assessed. Airway is patent although

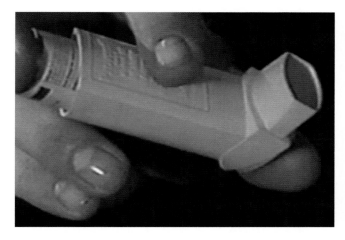

Figure 18-12. Bronchodilator inhaler (albuterol).

patient is exhibiting respiratory distress, C is assessed as adequate.

D (definitive care):
1. Terminate treatment.
2. Administer oxygen via full face mask, nasal hood, or nasal cannula at a flow of 5 to 6 liters/min.
3. Administer epinephrine or other appropriate bronchodilator via aerosol inhaler (albuterol) (Fig. 18-12) *or* IM/SC injection (0.3 mg [adult] or 0.15 mg [child]) of epinephrine. Dose may be repeated every 10 to 15 minutes if needed.
4. Observe the patient for 60 minutes before considering discharge. If relapse occurs, readminister 0.3 mg epinephrine via IM injection or aerosol. Summon outside medical assistance (911) if there is no response to treatment.
5. Administer histamine blocker to minimize relapse possibility (50 mg IM diphenhydramine [25 mg child] or 10 mg IM chlorpheniramine [5 mg child]).
6. Medical consultation. After medical consultation and observation the patient may be discharged or transferred to a hospital via ambulance with paramedical personnel.
7. Prescribe an oral histamine blocker and complete a thorough allergy evaluation before subsequent dental therapy.

Laryngeal edema. Laryngeal edema may be present when movement of air through the patient's nose and mouth cannot be heard or felt in the presence of spontaneous respiratory movements *or* when it is impossible to carry out artificial ventilation in the presence of a patent airway (tongue *not* causing obstruction). Partial obstruction of the larynx produces stridor (a characteristic high-pitched crowing sound), in contrast to the wheezing associated with bronchospasm. A partial obstruction may gradually or rapidly progress to total obstruction accompanied by the ominous "sound" of silence. The patient rapidly loses consciousness from lack of oxygen.

P→A→B→C. Position the unconscious patient supine. A, B, and C are assessed. If airway is maintained and the victim's chest is making spontaneous respiratory movements but no air is being exchanged, immediate and effective treatment is mandatory to save the victim's life.

D (definitive care):

1. Epinephrine. Administer 0.3 mg (0.15 mg for a child) epinephrine IM or SC. Epinephrine may be administered every 10 to 15 minutes as needed.
2. Activate emergency medical services (EMS). Summon emergency medical assistance and administer oxygen.
3. Maintain the airway. If it is partially obstructed, epinephrine may halt the progress of, or reverse the edema.
4. Additional drug management: histamine blocker IM or IV (50 mg diphenhydramine or 10 mg chlorpheniramine), corticosteroid IM or IV (100 mg hydrocortisone sodium succinate to inhibit and decrease edema and capillary dilation).
5. Perform cricothyrotomy. If the preceding steps have failed to secure a patent airway, an emergency procedure to create an airway is essential for survival. Figures 18-13 and 18-14 illustrate the anatomy of the region and the technique. Once established, the airway must be maintained, oxygen administered, and artificial ventilation used as needed. Monitor the patient's vital signs. The patient definitely requires hospitalization after transfer from the dental office by paramedical personnel.

Generalized Anaphylaxis. Generalized anaphylaxis is highly unlikely to develop in response to local anesthetic administration. Its management is included here, however, for completeness. The most common causes of death from anaphylaxis are parenterally administered penicillin and stinging insects (the *Hymenoptera:* wasps, hornets, yellow jackets, and bees).

Signs of allergy present. When signs and symptoms of allergy are present (e.g., urticaria, erythema, pruritus,

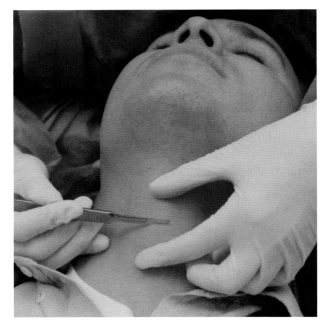

Figure 18-13. With fingers placed on the thyroid and cricoid cartilages, a horizontal incision is made through the cricothyroid membrane to gain access to the trachea.

and wheezing), they should signal an immediate diagnosis of allergy. The patient usually is unconscious.

P→A→B→C. Position the unconscious patient supine. A, B, and C are assessed and performed as indicated (Fig. 18-15).

D (definitive care):

1. Summon medical assistance. As soon as a severe allergic reaction is considered a possibility, emergency medical care should be summoned.
2. Administer epinephrine. The doctor should have previously called for the office emergency team. Epinephrine from the emergency kit (0.3 ml of 1:1000 for adults, 0.15 ml for children, and 0.075 ml for

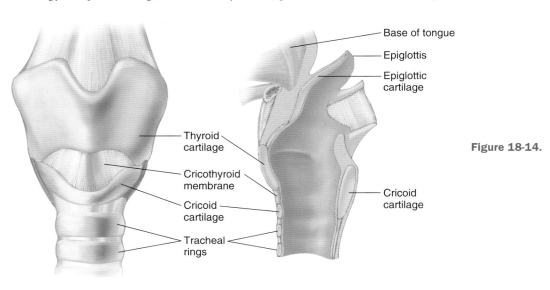

Base of tongue

Epiglottis

Epiglottic cartilage

Thyroid cartilage

Cricothyroid membrane

Cricoid cartilage

Tracheal rings

Cricoid cartilage

Figure 18-14.

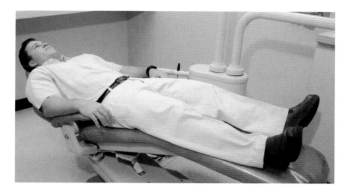

Figure 18-15. Positioning for basic life support.

infants) is administered IM as quickly as possible, or IV (if available, in a 1:10,000 solution). Because of the immediate need for epinephrine in this situation, a preloaded syringe of epinephrine is recommended for the emergency kit (Fig. 18-16). Epinephrine is the only injectable drug that should be kept in a preloaded form so as to prevent confusion when looking for it in this near-panic situation.

Should the clinical picture fail to improve or continue to deteriorate (increased severity of symptoms) within 10 minutes of the initial epinephrine dose, a second dose is administered. Subsequent doses may be administered as needed every 10 to 15 minutes, if the potential risk of epinephrine administration (excessive cardiovascular stimulation) is kept in mind and the patient is adequately monitored.

3. Administer oxygen.
4. Monitor vital signs. The patient's cardiovascular and respiratory status must be monitored continuously. Blood pressure and heart rate (at the carotid artery) should be recorded at least every 5 minutes, with closed chest compression started if cardiac arrest occurs.

During this acute, life-threatening phase of what is obviously an anaphylactic reaction, management consists of basic life support, the administration of oxygen and epinephrine, and continual monitoring of vital signs. Until an improvement in the patient's status is noted, no additional drug therapy is indicated.

5. Additional drug therapy. Additional drug therapy may be started once clinical improvement is noted (increased

blood pressure, decreased bronchospasm). This includes the administration of a histamine blocker and a corticosteroid (both drugs IM or, if possible, IV). Their function is to prevent a possible recurrence of symptoms and obviate the need for the continued administration of epinephrine. They are not administered during the acute phase of the reaction because they are too slow in onset and they do not do enough immediate good to justify their use at this time. Epinephrine and oxygen are the only drugs to administer during the acute phase of the anaphylactic reaction.

No signs of allergy present. If a patient receiving a local anesthetic injection loses consciousness and no signs of allergy are present, the differential diagnosis includes psychogenic reaction (vasodepressor syncope), overdose reaction, and allergic reaction involving only the cardiovascular system, among other possibilities.

P→A→B→C. Position the unconscious patient supine (see Fig. 18-15).
1. Terminate treatment.
2. Position patient. Management of this situation, which might prove to result from any of a number of causes, requires immediately placing the patient in the supine position with the legs elevated slightly.
3. Basic life support, as indicated (Fig. 18-17). A, B, and C are assessed and performed as indicated. Victims of vasodepressor syncope or postural hypotension rapidly recover consciousness once properly positioned with a patent airway. Patients who do not recover at this point should continue to have the elements of basic life support applied (breathing, circulation) as needed.

D. (definitive care):
1. Summon emergency medical services (EMS). If consciousness does not return rapidly after the institution of the steps of basic life support, EMS should be sought immediately.
2. Administer oxygen.
3. Monitor vital signs. Blood pressure, heart rate and rhythm, and respirations should be monitored at least every 5 minutes, with the elements of basic life support started at any time necessary.
4. Additional management. On arrival, the emergency medical personnel will seek to make a diagnosis of the cause of the loss of consciousness. If this is possible, appropriate drug therapy will be instituted, and the patient stabilized and then transferred to a local hospital emergency department.

In the absence of any definitive signs and symptoms of allergy, such as edema, urticaria, or bronchospasm, epinephrine and other drug therapy are not indicated. Any of a number of other situations may be the cause of the unconsciousness, for example, drug overdose, hypoglycemia, cerebrovascular accident, acute adrenal insufficiency, or cardiopulmonary arrest. Continued basic life support until medical assistance arrives is the most rational mode of management in this situation.

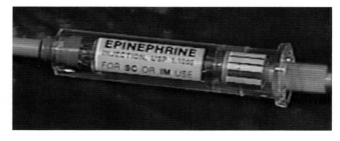

Figure 18-16. Syringe preloaded with 1:1000 epinephrine.

Airway

Head Tilt, Chin Lift

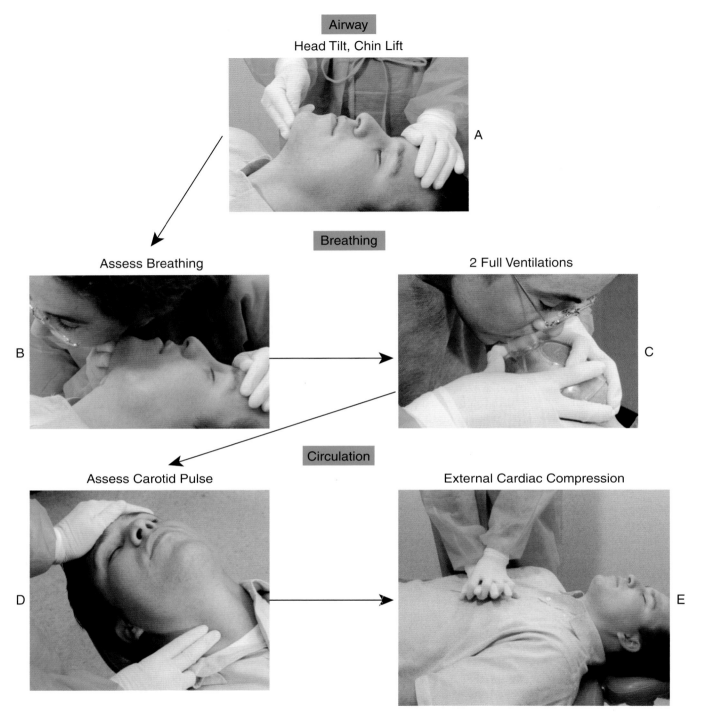

Figure 18-17. Summary of basic life support. **A,** Airway—head tilt, chin lift. **B,** Assess breathing. **C,** Two full ventilations. **D,** Assess carotid pulse. **E,** External chest compression—15 compressions: 2 ventilations.

SUMMARY

Systemic complications of local anesthetic drug administration and techniques are frequently preventable. Following is a summary of those procedures recommended to minimize their occurrence:

1. Preliminary medical evaluation should be completed before the administration of any local anesthetic.

2. Anxiety, fear, and apprehension should be recognized and managed before administration of a local anesthetic.

3. All dental injections should be administered with the patient supine or semisupine. Patients should not receive local anesthetic injections in the upright position unless special conditions dictate (e.g., severe cardiorespiratory disease).

4. Topical anesthetic should be applied before all injections for a minimum of 1 minute.

5. The weakest effective concentration of local anesthetic solution should be injected in the *minimum volume* compatible with successful anesthesia.

6. The anesthetic solution selected should be appropriate for the dental treatment contemplated (*duration of action*).

7. Vasoconstrictors should be included in all local anesthetics unless specifically contraindicated by the desired duration of effect or the patient's physical status.

8. Needles should be disposable, sharp, rigid, capable of reliable aspiration, and of adequate length for the contemplated injection techniques.

9. Aspirating syringes must *always* be used for all injections.

10. Aspiration should be carried out in at least two planes before injection.

11. Injection should be made slowly, a *minimum* of 60 seconds if depositing 1.8 ml of local anesthetic.

12. Observe the patient both during and after the administration for signs of undesirable reaction. *Never* give the injection and leave the patient alone while doing other procedures.

REFERENCES

1. Pallasch TJ: *Pharmacology for dental students and practitioners*, Philadelphia, 1980, Lea & Febiger.

2. Aldrete JA, Johnson DA: Evaluation of intracutaneous testing for investigation of allergy to local anesthetic agents, *Anesth Analg* 49:173-183, 1970.

3. Finder RL, Moore PA: Adverse drug reactions to local anesthesia, *Dent Clin North Am* 46(4):747-757, 2002.

4. Vinckier F: Local anesthesia in children, *Rev Belge Medec Dent* 55(1):61-71, 2000.

5. Malamed SF: Morbidity, mortality and local anesthesia, *Primary Dent Care* 6(1):11-15, 1999.

6. Meechan J: How to avoid local anaesthetic toxicity, *Br Dent J* 184(7):334-335, 1998.

7. Meechan J, Rood JP: Adverse effects of dental local anaesthesia, *Dent Update* 24(8):315-318, 1997.

8. Davis MJ, Vogel LD: Local anesthetic safety in pediatric patients, *NY State Dent J* 62(2):32-35, 1996.

9. Prince BS, Goetz CM, Rihn TL, et al: Drug-related emergency department visits and hospital admissions, *Am J Hosp Pharm* 49(7):1696-1700, 1992.

10. Kishikawa K, Namiki A, Miyashita K, et al: Effects of famotidine and cimetidine on plasma levels of epidurally administered lignocaine, *Anaesthesia* 45(9):719-721, 1990.

11. Shibasaki S, Kawamata Y, Ueno F, et al: Effects of cimetidine on lidocaine distribution in rats, *J Pharmacobio-dynam* 11(12):785-793, 1988.

12. Dailey PA, Hughes SC, Rosen MA, et al: Effect of cimetidine and ranitidine on lidocaine concentrations during epidural anesthesia for cesarian section, *Anesthesiology* 69(6):1013-1017, 1988.

13. de Jong RH: Bupivacaine preserves newborns' muscle tone, *JAMA* 237:53-54, 1977.

14. Steen PA, Michenfelder JD: Neurotoxicity of anesthetics, *Anesthesiology* 50:437-453, 1979.

15. Hazma J: Effect of epidural anesthesia on the fetus and the neonate, *Cah Anesthesiol* 42(2):265-273, 1994.

16. Shammas FV, Dickstein K: Clinical pharmacokinetics in heart failure: an updated review, *Clin Pharmacokinet* 15(2):94-113, 1988.

17. Hammermeister KE: Adverse hemodynamic effects of antiarrhythmic drugs in congestive heart failure, *Circulation* 81(3):1151-1153, 1990.

18. Pedersen NA, Jensen FS: Clinical importance of plasma cholinesterase for the anesthetist, *Ann Acad Med Singapore* 23(suppl 6):120-124, 1994.

19. Englesson S: The influence of acid-base changes on central nervous system toxicity of local anaesthetic agents, *Acta Anaesth Scand* 18:88-103, 1974.

20. Malagodi MH, Munson ES, Embro MJ: Relation of etidocaine and bupivacaine toxicity to rate of infusion in rhesus monkeys, *Br J Anaesth* 49:121-125, 1977.

21. Hersh EV, Helpin ML, Evans OB: Local anesthetic mortality: report of a case, *ASDC J Dent Child* 58(6):489-491, 1991.

22. Moore PA: Preventing local anesthetic toxicity, *J Am Dent Assoc* 123(3):60-64, 1992.

23. Yagiela JA: Local anesthetics. In Dionne RA, Phero JC, Becker DE eds: *Management of pain and anxiety in the dental office*, Philadelphia, 2002, WB Saunders.

24. Kaplan EL, editor: *Cardiovascular disease in dental practice*, Dallas, 1986, American Heart Association.

25. Adriani J, Campbell D: Fatalities following topical application of local anesthetics to mucous membrane, *J Am Med Assoc* 162:1527, 1956.

26. Wilburn-Goo D, Lloyd LM: When patients become cyanotic: acquired methemoglobinemia, *J Am Dent Assoc* 130(6):826-831, 1999.

27. Khan NA, Kruse JA: Methemoglobinemia induced by topical anesthesia: a case report and review, *Amer J Med Sci* 318(6):415-418, 1999.

28. Cooper HA: Methemoglobinemia caused by benzocaine topical spray, *South Med J* 90(9):946-946, 1997.

29. Smith M, Wolfram W, Rose R: Toxicity: seizures in an infant caused by (or related to) oral viscous lidocaine use, *J Emerg Med* 10:587-590, 1992.

30. Hess GP, Walson PD: Seizures secondary to oral viscous lidocaine, *Ann Emerg Med* 17:725-727, 1988.

31. Garrettson LK, McGee EB: Rapid onset of seizures following aspiration of viscous lidocaine, *J Pediatr* 30:413-422, 1992.

32. Rothstein P, Dornbusch J, Shaywitz BA: Prolonged seizures associated with the use of viscous lidocaine, *J Pediatr* 101:461-463, 1982.

33. Bartlett SZ: Clinical observations on the effects of injections of local anesthetics preceded by aspiration, *Oral Surg Oral Med Oral Pathol* 33:520, 1972.

34. Aldrete JA, Narang R, Sada T, et al: Reverse carotid blood flow: a possible explanation for some reactions to local anesthetics, *J Am Dent Assoc* 94:1142-1145, 1977.

35. Malamed SF: Allergic and toxic reactions to local anesthetics, *Dent Today* 22(4)114-121, April 2003.

36. Cheatham BD, Primosch RE, Courts FJ: A survey of local anesthetic usage in pediatric patients by Florida dentists, *J Dent Child* 59:401-407, 1992.

37. Malamed SF: Report of a case, unpublished data, 2002.

38. Munson ES, Tucker WK, Ausinsch B, et al: Etidocaine, bupivacaine, and lidocaine seizure thresholds in monkeys, *Anesthesiology* 42:471-478, 1975.

39. Rey E, Radvanyi-Bouvet MF, Bodiou C, et al: Intravenous lidocaine in the treatment of convulsions in the neonatal period: monitoring plasma levels, *Ther Drug Monit* 12(4):316-320, 1990.

40. Aggarwal P, Wali JP: Lidocaine in refractory status epilepticus: a forgotten drug in the emergency department, *Am J Emerg Med* 11(3):243-244, 1993.

41. Pascual J, Ciudad J, Berciano J: Role of lidocaine (lignocaine) in managing status epilepticus, *J Neurol Neurosurg Psychiatr* 55(1):49-51, 1992.

42. Jaffe AS: The use of antiarrhythmics in advanced cardiac life support, *Ann Emerg Med* 22:307-316, 1993.

43. Bruelle P, de La Coussaye JE, Eledjam JJ: Convulsions and cardiac arrest after epidural anesthesia: prevention and treatment, *Cah Anesthesiol* 42(2):241-246, 1994.

44. de La Coussaye JE, Eledjam JJ, et al: Cardiotoxicity of local anesthetics, *Cah Anesthesiol* 41(6):589-598, 1993.

45. Bachmann MB, Biscoping J, Schurg R, et al: Pharmacokinetics and pharmacodynamics of local anesthetics, *Anaesthesiol Reanim* 16(6):359-373, 1991.

46. Ryan CA, Robertson M, Coe JY: Seizures due to lidocaine toxicity in a child during cardiac catheterization, *Pediatr Cardiol* 14(2):116-118, 1993.

47. Rivera R, Segnini M, Baltodano A, et al: Midazolam in the treatment of status epilepticus in children, *Crit Care Med* 21(7):991-994, 1993.

48. Bertz RJ, Howrie DL: Diazepam by continuous intravenous infusion for status epilepticus in anticonvulsant hypersensitivity syndrome, *Ann Pharmacother* 27(3):298-301, 1993.

49. Lahat E, Aladjem M, Eshel G, et al: Midazolam in treatment of epileptic seizures, *Pediatr Neurol* 8(3):215-216, 1992.

50. Wroblewski BA, Joseph AB: Intramuscular midazolam for treatment of acute seizures or behavioral episodes in patients with brain injuries, *J Neurol Neurosurg Psychiatr* 55(4):328-329, 1992.

51. Hanley DF Jr, Pozo M: Treatment of status epilepticus with midazolam in the critical care setting, *Int J Clin Pract* 54(1):30-35, 2000.

52. Feldman HS, Arthur GR, Pitkanen M, et al: Treatment of acute systemic toxicity after the rapid intravenous injection of ropivacaine and bupivacaine in the conscious dog, *Anaesth Analg* 73(4):373-384, 1991.

53. de Jong RH: Vasoconstrictor. In de Jong RH, editor: *Local anesthetics*, St Louis, 1994, Mosby, pp 158-160.

54. Kellam SA, Smith JR, Scheffel SJ: Epinephrine absorption from commercial gingival retraction cords in clinical patients, *J Prosth Dent* 68(5):761-765, 1992.

55. American Dental Association: *Accepted dental therapeutics, 1984–1985*, Chicago, 1984, The American Dental Association.

56. Burr ML: Epidemiology of clinical allergy: introduction, *Monogr Allergy* 31:1-8, 1993.

57. Brown DT, Beamish D, Wildsmith JA: Allergic reaction to an amide local anaesthetic, *Br J Anaesth* 53:435-437, 1981.

58. Aldrete JA, O'Higgins JW: Evaluation of patients with history of allergy to local anesthetic drugs, *South Med J* 64:1118-1121, 1971.

59. Jackson D, Chen AH, Bennett CR: Identifying true lidocaine allergy, *J Am Dent Assoc* 125(10):1362-1366, 1994.

60. Doyle KA, Goepferd SJ: An allergy to local anesthetics? The consequences of a misdiagnosis, *ASDC J Dent Child* 56(2):103-106, 1989.

61. Haas DA: An update on local anesthetics in dentistry, *J Can Dent Assoc* 68(9):546-551, 2002.

62. Schwartz HJ, Sher TH: Bisulfite sensitivity manifesting as allergy to local dental anesthesia, *J Allergy Clin Immunol* 75(4):525-527, 1985.

63. Seng GF, Gay BJ: Dangers of sulfites in dental local anesthetic solutions: warnings and recommendations, *J Am Dent Assoc* 113(5):769-770, 1986.

64. Perusse R, Goulet JP, Turcotte JY: Sulfites, asthma and vasoconstrictors, *Can Dent Assoc J* 55:55-56, 1989.

65. Shojaie AR, Haas DA: Local anesthetic cartridges and latex allergy: a literature review, *J Can Dent Assoc* 68(10):622-626, 2002.

66. Perusse R, Goulet JP, Turcotte JY: Contraindications to vasoconstrictors in dentistry: Part II. Hyperthyroidism, diabetes, sulfite sensitivity, cortico-dependent asthma, and pheochromocytoma, *Oral Surg Oral Med Oral Pathol* 74:687-691, 1992.

67. Bruze M, Gruvberger B, Thulin I: PABA, benzocaine, and other PABA esters in sunscreens and after-sun products, *Photodermatol Photoimmunol Photomed* 7(3):106-108, 1990.

68. Malamed SF: *Medical emergencies in the dental office*, ed 5, St Louis, 2000, Mosby.

69. Peter R: Sudden unconsciousness during local anesthesia, *Anesth Pain Control Dent* 2(3):140-142, 1993.

70. Chandler MJ, Grammer LC, Patterson R: Provocative challenge with local anesthetics in patients with a prior history of reaction, *J Allergy Clin Immunol* 79(6):883-886, 1987.

71. Riedenburg MM, Lowenthal DT: Adverse nondrug reaction, *N Engl J Med* 279:678-679, 1968.

72. Hodgson TA, Shirlaw PJ, Challacombe SJ: Skin testing after anaphylactoid reactions to dental local anesthetics. A comparison with controls, *Oral Surg Oral Med Oral Pathol* 75(6):706-711, 1993.

73. Rozicka T, Gerstmeier M, Przybilla B, et al: Allergy to local anesthetics: comparison of patch test with prick and intradermal test results, *J Am Acad Dermatol* 16(6):1202-1208, 1987.

74. Escolano F, Aliaga L, Alvarez J, et al: Allergic reactions to local anesthetics, *Rev Esp Anesesiol Reanim* 37(3):172-175, 1990.

75. Canfield DW, Gage TW: A guideline to local anesthetic allergy testing, *Anesth Prog* 34(5):157-163, 1987.

76. Swanson JG: An answer for a questionable allergy to local anesthetics, *Ann Emerg Med* 17(5):554, 1988.

77. Malamed SF: The use of diphenhydramine HCl as a local anesthetic in dentistry, *Anesth Prog* 20:76-82, 1973.

78. Ernst AA, Anand P, Nick T, et al: Lidocaine versus diphenhydramine for anesthesia in the repair of minor lacerations, *J Trauma* 34(3):354-357, 1993.

79. Quarnstrom F, Milgrom P: Clinical experience with TENS and TENS combined with nitrous oxide-oxygen, *Anesth Prog* 36:66-69, 1989.

80. Donaldson D, Quarnstrom F, Jastak T: The combined effect of nitrous oxide and oxygen and electrical stimulation during restorative dental treatment, *J Am Dent Assoc* 118:733-736, 1989.

81. Oh VM: Treatment of allergic adverse drug reactions, *Singapore Med J* 30(3):290-293, 1989.

82. Adkinson FN Jr, Yuninger JW, Busse WW, et al: *Middleton's allergy: principles and practice*, ed 6, St Louis, 2003, Mosby.

83. Stafford CT: Life-threatening allergic reactions. Anticipating and preparing are the best defenses, *Postgrad Med* 86(1):235-242, 245, 1989.

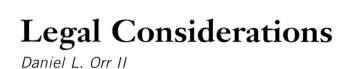

Legal Considerations

Daniel L. Orr II

CHAPTER
19

There are several legal theories by means of which plaintiffs may proceed against defendant healthcare professionals.

For instance, contract law has provided a basis for suits in which a healthcare professional is accused of guaranteeing a result from treatment. When the result is not to the plaintiff's satisfaction, remedy may be sought in court. Plaintiff suits based in contract law against health providers are rare.

Recent history has seen a disturbing and dramatic increase in the number of suits filed under criminal law theories by government prosecutors for both alleged fraudulent activity on the part of the healthcare provider and for plaintiff morbidity or mortality damage. Prosecutors attacking healthcare providers criminally must be able to prove that a criminal mind *(mens rea)* exists and that society has been injured.

However, the legal theory covering most healthcare professional lawsuit activity is that of the tort. A *tort* is a private civil wrong not dependent on a contract. The tort may or may not lead to further criminal prosecution. Classically, a viable suit in tort requires perfection of four essential elements: duty, a breach of duty, proximate cause, and damage. A healthcare professional may successfully defend a suit in tort by proving that no duty existed, no breach of duty occurred, the healthcare professional's conduct was not the cause of damage, or no damage exists.

Briefly, the healthcare professional owes a duty to a patient if the practitioner's conduct created a foreseeable risk to the patient. Generally, a duty is created when a patient and practitioner personally interact for healthcare purposes. Face-to-face interaction at the practitioner's place of practice most likely fulfills the requirement of a created duty, whereas interaction over the telephone, Internet, and so on may not be as clear-cut about establishment of duty.

A breach of duty occurs when the healthcare professional fails to act as a reasonable healthcare provider, which in medical or dental malpractice cases is proved to the jury by comparing the defendant's conduct with the reasonable conduct of a similarly situated healthcare professional. Testimony for this aspect of a suit for malpractice is developed by expert witnesses. Exceptions to the rule requiring experts are cases in which no consent was given or obtained for an elective procedure or cases in which the defendant's conduct is obviously erroneous and speaks for itself *(res ipsa loquitur)*, such as wrong-sided surgery. In addition, some complications are defined as malpractice per se by statute, such as unintentionally leaving a foreign body in a patient after a procedure.

The experts testifying as to the alleged breach of duty argue about standard of care. It is often mistakenly assumed that the standard of the practitioner's community is the one to which he or she will be judged. Today, the community standard is the national standard. If there are specialists reasonably accessible to the patient, the standard is the national standard for specialists, whether the practitioner is a specialist or not.

The standard of care also may be illustrated by the professional literature. Healthcare professionals are expected to be aware of current issues in the literature, such as previously unreported complications to local anesthetics. Often articles also proffer preventative suggestions and review treatment options.

Simply because an accepted writing recommends conduct other than that which the healthcare provider used is not necessarily indicative of a breach of duty. For instance, specific drug use other than that which is recommended by the generic *Physicians' Desk Reference* is commonplace and legally acceptable as long as the healthcare provider can articulate a reasonable purpose for his or her conduct. Part of this reasoning may likely include a benefit–risk analysis for various treatment options for a specific patient.

Proximate cause is the summation of actual cause and legal cause. Actual cause exists if a chain of events factually flows from the defendant's conduct to the plaintiff's injury. Legal cause is present if actual cause exists and if the plaintiff's attorney can prove that the harm sustained was foreseeable or not highly extraordinary in hindsight.

Damage is the element of the cause of action usually most easy to identify because it is most often manifested physically. Simply because damage is present does not mean malpractice has been committed, but damage must be present to fulfill all the elements of the tort.

The nation has seen a dramatic rise not only in tort-based malpractice lawsuits over the past several years, but also in the predictable sequelae of such legal action. Trauma centers have closed, doctors are actively and passively leaving lawsuit-friendly communities or states (e.g., by limiting their practice or opting for early retirement), and patient consumers are now starting to directly feel the loss of healthcare professional availability and other consequences of a litigation system that has never been busier.

The administration of local anesthetics is not a procedure immune from the liability crisis. When it is estimated that more than 300 million local anesthetic administrations are performed annually in the United States, at times the administration of local anesthesia, although extremely safe, results in unintended damage to the patient. If the elements of duty, breach of duty, and proximate cause accompany that damage, malpractice may have been committed. However, complications most often occur without any fault on the part of the local anesthetic administrator. In these situations, most complications are still foreseeable, and because they are predictable, the reasonable practitioner should be aware of optimal immediate and long-term treatment for the complications of local anesthetic administration.

The purpose of this chapter is not to describe in great detail the prevention or treatment of various local anesthetic complications, but to simply mention foreseeable complications and comment on the standard of care with regard to appropriate prevention and treatment. Obviously, some complications are common and others are rare, and frequency is an issue that is considered in legal evaluation of a case. In any case, the healthcare professional administering potent local anesthetics by definition tells the public that it can trust in that professional while in his or her care. When pretreatment questions arise, it is the healthcare professional's duty to investigate controversial or unknown areas to minimize the risk and maximize the benefits of his or her therapeutic decisions. When foreseen or unforeseen complications arise, the healthcare provider must be able to act in a reasonable manner for treatment of these untoward events.

Adequate legal response to a local anesthetic complication or emergency is often equivalent to adequate dental or medical response. However, when damage persists, plaintiff attorneys argue that the dental or medical response was not an adequate legal response and seek damages. The fact that the treatment rendered by the practitioner is recognized by the majority of his or her colleagues as optimal may not convince a jury when the plaintiff can find an expert who opines the opposite opinion. However, damage alone does not prove malpractice. The tort can be successfully defended by showing no duty, no breach of duty, or no proximate cause. In many cases, no matter what the complication discussed in this chapter, these legal defenses are the same in theory and applicable across the board, although the dental or medical responses are more specific to the precise situation.

If one is uncomfortable with any of the situations mentioned in this chapter, further individual research in that area may be warranted.

In addition to the civil, or tort, remedies available to the plaintiff patient, a healthcare practitioner also may have to defend conduct in other fora. Depending on the disposition of the plaintiff and his or her representative, the healthcare practitioner's conduct may be predictably evaluated not only civilly, but perhaps criminally or via other state agencies, such as licensing boards, better business bureaus, and so on. Although theoretically the arguments presented by the competing sides in these varying fora are the same no matter what the environment, there are very real differences involved. In particular, the penalties, and thus the burden of proof, are significantly different.

If the case is taken to a state agency, which is typically the board that issues the healthcare professional's license, the rules of evidence are not onerous as far as admission by the plaintiff. Essentially, the regulatory agency can accept any evidence it deems relevant, including hearsay, which means the defendant may not have the right to face an accuser. The burden of proof, which typically rests with the moving party or plaintiff, may even be arbitrarily switched to the defendant by the agency. The rules of evidence are so liberal in state agency fora because the issuance of an agency professional license is a privilege and not a right. The significance of proper representation and preparation if one is called before a regulatory agency cannot be understated when one considers the very real possibility of the loss of a license and subsequent loss of ability to practice.

If one is summoned to a civil forum, the rules of evidence and burden of proof are more strictly defined. Rules of evidence are subject to state and federal guidelines, although this is an area that is not black and white and attorneys are frequently necessary to zealously argue for or against admission of evidence. In a civil forum, the burden of proof generally remains with the plaintiff, and the plaintiff is required to prove the allegations by a preponderance of the evidence. Expressed mathematically, a preponderance is anything more than 50%. This essentially means that anything that even slightly tips the scales in the plaintiff's favor means the plaintiff has met the burden and thus may prevail.

In criminal cases, which again may be initiated for exactly the same conduct that may place the defendant in other fora, the burden of proof rests squarely with the prosecution (for example, the state or federal government). In addition, the burden is met only by proof that is beyond a reasonable doubt, not simply a preponderance of the evidence. Although the definition of reasonable doubt is open to argument, reasonable doubt is a more difficult standard to meet that is found in either agency or civil fora.

CONSENT

The consent process is an essential part of patient treatment for healthcare professionals. Essentially, consent involves explaining to the patient the advantages and disadvantages of different treatment options, including the benefits and risks of no treatment at all. Often treatment planning results in several viable options that may be recommended by the doctor. The patient then makes an informed decision as to which option is most preferable to that patient, and treatment may begin.

Consent is essential because many of the procedures doctors perform would be considered illegal in other settings; for example, an incision developed by a doctor during surgery versus an equivalent traumatic wound placed in a criminal battery.

Consent may be verbal or written, but when a controversy presents at a later date a written consent is extremely beneficial (Fig. 19-1). In fact, because many times consent is the standard of care for a procedure, the lack of a written consent may reduce the fact finding to a "he said/she said" scenario. This circumstance may greatly diminish the plaintiff's burden of proving the allegations and may even shift the burden of proof to the defendant.

When treating the mentally challenged or children under the age of majority, consent from a legal guardian is necessary for elective procedures.

Consent obtained before one procedure may not be assumed for the same procedure at a different time or a different procedure at the same time. In addition, consent obtained for one healthcare provider may not be transferable to another healthcare provider, such as a partner doctor or an employee dental hygienist or registered nurse.

Consent is not necessary at times. When treating a patient in an emergency setting, such as a spontaneously or traumatically unconscious patient, consent is implied. However, when possible, consent may be obtained from a legal guardian. The possibility of obtaining consent from a guardian before an emergency procedure is generally time dependent. In an urgent situation, time may be available to discuss treatment options with a guardian. However, during a more emergent situation, taking time to discuss treatment options may actually compromise the patient.

Generally, emergencies in nondental or nonmedical settings do not require consent secondary to "Good Samaritan" statutes, which apply to "rescues." However,

a source of liability even when being a "Good Samaritan" is reckless conduct. Reckless conduct in a rescue situation involves leaving the victim in a situation that is worse than when the rescuer found the victim. An example of such conduct would be if a rescuer offers to transport a victim to a hospital for necessary treatment and then abandons the victim further from a hospital than where the victim was initially found.

It is a recognized legal principle that a patient may not consent to malpractice. The patient who offers to sign a "waiver" to convince a practitioner to provide treatment, for instance, will not likely be held to that waiver if malpractice is adjudicated to exist.

Is consent necessary with regard to local anesthetic administration?

Some patients prefer not to be given any local anesthesia, even for significant operative procedures. If a patient is forced to have a local anesthetic without consent, technically a battery has occurred.

At times, local anesthetic administration is all that is necessary for certain diagnostic or therapeutic procedures such as differential diagnosis or treatment of atypical facial pain syndromes.

Finally, local anesthetic administration involves injecting or otherwise administering potent pharmaceutical agents. Either these agents or the means used to administer them may inadvertently damage a patient. Any conduct by a healthcare professional that may reasonably be expected to predictably result in damage requires consent.

HEALTH INSURANCE PORTABILITY AND ACCOUNTABILITY ACT OF 1996[1]

The Health Insurance Portability and Accountability Act (HIPAA) of 1996 was signed into law by former President Bill Clinton on August 21, 1996. Conclusive regulations were issued on August 17, 2000, to be instated by October 16, 2002. HIPAA requires that the transactions of all patient healthcare information be formatted in a standardized electronic style. In addition to protecting the privacy and security of patient information, HIPAA includes legislation on the formation of medical savings accounts, the authorization of a fraud and abuse control program, the easy transport of health insurance coverage, and the simplification of administrative terms and conditions.

HIPAA encompasses three primary areas, and its privacy requirements can be broken down into three types: privacy standards, patients' rights, and administrative requirements.

Privacy Standards

A central concern of HIPAA is the careful use and disclosure of protected health information (PHI), which generally is electronically controlled health information that is able to be distinguished individually. PHI also refers to verbal communication, although the HIPAA Privacy

INFORMED CONSENT

I hereby request that _____ provide treatment for me for the following condition: _____.
I have been afforded the time and opportunity to discuss this proposed treatment, the alternatives, and risks with _____, and I understand:

     1. The means of treatment will be: _____

     _____

     2. The alternative means of treatment are: _____

     _____

     3. The advantages of proposed treatment over alternative treatment are:

     _____

     _____

     4. That all treatments including the one proposed have some risks. The risks of importance involved in my treatment have been explained to me, and they are: _____

     _____

     5. The risks of nontreatment are:_____

     _____

_____
Signature of Patient

_____
Date

_____
Signature of Witness

_____
Signature of Healthcare Practitioner

Figure 19-1. Sample informed consent form.

Rule is not intended to hinder necessary verbal communication. The United States Department of Health and Human Services (USDHHS) does not require restructuring, such as soundproofing, architectural changes, and so forth, but some caution is necessary when exchanging health information by conversation.

An Acknowledgment of Receipt Notice of Privacy Practices, which allows patient information to be used or divulged for treatment, payment, or healthcare operations

(TPO), should be procured from each patient. A detailed and time-sensitive authorization also can be issued, which allows the dentist to release information in special circumstances other than TPOs. A *written consent* is also an option. Dentists can disclose PHI *without* acknowledgment, consent, or authorization in very special situations; for example, perceived child abuse, public health supervision, fraud investigation, or law enforcement with valid permission (e.g., a warrant). When divulging PHI, a dentist must try to disclose only the *minimum necessary* information, to help safeguard the patient's information as much as possible.

Dental professionals must adhere to HIPAA standards because healthcare providers (as well as healthcare clearinghouses and healthcare plans) who convey *electronically* formatted health information via an outside billing service or merchant are considered *covered entities*. Covered entities may be dealt serious civil and criminal penalties for violation of HIPAA legislation. Failure to comply with HIPAA privacy requirements may result in civil penalties of up to $100 per offense with an annual maximum of $25,000 for repeated failure to comply with the same requirement. Criminal penalties resulting from the illegal mishandling of private health information can range from $50,000 and/or 1 year in prison to $250,000 and/or 10 years in prison.

Patients' Rights

HIPAA allows patients, authorized representatives, and parents of minors, as well as minors, to become more aware of the health information privacy to which they are entitled. These rights include, but are not limited to, the right to view and copy their health information, the right to dispute alleged breaches of policies and regulations, and the right to request alternative forms of communicating with their dentist. If any health information is released for any reason other than TPO, the patient is entitled to an account of the transaction. Therefore dentists must keep accurate records of such information and provide them when necessary.

The HIPAA Privacy Rule determines that the parents of a minor have access to their child's health information. This privilege may be overruled; for example, in cases where there is suspected child abuse or the parent consents to a term of confidentiality between the dentist and the minor. The parents' rights to access their child's PHI also may be restricted in situations when a legal entity, such as a court, intervenes and when a law does not require a parent's consent. For a full list of patient rights provided by HIPAA, a copy of the law should be acquired and well understood.

Administrative Requirements

Complying with HIPAA legislation may seem like a chore, but it does not need to be so. It is recommended that healthcare professionals become appropriately familiar with the law, organize the requirements into simpler tasks, begin compliance early, and document their progress in compliance. An important first step is to evaluate the current information and practices of the dental office.

Dentists should write a *privacy policy* for their office, a document for their patients detailing the office's practices concerning PHI. The ADA's *HIPAA Privacy Kit* includes forms that the dentist can use to customize his or her privacy policy. It is useful to try to understand the role of healthcare information for patients and the ways in which they deal with the information while they are visiting the dental office. Staff should be trained and familiar with the terms of HIPAA and the office's privacy policy and related forms. HIPAA requires a designated *privacy officer*, a person in the practice who is responsible for applying the new policies in the office, fielding complaints, and making choices involving the minimum necessary requirements. Another person with the role of *contact person* will process complaints.

A *Notice of Privacy Practices*—a document detailing the patient's rights and the dental office's obligations concerning PHI—also must be drawn up. Furthermore, any role of a third party with access to PHI must be clearly documented. This third party is known as a *business associate* (BA) and is defined as any entity who, on behalf of the healthcare provider, takes part in any activity that involves exposure of PHI. The *HIPAA Privacy Kit* provides a copy of the USDHHS "Business Associate Contract Terms," which provides a concrete format for detailing BA interactions (Fig. 19-2).

The main HIPAA privacy compliance date, including all staff training, was April 14, 2003, although many covered entities who submitted a request and a compliance plan by October 15, 2002, were granted 1-year extensions. Local branch of the ADA may be contacted for details. It is recommended that dentists prepare their offices ahead of time for all deadlines, which include preparing privacy polices and forms, business associate contracts, and employee training sessions (Fig. 19-3).

For a comprehensive discussion of all of these terms and requirements, a complete list of HIPAA policies and procedures, and a full collection of HIPAA privacy forms, the American Dental Association for a *HIPAA Privacy Kit* should be contacted. The relevant ADA website is *www.ada.org/goto/hipaa*. Other websites that may contain useful information about HIPAA are:

- USDHHS Office of Civil Rights: *www.hhs.gov/ocr/hipaa*
- Work Group on Electronic Data Interchange: *www.wedi.org/SNIP*
- Phoenix Health: *www.hipaadvisory.com*
- USDHHS Office of the Assistant Secretary for Planning and Evaluation: *http://aspe.os.dhhs.gov/admnsimp/*

THIRD PARTIES

It should appear obvious that when any untoward reaction occurs, including during local anesthetic administration, the complication will be more ideally treated by a responsive team trained to handle such events rather than just the local anesthetic administrator.

In addition to having additional trained hands, third parties are also witnesses and can testify to events leading to, during, and after the event in question and may be invaluable in describing an event, including psychogenic patient phenomena.

BUSINESS ASSOCIATE CONTRACT

This contract between the office of Dr. _____ (the *entity*) and _____ (the *business associate*) discloses the conditions to satisfactorily ensure compliance with the Privacy Rule of the Health Insurance Portability and Accountability Act (HIPAA).

During the contract period the business associate must observe the following responsibilities with respect to protected health information:

1. A business associate must limit requests for protected health information on behalf of the covered entity to that which is reasonably necessary to accomplish the intended purpose, a covered entity is permitted to reasonably rely on such requests from a business associate of another covered entity as the minimum necessary.

2. Make information available including information held by business associate as necessary to determine compliance by the covered entity.

3. Fulfill an individual's rights to access and amend his or her protected health information contained in a designated record set, including information held by a business associate, if appropriate, and receive an accounting of disclosures by a business associate.

4. Mitigate, to the extent practicable, any harmful effect that is known to the covered entity of an impermissible use or disclosure of protected health information by its business associate.

5. A business associate cannot use protected health information for his or her own purposes. This includes, but is not limited to, selling protected health information to third parties for the third party's own marketing activities, without authorization.

6. The covered entity is required to ensure, in whatever reasonable manner deemed effective by the covered entity, the appropriate cooperation by his or her business associate in meeting these requirements.

7. If the covered entity discovers a material breach of violation of the contract by the business associate, it will take reasonable steps to cure the breach or end the contract with the business associate. If termination is not feasible the covered entity will report the problem to the Department of Health and Human Services Office for Civil Rights.

Figure 19-2. Sample Business Associate Contract for compliance with the privacy rule of the Health Insurance Portability and Accountability Act.

OVERDOSE

The term *local anesthesia* actually describes such a drug's desired effect, not what actually occurs physiologically. Administration of a local anesthetic may or may not produce the desired depression of area nerve function, but it definitely produces systemic effects. One must be prepared to articulate systemic considerations with regard to the injection of these "local" agents.

Dosages of local anesthetic drugs administered to patients are most properly given and recorded in milligrams, not in milliliters, cartridges, ccs, and so forth. The most obvious limiting factor to the administration of certain doses of local anesthetics to a patient is the patient's weight. Other factors that should be considered include medical history, particularly cardiovascular disease, and previous demonstration of sensitivity to normal dosing. Presence of acute or chronic infection and concomitant administration of other oral, parenteral, or inhaled agents also may alter the textbook recommendations for local anesthetic dosages. The reasonable practitioner should be able to readily determine the proper dosage levels to be administered to patients before administration. At times, one local anesthetic formulation may be significantly more advantageous than another. The minimal amount of local anesthetic, and vasoconstrictor contained

OFFICE STAFF TRAINING REGISTRY

I hereby certify that the following employees of the below named dental office have received the office policy regarding the Health Insurance Portability and Accountability Act (HIPAA) Privacy Rule.

Privacy Officer_____ Date_____

       Dental Office _____

       Address_____

       _____

       City _____ State_____

I understand the office privacy policy and procedures needed to protect the private health information of patients and will access only information that is reasonably needed to carry out my duties.

Name   **Date**

Figure 19-3. Sample staff training registry for all employees to sign verifying receipt of the office policy to comply with the privacy rule of the Health Insurance Portability and Accountability Act.

therein, if applicable, necessary to achieve operative anesthesia should be used. An inability to properly determine the dosage for most patients is below the standard of care.

Overdose may occur without error by the healthcare professional, such as in a previously undiagnosed hypersensitive patient or in a patient who gives an incomplete medical history. Intravascular injection can occur even with

judicious negative aspiration through an appropriate needle and after slow injection, and may result in overdose.

Generally, the initial presentation of overdose is physiological excitement, which is followed by depression. Treatment protocols vary depending on the timing of the diagnosis of overdose. Rapid accurate evaluation is beneficial as opposed to a delayed diagnosis and speaks favorably for the responsible healthcare provider. It is much more desirable to treat syncope secondary to overdose than cardiac arrest, which may follow undiagnosed syncope and respiratory arrest.

Adding to the diagnostic challenge is the fact that there is often more than one chemical within the local anesthetic solution that may cause overdose; for example, lidocaine and epinephrine. Latency and duration of overdose of the different components of the local anesthetic solution is something else about which the operator must be cognizant.

However, no matter the particular manifestation or whether fault is or is not included in the etiology of any situation of overdose, the reasonable practitioner needs to be prepared to effectively handle the overdose. An inability to reasonably treat complications that are foreseeable, such as overdose, is a breach of duty.

If an overdose occurs, results can range from no damage whatsoever to death and often depend on the preparedness of the practitioner for this foreseeable emergency.

ALLERGY

Related to overdose, but not a dose-dependent manifestation of local anesthetic administration, allergic reactions also are foreseeable, although relatively rare, particularly for severe allergic responses such as anaphylaxis.

An accurate medical history is mandatory in minimizing the occurrence of allergy. Patients, in part secondary to doctors who do not take the time to explain the difference between allergy, overdose, and sensitivity, often list any adverse drug reaction as an "allergy." Inaccurate reporting of drug-related allergy by patients is not rare. In fact, more than half of patient-reported allergies are not allergies at all, but some other reaction that may not have even been drug related.

The healthcare professional's duty when administering local anesthetics includes avoiding known allergenic substances, including the local anesthetic in particular, and also any chemical additions to the local anesthetic solution. If an allergic reaction occurs (whether fault is present or not), the healthcare provider must be able to treat it in a reasonable manner. Reasonable treatment may be the difference between resultant transient rhinorrhea and death.

INSTRUMENTS

Syringe

A compromised syringe may still be able to be used to administer a local anesthetic. But if, for instance, the syringe cannot be controlled in a normal manner (e.g., secondary to an ill-fitting thumb ring), any damage from such a lack of control is foreseeable and a breach of duty. A properly prepared and functioning syringe is mandatory

for safe local anesthetic administration. Factors to be aware of in evaluating a syringe include all components of the syringe: the thumb ring, slide assembly, harpoon, threads that engage the needle, and so forth.

Local Anesthetic Cartridge

Originally cartridges were much different than they are now. Problems that have been identified through the years include the fact that chemicals can leach from or into the solution within the cartridge and that the contents are subject to extremes of heat or cold or prolonged shelf life. Cartridge are now coated with a protective film, thus helping prevent any shattered glass effect from cartridge fracture, which can occur with even normal injection pressures.

Local Anesthetic Needle

Disposable needles have been the norm for decades, and although they prevent many problems formerly manifested with reusable needles, malfunction can still occur. Needle breakage can occur with or without fault from the operator. Absent intentional bending and hubbing of the needle into loose mucosa, underlying muscle, and bone, needles still occasionally break secondary to other reasons, such as a patient who grabs the operator's hand during an injection, and so on. In addition, latent manufacturing defects occasionally are noted during routine inspection of the needle before local anesthetic administration. In addition to needle barbs, the author has also discarded preoperatively inspected needles with defects such as patency in the side of needles, needles that were partially or totally occluded, needles loose within the plastic hub, and needles with plastic hubs that did not engage the metal threads of the syringe effectively.

Once again, broken needle instrument damage is foreseeable, as are other instrument failures. The prudent operator will be prepared to handle this complication and prevent further morbidity by means such as a throat pack, not hubbing the needle, and having a prepared assistant who can pass a hemostat to the operator in a fashion that does not require the operator to take his or her eyes from the field. If a needle is lost in tissue, protocols have been established for retrieval of such foreign bodies, and if the operator is not comfortable with these procedures, an expeditious referral should be considered.

Contamination of the local anesthetic solution or delivery system (e.g., the needle) will likely produce complications and thus should be assiduously avoided. It is reasonable to expect a practitioner to be able to intelligently describe in some detail the methods used to minimize any potential contamination, if called on to do so. Limiting contamination has the added benefit of not compromising the health of the practitioner or any member of his or her team.

Any damage resulting from unorthodox use of the syringe, needle, or cartridge associated with damage also opens the argument that a breach of the standard of care and thus breach of duty occurred.

ALTERNATIVE DELIVERY SYSTEMS OR TECHNIQUES

At times practitioners may elect to use alternative delivery systems or techniques, such as periodontal ligament, intraosseous, or extraoral injections via specialized armamentaria. The standard of care, which includes the reasoning that, all things considered, a practitioner will choose the best treatment for his or her patient, certainly includes these alternate local anesthetic delivery systems or techniques.

As with any other routine or less than routine clinical treatment plan, the practitioner should be able to intelligently articulate reasoning for the decision. This is mandatory not only if a disgruntled patient seeks legal recourse, but also for nonlitigious patients who simply want to know why they have "never seen that before."

Although a drug or equipment manufacturer's promotional material may be helpful in identifying advantages of new drugs or equipment, it is incumbent on the healthcare professional to also make an independent and reasonable effort to identify potential disadvantages to new modalities.

LOCAL REACTIONS TO LOCAL ANESTHETIC ADMINISTRATION

Topical or injected local anesthetics can cause reactions, from erythema to tissue sloughing, in local areas secondary to several factors, including multiple needle penetrations, hydraulic pressure within the tissues, or a direct tissue reaction to the local anesthetic. Topical anesthetics in particular are generally more toxic to tissues than injected solutions, and dosages must be carefully administered. For instance, allowing the patient to self-administer prescription-strength topical anesthetics at home certainly could be criticized if an adverse reaction occurred.

Local tissue reactions may be immediate or delayed by hours or days; thus it is mandatory in this situation, as it is in others, that the patient have access to a professional familiar with such issues even during off hours. Simply letting patients fend for themselves or advising them to go to the emergency room may not be optimal care.

Finally, one should be able to reasonably justify the use of topical anesthetics for intraoral injection purposes because some authors have opined that these relatively toxic agents are not objectively effective.

Psychological considerations on the part of the patient may be adequate if dosage is carefully monitored.

LIP CHEWING

Local tissue maceration secondary to lip chewing most often occurs in children after an inferior alveolar nerve injection. Tissue maceration also may be seen in patients whose mental status has been compromised by sedatives, general anesthetics, or central nervous system trauma, or during development. A prudent practitioner advises any patient who may be prone to such an injury, and that patient's guardian, to be aware of the complication. If this complication is not prevented, it must be properly treated after being diagnosed.

SUBCUTANEOUS EMPHYSEMA

Emphysema or air embolism can occur when air is introduced into tissue spaces. This complication usually occurs after incisions have been made through skin or mucosa but also can occur via needle tracts, particularly when air pressure sprays, pneumatic handpieces, and so forth are used near the needle tract. The sequelae of air embolism are usually fairly benign even though disconcerting to the patient. An unrecognized and progressive embolism can be life threatening. A progressive embolism is a situation where the practitioner, preparing for the worst-case scenario, would not be criticized for not only summoning paramedics, but also accompanying the patient to the hospital.

VASCULAR PENETRATION

Even with the most careful technique, excessive bleeding can occur when vessels are partially torn by needles. The fact that aspirating syringes are used reveals that placing needles into soft tissues is indeed a blind procedure. At times, the goal of an injection is intravenous or intraarterial placement. This is not typically the case with the use of local anesthetics for pain control, and a positive aspiration necessitates additional measures be taken for a safe injection. The prepared healthcare professional should be able to articulate exactly what the goal of the administration of a local anesthetic is and how that is technically accomplished. For instance, why was a particular anesthetic and needle chosen? What structures might be encountered by the needle during the administration of a block? In addition, what measures are taken if a structure is inadvertently compromised by a needle? Even with optimal preparation, vascular compromise can result in tumescence, ecchymosis, or overt hemorrhage that should be addressed. These conditions can be magnified by bleeding dyscrasia. The medical history may reveal certain prescriptions that may alter bleeding time, which may indicate the need for hematological consultation preoperatively.

NEURAL PENETRATION

Just as there is a rich complex of vessels in the head and neck area, so it is with nerves. Neural anatomy can vary considerably from the norm, and penetration of a nerve by a needle can occasionally occur even in the most careful and practiced hands. Permanent changes in neural function can occur with a single needle stick; although this complication does not necessarily imply a deviation from the standard of care, the practitioner must be prepared to treat the complication as optimally as possible.

Lingual nerve injury is an area that has been zealously contested in the courts during recent years. Typically, the rare instances of loss or change in lingual nerve function have occurred during mandibular third molar surgery. Plaintiff experts readily opine that but for negligence (e.g., malpractice), this injury does not occur, period. In these experts' opinions, the only way lingual nerves are damaged is secondary to unintentional manipulation with a surgical blade, periosteal elevator, bur, and so on, when the operator is in an anatomical area where he or she should not be. In spite of the fact that defense experts routinely counter these plaintiff opinions, occasionally juries rule for the plaintiff, and lingual nerve awards have exceeded $1 million.

Although lingual nerve injury occasionally occurs secondary to unintentional contact with surgical blades, periosteal elevators, burs, and so on, when an operator unintentionally enters into unintended anatomical areas, it is more likely that the injury was secondary to other means. For instance, lingual nerve anatomy has been shown to be widely variant from the average position lingual to the lingual plate in the third molar area. Lingual nerve position has been shown to vary from within unattached mucosal tissue low on the lingual aspect of the lingual plate to firmly adherent within lingual periosteum high on the lingual plate to within the soft tissues over buccal cusps of impacted third molars.

Permanent lingual nerve injury also occurs in the absence of third molar surgery and secondary to needle penetration during inferior alveolar or lingual nerve blocks. Lingual nerve injury also can occur secondary to pressure placed on the nerve during operative procedures (e.g., with lingual retractors).

A higher incidence of lingual nerve injury is demonstrated with certain local anesthetic solution formulations over others. The practitioner whose patient develops a paresthesia after the practitioner's routine use of, for instance, 4% local anesthetic solutions instead of 2% solutions, must be prepared to answer questions such as

why solutions that are twice as toxic as others that are generally equally effective are routinely used. Obviously, the suggestion here is that no treatment is rote or routine but is developed on a patient-by-patient basis after a thoughtful risk-benefit analysis.

Finally, lingual nerve injury also can occur without any professional treatment whatsoever. Paresthesia can occur with mastication, and anesthesia can occur spontaneously. Both these conditions may be rectified by dealing with the pathology associated with the change in function, such as by removing impacted third molars or freeing the lingual nerve from an injury-susceptible position within the periosteum.

However, no matter what the etiology, the prudent operator must be prepared to address neural injury effectively when it occurs.

CHEMICAL NERVE INJURY

It is not surprising that potent chemicals such as local anesthetics occasionally compromise nerve function to a greater degree than they are designed to do. After all, local anesthetics are specifically formulated in an effort to alter nerve function, albeit reversibly. Just as systemic toxicity varies from one local anesthetic to another, so limited nerve or local toxicity may at times alter nerve function in a way not typically seen. Deposition of local anesthetic solutions directly on a nerve trunk or too near a nerve trunk in a susceptible patient may result in long-term or permanent paresthesia. Local anesthetic toxicity generally increases as potency increases. In addition, occasionally other nerves in the head and neck are affected by local anesthetic deposition, such as transient amaurosis seen after maxillary or mandibular nerve blocks when the optic nerve is affected. One should not be particularly surprised at the various neural manifestations of these potent agents when one considers that toxic overdose is actually a compromise of higher neural functions. Anyone who chooses to utilize agents designed to relieve pain directly on or near nerve tissue must be prepared to treat adequately even the rare complications seen. Adequate treatment may range from reassuring a patient who has temporarily lost vision to treating or referring for treatment a permanent anesthesia resulting from an adverse chemical compromise of the nerve from the local anesthetic solution or other agents.

LOCAL ANESTHETIC DRUG INTERACTIONS

Use of other local or systemic agents certainly predictably affects and alters the latency, effect, duration, and overall metabolism of local agents. Modern polypharmacy only complicates the situation. However, there are specific well-known drug interactions that the healthcare professional must be aware of in addition to general principles for generalized drug classes. Oral contraceptives, β-blockers, calcium channel blockers, angiotensin converting enzyme inhibitors, other cardiovascular prescriptions including antihypertensives and anticoagulants, thyroid medications, antihistamines, antibiotics, anabolics or corticosteroids, psychogenic medications, and various street drugs all may be considered common to the routine dental population.

Drugs interact with various receptor sites, and drug therapy is based on either potentiation or inhibition of normal physiological responses to stimuli. Ideally, no unwanted systemic reactions occur with local anesthetic and local nerve tissues are reversibly inhibited for a relatively brief period of time, after which the tissues regain full function. Concomitant use of other agents can change the usually predicable course of a local anesthetic and vice versa.

For instance, the commonly used β-blocker propranolol has been shown to create a chemically induced decrease in liver function (e.g., hepatic blood flow), which can decrease lidocaine metabolism by as much as 40%. Chronic alcohol use induces enzymes dramatically. Methemoglobinemia has been reported from topical local anesthetics.

Therapeutic areas of special concern arise in patients who are obviously ill, report significant medical history, report significant drug use (whether prescribed, over the counter, or herbal), and are at the extremes of age. The incidence of adverse local anesthetic drug interaction increases with patients who report risk factors, particularly cardiovascular risk factors, as opposed to the general population. One must develop the knowledge to optimally treat such patients with increased potential for adverse drug reactions before treatment.

PSYCHOGENIC REACTIONS

At times the practitioner may have to deal with psychogenic reactions that may be mild or severe. For instance, excitement is the initial manifestation of a toxic overdose, whether noted or not. Excitement also may be secondary to nothing other than stress from being in a situation with which the patient is not comfortable. Excitement may be manifested, for instance, by controlled or uncontrolled agitation, disorientation, hallucination, or somnolence by the patient.

Such reactions may be potentiated by pharmaceuticals administered by the healthcare professional acutely or by authorized or unauthorized agents taken by the patient before an appointment. The incidence of such reactions is increased with the increased utilization of pharmaceuticals, particularly those that may affect the central nervous system, such as local anesthetics.

These reactions can occur with children, adolescents, adults, or aged individuals.

Psychogenic reactions are often frustrating to diagnose and treat. It may be difficult to determine if the reaction is secondary to an administered drug, including local anesthesia or other causes.

Treatment may require restraint if the patient is in danger of inflicting harm on himself or herself, as might be seen in an epileptic seizure.

Fortunately, most of these reactions are short term, often lasting only moments. However, at times, they may last days and require hospitalization.

Although many practitioners diagnose such an event, prudence requires that one be aware of the etiology and treatment of such reactions. Even when psychogenic reactions are handled appropriately, patients may assume the healthcare professional "did something wrong" and seek the advice of an attorney.

Eroticism

Occasionally a singularly troublesome psychogenic reaction to potent agents is observed in which the patient reacts with sexual affections that may or may not be recalled at a later time. Historically, such reactions were fairly common during administration of cocaine solutions.[2]

Generally speaking, these reactions appear to be rare and usually of relatively short duration. However, as with other psychogenic or hysterical phenomena, rapid diagnosis and treatment is optimal.

Although concomitant use of agents such as nitrous oxide or administration of minor tranquilizers generally may be of benefit during local anesthesia, these and many other agents also have been reported to produce erotic hallucination or behavior in patients so predisposed.

In the case of eroticism, the practitioner who has administered local or other agents without a neutral third-party present when such reactions occur will have more difficulty exonerating conduct than the practitioner with witnesses to the reaction. In addition, with regard to eroticism, it is usually optimal to have witnesses of the same sex as the patient.

Occasionally a patient may request to speak with or to be treated privately by the healthcare practitioner. Absent unusual circumstances (e.g., treating a close relative), practitioners may want to consider avoidance of situations such as treating an emergency patient alone after hours or even speaking to a patient behind closed doors.

POSTPROCEDURE EVALUATION

An evaluation of the patient is necessary any time potent agents are utilized. This evaluation consists of at least a preoperative assessment, continuous examination during treatment when the drugs utilized are at peak effect, and a postoperative appraisal.

Although most adverse reactions to local anesthetics occur rapidly, delayed sequelae are possible. Just as patients who have been administered agents by intravenous, inhalation, oral, or other routes are evaluated postprocedure, so should patients who have been administered local anesthetics. Any question about a less than optimal time-related recovery from local anesthesia should be addressed before releasing the patient from direct care.

For instance, it is widely accepted that patients may drive after administration of local anesthesia for dental purposes. Occasionally, a postprocedure concern developing secondary to local anesthesia or other procedures may dictate that a patient who was not accompanied should obtain assistance before leaving the place of treatment. Patients whose employment requires higher than normal mental or physical performance may be cautioned about the potential effects of local anesthetic administration. As an example, United States Air Force and United States Navy pilots are restricted from flying for 24 hours after local anesthetic administration.

After the patient is released, some practitioners routinely call the patient several hours after treatment has been terminated to assure recovery is uneventful. Such calls usually are welcomed by patients as a sign that their healthcare provider is truly concerned about their welfare. Occasionally, the practitioner's call may enable one to address a developing concern or objective complication in the early hours.

RESPONDIAT SUPERIOR

Respondiat superior (let the superior reply), or vicarious liability, is the legal doctrine that holds an employer responsible for an employee's conduct during the course of employment. The common law principle that all have a duty to conduct themselves so as to not harm another thus also applies to employees assigned tasks by an employer. Respondiat superior is in part justified by the assumption that the employer has the right to direct the actions of employees. For the healthcare professional, responsibility may exist for clerical staff, surgical or other assistants, dental hygienists, lab technicians, and so forth. At times vicarious liability extends between employer doctors and employee doctors if the employee doctors are agents of the employer doctor within a practice.

Respondiat superior does not relieve the employee from responsibility for employee conduct, but enables a plaintiff to also litigate against the employer.

An employer is not responsible for employee conduct that is not related to the employment. What employee conduct is related to the job is an arguable proposition, as are most legal issues. For instance, the question of whether an employer is responsible for employee conduct outside the normal work place is open to a case-by-case evaluation. Conduct during trips to and from the work place may or may not be related to employment. For example, an employer probably is not responsible for employee conduct when driving home from the place of employment. However, if the employer asked the employee to perform a task on the way home, responsibility for that employee conduct may attach.

An employer may not be responsible for an independent contractor. One test to evaluate the relationship between one employer and another is if the employer has the authority to direct how a task is done, as opposed to simply requesting that a task be completed. For instance, a dentist may request that a plumber make repairs but will not likely direct how the repairs are to be accomplished. The same dentist will also request that a dental hygienist perform hygiene duties, but the dentist has the ability to instruct how the duties will be performed.

Both dentists and dental hygienists routinely accomplish the administration of local anesthesia. Generally speaking, and subject ultimately to state statutes, although a dental hygienist may be an independent contractor according to many elemental definitions, the dental hygienist generally is not an independent contractor with regard to the provision of healthcare services, which includes the administration of local anesthetics. Thus the employee dentist is likely responsible for any negligent conduct that causes damage to a patient during the course of hygiene treatment.

With regard to the degree of supervision, one must consult the state statutes. Often verbiage such as *direct* or *indirect supervision* is used; understanding the definition of these or other terms used is paramount for both the supervising or supervised healthcare provider.

STATUTE VIOLATION

Violation of a state or federal statute leads to an assumption of negligence if damage to a patient occurs. In other words, the burden of proof now shifts to the defendant to prove that the statute violation was not such that it caused any damage claimed.

Two basic types of statutes exist, malum in se and malum prohibitum. *Malum in se* (bad in fact) statutes restrict behavior that in and of itself is recognized as harmful, such as driving while inebriated. *Malum prohibitum* (defined as bad) conduct in and of itself may not be criminal, reckless, wanton, and so on, but is regulated simply, for instance, to promote social order. Driving at certain speeds is an example of a malum prohibitum statute. The difference between legally driving at 15 mph in a school zone and criminally driving at 16 mph in a school zone is not the result of a criminal mind, but a social regulatory decision.

For instance, if one is speeding while driving, several sequelae may result when that statute violation is recognized. First, the speeder simply may be warned to stop speeding. Second, the speeder may be issued a citation and have to appear in court, argue innocence, pay a fine if found guilty, attend traffic school, and so on. Third, additional civil or criminal sanctions may apply if the speeder's conduct causes damage to others. Fourth, the situation may be compounded civilly or criminally if multiple statute violations are present, such as speeding and driving recklessly or driving while intoxicated.

Occasionally statute violation is commendable. For instance, a driver may swerve to the "wrong" side of the center line to avoid a child who suddenly runs into the street from between parked cars. At times, speeding may be considered a heroic act, such as when a driver is transporting a patient to a hospital during an emergency. However, even if the speeder feels he or she somehow is contributing to the public welfare, the statute violation is still subject to review.

For healthcare professionals, for instance, administration of local anesthetic without a current health professional license or Drug Enforcement Administration certification is likely a violation of statute. If the type of harm sustained by the patient is the type that would have been prevented by obeying the statute, additional liability may attach to the defendant.

Conversely, an example of a beneficial statute violation occurred when a licensee did not fulfill mandatory basic CPR (cardiopulmonary resuscitation) certification, but chose to complete ACLS (advanced cardiac life support) certification instead. When admonished by the state board that a violation of statute had occurred, potentially putting the pubic at greater risk, the licensee pointed out to the regulatory board that ACLS certification is actually more beneficial to the public than CPR. The licensing board then changed the statute to allow CPR or ACLS certification as a requirement to maintain a license.

Generally, employers are not responsible for statute violations of employees. An exception to this guideline is in the health professions. When employees engage in the practice of dentistry or medicine, even without the knowledge or approval of the employer, that employee and the employer may both be held liable for damage. Employer sanctions may be magnified, such as loss of one's professional license, if an employee practices dentistry or medicine with employer knowledge.

Finally, at times some types of specific conduct are defined statutorily as malpractice per se. For instance, unintentionally leaving a foreign body in a patient after a procedure may be deemed malpractice per se. In these types of cases, theoretically simply the plaintiff's demonstration of the foreign body, via radiograph, and a secondary procedure to remove the foreign body may be all that is necessary to establish malpractice.

IF MALPRACTICE EXISTS

Although attorneys and doctors do not always agree on when the requirements of malpractice have been fulfilled, occasionally the healthcare professional may feel he or she has made a mistake that has damaged a patient. As can be easily and successfully argued, the simple fact that a patient has damage, even significant damage, does not fulfill all the requirements of the tort of malpractice.

However, it is likely that malpractice has occurred if the practitioner determines that a duty existed, the duty was breached, and that breach was the proximate cause of the damage. In this instance, the healthcare professional is likely ethically, if not yet legally, responsible for making the patient "whole." If damage is minimal (e.g., transient ecchymosis), nominal recompense, perhaps even an apology, may be all that is necessary. However, if the damage is significant, then significant recompense may be required.

Certainly any significant damage whatsoever from malpractice necessitates that the healthcare professional contact his or her liability carrier as soon as possible. The same holds true, even if damage is not evident, when the healthcare professional receives notice of patient dissatisfaction, often in the form of a request for records. The liability insurance carrier's representative helps evaluate the situation and provide valuable insight from a significant experience pool. In all likelihood, the carrier will be more successful in negotiating a settlement to any case that is controversial as far as damages. The practitioner should be very cautious about undertaking any such negotiations without the carrier's input. Such unauthorized negotiations or similar conduct (e.g., not informing the carrier about a potential complaint in a timely fashion) may even cause liability coverage to become the practitioner's sole responsibility. At times, if the practitioner and patient still have a good working relationship, the carrier allows the practitioner to negotiate a reasonable settlement. This course of action is advantageous in that the patient receives immediate financial aid that may be necessary for additional expenses or time off from work and litigation-driven financial damage is limited. In addition, the plaintiff patient is not required to overcome the assumption that the healthcare provider acted reasonably and to prove malpractice, which may be very difficult.

No matter whether or not the damage is secondary to negligence, the practitioner must still try to treat the patient optimally. Hopefully the patient will not independently seek treatment elsewhere because this course of action may simply prolong recovery and aggravate future legal considerations. If, on the other hand, referral is beneficial, the practitioner should facilitate that referral for the patient and not just send the patient out to fend alone. After a referral is made, continued care as needed for the patient is advisable if possible.

Once legal action has been initiated, it may be wise to refuse further treatment for the patient because the patient has now expressed the opinion that the practitioner's conduct was below the level of the standard of care and has resulted in damage. It is an unfortunate circumstance when a plaintiff patient realizes that the perceived malpractice did not exist and is unable to continue care with the practitioner most familiar with the intricacies of that patient's individual circumstances.

Many patients shortsightedly and unintentionally limit their healthcare options by pursuing malpractice actions. Most malpractice cases take years to resolve and involve great expense for both the defendant and plaintiff. Ultimately, the vast majority of alleged malpractice claims result in adjudication in favor of the defendant doctor.

No matter who prevails in a malpractice claim, for both the defendant and plaintiff the victory is often pyrrhic when the temporal, social, and economic costs are considered.

SUMMARY

Just as administration of local anesthetics may undergo change with time secondary to new drugs, instrumentation, and knowledge bases, so too is the law subject to variation over time. For instance, the philosophy of detailed versus general informed consent has undergone several permutations over the years. The decision of one court in a contractual, criminal, or civil tort proceeding may be appealed by the losing party and eventually reversed by another court secondary to a new fact pattern or simply from re-evaluation of the same fact pattern under different legal formulae. However, one thing that never changes is that reasonable and responsible healthcare practitioners will continue to be informed as to the current standard of care and attempt to optimize their decision making and treatment planning for patients on an individual basis after a realistic risk-benefit analysis. The opinions printed in this chapter and this text are meant as guidelines and may be subject to modification on an individual patient treatment basis by knowledgeable practitioners and informed patients.

REFERENCES

1. HIPAA Privacy Kit, *http://www.ada.org/prof/prac/issues/topics/hipaa/index.html.*
2. Fischer G, Reithmuller RH: *Local anesthesia in dentistry,* ed 2, Lea & Febiger, 1914, Philadelphia.

SUGGESTED READINGS

Arroliga ME, Wagner W, Bobek MB, et al: A pilot study of penicillin skin testing in patients with a history of penicillin allergy admitted to a medical ICU, *Chest* 118:1106-1108, 2000.

Associated Press: Jury acquits Pasadena dentist of 60 child endangering charges, Mar 5, 2002.

Bax NDS, Tucker GT, Lennard MS, et al: The impairment of lignocaine clearance by propranolol: major contribution from enzyme inhibition, *Br J Clin Pharm* 19:597-603, 1985.

Burkhart CG, Burkhart KM, Burkhart AK: The Physicians' Desk Reference should not be held as a legal standard of medical care, *Arch Pediatr Adolesc Med* 152:609-610, 1998.

Cohen JS: Adverse drug effects, compliance, and initial doses of antihypertensive drugs recommended by the Joint National Committee vs the Physicians' Desk Reference, *Arch Intern Med* 161:680-685, 2001.

Cohen JS: Dose discrepancies between the Physicians' Desk Reference and the medical literature, and their possible role in the high incidence of dose-related adverse drug events, *Arch Intern Med* 161:757-764, 2001.

College C, Feigal R, Wandera A, et al: Bilateral versus unilateral mandibular block anesthesia in a pediatric population, *Pediatr Dent* 22:653-657, 2000.

Covino BG, Vassallo HG: *Local anesthetics: mechanisms of action and clinical use,* New York, Grune & Stratton, 1976.

Daublander M, Muller R, Lipp MD: The incidence of complications associated with local anesthesia in dentistry, *Anesth Prog* 44:432-441, 1997.

Dyer C: Junior doctor is cleared of manslaughter after feeding tube error, *Br Med J* 325:414, 2003.

Evans IL, Sayers MS, Gibbons AJ, et al: Can warfarin be continued during dental extraction? Results of a randomized controlled trial, *Br J Oral Maxillofac Surg* 40:348-352, 2002.

Faria MA: *Vandals at the gates of medicine,* Macon, Ga, 1994, Hacienda Publishing.

Gill CJ, Orr DL: A double-blind crossover comparison of topical anesthetics, *J Am Dent Assoc* 98:213-214, 1979.

Gilman CS, Veser FH, Randall D: Methemoglobinemia from a topical oral anesthetic, *Acad Emerg Med* 4:1011-1013, 1997.

Goldenberg AS: Transient diplopia as a result of block injections. Mandibular and posterior superior alveolar, *NY State Dent J* 63:29-31, 1997.

Lang MS, Waite PD: Bilateral lingual nerve injury after laryngoscopy for intubation, *J Oral Maxillofac Surg* 59:1497-1499, 2001.

Lee TH: By the way, doctor . . . My hair has been thinning out for the past decade or so, but since my doctor started me on Lipitor (atorvastatin) a few months ago for high cholesterol, I swear it's been falling out much faster. My doctor discounts the possibility, but I looked in the Physicians' Desk Reference (PDR) and alopecia is listed under "adverse reactions." What do you think? *Harv Health Lett* 25:9, 2000.

Lustig JP, Zusman SP: Immediate complications of local anesthetic administered to 1,007 consecutive patients, *J Am Dent Assoc* 130:496-499, 1999.

Lydiatt DD: Litigation and the lingual nerve, *J Oral Maxillofac Surg* 61:297-299, 2003.

Malamed SF, Gagnon S, Leblanc D: Efficacy of articaine: a new amide local anesthetic, *J Am Dent Assoc* 131:635-642, 2000.

Meechan JG, Intra-oral topical anesthetics: a review, *J Dent* 28:1-14, 2000.

Meechan JG, Cole B, Welbury RR: The influence of two different dental local anaesthetic solutions on the haemodynamic responses of children undergoing restorative dentistry: a randomised, single-blind, split-mouth study, *Br Dent J* 190:902-904, 2001.

Meyer FU: Complications of local dental anesthesia and anatomical causes, *Anat Anz* 181:105-106, 1999.

Moore PA: Adverse drug interactions in dental practice: interactions associated with local anesthetics, sedatives, and anxiolytics. Part IV of a series, *J Am Dent Assoc* 130:441-454, 1999.

Mullen WH, Anderson IB, Kim SY, et al: Incorrect overdose management advice in the Physicians' Desk Reference, *Ann Emerg Med* 29:255-261, 1997.

Olson WK: *The litigation explosion, what happened when America unleashed the lawsuit,* New York, 1991, Penguin.

Orr DL: Conversion part I. Pract Reviews, *Oral Maxillofac Surg* 8,7 audiocassette, 1994.

Orr DL: Conversion part II. Pract Reviews, *Oral Maxillofac Surg* 8,8 audiocassette, 1994.

Orr DL: Conversion phenomenon following general anesthesia, *J Oral Maxillofac Surg* 43:817-819, 1985.

Orr DL: Intraseptal anesthesia, *Compend Cont Educ Dent* 8:512, 1987.

Orr DL: Medical malpractice. Pract Reviews, *Oral Maxillofac Surg* 3,4 audiocassette, 1988.

Orr DL: Paresthesia of the second division of the trigeminal nerve secondary to endodontic manipulation with N2, *J Headache* 27:11-22, 1987.

Orr DL: Paresthesia of the trigeminal nerve secondary to endodontic manipulation with N2, *J Headache* 25(6):334-336, 1985.

Orr DL: PDL injections, *J Am Dent Assoc* 114:578, 1987.

Orr DL: Pericardial and subcutaneous air after maxillary surgery, *Anesth Analg* 66:921, 1987.

Orr DL: Protection of the lingual nerve, *Br J Oral Maxillofac Surg* 36:258, 1998.

Orr DL: Reduction of ketamine induced emergence phenomena, *J Oral Maxillofac Surg* 41:1, 1983.

Orr DL: The broken needle: report of case, *J Am Dent Assoc* 107:403-604, 1983.

Penarrocha-Diago M, Sanchis-Bielsa JM: Opthalmologic complications after intraoral local anesthesia with articaine, *Oral Surg Oral Med Oral Pathol Oral Radiol Endod* 90:11-14, 2000.

Pogrel MA, Schmidt BL, Sambajon V, et al: Lingual nerve damage due to inferior alveolar nerve blocks: a possible explanation, *J Am Dent Assoc* 134:195-199, 2003.

Pogrel MA, Thamby S: Permanent nerve involvement resulting from inferior alveolar nerve blocks, *J Am Dent Assoc* 131:701-707, 2000.

Rawson RD, Orr DL: Vascular penetration following intraligamental injection, *J Oral Maxillofac Surg* 43:600-604, 1985.

Sawyer RJ, von Schroeder H: Temporary bilateral blindness after acute lidocaine toxicity, *Anesth Analg* 95:224-226, 2002.

Webber B, Orlansky H, Lipton C, et al: Complications of an intra-arterial injection from an inferior alveolar nerve block, *J Am Dent Assoc* 132:12702-12704, 2001.

Wilkie GJ: Temporary uniocular blindness and opthalmoplegia associated with a mandibular block injection. A case report, *Aust Dent J* 45:231-233, 2000.

Younessi OJ, Punnia-Moorthy A: Cardiovascular effects of bupivacaine and the role of this agent in preemptive dental analgesia, *Anesth Prog* 46:56-62, 1999.

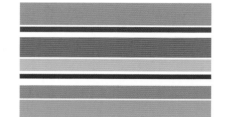

Future Trends in Pain Control

CHAPTER
20

Although local anesthesia remains the backbone of pain control in dentistry, research has continued, in both medicine and dentistry, to seek new and better means of managing pain associated with many surgical treatments. Much of this research has focused on improvements in the area of local anesthesia—safer needles and syringes, more successful techniques of regional nerve block, such as the anterior middle superior alveolar (AMSA) and P-ASA (Chapter 13), and newer drugs. Several of these advances have been discussed at some depth in the preceding chapters: intraosseous anesthesia (Chapter 15), and the self-aspirating, pressure, safety syringes, and computer-controlled local anesthetic delivery systems (Chapter 5).

Considerable interest has focused on improvements in drugs that are injected to block pain impulses from reaching the brain. Several have been mentioned previously: *centbucridine* (Chapter 2) and *articaine* (Chapter 4). They are just two of the newly developed local anesthetics that possess potentially useful characteristics; others include *ropivacaine*, an amide local anesthetic that has gained considerable utility in the area of regional anesthesia,[1] and levobupivacaine.[2–4]

Also in the realm of local anesthetic improvements, initially in medicine but of potential interest in dentistry as well, have been efforts to increase the ability of the anesthetic to cross (diffuse through) a relatively impervious barrier, such as intact skin. *EMLA* (eutectic mixture of local anesthetics) is one agent that has been used, with considerable success, in many areas of medicine requiring the insertion of needles into skin. Interest in the use of EMLA in dentistry has increased; the drug is discussed more completely in Chapter 4. In addition, the desire to speed the onset of anesthesia and make the administration of local anesthetics (into the skin or any tissue) more comfortable for the patient has given rise to the concept of altering the *pH* of the anesthetic solution. *Hyaluronidase* has been added to local anesthetic solutions because it permits injected solutions to spread and penetrate tissues more effectively than plain solutions.

Most of the drugs mentioned in the preceding are attempts at making the injection of local anesthetics into tissue more comfortable for the patient. This is important because most adverse reactions to local anesthetics arise *not as a reaction to the drug being administered, but as a response to the act of administering the drug.* The use of a needle to deliver local anesthetics (and other) drugs into tissues increases the likelihood of development of psychogenic reactions. This is true not only in dentistry but also in medical specialties that frequently involve local anesthetic administration (e.g., dermatology or ophthalmology).

Because of reactions to needle delivery of local anesthetics, the use of alternative techniques of pain control has been of interest in dentistry for many years. Previous editions of this textbook have followed the development of the technique of electronic dental anesthesia (EDA) (the modification of TENS [transcutaneous electrical nerve stimulation] for dental use). Its popularity in dentistry has diminished; however, EDA still retains some interest within pediatric dentistry.[5–7]

An area of nascent interest is the possibility of reversing local anesthesia at the conclusion of a dental procedure. Similar in concept to reversal of opioid analgesics with naloxone[8] and of benzodiazepines with flumazenil,[9] current research is looking into several drugs that could be injected, at the conclusion of the dental procedure, into the original site of local anesthetic administration and that would work to significantly decrease the duration of posttreatment anesthesia. Although not indicated for use in surgical procedures where postoperative pain control is of significant benefit to the patient, shortening the duration of soft-tissue anesthesia is appreciated by patients undergoing most typical dental treatments in which there is no posttreatment discomfort. Several clinical trials were proceeding as of September 2003. It is expected that it will be approximately 5 years before a local anesthetic reversal agent becomes clinically available in the event that these studies demonstrate the utility of this procedure.

LOCAL ANESTHETICS

Centbucridine

Centbucridine, a quinoline derivative, was first discussed in the second edition of this book as a drug with five to eight times the potency of lidocaine and with an equally rapid onset and equivalent duration of action. Significantly, it does not affect the central nervous system (CNS) or cardiovascular system (CVS) adversely except when administered in very large doses.[10] Most of the research on this drug has been conducted in India.

Centbucridine has been used in subarachnoid and extradural anesthesia,[11] intravenous regional anesthesia,[12] and intraocular surgery.[13] In the only reported dental trial with centbucridine, Vacharajani and associates compared the efficacy of an 0.5% centbucridine concentration with that of 2% lidocaine for dental extractions in 120 patients.[14] They reported a degree of analgesia attained with centbucridine that compared well with that obtained with lidocaine. Centbucridine was well tolerated, with no significant changes in cardiovascular parameters and no serious side effects. When administered to overdose, centbucridine functions, unlike lidocaine, as a true stimulant of the central nervous system.[15]

Developments Since the Fourth Edition of This Book. Since the fourth edition of this textbook, in 1997, little research has been published relative to centbucridine. The only trial of centbucridine in dentistry showed it to be as effective, in an 0.5% concentration, as lidocaine 2%.[14]

Ropivacaine

Ropivacaine is a long-acting amide anesthetic, similar to bupivacaine and etidocaine in duration of activity. It is similar structurally to mepivacaine and bupivacaine (Fig. 20-1), but is unique in that ropivacaine is prepared as an isomer rather than a racemic mixture. Ropivacaine has a greater margin of safety between convulsive and lethal doses than does bupivacaine[16] and also a lower dysrhythmogenic potential than bupivacaine.[17] The elimination half-life of ropivacaine is 25.9 minutes, which is considerably shorter than that of other amides.[18] Ropivacaine has demonstrated decreased cardiotoxicity relative to bupivacaine, but its clinical duration of action is approximately 20% shorter.[19,20] The primary use of ropivacaine in anesthesiology has been for regional nerve block, primarily epidural.

Developments Since the Fourth Edition of This Book. Ernberg and Kopps administered ropivacaine via infiltration and inferior alveolar nerve block to 30 subjects.[21] At a 0.75% concentration ropivacaine provided pulpal anesthesia after inferior alveolar nerve block within 10 minutes and lasted from 2 to 6 hours, with mandibular soft-tissue anesthesia lasting from 5 to 9 hours.

Eutectic Mixture of Local Anesthetics

Intact skin is an impervious barrier to the penetration of drugs, including topical anesthetics. Yet once skin is damaged, as occurs in sunburn or injury, anesthetic drugs such as Solarcaine could be applied topically for the relief of pain. For years a drug or technique was sought that would permit needles to be inserted painlessly through intact skin. The development of an oil-in-water emulsion containing high concentrations of lidocaine and prilocaine in base form resulted in *EMLA*

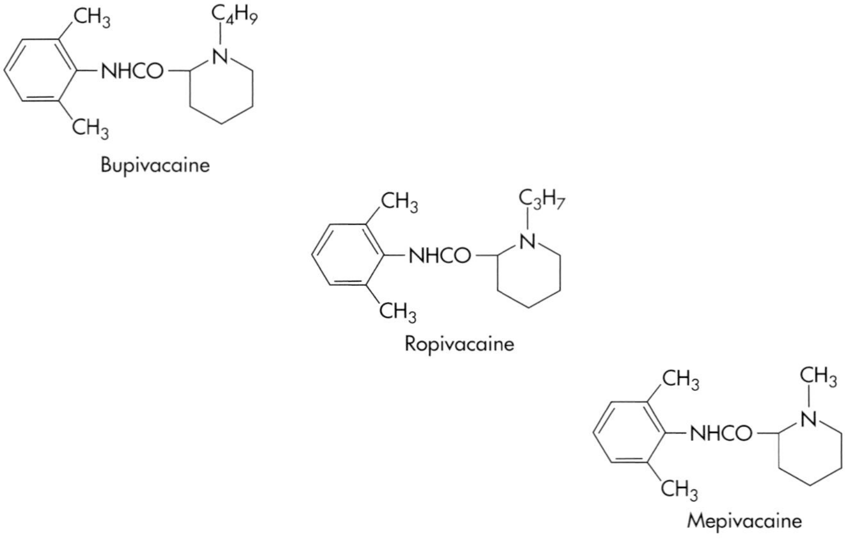

Figure 20-1. Chemical structures of bupivacaine, ropivacaine, and mepivacaine.

(eutectic mixture of local anesthetics), which has been shown to provide anesthesia of intact skin profound enough to permit venipuncture to be performed painlessly.[22–24]

EMLA consists of a 5% cream containing 25 mg/g lidocaine and 25 mg/g prilocaine. It is applied to the skin for at least 1 hour before the anticipated procedure. The cream is covered with an occlusive dressing. Since its introduction in the United States, research has demonstrated the effectiveness of EMLA in many aspects of pediatrics, including venipuncture, vaccination,[25] suture removal, lumbar puncture, minor otological surgery, minor gynecological and urological procedures, and dermatological surgery, including split-thickness skin graft harvesting, argon laser treatments, postherpetic neuralgia, débridement of infected ulcers, and inhibition of itching and burning in adults.[26]

The potential for toxic local anesthetic blood levels developing with EMLA is minimal. Peak plasma anesthetic concentrations occurring 180 minutes after application have been low.[27] The use of EMLA in infants under the age of 6 months is contraindicated because of the possibility of a metabolite of prilocaine inducing methemoglobinemia.[22] Adverse responses noted included transient and mild skin blanching and erythema. There is one report of an allergic contact dermatitis developing in response to EMLA application to the skin.[28]

Developments Since the Fourth Edition of This Book. EMLA is now available in North America (Canada, 1991; United States, 1993). It has gained acceptance as an effective means of minimizing or eliminating the pain associated with percutaneous needle insertion. Although useful in all age groups, EMLA has been readily accepted in pediatric populations. The intraoral application of EMLA as a topical anesthetic appears to provide anesthesia as effective as traditional topical formulations, but it does need an extended period of application, which is a significant drawback.[32] Whether EMLA is capable of providing clinically effective pulpal anesthesia, in either primary or permanent teeth, is questionable. Munshi and associates evaluated the effectiveness of EMLA for extraction of mobile primary teeth, root stumps, and pulpal therapy procedures in primary teeth, and concluded that "EMLA could to some extent eliminate the use of the needle in the procedures performed, especially in pediatric dentistry."[33] Dental application of EMLA is discussed in Chapter 4.

pH Alterations

The administration of local anesthetics into skin and, to a lesser degree, oral mucous membranes is frequently uncomfortable. Although many factors are involved in this—including the speed of injection, volume of solution, density of the tissues, and a lot of psychology—the acidic pH of the anesthetic solution plays a significant role in provoking discomfort during local anesthetic injections. The pH of a "plain" local anesthetic solution is approximately 5.5, whereas that of a vasopressor-containing solution is about 4.5. The addition of substances to the anesthetic that alkalinize the solution should make the drug's administration more comfortable. In addition, at a higher pH the anesthetic drug should have a more rapid onset of action and greater potency.

Two strategies have been used to achieve this effect: the addition of sodium bicarbonate to the anesthetic solution and the addition of carbon dioxide. Carbonation of local anesthetics is not really new; its use was described as early as 1965.[34]

The addition of *sodium bicarbonate* to a local anesthetic solution immediately before injection alkalinizes the solution, increasing the number of uncharged base molecules (RN). Because it is this uncharged ionic form of the drug that is lipid soluble and able to diffuse through the nerve membrane, a formulation of lidocaine with epinephrine plus sodium bicarbonate (pH 7.2) provides a more rapid onset of anesthetic block (onset = 2 minutes) than commercially prepared (pH 4.55) lidocaine plus epinephrine (onset = 5 minutes).[35–37] However, if the pH of the solution is too high, local anesthetic will precipitate out as the drug base. The stability of the local anesthetic decreases as pH increases, leading to considerably shorter shelf-lives. Stewart and associates demonstrated that a solution of lidocaine 1% with epinephrine 1:100,000 and sodium bicarbonate (80 mEq/L) provided the same depth and area of anesthesia after 1 week of storage as that provided by a freshly prepared solution.[38] However, the preparation of such solutions into dental cartridges with a 2- to 3-year shelf-life seems impractical at this point. Alkalinization of epinephrine-free anesthetic solutions proffers no benefit.[36] Clinical trials in blepharoplasty and rhinoplasty found a more rapid onset of clinical action and increased patient comfort along with no discernible difference in hemostasis or duration of action.[37,39] Recommendations for preparation of the local anesthetic with bicarbonate appear divided between 1 part 4.2% bicarbonate with 10 parts local anesthetic,[36,40] and 1 part 8.4% bicarbonate in 5 parts local anesthetic.[37,39]

Carbon dioxide (CO_2) enhances diffusion of local anesthetic through nerve membranes, providing a more rapid onset of nerve block. As CO_2 diffuses through the nerve membrane, intracellular pH is decreased, raising the intracellular concentration of charged cations (RNH$^+$), the form of the anesthetic that attaches to receptor sites in sodium channels. Because the cationic form of the drug does not readily diffuse out of the nerve, the anesthetic becomes concentrated within the nerve trunk (termed *ion trapping*), providing a longer duration of anesthesia.[41] The problem clinically has been that if the carbonated local anesthetic agent is not injected almost immediately after opening the vial, the CO_2 will diffuse out of solution, significantly diminishing its effectiveness. The anesthetic drug must be administered within a short time after preparing the syringe.

Developments Since the Fourth Edition of This Book.
The use of alkalinized local anesthetics has received considerable attention in medicine where skin surgery is performed. Sodium bicarbonate has received most of the attention, because it is easier to work with than CO_2. Most studies have concluded that pain on injection is diminished and speed of onset increased, with no deleterious effect on either duration of action or area of anesthesia.[42] The only published dental study (1991) reported no clinical difference between lidocaine hydrochloride and lidocaine hydrocarbonate solutions with 1:100,000 epinephrine when administered via inferior alveolar nerve block.[43]

Hyaluronidase

Hyaluronidase is an enzyme that breaks down intracellular cement. It has been advocated as an additive to local anesthetics because it permits injected solutions to spread and penetrate tissues.[44]

The primary use of hyaluronidase has been in plastic surgery, dermatology, and ophthalmologic procedures, primarily in retrobulbar nerve blocks, where it has been demonstrated to speed both the onset of anesthesia and the area of anesthesia significantly when compared with non–hyaluronidase-containing anesthetic solutions.[45–47] The duration of anesthesia is slightly decreased when hyaluronidase is added, but the benefits associated with its addition more than outweigh this minor inconvenience.[47]

The use of hyaluronidase in dental local anesthetic solutions has been discussed for many years. The first paper in dental literature discussing the use of hyaluronidase in local anesthetics appeared in 1949,[48] but there has been no mention of hyaluronidase in dental literature in recent years. However, a considerable number of dentists in the United States and elsewhere do add hyaluronidase to their anesthetic solutions and anecdotally report a considerably more rapid onset of nerve block anesthesia and an increase in success rate, especially in the inferior alveolar nerve block. The negative factor of a decreased duration of anesthesia is considered a minor inconvenience because the duration provided when a vasopressor-containing solution is used is more than adequate to permit completion of the procedure painlessly.

Hyaluronidase is available as Wydase (Wyeth-Ayerst) in a lyophilized powder and a stabilized solution. It is added to the anesthetic cartridge just before administration by removing approximately one eighth of the anesthetic solution and refilling the cartridge with hyaluronidase.

Allergic reactions have been reported after hyaluronidase administration.[49]

Developments Since the Fourth Edition of This Book.
First discussed in the fourth edition, hyaluronidase is mentioned again because of a seemingly consistent interest in its use among dentists communicating on the Internet. Caution is advised before considering the use of hyaluronidase in dental local anesthetics. Clinical research trials to demonstrate the efficacy, safety, and proper dosage of this combination should be completed before its widespread use.

Ultra–long-acting Local Anesthetics

Tetrodotoxin (TTX) and *saxitoxin* (STX) are classified as biotoxins. Found in the puffer fish (TTX) and certain species of dinoflagellates (STX), they specifically block sodium channels on nerve membranes when applied to the outer membranous surface and thus produce conduction blockade. Although these agents are about 250,000 times as potent as procaine in providing conduction blockade of isolated nerve preparations,[50] they both are highly toxic and can not pass readily through the epineurium surrounding peripheral nerves; therefore they provide little or no conduction blockade of the sciatic nerve.[51] However, when administered via subarachnoid block in sheep, they have induced spinal anesthesia of almost 24 hours' duration.[52] Unfortunately, both TTX and SSX are extremely difficult to synthesize and are not very stable in aqueous solutions, thereby significantly limiting their usefulness. There is little likelihood that they will be of any clinical value in anesthesiology or dentistry in the near future.

Developments Since the Fourth Edition of This Book.
There are no significant developments in the areas of anesthesiology or dentistry. TTX and SSX are mentioned as items of potential interest.

ELECTRONIC DENTAL ANESTHESIA

The use of electricity as a therapeutic modality in medicine and dentistry is not new. The first recorded report of electrotherapy dates from 46 AD, when Scribonius Largus, physician to the emperor Claudius, used the torpedo fish to relieve the pains of gout.[53] Electricity continued to be used into the eighteenth century, when interest in its therapeutic potential reached new heights. With the ability to produce electricity, devices were designed to treat a wide range of disorders in the human body. Textbooks in the late eighteenth and early nineteenth centuries illustrated the technique of electrotherapy for managing ulcers and toothaches (Fig. 20-2).[54,55] It must be remembered that local anesthetics were not available at this time. Unfortunately, "electroquackery" also became popular during the late eighteenth century. Elisha Perkins, a Connecticut physician, created "Perkins Patent Tractors," two brass and iron rods about 3 inches long, rounded at one end and pointed at the other. He claimed that by moving these devices downward from the site of pain to the patient's extremities he could draw disease out of the body.[56] Sales of the tractors netted enormous wealth for Perkins, but feeling was so strong against him and his tractors that the

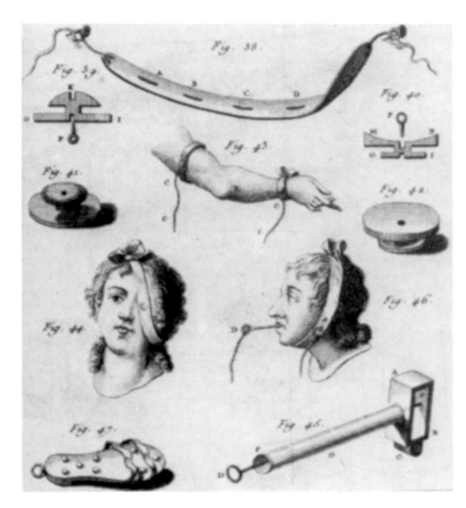

Figure 20-2. Electrodes available in 1786.

Connecticut Medical Society expelled him from membership in 1796.

In 1883 Erb wrote, "At the present time we possess in the electrical current one of the most certain and brilliant remedies for neuralgia, although we must admit that much progress has not been made in our knowledge concerning its mode of action in these forms of disease."[57]

References to electroanalgesia continued into the early twentieth century, but after this time there was scarce mention of the use of electrical stimulation for pain relief in either the medical or dental literature.[58] This gap extended into the mid-1960s, when interest in the field of electronic anesthesia was renewed. One example (circa 1970) of "new" electroanesthesia equipment was the Desensor handpiece (Fig. 20-3), a high-speed device that carried low-voltage electrical current through a bur directly onto the tooth being treated. Its lack of consistent reliability led to its rapid demise.

The use of transcutaneous electrical nerve stimulation (TENS) and its dental progeny, EDA, has developed since the mid-1960s into techniques that have considerable utility in the management of pain (Fig. 20-4).

Only time will tell whether EDA represents another fad, which will die out only to reappear at some other time in the future, or will prove valuable enough to gain a strong foothold in the dental armamentarium for pain control.

Mechanism of Action

At the low-frequency setting of 2 Hz (hertz or cycles per second), which is most often used in the *management of chronic pain*, TENS produces measurable changes in the

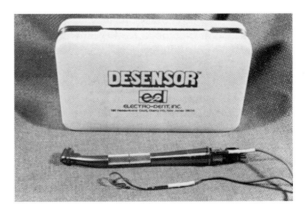

Figure 20-3. Electroanesthesia handpiece, circa 1970.

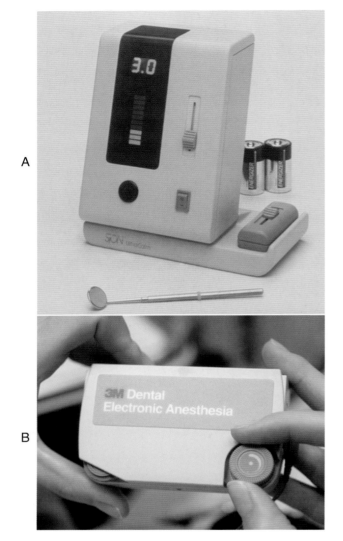

Figure 20-4. **A** and **B**, Electronic dental anesthesia (EDA) unit, circa 1980.

period. Opioid-agonist analgesics prescribed for posttreatment pain are rarely necessary when TENS or EDA has been used during or after treatment.

The mechanism by which EDA operates to prevent *acute pain* during surgery or dentistry is somewhat different. It is felt that the Melzack and Wall gate control theory of pain provides an adequate explanation for the prevention of acute pain provided by EDA.[61] Used at a higher frequency (≥120 Hz), EDA causes the patient to experience a sensation most often described as "vibrating," "throbbing," "pulsing," or "twitching." This involves the stimulation of larger-diameter nerves (A fibers), which transmit the sensations of touch, pressure, and temperature. If the patient can maintain a minimum "threshold" intensity of A fiber stimulation, the pain impulse produced by the high-speed drill, scalpel, or curette that is transmitted to the CNS more slowly along the smaller A-delta and C fibers will come on a "closed" gate and be unable to reach the brain, where it is translated into physical pain. Thus large-fiber input is said to inhibit central transmission of the overall effects of small-fiber input. When the pain impulse fails to reach the brain, the sensation of pain does not occur.

Blood levels of serotonin and endorphins likewise are elevated during high-frequency stimulation and probably play a secondary, albeit important, role in providing acute pain control during most dental treatment.

Electrotherapy in Medicine

During the 1960s neurosurgeons began the use of implanted electrodes in the spinal cord as an alternative to cordotomy in patients with chronic debilitating back pain. Neurosurgical procedures, although effective, did not possess an exceptionally high success rate in eliminating the chronic pain being experienced.

In 1967 Shealy and associates reported that intractable pain could be suppressed without the need for an irreversible surgical procedure through direct stimulation of the dorsal column of the spinal cord.[62] The success rate of this technique was satisfactory, and the use of direct electrical stimulation became a more accepted mode of therapy for patients with chronic debilitating pain.

In the early 1970s Shealy[63] and Long,[64] working with electrode pads placed on the patient's skin over the spinal cord, were able to eliminate pain without the need for implanting electrodes into the cord. Thus the technique of TENS was founded.

Today TENS is an accepted treatment modality in the management of an ever-growing variety of chronic pain disorders (Box 20-1). However, TENS has had its greatest acceptance in the realm of sports medicine.[65] The application of a low-frequency electrical current to an area that has been injured recently can be of benefit to the patient in two ways:

1. First, it acts to increase tissue perfusion produced by capillary and arteriolar dilation while stimulating the

blood levels of l-tryptophan, serotonin, and β-endorphins. l-tryptophan, a precursor of serotonin, is present in the blood in decreasing amounts as the duration of TENS increases. By contrast, serotonin levels in the blood increase with time.[59] Serotonin possesses analgesic actions, elevating the pain reaction threshold. At the same time, levels of β-endorphins and enkephalins in the cerebral circulation also increase. β-Endorphins and enkephalins are potent analgesics produced by the body in response to certain types of stimulation.[60] It appears that elevated blood levels of these chemicals are not achieved for a period of about 10 minutes after the start of TENS or EDA stimulation—findings that provide a clearer understanding of the mechanism whereby TENS may aid in the management of chronic pain. Because blood levels of serotonin and β-endorphins remain elevated for several hours after the termination of TENS therapy, patients benefit from this residual analgesic action in the immediate posttreatment

BOX 20-1

Medical Uses of Transcutaneous Electrical Nerve Stimulation

Causalgia
Phantom limb pain
Postherpetic neuralgia
Intractable cancer pain
Lower back pain
Spinal cord injury
Ileus
Peripheral nerve injury
Bursitis
Parturition
Polycythemia vera
Cervical back pain
Postoperative pain
Diabetic ulceration

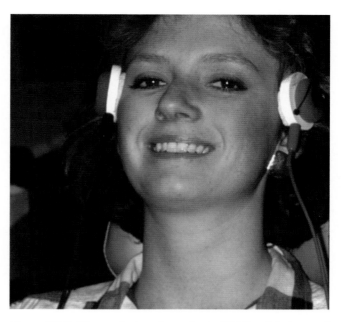

Figure 20-5. Electronic dental anesthesia (EDA) unit being used for temporomandibular joint/myofascial pain dysfunction (TMJ/MPD) treatment. The electrodes are placed bilaterally over the TMJs.

contraction of skeletal muscles. The net effect of these two processes is to provide a pumping action in the area of application of the current. Therapeutically, a 1-hour treatment at a low frequency (2.5 Hz) helps to decrease edema (skeletal muscle-stimulating effect) and the increased perfusion and skeletal muscle stimulation act to "cleanse" the area of tissue-injury breakdown products. The use of TENS in this manner speeds the recovery process, enabling the athlete to return to the field of play sooner.

2. A second benefit in the recovery from injury is the analgesic action it possesses. Low-frequency stimulation for longer than 10 minutes produces elevated blood levels of serotonin and endorphins. These increased levels persist for several hours after the termination of TENS, helping to block the pain "cycle" that has been partially responsible for the chronicity of the pain experienced by the patient. Once this pain cycle is broken, it becomes considerably easier to keep the patient comfortable.

Transcutaneous Electrical Nerve Stimulation in Dentistry

Temporomandibular Joint (TMJ) or Myofascial Pain Dysfunction (MPD).

TENS has been used with great success in dentally related chronic pain in the management of temporomandibular joint (TMJ) problems for many years. Until recently the management of TMJ pain and dysfunction with TENS was almost exclusively limited to physical therapists. In recent years dentistry has begun to incorporate TENS into its armamentarium for the treatment of these patients. Meizels,[66] Clark and associates,[67] and Geissler and McPhee[68] have all demonstrated the efficacy and ease of using this technique for TMJ and myofascial pain dysfunction (MPD) syndrome. For the management of limited mandibular opening secondary to TMJ problems, EDA has been used in a manner similar to that described in the preceding in medicine; that is, low-frequency extraoral stimulation of the area. Clark and associates,[67] Christensen,[69] and others who have been working with EDA for TMJ/MPD patients have had significant success rates (increased range of motion and decreased discomfort) compared with those achieved with placebo (Fig. 20-5).

Acute Dental Pain.

The success of EDA in the management of acute pain associated with dental treatment has not been as great as with chronic pain.

To manage acute pain, higher frequency of electronic stimulation is necessary. The most often used frequency for acute pain management has been 120 Hz, although one EDA unit provided 16,000 Hz (Fig. 20-6).

The areas that received greatest interest were restorative dentistry, periodontal procedures, fixed prosthodontics, and endodontics, although clinical trials have been pursued in other areas (removable prosthodontics, oral surgery, and orthodontics).

Using EDA alone (no local anesthesia or sedation) in *restorative dentistry*, Clark and associates demonstrated a statistically significant success rate when EDA was used (13 of 14) versus a placebo EDA unit (4 of 7).[67] Hochman, using a much larger patient sample, had a success rate of 76% in 473 restorative dentistry procedures.[70] Patients, using a visual analogue scale, evaluated the degree of pain control achieved, from 0% (painful) to 100% (no pain). Those indicating pain relief of better than 90% were considered successes. Malamed and associates demonstrated a success rate of 80% in 109 restorative

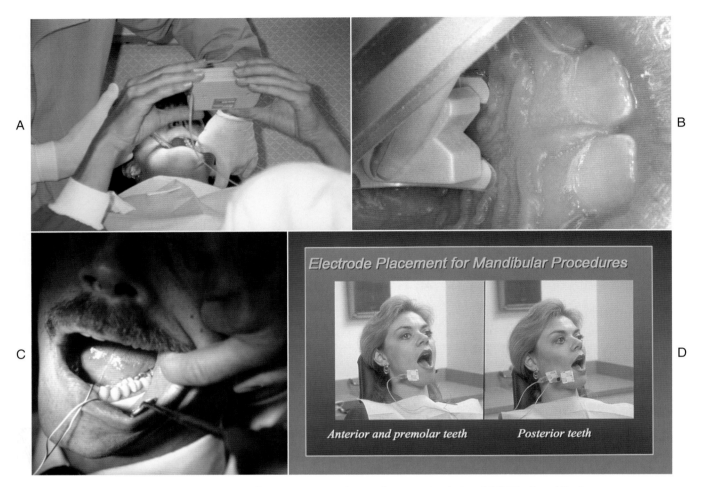

Figure 20-6. Intraoral use of transcutaneous electrical nerve stimulation (TENS), **A** and **B,** for comfortable administration of local anesthesia and, **C** and **D,** for treatment without need for local anesthesia.

procedures in both arches.[71] Success rates for restorative dentistry utilizing EDA approach those seen with local anesthesia. Mellor, comparing local anesthesia with EDA for restorative dentistry, found that 60% of patients (*n* = 25) preferred EDA to local anesthesia, whereas 28% had no preference.[72] The degree of pain control obtained by both techniques was evaluated as equal.

EDA has had its greatest success to date in periodontal procedures. The procedures being considered are *nonsurgical periodontics* (e.g., root planing, curettage, and subgingival scaling). Periodontal and other surgical procedures are discussed in the following. Success rates in excess of 90% for EDA alone have been found by Clark (100%) and Malamed (97%). Hochman reported an 83% success rate in 71 patients undergoing "scaling and prophylaxis."[70] The use of EDA as an alternative to local anesthesia in nonsurgical periodontics appears well founded. This may be of special interest in those countries, states, and provinces where dental hygienists are not permitted to inject local anesthetics.

In *fixed prosthodontics*, results to date for EDA have not been as impressive as in restorative and periodontal procedures, a success rate of 53% in 29 procedures being reported by Hochman.[70] Fixed prosthodontics is an area in which EDA usually can provide adequate pain control for the preparation of the tooth. Most failures in the past have occurred when the gingival retraction cord was being placed, or after that, when the impression was being taken (because of the need to remove the intraoral electrode pads from the patient's mouth during the period of impression taking). Modifications in EDA technique, using more adhesive and less obtrusive electrodes or extraoral electrodes, have provided a satisfying increase in its success rate and patient acceptance in fixed prosthodontics.

In *endodontics*, Clark and associates reported a 0% success rate (*n* = 4).[67] Until recently the author also had met with little success using EDA alone for pain control in the pulpally involved tooth. However, when EDA is employed as an adjunctive technique to local anesthesia or sedation (preferably inhalation sedation with N_2O/O_2), the author has achieved considerable success in extirpating the pulps of some very difficult to anesthetize teeth (mandibular molars). Although much more work needs to be done in the area of EDA and endodontics, EDA can provide the doctor with one more technique of pain control when seeking to open up the pulp chamber of the infected tooth.

Clark and associates were able to remove comfortably 50% (two of four) of nonimpacted teeth with EDA versus 0% with a placebo EDA unit.[67] EDA can be used effectively in *simple exodontia* and other surgical (e.g., periodontal or endodontic) procedures; however, the immediate cessation of anesthesia when the unit is turned off after the procedure may leave the patient with little postsurgical pain control if the surgical procedure is of short duration. Fortunately, a degree of pain relief is present after surgery because the blood levels of serotonin and β-endorphins remain elevated (for several hours) after the unit has been turned off. If the procedure was very short (<10 minutes), there will be little or no increased blood level of these chemicals and the patient may experience immediate posttreatment pain.

The elevated serotonin and β-endorphin levels after EDA greatly benefit the patient undergoing restorative, crown-and-bridge, or periodontal procedures, in which there may normally be a slight degree of soreness in the immediate posttreatment period. After lengthy surgical procedures in which EDA was used, the author has been impressed with the general lack of discomfort experienced by the patient. Considerable work is presently being undertaken to determine the efficacy of EDA as a postsurgical pain prevention modality in dentistry.

Two other areas in which EDA has been used with success in dentistry include the following:
1. Providing pain control for the administration of local anesthetics. EDA produces excellent soft-tissue anesthesia. It may be used when local anesthetic injections must be given, as in multiple palatal infiltrations to achieve hemostasis. Meechan and associates compared patient discomfort during inferior alveolar nerve block using no pretreatment, topically applied benzocaine, and EDA.[1-3,73] Pain scores were significantly decreased with TENS compared with both no pretreatment and topical anesthetic.
2. Reversing local anesthesia. After successful inferior alveolar nerve block with lidocaine with epinephrine, soft-tissue anesthesia of approximately 5 hours is to be expected but perhaps not welcomed by the patient. EDA (applied unilaterally) at its low-frequency setting (thereby maximizing vasodilation and muscle contraction) for a period of 10 to 15 minutes can successfully remove a large volume of residual anesthetic solution and thereby partially or totally reverse the anesthetic effect.

Electronic Dental Anesthesia Plus Sedation.   The studies reported in the preceding have involved the use of EDA as an alternative to local anesthesia. No other technique of pain control or sedation was used. Quarnstrom has demonstrated significantly higher success rates when EDA was used in combination with nitrous oxide-oxygen inhalation sedation (N_2O/O_2) than when either technique was used alone.[74,75] He reported success rates of 32% for EDA alone and 39% for N_2O/O_2 alone, whereas an overall success rate of 86% was achieved with a combination of the two techniques. EDA and N_2O/O_2 complement each other well (as does the combination of local anesthesia and N_2O/O_2).

Where local anesthesia is less than 100% successful in blocking transmission of pain impulses to the brain, N_2O/O_2 may increase the pain reaction threshold to a point that no pain is interpreted by the patient. Yet when local anesthesia fails entirely, merely adding N_2O/O_2 does not provide adequate pain relief.

This same interaction occurs with EDA and N_2O/O_2. These three techniques are extremely complementary and may be used with impunity in combination. However, potential contraindications to each procedure should always be considered before it is used clinically.

Electronic Dental Anesthesia in Pediatric Dentistry.   Electronic dental anesthesia requires a considerable degree of patient cooperation and participation to be successful. Patients are responsible for determining when "threshold" has been achieved and must be made to understand that they must increase their level of stimulation should they experience any pain during the dental procedure. With this in mind, the use of EDA in younger populations, although not contraindicated, requires a more intensive evaluation of patients' abilities to both understand the concept of EDA and their ability to perform their tasks properly.

te Duits and associates used EDA on 27 children between the ages of 6 and 12 years for restorative dentistry.[76] Two opposing teeth were treated, one with local anesthesia, the other with EDA. There was no overall significant difference in pain perception between the two modalities of treatment, regarding dentin sensitivity and rubber dam clamp placement. When asked for a preference of techniques, 78% chose EDA over local anesthesia.

Munshi and associates reported on 40 children, ranging in age from 5 to 12 years, who received EDA for minor extractions, restorations, and pulpal therapy.[5] They concluded that EDA, "besides offering safety and psychological advantages, may also be a promising alternative to the conventional methods of local anesthesia."[5]

Electronic Dental Anesthesia Indications

The most significant indication for the utilization of EDA as a technique in pain control is *needle phobia* (fear of injections). Patients who state that they "hate shots" but once numb are "okay" are ideal candidates for EDA. The combination of the technique's success rate and a positive placebo response in this patient group (they want it to work) provides a unique situation for a successful procedure, in stark contrast to the situation in the dental phobic who is fearful of all aspects of dentistry, including EDA.

Other indications for EDA, either alone or in combination with local anesthetics and N_2O/O_2, include the following:
1. Ineffective local anesthesia
2. Instances where local anesthetics cannot be administered (e.g., with a history of true, documented reproducible allergy)

The most likely dental procedures to prove successful with EDA are the following (in descending order of anticipated success):
1. TMJ/MPD (chronic pain)
2. Administration of local anesthesia
3. Nonsurgical periodontal procedures (acute pain)
4. Restorative dentistry (acute pain)
5. Fixed prosthodontic procedures (acute pain)
6. Endodontics (recommended in conjunction with local anesthesia or N_2O/O_2)

Electronic Dental Anesthesia Contraindications

Specific medical contraindications to the use of EDA are those stated for TENS (ASA IVs remain contraindications for all modes of dental care, including EDA):
1. Cardiac pacemakers
2. Neurological disorders
   a. Status post–cerebrovascular accident (stroke)
   b. History of transient ischemic attacks
   c. History of epilepsy
3. Pregnancy
4. Immaturity (inability to understand the concept of patient control of pain)
   a. Very young pediatric patient
   b. Older patients with senile dementia
   c. Language communication difficulties

Perhaps the most significant nonmedical contraindication to the use of EDA are patients who are *dental phobics*—that is, fearful of everything dental: the smells, sounds, and sensations involved with therapeutic interventions in the mouth. To them everything a dentist does represents a threat. EDA is looked on by them as just one more thing to fear. The likelihood of success in such circumstances is negligible. In Hochman's study of 600 patients, in which the level of "concern" toward this new technique (EDA) was evaluated, patients who considered themselves as "trusting," "ambivalent," or "slightly anxious" had an EDA success rate of 73%, whereas those rating themselves as "extremely apprehensive" had a success rate of 53%.[70] With EDA (as with most dental therapies), patient selection is an important component of success.

Also somewhat confusing to the doctor are the few patients who undergo a very successful EDA treatment (e.g., no pain experienced), but when asked which pain control technique, EDA or local anesthesia, they would prefer if required to undergo the same type of dental care at the next visit, state that they would choose local anesthesia. When questioned, these patients often mention that although they did not experience any pain, they disliked EDA for one of two reasons:
1. The "feeling" involved in the EDA was too intense, bordering on uncomfortable.
2. They were unable to "relax" with EDA. After a local anesthetic injection (which they disliked intensely) they were at least able to relax because they knew that they would not experience any further pain during their treatment. However, with EDA they had to remain alert throughout the entire procedure, ready to increase the level of stimulation if they became uncomfortable.

Electronic Dental Anesthesia Advantages

The advantages of using electronic dental anesthesia over injectable local anesthetics include the following:
1. No need for needle
2. No need for injection of drugs
3. Patient is in control of the anesthesia
4. No residual anesthetic effect at the end of the procedure
5. Residual analgesic effect remains for several hours

Electronic Dental Anesthesia Disadvantages

1. Cost of the unit
2. Training
3. "Learning curve:" initial success may be low but increases with experience
4. Intraoral electrodes: weak link in the entire system. The availability of extraoral electrodes on some units has lessened this disadvantage; however, clinical experience with extraoral electrodes has demonstrated that the depth of anesthesia obtained may not always be as great as that with intraoral electrodes.

Developments Since the Fourth Edition of This Book. Several of the manufacturers of EDA units have ceased marketing to dentistry because of the lack of interest in this technique among most dentists. However, the use of TENS in the management of chronic pain, specifically TMJ/MPD, has continued to increase.

It is obvious that dentists throughout the world are unwilling to abandon local anesthesia as their primary technique of pain control. However, EDA has been shown to be an effective method of minimizing patient discomfort *during* the injection of local anesthetics. This could prove to be one of the more important uses of this technique in dentistry, although the proper application of topical anesthetics, coupled with slow injection of the local anesthetic solution, does minimize (or eliminate) any patient perception.

Postsurgical pain and swelling can be minimized through the use of EDA *after* surgical procedures. The use of EDA at a low-frequency setting for 30 to 60 minutes at the completion of surgery provides a more comfortable postoperative recovery for many patients.

The administration of N_2O/O_2 in conjunction with EDA adds to the success of EDA.

REFERENCES

1. McClellan KJ, Faulds D: Ropivacaine: an update on its use in regional anaesthesia, *Drugs* 60(5):1065-1093, 2000.
2. Mather LE, Chang DH: Cardiotoxicity with modern local anesthetics. Is there a safer choice? *Drugs* 61(3):333-342, 2001.
3. McLeod GA, Burke D: Levobupivacaine, *Anaesthesia* 56(4):331-341, 2001.
4. Foster RH, Markham A: Levobupivacaine: a review of its pharmacology and use as a local anaesthetic, *Drugs* 59(3):551-579, 2000.
5. Munshi AK, Hegde AM, Girdhar D: Clinical evaluation of electronic dental anesthesia for various procedures in pediatric dentistry, *J Clin Pediatr Dent* 24(3):199-204, 2000.
6. Baghdadi ZD: A comparison of parenteral and electronic dental anesthesia during operative procedures in children, *Gen Dent* 48(2):150-156, 2000.
7. Wilson S, Molina Lde L, Preisch J, et al: The effect of electronic dental anesthesia on behavior during local anesthetic injection in the young, sedated dental patient, *Pediatr Dent* 21(1):12-17, 1999.
8. Kattwinkel J, Niermeyer S, Nadkarni V, et al: An advisory statement from the Pediatric Working Group of the International Liaison Committee on Resuscitation, *Pediatrics* 103(4):456, 1999.
9. Dart eC, Goldfrank LA, Chyka PA, et al: Combined evidence-based literature analysis and consensus guidelines form stocking emergency antidotes in the United States, *Ann Emerg Med* 36(2):126-132, 2000.
10. Gupta PP, Tangri AN, Saxena RC, et al: Clinical pharmacology studies on 4-N-butylamino-1,2,3,4,-tetrahydroacridine hydrochloride (centbucridine), a new local anaesthetic agent, *Indian J Exp Biol* 20:344-346, 1982.
11. Suri YV, Singhal AP, Phadke VK, et al: Double blind study on centbucridine for subarachnoid and extradural anaesthesia, *Indian J Med Res* 76:875-881, 1982.
12. Suri YV, Patnaik GK, Nayak BC, et al: Evaluation of centbucridine for intravenous regional anaesthesia, *Indian J Med Res* 77:722-727, 1983.
13. Beri S, Biswas NR, Shende DR, et al: Injectable centbucridine and lidocaine hydrochloride for intraocular surgery, *Ophthalmol Surg Lasers* 28(12):1027-1029, 1997.
14. Vacharajani GN, Parikh N, Paul T, et al: A comparative study of centbucridine and lidocaine in dental extraction, *Int J Clin Pharmacol Res* 3:251-255, 1983.
15. Samsi AB, Bhalerao RA, Shah SC, et al: Evaluation of centbucridine as a local anaesthetic, *Anesth Analg* 62:109-111, 1983.
16. Reiz S, Haggmark S, Johansson G, et al: Cardiotoxicity of ropivacaine: a new amide local anesthetic, *Acta Anaesthesiol Scand* 33:93-98, 1989.
17. Arthur GR, Feldman HS, Covino BG: Comparative pharmacokinetics of bupivacaine and ropivacaine, a new amide local anesthetic, *Anesth Analg* 67:1053-1058, 1988.
18. Arthur GR, Covino BG: What's new in local anesthetics? *Anesthesiol Clin North Am* 6:357-370, 1988.
19. Brown DL, Carpenter RL, Thompson GE: Comparison of 0.5% ropivacaine and 0.5% bupivacaine for epidural anesthesia in patients undergoing lower-extremity surgery, *Anesthesiology* 72:633-636, 1990.
20. Moller RA, Covino BG: Effect of progesterone on the cardiac electrophysiologic alterations produced by ropivacaine and bupivacaine, *Anesthesiology* 77:735-741, 1992.
21. Ernberg M, Kopp S: Ropivacaine for dental anesthesia: a dose-finding study, *J Oral Maxillofac Surg* 60(9):9004-1010, discussion 1010-1011, 2002.
22. Buckley MM, Benfield P: Eutectic lidocaine/prilocaine cream. A review of the topical anaesthetic/analgesic efficacy of a eutectic mixture of local anaesthetics (EMLA), *Drugs* 46(1):126-151, 1993.
23. Brodin A, Nyqvist-Mayer A, Wadsten T, et al: Phase diagram and aqueous solubility of the lidocaine-prilocaine binary system, *J Pharm Sci* 73:481-484, 1984.
24. Evers H, von Dardel O, Juhlin L, et al: Dermal effects of compositions based on the eutectic mixture of lignocaine and prilocaine (EMLA): studies in volunteers, *Br J Anaesth* 57:997-1005, 1985.
25. Taddio A, Nulman I, Goldbach M, et al: Use of lidocaine-prilocaine cream for vaccination pain in infants, *J Pediatr* 124(4):643-648, 1994.
26. Lycka BA: EMLA: a new and effective topical anesthetic, *J Dermatol Surg Oncol* 18(10):859-862, 1992.
27. Buckley MM, Benfield P: Eutectic lidocaine/prilocaine cream: a review of the topical anaesthetic/analgesic efficacy of an eutectic mixture of local anaesthetics (EMLA), *Drugs* 46(1):126-151, 1993.
28. van den Hove J, Decroix J, Tennstedt D, et al: Allergic contact dermatitis from prilocaine, one of the local anaesthetics in EMLA cream, *Contact Dermatitis* 30(4):239, 1994.
29. Svennson P, Petersen JK: Anesthetic effect of EMLA occluded with Orahesive oral bandages on oral mucosa, *Anesth Prog* 39:79-82, 1992.
30. Vickers ER, Punnia-Moorthy A: Pulpal anesthesia from an application of a eutectic topical anesthetic, *Quint Int* 24(8):547-551, 1993.
31. Meechan JG, Donaldson D: The intraoral use of EMLA cream in children: a clinical investigation, *ASDC J Dent Child* 61(4):260-262, 1994.
32. Vickers ER, Punnia-Moorthy A: A clinical evaluation of three topical anaesthetic agents, *Austral Dent J* 37(4):267-270, 1992.
33. Munshi AK, Hedge AM, Latha R: Use of EMLA: is it an injection free alternative? *J Clin Pediatr Dent* 25(3):215-219, 2001.
34. Bromage PR: A comparison of the hydrochloride and carbon dioxide salts of lidocaine and prilocaine in epidural analgesia, *Acta Anaesthesiol Scand* Suppl 16:55-69, 1965.
35. DiFazio CA, Carron H, Grosslight KR, et al: Comparison of pH-adjusted lidocaine solutions for epidural anaesthesia, *Anaesth Analg* 65:760-764, 1986.
36. Berrada R, Chassard D, Bryssine S, et al: In vitro effects of alkalinization of 0.25% bupivacaine and 2% lidocaine, *Ann Fr Anesth Reanim* 13(2):165-168, 1994.
37. Metzinger SE, Rigby PL, Bailey DJ, et al: Local anesthesia in blepharoplasty: a new look? *South Med J* 87(2):225-227, 1994.

38. Stewart JH, Chinn SE, Cole GW, et al: Neutralized lidocaine with epinephrine for local anesthesia—II, *J Derm Surg Oncol* 16(9):842-845, 1990.

39. Metzinger SE, Bailey DJ, Boyce RG, et al: Local anesthesia in rhinoplasty: a new twist? *Ear Nose Throat J* 71(9):405-406, 1992.

40. Redd DA, Boudreaux AM, Kent RB III: Towards less painful local anesthesia, *Ala Med* 60(4):18-19, 1990.

41. Bokesch PM, Raymond SA, Strichartz GR: Dependence of lidocaine potency on pH and PCO_2, *Anesth Analg* 66:9-17, 1987.

42. Davies RJ: Buffering the pain of local anesthetics: a systematic review, *Emerg Med* 15(1):81-88, 2003.

43. Chaney MA, Kerby R, Reader A, et al: An evaluation of lidocaine hydrocarbonate compared with lidocaine hydrochloride for inferior alveolar nerve block, *Anesth Prog* 38:212-216, 1991.

44. Courtiss EH, Ransil BJ, Russo J: The effects of hyaluronidase on local anesthesia: a prospective, randomized, controlled, double-blind study, *Plast Reconstr Surg* 95(5):876-883, 1995.

45. Johansen J, Kjeldgärd M, Croydon L: Retrobulbar anaesthesia: a clinical evaluation of four different anaesthetic mixtures, *Acta Ophthalm* 71(6):787-790, 1993.

46. Watson D: Hyaluronidase, *Br J Anaesth* 71(3):422-425, 1993.

47. Clark LE, Mellette JR Jr: The use of hyaluronidase as an adjunct to surgical procedures, *J Dermatol Surg Oncol* 20(12):842-844, 1994.

48. Looby JP, Kirby CK: Use of hyaluronidase with local anesthetic agents in dentistry, *J Am Dent Assoc* 38:1-4, 1949.

49. London NJ, Osman FA, Ramagopal K, et al: Hyaluronidase (Hylase): a useful addition in haematoma block? *J Accident Emerg Med* 13(5):337-338, 1996.

50. Covino BG, Vassallo HG: *Local anesthetics: mechanisms of action and clinical use*, New York, 1976, Grune & Stratton.

51. Adams HJ, Blair MR Jr, Takman VH: The local anaesthetic activity of tetrodotoxin alone and in combination with vasoconstrictors and local anaesthetics, *Anaesth Analg* 55:568-573, 1976.

52. Akerman GR, Feldman HS, Norway SB: Acute IV toxicity of LEA-103, a new local anesthetic, compared to lidocaine and bupivacaine in the awake dog, *Anesthesiology* 65:182, 1986.

53. Scribonius Largus: *De compositione medicamentorum*, Liber CLXII, Paris, 1528, C Wechel.

54. Wesley J: *The desideratum: or electricity made plain and useful*, London, 1760, W Flexney.

55. Ferguson J: *An introduction to electricity*, London, 1770.

56. Malamed SF, Joseph C: Electricity in dentistry, *J Calif Dent Assoc* 15:12-14, 1987.

57. Erb W: *Handbook of electrotherapeutics*, New York, 1883, W Wood.

58. Sturridge E: *Dental electro-therapeutics*, ed 2, Philadelphia, 1918, Lea & Febiger.

59. Silverstone L: Electronic dental anesthesia, *Dent Pract* 27:4-6, 1989.

60. Hughes J, Smith TW, Kosterlitz HW: Identification of two related pentapeptides from the brain with potent opiate agonist activity, *Nature* 258:577-580, 1975.

61. Melzack R, Wall PD: Pain mechanisms: a new theory, *Science* 150:971-979, 1965.

62. Shealy CN, Mortimer JT, Reswick JB: Electrical inhibition of pain by stimulation of the dorsal column: preliminary clinical report, *Anesth Analg* 45:489-491, 1967.

63. Shealy CN: Transcutaneous electrical stimulation for control of pain, *Clin Neurosurg* 21:269-277, 1974.

64. Long DM: External electrical stimulation as a treatment of chronic pain, *Minn Med* 57:195-198, 1974.

65. Smith MJ, Hutchins RC, Hehenberger D: Transcutaneous neural stimulation use in postoperative knee rehabilitation, *Am J Sport Med* 11:75-82, 1983.

66. Meizels P: H-wave and TMJ treatment, *J Calif Dent Assoc* 15:42-44, 1987.

67. Clark MS, Silverstone LM, Lindemuth J, et al: An evaluation of the clinical analgesia/anesthesia efficacy on acute pain using the high frequency neural modulator in various dental settings, *Oral Surg* 63:501-505, 1987.

68. Geissler PR, McPhee PM: Electrostimulation in the treatment of pain in the mandibular dysfunction syndrome, *J Dent* 14:62-64, 1986.

69. Christensen GJ: Electronic anesthesia: research and thoughts, *J Calif Dent Assoc* 15:46-48, 1987.

70. Hochman R: Neurotransmitter modulator (TENS) for control of dental operative pain, *J Am Dent Assoc* 116:208-212, 1988.

71. Malamed SF, Quinn CL, Torgerson RT, et al: Electronic dental anesthesia for restorative dentistry, *Anesth Prog* 36:195-198, 1989.

72. Mellor AC: A comparison of injectable local anesthesia and electronic dental anesthesia in restorative dentistry, *Anesth Pain Control Dent* 2(3):177-179, 1993.

73. Meechan JG, Gowans AJ, Welbury RR: The use of patient-controlled transcutaneous electrical nerve stimulation (TENS) to decrease the discomfort of regional anaesthesia in dentistry. A randomized controlled clinical trial, *J Dent* 26(5):417-420, 1998.

74. Quarnstrom FC: Electrical anesthesia, *J Calif Dent Assoc* 16:35-40, 1988.

75. Quarnstrom FC: Clinical experience with TENS and TENS combined with nitrous oxide-oxygen, *Anesth Prog* 36:66-69, 1989.

76. teDuits E, Goepferd S, Donly K, et al: The effectiveness of electronic dental anesthesia in children, *Pediatr Dent* 15(3):191-196, 1993.

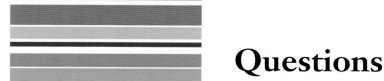

Questions

CHAPTER
21

LOCAL ANESTHETICS

QUESTION: Why is it said that intravascular administration of local anesthetics is dangerous when physicians frequently administer intravenous (IV) lidocaine to correct serious cardiac dysrhythmias?

The intravenous administration of local anesthetics is potentially hazardous at all times and in all patients. However, IV local anesthetics, such as lidocaine and procainamide, do have an important place in the management of various ventricular dysrhythmias, such as premature ventricular contractions and ventricular tachycardia. Several factors, including weighing the risk versus the benefit, must be considered whenever local anesthetics are to be administered "safely" intravenously.

1. *The patient's physical status.* Patients receiving IV lidocaine or other antidysrhythmic drugs have potentially life-threatening cardiac dysrhythmias. The myocardium is highly irritable (usually secondary to ischemia), which is one of the reasons for the dysrhythmia's presence. Local anesthetics are myocardial depressants. By depressing myocardial activity they decrease the incidence of dysrhythmias. Patients with normal cardiac rhythms receiving IV local anesthetics also have their myocardium depressed; their cardiac function may be impaired by the local anesthetic in this circumstance.

2. *The form of lidocaine used.* Lidocaine for IV use in the management of ventricular dysrhythmias, so-called cardiac lidocaine, is prepared in single-use ampules. These ampules contain only lidocaine and sodium chloride. The typical dental cartridge of lidocaine contains lidocaine, distilled water, vasopressor, sodium bisulfite, and sodium chloride. IV injection of these ingredients, in and of itself, might precipitate unwanted cardiovascular responses rather than terminate them.

3. *The rate of injection.* Lidocaine for antidysrhythmic use is titrated slowly into the cardiovascular system to achieve a therapeutic blood level in the myocardium. Typically, a dose of 1.0 to 1.5 mg/kg is administered slowly under electrocardiographic monitoring, titrating to clinical effect. In the typical dental practice a 1.8-ml cartridge of lidocaine (36 mg) is deposited in 15 seconds or less. The rate at which the drug is administered intravenously has a significant bearing on the peak blood level of the drug. Overly rapid IV administration results in lidocaine blood levels that quickly enter into the overdose range, whereas a more slowly administered dose results in blood levels well within the therapeutic range for terminating dysrhythmias.

4. *Risk versus benefit.* An overdose reaction is always a possibility whenever IV lidocaine is administered. Even under controlled conditions in a hospital, adverse reactions related to overly high blood levels do develop. The risk of administering local anesthetics intravenously always must be weighed against the potential benefit to be gained from their use. For high-risk patients with a specific life-threatening dysrhythmia, the benefit clearly outweighs the risk. For dental patients seeking relief from intraoral pain, IV local anesthetic administration confers no benefit yet adds many risks.

QUESTION: What shall I do when a patient claims to be allergic to a local anesthetic?

Believe the patient! Do not use any form of local anesthetic (especially topical anesthetic preparations) on this patient. Seek to determine what actually happened to the patient to prompt such a claim. (A detailed discussion of this problem is found in Chapter 18.)

No. When used properly, all currently available local anesthetics are highly effective and safe. "Used properly" is the key phrase. Aspiration before injection (to minimize the risk of intravascular administration) and slow administration of the drug are vital. A medical history and physical evaluation, to determine potential contraindications to specific local anesthetics or additives, must be completed before their use. Maximum dosage of a drug should be determined for a given patient and not exceeded. Charts for the most commonly used local anesthetics are found in Chapters 4 and 18. The figures cited are maximum recommended doses. They should be decreased in patients with certain medical complications and older individuals. Most systemic reactions to local anesthetics are entirely preventable. Overdose reactions that have led to death are frequently the result of the administration of too large a dose to a younger, lighter-weight, well-behaved patient requiring multiple quadrants of dental care, or after accidental IV administration. Psychogenic reactions, by far the most common adverse response to local anesthetic administration, may be virtually eliminated through increased rapport with the patient, use of an atraumatic injection technique (Chapter 11), placement of the patient in a supine position during injection, and ample doses of empathy.

Two factors are particularly important:
1. The duration of pain control necessary to complete the procedure and the need for posttreatment pain control (e.g., after surgical procedures). Box 4-1 lists currently available local anesthetics by their estimated duration of action.
2. The patient's physical status (e.g., ASA classification), hypersensitivity, methemoglobinemia, or sulfur allergy, which may preclude the use of some drugs

For most patients the duration of desired pain control is the ultimate deciding factor in local anesthetic selection, because there is usually no contraindication to the administration of any particular agent.

It is suggested that a number of local anesthetics be available at all times. The nature of the dental practice dictates the number and types of local anesthetics needed. In a typical dental practice the selection of a drug is based on the desired duration of anesthesia; for example, less than 30 minutes, approximately 60 minutes, in excess of 90 minutes. One local anesthetic preparation from each group, necessitated by the nature of the doctor's practice, should be available. For example, the pediatric dentist has little need or desire for long-acting local anesthetics, such as bupivacaine, whereas the oral and maxillofacial surgeon may have little need for shorter-acting drugs such as mepivacaine plain, but a greater need for bupivacaine. Remember that not all patients have similar local anesthetic requirements, and the same patient may require a different local anesthetic for a dental procedure of a different duration. In general, amide local anesthetics are preferred to the esters because of their decreased incidence of allergy.

Yes, if the topical anesthetic preparation is applied to mucous membrane for an adequate length of time.[1] The American Dental Association recommends a 1-minute application.[2] The Food and Drug Administration recommends application for a minimum of 1 minute. Gill and Orr recommend application for 2 to 3 minutes.[3] Topical anesthetics containing benzocaine are not absorbed from their site of application into the cardiovascular system. Therefore risk of overdose is minimal when benzocaine-containing topical anesthetic preparations are used. Because of the rapid absorption of some topically applied local anesthetics such as lidocaine, it is recommended that their use be restricted to the following situations:
1. Locally, at the site of needle puncture before injection
2. For scaling or curettage, over no more than three or four teeth at a time

Pressurized sprays of topical anesthetics cannot be recommended unless they release a metered dose of the drug, not a steady uncontrolled dose. Sterilization of the spray nozzle must be possible if a spray is used. Many pressurized topical anesthetic sprays are available in metered form with disposable spray nozzles.

EMLA (eutectic mixture of local anesthetics), a combination of lidocaine and prilocaine, designed to provide cutaneous anesthesia before venipuncture, has been employed in dentistry with some degree of success.[4,5]

VASOCONSTRICTORS

Yes. Use of local anesthetics with vasopressors should be avoided or kept to an absolute minimum in the following cases:[6-8]
1. Patients with blood pressure in excess of 200 mmHg systolic or 115 mmHg diastolic
2. Patients with uncontrolled hyperthyroidism

3. Patients with severe cardiovascular disease
    a. Less than 6 months after myocardial infarction
    b. Less than 6 months after cerebrovascular accident
    c. Daily episodes of angina pectoris or unstable (preinfarction) angina
    d. Cardiac dysrhythmias despite appropriate therapy
    e. Postcoronary artery bypass surgery, less than 6 months
4. Patients who are undergoing general anesthesia with halogenated agents
5. Patients receiving nonspecific β-blockers, monoamine oxidase inhibitors, or tricyclic antidepressants

Patients in categories 1 to 3a through 3d are classified as ASA IV risks and are *not* normally considered candidates for elective or emergency dental treatment in the office. (Refer to Chapter 3 for a more detailed discussion; also see the next question.)

QUESTION: Often medical consultants recommend against inclusion of a vasopressor in a local anesthetic for a cardiovascular risk patient. Why? And what can I do to achieve effective pain control?

As indicated, there are several instances in which it is prudent to avoid the use of vasopressors in local anesthetics. Most of these situations (high blood pressure, severe cardiovascular disease) also represent absolute contraindications to elective dental care because of the greater potential risk to the patient. If a dental patient with cardiovascular disease is deemed treatable (ASA II or III), then local anesthetics for pain control are indicated. The patient's physician often states that, although local anesthetics can be used, epinephrine should be avoided.

QUESTION: When should epinephrine be avoided?

One of the few valid reasons for avoiding epinephrine is the patient with cardiac rhythm abnormalities that are unresponsive to medical therapy. The presence of dysrhythmias (especially ventricular) usually indicates an irritable or ischemic myocardium. Epinephrine, either exogenous or endogenous, increases myocardial sensitivity even more, predisposing this patient to a greater frequency of dysrhythmias or to more significant types of dysrhythmias, such as ventricular tachycardia or ventricular fibrillation. In these patients epinephrine-containing local anesthetics should be avoided if at all possible. However, many cardiologists today do not even consider the ischemic myocardium a valid reason for excluding vasoconstrictors from local anesthetics, provided the dose of epinephrine administered is minimal and intravascular administration is avoided.

It is my recommendation that with a patient who is deemed able to tolerate the stresses involved in their planned dental treatment, a vasoconstrictor should be included in the local anesthetic if there is a reason for its inclusion (e.g., depth or duration of anesthesia, need for hemostasis). As Bennett has stated, the greater the medical risk of a patient, the more important effective control of pain and anxiety becomes.[9]

QUESTION: Why do many physicians still recommend against the use of epinephrine (and other vasopressors) in cardiovascular risk patients?

Most physicians never, or at best rarely, use epinephrine in their practice. The only physicians doing so on a regular basis are anesthesiologists, emergency medicine specialists, and surgeons. As used in medicine, epinephrine is almost always used in emergency situations. At those times the dose is considerably higher than that used in dentistry. The average emergency dose of intramuscular (IM) or IV epinephrine (used in a 1:1000 or 1:10,000 concentration) for anaphylaxis or cardiac arrest is 0.3 to 1 mg, whereas one dental cartridge with 1:100,000 epinephrine contains only 0.018 mg.

Therefore it is understandable that many physicians, lacking an intimate knowledge of the practice of dentistry, think of epinephrine in terms of the doses used in emergency medicine and not in the much more dilute forms used for anesthesia in dentistry.

An example follows. In a hospital situation, a patient with a serious cardiovascular problem (ASA IV) who requires a surgical procedure (e.g., emergency appendectomy) may be considered too great a risk for general anesthesia. Many anesthesiologists opt to use a regional local anesthetic (spinal) block with an IV antianxiety agent (diazepam or midazolam) for sedation in place of general anesthesia. The local anesthetic usually contains a vasopressor such as epinephrine in a 1:100,000 or 1:200,000 concentration, added primarily to decrease the rate at which the local anesthetic is absorbed into the cardiovascular system but also to minimize bleeding and prolong the duration of clinical action.

QUESTION: Why is the use of vasopressors in local anesthetics recommended for cardiac risk patients?

Pain is stressful to the body. During stress, endogenous catecholamines (e.g., epinephrine or norepinephrine) are released from their storage sites into the cardiovascular system at a level approximately 40 times greater than at the resting level. (Refer to Chapter 3 for a review of the pharmacology of this group of drugs.)

Release of epinephrine and norepinephrine into the blood increases the cardiovascular workload; thus the myocardial oxygen requirement increases. In patients with compromised (partially occluded) coronary arteries, this greater myocardial oxygen requirement may not be met, with the subsequent development of ischemia, leading to dysrhythmias, anginal pain (if ischemia is transient), or myocardial infarction (if prolonged). Increased cardiac workload also may lead to acute exacerbation of congestive heart failure. Elevated catecholamine levels can produce a dramatic increase in blood pressure, which can precipitate another life-threatening situation (cerebrovascular accident [CVA, "brain attack"]).

Therefore the goal is to minimize endogenous catecholamine release during dental therapy. The stress reduction protocol is designed to accomplish this. A local anesthetic without vasopressor produces pulpal anesthesia of shorter duration than the same drug with a vasopressor. Profound pain control of adequate duration is less likely to be achieved when a vasopressor is excluded from a local anesthetic solution. If the patient experiences pain during treatment, an exaggerated stress response is observed.

With the proper use (aspiration and slow injection) of a local anesthetic with minimum concentration of exogenous vasopressor (e.g., 1:100,000 or 1:200,000), pain control of longer duration is virtually guaranteed and the exaggerated stress response is avoided. Levels of catecholamine in the blood are elevated when exogenous epinephrine is administered, but these levels usually are not clinically significant.

An often-repeated and essentially true statement is that the cardiovascularly impaired patient is more at risk from endogenously released catecholamines than from exogenous epinephrine administered in a proper manner.

QUESTION: Can I administer a local anesthetic with a vasopressor even if a physician has advised against it?

Yes. A medical consultation is a request for advice from you to a person with more knowledge of the matter being discussed. You should not always heed this advice if you feel it may be inaccurate. If any doubt persists in your mind concerning proper treatment protocol after this initial consultation, additional opinions should be sought, preferably from a specialist in the "area" of concern, such as a cardiologist, anesthesiologist, or dental expert in local anesthesia. Of course, there are patients for whom exogenous catecholamines may prove too great a risk, in which case "plain" local anesthetic solutions are administered.

It always must be remembered that the primary responsibility for the care and well-being of a patient rests solely in the hands of the person who performs the treatment, not the one who gives advice.

An incident concerning a medical consultation is worth relating. A periodontal graduate student was planning four quadrants of osseous surgery on a patient whose medical history was within normal limits except for a torticollis for which she was receiving imipramine, a tricyclic antidepressant. A written consultation was sent to the patient's physician requesting that the patient be taken off the imipramine before the surgical procedure. The response, not surprisingly, was that the patient could not be taken off the drug, as it had taken more than a year to get her medical condition stabilized. Moreover, it was

recommended that epinephrine be avoided during this patient's surgery. It was decided to contact the physician directly to discuss the matter and attempt to explain the importance of epinephrine during the surgical procedure. In the ensuing conversation it was agreed that epinephrine could be used, but in a limited dose, and that the patient was to be monitored (vital signs) throughout the procedure. The surgery was carried off without incident.

The lesson to be learned from this episode is that the wording of the original consult was too constricting, or indeed might have been construed as threatening, to the physician. Whenever possible, direct contact and discussion with both parties explaining their needs should be obtained, because this is more likely to lead to a satisfactory compromise and to better and safer patient management.

QUESTION: If epinephrine is used in cardiac risk patients, is there a maximum dose?

Yes. Bennett recommends, and I concur, that the maximum dose of epinephrine in a cardiac risk patient should be 0.04 mg.[9] This equates to roughly
- One cartridge of 1:50,000 epinephrine
- Two cartridges of 1:100,000 epinephrine
- Four cartridges of 1:200,000 epinephrine

I do *not* recommend the use of 1:50,000 epinephrine for pain control purposes. (Further information on dental management of the cardiovascular risk patient is available.)[10-12]

QUESTION: What about epinephrine-containing gingival retraction cord?

Racemic epinephrine gingival retraction cord should *never* be used in cardiovascular risk patients, and it is my opinion that it should not be used for any patient. Gingival retraction cord contains 8% racemic epinephrine. Half of this is the levorotatory form, which provides a concentration of active epinephrine of 4% (or 40 mg/ml). This is *40 times* the concentration used in the management of anaphylaxis or cardiac arrest. Absorption of epinephrine through mucous membrane into the cardiovascular system is normally rapid but is even more so with active bleeding, such as that occurring after subgingival tooth preparation. Levels of epinephrine in the blood rise rapidly, leading to cardiovascular manifestations of epinephrine overdose (p. 318).

This increase in cardiovascular activity may prove to be life-threatening in patients with preexisting clinically evident or subclinical cardiovascular disease.

QUESTION: If I elect not to use a vasopressor for a patient, which local anesthetics are clinically useful?

The clinically available local anesthetics are listed by their duration of action in Box 4-1. Mepivacaine 3% can provide up to 40 minutes of pulpal anesthesia (via nerve block) for the average patient, whereas prilocaine 4% via nerve block can provide up to 60 minutes.

SYRINGES

QUESTION: What kind of syringe is recommended?

Although a wide variety is available, there are two factors of primary importance in their selection.
1. A syringe must be capable of aspiration. *Never* use a syringe that does not permit aspiration.
2. A syringe must be sterilizable, unless it is disposable.

In addition, with the introduction of so-called *safety syringes*, it is my recommendation that every consideration be given to the use of a syringe that is designed to minimize the risk of accidental needle stick after injection is completed. Although the unit cost of the disposable safety syringe increases office expenses, the decreased liability faced by the doctor in needle-stick injuries should more than cover this consideration.

QUESTION: Do computer-controlled, local anesthetic delivery systems (CCLADs) work well enough to justify their purchase?

Yes. In most instances CCLADs enable the patient to receive effective local anesthesia in an entirely pain-free manner. Response from dentists using CCLADs varies from those who are extremely ecstatic to those who do not feel they are worth the expense. The majority of responses are favorable. In my experience CCLADs make it easier to more comfortably deliver those injection that are "difficult" to administer painlessly. These include all palatal injections and the periodontal ligament (PDL) techniques.

NEEDLES

QUESTION: What gauge and length of needles are recommended for injection?

Selection of a needle depends on several factors, foremost among which are the aspiration potential of the injection and estimated depth of soft-tissue penetration.
1. A long needle is recommended for the inferior alveolar, Gow-Gates mandibular, Vazirani-Akinosi mandibular, ASA (infraorbital), buccal, and maxillary nerve blocks in adults.
2. A short needle is recommended for the posterior superior alveolar, mental, and incisive nerve blocks; maxillary infiltration (supraperiosteal injection); palatal nerve blocks and infiltration; and periodontal ligament and intraseptal injections.

In earlier editions I specified the gauge of the needle for each injection. A 25-gauge needle was recommended

for number 1, a 27-gauge needle for number 2. This remains my recommendation today.

If only two needles were to be available in my dental office, I would opt for a 25-gauge long and a 27-gauge short. I have absolutely no need or desire to ever use a 30-gauge needle for an intraoral injection. However, this is not the case in dentistry in the United States. Information received from needle manufacturers indicates that the most commonly purchased needles in dentistry in the United States are the 27-gauge long and 30-gauge short.

I do not recommend a 30-gauge short, but it may be used for local infiltration to produce hemostasis.

CARTRIDGES

QUESTION: Why do you (the author) call this a cartridge when everyone else calls it a carpule?

Carpule is a proprietary name for the glass cartridge. The name is trademarked by the Cook-Waite Corporation (now Kodak).

QUESTION: Can glass cartridges be autoclaved?

No. Autoclaving of glass cartridges destroys their seals. The heat of autoclaving also degrades the heat-labile vasopressor.

QUESTION: Should local anesthetic cartridges be stored in alcohol or cold sterilizing solution?

No. Alcohol or cold sterilizing solution diffuses into the cartridge. Injection of these into tissues may produce burning, irritation, or paresthesia. (The care and handling of local anesthetic cartridges are discussed in Chapter 8.)

QUESTION: Are cartridge warmers effective in making local anesthetic solutions more comfortable on injection?

No. Most cartridge warmers make the local anesthetic solution too warm, leading to increased discomfort on injection and possible destruction of the heat-sensitive vasopressor. Cartridges stored at room temperature produce no discomfort to patients and are greatly preferred.

QUESTION: Why do some patients complain of a burning sensation when a local anesthetic is injected?

Because of its pH, any local anesthetic may cause a slight burning sensation during the initial injection. The pH of a plain solution is in the 5.5 to 6.0 range, that of a vasopressor-containing solution in the mid-3 to mid-4 range. Other causes include an overly warm solution, the presence of alcohol or cold sterilizing solution within the cartridge, or solution with a vasopressor at or near its expiration date.

QUESTION: What causes local anesthetic solution to run down the outside of the needle into a patient's mouth?

Improper preparation of the armamentarium is to blame here. (See Chapter 9.) The recommended sequence for preparation is as follows (using a metal syringe and disposable needle):
1. Place the cartridge in the syringe.
2. Embed the aspirating harpoon.
3. Place the needle on the syringe.

This sequence provides a perfectly centric perforation of the rubber diaphragm by the needle, with a tight seal formed around the needle. No leakage of anesthetic occurs.

When the needle is placed onto the syringe first, followed by the cartridge, it is possible for the perforation of the diaphragm to be ovoid, not round. The ovoid perforation does not seal itself as well around the metal needle, leading to leakage of anesthetic around this area as the anesthetic drug is injected.

QUESTION: What causes cartridges to break during injection?

1. Damage during shipping. Visually check cartridges before use.
2. Using excessive force to engage the aspirating harpoon in the rubber stopper. Proper preparation of the needle, cartridge, and syringe (see previous question) precludes breakage caused by excessive force. When the needle is placed onto the syringe before the cartridge it is necessary to "hit" the plunger to embed the harpoon into the rubber stopper. This may cause a cartridge to shatter.
3. Attempting to force a cartridge with an extruded plunger into the syringe.
4. Using a syringe with a bent aspirating harpoon.
5. Bent needle with an occluded lumen. Always expel a small volume of anesthetic from the syringe before inserting the needle into the patient's mouth to ensure patency of the needle.

TECHNIQUES OF REGIONAL ANESTHESIA IN DENTISTRY

QUESTION: What should always be done before local anesthetic administration in a patient?

Review of the patient's medical history questionnaire (visually or verbally) and a physical examination, including vital signs and visual inspection, are recommended when a patient is seen for the first time or after a long absence from the office. This identifies possible contraindications to the use of local anesthetics or vasopressors and in general determines a patient's ability to tolerate physically and psychologically the stresses of dental care without undue risk.

QUESTION: What are the medical contraindications to use of local anesthetics and vasopressors?

These are discussed in Chapter 4 and in excellent review articles by Perusse, Goulet, and Turcotte.[6–8]

QUESTION: Should a patient be advised that a local anesthetic injection will hurt before the injection is started?

No. Local anesthetic injections need not hurt. Careful adherence to the atraumatic injection protocol described in Chapter 11 can make virtually all injections, including palatal, painless.

QUESTION: Is any chair position best for administration of local anesthetics?

Yes, absolutely! Because the most commonly observed adverse reactions to local anesthetics are psychogenic, the position of choice during intraoral injections is one in which the patient's chest and head are parallel to the floor with the feet slightly elevated. Presyncopal episodes may still occur (pallor, light-headedness), but actual loss of consciousness is extremely unlikely to develop with the patient in this position.

After completion of several mandibular injections (inferior alveolar, Gow-Gates mandibular, and Vazirani-Akinosi mandibular nerve blocks), it is suggested that the patient be returned to a comfortable, more upright position during the ensuing 5 to 10 minutes. This change in patient position appears to help speed the onset of mandibular block anesthesia.

QUESTION: Why do you (the author) recommend regional block anesthesia in the maxilla instead of infiltration (supraperiosteal) anesthesia?

Regional block anesthesia in the maxilla is preferred to infiltration whenever more than two teeth are to be treated. Its advantages include the following:
1. Fewer penetrations of tissue, thus less likelihood of postinjection problems
2. Smaller volume of local anesthetic (e.g., than for multiple infiltrations of the same area), thereby decreasing the risk of systemic reactions such as overdose
3. Clinically adequate anesthesia more likely when infiltration is ineffective because of the presence of infection

QUESTION: Do palatal injections always hurt?

No. Careful adherence to the protocol for atraumatic injections can do much to minimize any discomfort associated with palatal anesthesia. In addition, the following are important:
1. Topical anesthesia
2. Pressure anesthesia

3. Control of the needle
4. Slow deposition of solution
5. Positive attitude by the administrator

Interestingly, an area of considerable interest among practicing dentists is palatal anesthesia and how to increase patient comfort. Over the years I have received many devices designed by dentists in an attempt to minimize or eliminate pain during palatal injections, and I have also been told of many techniques. These include vibrating wands, letting the needle trace along the palate for a second or two so they know it is coming and is not a "shock," and avoiding the use of palatal injections unless they are absolutely necessary.

The clinical introduction of CCLADs (see the preceding and Chapter 5) permits the delivery of local anesthetic injections in any area of the oral cavity in a pain-free manner in most situations.

QUESTION: Why do I miss inferior alveolar nerve blocks more often than any other injection?

Of all nerve blocks in dentistry and, with few exceptions, in medicine too, the inferior alveolar is the most elusive of consistent success. A success rate, bilaterally, of 85% or greater indicates that one's technique is basically correct. However, many factors can affect this rate of success:
1. *Anatomical variation.* It is well known that if there is any one aspect of human anatomy that is consistent it is its inconsistency. Strict adherence to injection technique does not always produce adequate inferior alveolar anesthesia.
2. *Technical errors.* The most common technical error I observe with the inferior alveolar nerve block is insertion of the needle too low on the medial side of the ramus (below the mandibular foramen). A second common technical error is insertion of the needle too far anteriorly (laterally) on the medial side of the ramus (thus contacting bone quite soon after penetration).
3. *Accessory innervation.* When isolated regions of mandibular teeth remain sensitive when all other areas are insensitive, the possibility of accessory innervation should be considered. The technique used in eliminating this problem (which is usually produced by the mylohyoid nerve) is described in Chapter 14.

QUESTION: Why do I have a much higher failure rate with inferior alveolar nerve blocks on one side than on the other?

Because of significantly different operator positions during the administration of the inferior alveolar nerve block on contralateral sides of the mouth, it is not uncommon for some doctors to encounter significant variation in their success rate. The inferior alveolar is the only intraoral nerve block for which significant differences in success

rates are noted on opposite sides of the mouth. Although basic protocols are the same on the right and left side, the view of the target area by the administrator, the angle of needle entry, and other factors may be responsible for an increased failure rate on one side. The solution to this problem is to evaluate critically one's technique on the less successful side and seek to correct it without interfering in the success on the opposite side. Patience is often necessary.

QUESTION: How can I achieve adequate pain control when gaining access in pulpally involved teeth?

The recommended sequence of injection techniques for pulpally involved teeth follows:
1. Local infiltration, if possible and not contraindicated
2. Regional nerve block
3. PDL injection, if not contraindicated by the presence of infection
4. Intraosseous injection
5. Intraseptal injection
6. Intrapulpal injection
7. Psychosedation, if pain control techniques have proved unsuccessful in completely blocking pain impulses from reaching brain
8. Electronic dental anesthesia
9. Prayer . . . when nothing else works! However, with the introduction of intraosseous anesthesia, this step is rarely if ever needed.

For all teeth in the mouth, with the probable exception of mandibular molars, clinically adequate pain control for pulpal extirpation can be obtained with either local infiltration or nerve block injection. Difficulties arise most often in the mandibular molars. A working knowledge of alternative mandibular anesthesia techniques, such as the Gow-Gates mandibular block or the Vazirani-Akinosi mandibular block, increases the likelihood of obtaining anesthesia. In addition, the use of intraosseous anesthesia greatly increases success rates in mandibular molars.

Mandibular premolars and anterior teeth can be anesthetized adequately for pulpal extirpation with the incisive nerve block.

QUESTION: What special concerns are involved with local anesthesia in pediatric dentistry?

Pain control generally is easier to achieve in pediatric dentistry. However, there are two concerns that always should be considered:
1. *Increased potential for overdose* exists because (most) children are smaller and weigh less than adults. Use milligram-per-weight formulas to minimize doses in children.
2. *Prolonged anesthesia* can lead to traumatization of the lips and tongue, unless shorter-duration drugs are used and both patient and parent are warned of this possible complication.

A third concern relates to injection technique and the appropriate needle to be used in specific techniques. A long dental needle is recommended for the injections described in this book for which a considerable thickness of soft tissue is to be penetrated. The rationale for this is the rule of thumb that "a needle should not be inserted into tissue all the way to its hub, unless it is absolutely necessary for the success of that injection." If it is possible for an injection technique to be administered in a child with a short (~20-mm length) needle within the parameters of this rule, then use of this needle is warranted. Psychologically, the sight of a long needle is more traumatic than is the sight of a short needle (in point of fact, needles and syringes should always be kept out of a patient's line of sight, if possible).

QUESTION: What is the recommended method of achieving hemostasis in surgical areas?

The recommended technique is *local infiltration* of a vasopressor-containing anesthetic into the region of the surgery. Only small volumes are necessary for this purpose. Epinephrine in a concentration of 1:100,000 is recommended (although 1:50,000 also may be used).

REFERENCES

1. Meechan JG: Intra-oral topical anaesthetics: a review, *J Dent* 28:1-14, 2000.
2. American Dental Association Council on Dental Therapeutics: *Accepted dental therapeutics*, Chicago, 1984, The American Dental Association.
3. Gill CJ, Orr DL: A double blind crossover comparison of topical anesthetics, *J Am Dent Assoc* 98:213, 1979.
4. Gunter JB: Benefits and risks of local anesthetics in infants and children, *Paediatr Drugs* 4:649-672, 2002.
5. Bernardi M, Secco F, Benech A: Anesthetic efficacy of a eutectic mixture of lidocaine and prilocaine (EMLA) on the oral mucosa: prospective double-blind study with a placebo, *Minerv Somatol* 48:39-43, 1999.
6. Perusse R, Goulet J-P, Turcotte J-Y: Contraindications to vasoconstrictors in dentistry: Part I. Cardiovascular diseases, *Oral Surg* 74(5):692-697, 1992.
7. Perusse R, Goulet J-P, Turcotte J-Y: Contraindications to vasoconstrictors in dentistry: Part II. Hyperthyroidism, diabetes, sulfite sensitivity, cortico-dependent asthma, and pheochromocytoma, *Oral Surg* 74:587-691, 1992.
8. Perusse R, Goulet J-P, Turcotte J-Y: Contraindications to vasoconstrictors in dentistry: Part III. Pharmacologic interactions, *Oral Surg* 74:592-697, 1992.
9. Bennett CR: *Monheim's local anesthesia and pain control in dental practice*, ed 7, St Louis, 1984, Mosby.
10. Anonymous: *Cardiovascular effects of epinephrine in hypertensive dental patients*, Evidence Report: Technology Assessment (Summary) 48:1-3, 2002.
11. Silvestre FJ, Verdu MJ, Sanchis JM, et al: Effects of vasoconstrictors in dentistry on systolic and diastolic arterial pressure, *Medicina Oral* 6:17-63, 2001.
12. Yagiela JA, Adverse drug interactions in dental practice: interactions associated with vasoconstrictors. Part V of a series, *J Am Dent Assoc* 130:701-709, 1999.

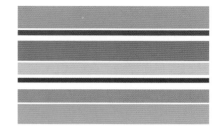

Appendix A:
Overview of CDC
Hand Hygiene Guidelines

The Centers for Disease Control and Prevention (CDC) recently released new recommendations for hand hygiene in healthcare settings. Hand hygiene is a term that applies to either hand washing, use of an antiseptic hand rub, or surgical hand antisepsis. Evidence suggests that hand antisepsis, the cleansing of hands with an antiseptic hand rub, is more effective in reducing nosocomial infections than plain hand washing.

GUIDELINES FOR THE CARE OF ALL PATIENTS

- Continue to wash hands with either a nonantimicrobial or an antimicrobial soap and water whenever the hands are visibly soiled.
- Use an alcohol-based hand rub to routinely decontaminate the hands in the following clinical situations: (*Note:* If alcohol-based hand rubs are not available, the alternative is hand washing.)
  - Before and after client contact
  - Before donning sterile gloves when inserting central intravascular catheters
  - Before performing nonsurgical invasive procedures (e.g., urinary catheter insertion, nasotracheal suctioning)
  - After contact with body fluids or excretions, mucous membranes, nonintact skin, and wound dressings
  - If moving from a contaminated body site (rectal area or mouth) to a clean body site (surgical wound, urinary meatus) during client care
  - After contact with inanimate objects (including medical equipment) in the immediate vicinity of the client)
  - After removing gloves
  - Before eating and after using a restroom, wash hands with a non–antimicrobial or an antimicrobial soap and water
- Antimicrobial-impregnated wipes (e.g., towelettes) are not a substitute for using an alcohol-based hand rub or antimicrobial soap.
- If exposure to *Bacillus anthracis* is suspected or proved, wash hands with a non–antimicrobial or an antimicrobial

soap and water. The physical action of washing and rinsing hands is recommended because alcohols, chlorhexidine, iodophors, and other antiseptic agents have poor activity against spores.

METHOD FOR DECONTAMINATING HANDS

When using an alcohol-based hand rub, apply product to palm of one hand and rub hands together, covering all surfaces of hands and fingers, until hands are dry. Follow the manufacturer's recommendations regarding the volume of product to use.

GUIDELINES FOR SURGICAL HAND ANTISEPSIS

- Surgical hand antisepsis reduces to a minimum the resident microbial count on the hands.
- The CDC recommends using an antimicrobial soap, and to scrub hands and forearms for the length of time recommended by the manufacturer, usually 2 to 6 minutes. The Association of Operating Room Nurses recommends 5 to 10 minutes. Refer to agency policy for time required.
- When using an alcohol-based surgical hand scrub product with persistent activity, follow the manufacturer's instructions. Before applying the alcohol solution, prewash hands and forearms with a non–antimicrobial soap and dry hands and forearms completely. After application of the alcohol-based product as recommended, allow hands and forearms to dry thoroughly before donning sterile gloves.

GENERAL RECOMMENDATIONS FOR HAND HYGIENE

- Use hand lotions or creams to minimize the occurrence of irritant contact dermatitis associated with hand antisepsis or hand washing.

- Do not wear artificial fingernails or extenders when having direct contact with clients at high risk (e.g., those in intensive care units or operating rooms).
- Keep natural nails tips less than $\frac{1}{4}$-inch long.
- Wear gloves when contact with blood or other potentially infectious materials, mucous membranes, and nonintact skin could occur.
- Remove gloves after caring for a client. Do not wear the same pair of gloves for the care of more than one client, and do not wash gloves between uses with different clients.
- Change gloves during client care if moving from a contaminated body site to a clean body site.

(Data from Centers for Disease Control and Prevention: *Morbidity and Mortality Weekly Report MMWR* 51(RR16):1-44, 2002 *www.cdc.gov/handhygiene.*)

INDEX

BOX 4-1

Approximate Duration of Action of Local Anesthetics

SHORT DURATION (pulpal anesthesia approximately 30 minutes)
Lidocaine HCl 2%
Mepivacaine HCl 3%
Prilocaine HCl 4% (by infiltration)

INTERMEDIATE DURATION (pulpal anesthesia approximately 60 minutes)
Articaine HCl 4% + epinephrine 1:100,000
Articaine HCl 4% + epinephrine 1:200,000
Lidocaine HCl 2% + epinephrine 1:50,000
Lidocaine HCl 2% + epinephrine 1:100,000
Mepivacaine HCl 2% + levonordefrin 1:20,000
Mepivacaine HCl 2% + epinephrine 1:100,000
Prilocaine HCl 4% (via nerve block only)
Prilocaine HCl 4% + epinephrine 1:200,000

LONG DURATION (pulpal anesthesia approximately 90+ minutes)
Bupivacaine HCl 0.5% + epinephrine 1:200,000

TABLE 4-2
Contraindications for Local Anesthetics

Medical Problem	Drugs to Avoid	Type of Contraindication	Alternative Drug
Local anesthetic allergy, documented	All local anesthetics in same chemical class (e.g., esters)	Absolute	Local anesthetics in different chemical class (e.g., amides)
Bisulfite allergy	Vasoconstrictor-containing local anesthetics	Absolute	Any local anesthetic without vasoconstrictor
Atypical plasma cholinesterase	Esters	Relative	Amides
Methemoglobinemia, idiopathic or congenital	Prilocaine	Relative	Other amides or esters
Significant liver dysfunction (ASA III-IV)	Amides	Relative	Amides or esters, but judiciously
Significant renal dysfunction (ASA III-IV)	Amides or esters	Relative	Amides or esters, but judiciously
Significant cardiovascular disease (ASA III-IV)	High concentrations of vasoconstrictors (as in racemic epinephrine gingival retraction cords)	Relative	Local anesthetics with epinephrine concentrations of 1:200,000 or 1:100,000 or mepivacaine 3% or prilocaine 4% (nerve blocks)
Clinical hyperthyroidism (ASA III-IV)	High concentrations of vasoconstrictors (as in racemic epinephrine gingival retraction cords)	Relative	Local anesthetics with epinephrine concentrations of 1:200,000 or 1:100,000 or mepivacaine 3% or prilocaine 4% (nerve blocks)